250 CASES IN CLINICAL MEDICINE

Dedicated to

The memory of my paternal grandparents
Bantwal Vaikunta and Sharada Baliga
who not only had the courage to actively participate in India's freedom movement but also to eat food with the so-called 'untouchables' in the 1920s when it was anathema to do so

The memory of my maternal grandparents
Kochikar Sanjiv and Girija Pai
who actively participated in the underground movement during India's pursuit for freedom

The memory of my father
Ram Krishna Baliga
who envisioned the Electronic City in Bangalore, India, in the 1970s, making it a modern-day global powerhouse

. My mother
Shanthi Baliga
who to this day continues to pursue her lifetime social mission, which includes emancipation of women and providing for indigent children

My wife
Jayashree
for her solid support over the last two decades

My siblings **Narendra and Lathika**
for their help all along

My children **Anoop and Neena**

250 CASES IN CLINICAL MEDICINE

RAGAVENDRA R BALIGA
MD MBA DNB FRCP(EdIN) FACP FACC

Professor of Internal Medicine
Vice-Chief and Assistant Division Director, Division of Cardiovascular
Medicine, The Ohio State University Medical Center
Consultant Cardiologist, Stephen M. Ross Heart Hospital,
Columbus, Ohio
Editor-in-Chief, Heart Failure Clinics of North America
Associate Editor, American College of Cardiology Cardiosource
Journal Scan

FOURTH EDITION

ELSEVIER   Edinburgh London New York Oxford
Philadelphia St Louis Sydney Toronto 2012

SAUNDERS
ELSEVIER

First edition 1997
Second edition 1999
Third edition 2002

ISBN 9780702033865
International ISBN 9780702033858

British Library Cataloguing in Publication Data
A catalogue record for this book is available from the British Library

Library of Congress Cataloging in Publication Data
A catalog record for this book is available from the Library of Congress

Printed in China

Preface: 'connecting-the-dots'

The current edition of the book has been updated to reflect the new expectations of the Royal College of Physicians and its examiners. The practice of clinical medicine requires 'connecting-the-dots' across pieces of information; that is, it requires utilization of both verbatim memory and gist memory (JAMA, 2009;302:1332–1333). Verbatim memory involves mere recollection of facts (e.g. causes of pleural fluid) whereas gist memory involves interpretation (e.g. that a very low pleural fluid glucose in a patient with inflamed joints indicates that rheumatoid arthritis may be the cause of pleural effusion). Clinical examinations have been redesigned to reflect the day-to-day practice of clinical medicine. Therefore, success in clinical examinations requires development of both forms of memory. Astute clinicians utilize such gist-based reasoning to arrive at the right diagnosis, and their clinical reasoning is superior because they are able to recognize the gist of clinical symptoms: clinical examinations are designed to identify this competency. This edition has been updated keeping in mind these new expectations. More cases now have representative pictures to enhance gist memory to help a prospective candidate to 'connect-the-dots' in the examination situation in a timely fashion; the text provides material to improve verbatim memory.

HOW TO USE THIS BOOK

Although this book is designed for the clinical examination it is best utilized at least 6 months before the Part 1 MRCP written examination and at least a year before the PACES clinical examination. Simultaneous development of both gist and verbatim memory requires a lot of practice and, therefore, this book is best utilized at the bedside after seeing an index case. To improve gist memory by only seeing patients (without using this book) is like embarking on a trans-Atlantic flight without a flight plan, but merely to read books without seeing adequate numbers of patients is like a plane not taking off at all. Each candidate is encouraged not only to see at least three to four representative patients of each case but also to present each patient to a colleague who has passed the examination or a consultant physician (i.e. each case should have been presented by the candidate at least three to four times before the examination); *style matters* as much as substance and this requires practise, practise and more practise.

This book should continue to be useful for MBBS, PLAB, LRCP, MRCP (UK), MRCPI, postgraduate clinical examinations in the US, Australia (FRACP) and Canada (FCCP), and MD (New Zealand, Malaysia, Singapore, India, Pakistan, Sri Lanka and Bangladesh). The current organization of this book should also be appropriate for medical students in the US taking the USMLE and for the American Board of Internal Medicine Examination (ABIM). Cases for examinations are drawn from the same pool for both undergraduate and postgraduate examinations, although in the latter the candidate's performance has to be faultless and he or she will be expected to know certain aspects in greater detail.

Each case is discussed under a number of headings.

Instruction: this allows the candidate to know what sort of instruction or command may be expected from an examiner.

Salient features: this section includes important features in each case including aspects in history, physical signs, guidelines on how to proceed when faced with these signs and what to tell the examiner, in order to satisfy the examiner that the candidate is 'safe and sound' to be a competent clinician.

Diagnosis: most candidates are unable to present their diagnosis in a succinct manner, although they are able to elicit the clinical signs. This heading has been included to help candidates to present their diagnosis in a crisp and confident fashion.

Questions: this section supplies the questions (with answers) that a candidate can expect in a given case. These are also useful for the viva component of the examination.

Endnotes: many of the cases have endnotes giving historical aspects relevant to that particular case, and some have key review references. Although examiners will not deduct marks for ignorance of things that have little relevance to patient welfare, candidates who know the facts can expect a congratulatory glow to pervade the examiner, so that the rest of the questions may be softened accordingly.

R R B

Commissioning Editor: **Pauline Graham**
Development Editor: **Helen Leng**
Copy Editor: **Jane Ward**
Project Managers: **Jess Thompson and Andrew Riley**
Designer/Design Direction: **Kirsteen Wright**
Illustration Manager: **Merlyn Harvey**
Illustrators: **Ethan Danielson and Richard Prime**

Acknowledgements

I would like to thank Pauline Graham, Commissioning Editor for inviting me to update this book and putting up with my expectations and balance the budget allocated to this book by her superiors, Helen Leng, Development Editor at Elsevier, for her patience and gentle but relentless prodding to meet deadlines of this project. I thank Jess Thompson and Andrew Riley for doing an outstanding job of managing the editing, proofing and printing stages.

Finally I thank Geoffrey Gatts, my administrative assistant for his help.

Figure sources

The author would like to thank those who have provided the illustrations for this edition.

Figs 1.2, 5.3, 34.1, 188.1: Zipes DP, Libby P, Bonow RO, Braunwald E. Braunwald's heart disease. Philadelphia, PA: Saunders, 2007.

Figs 3.1, 28.1, 31.2, 103.1, 104.1, 105.1, 111.1, 116.1, 249.1: Adam A, Dixon AK, Grainger RG, Allison DJ. Grainger and Allison's diagnostic radiology, 5th edn. Edinburgh: Churchill Livingstone, 2008.

Fig. 16.2: Krum H. Optimising management of chronic heart failure. Lancet 2009;374:1808.

Figs 17.2, 62.2, 118.1, 120.1, 159.1, 216.1: Goldman L, Ausiello DA. Cecil medicine, 23rd edn. Philadelphia, PA: Saunders, 2007.

Fig. 71.1: Andreoli TE. Cecil medicine, 4th edn. Philadelphia, PA: Saunders, 1997.

Fig. 20.1: Hayek E, Gring CN, Griffin BP. Mitral valve prolapse Lancet 2005;365:507–18.

Fig. 21.2, 29.1: Perloff JK. Clinical recognition of congenital heart disease, 5th edn. Philadelphia, PA: Saunders.

Fig. 23.2: Elliott P, McKenna WJ. Hypertrophic cardiomyopathy Lancet 2004;363:1881–91.

Fig. 25.2, 33.2, 135.1, 135.2, 159.1, 183.1, IX.1B, 233.1: Kliegman RM, Behrman RE, Jenson HB, Stanton BF. Nelson textbook of pediatrics, 18th edn. Philadelphia, PA: Saunders, 2007.

Fig. 26.1, 35.1, 96.1, 97.1, 99.1, 100.1, 107.1, 108.1, 123.1: Mettler FA. Essentials of radiology, 2nd edn. Philadelphia, PA: Saunders-Elsevier, 2004.

Fig. 27.2, 142.1: Carey WD for the Cleveland Clinic. Current clinical medicine 2009. Philadelphia, PA: Saunders, 2009.

Fig. 33.1: Troughton RW, Asher CR, Klein AL. Pericarditis. Lancet 2004;363:717–27.

Figs 34.1, 98.2, 101.1, 109.1: Albert RK, Spiro SG, Jett JR. Albert: Clinical respiratory medicine, 3rd edn. Philadelphia, PA: Mosby, 2008.

Fig. 36.1: Compston A, Confavreux C, Lassmann H et al. McAlpine's multiple sclerosis, 4th edn. Edinburgh: Churchill Livingstone, 2005.

Figs 49.1, 60.1, 64.1, 64.2, 66.1, 68.1, 69.1, 83.1, 83.2: Bradley WG, Daroff RB, Fenichel G, Jankovic J. Neurology in clinical practice, 5th edn. Oxford: Butterworth-Heinemann, 2008.

Fig. 56.1: Pareyson D, Marchesi C. Diagnosis, natural history, and management of Charcot–Marie–Tooth disease. Lancet Neurol 2009;8:654–67.

Figs 57.1, 70.1, 183.2, VIII.1, 206.1, 249.1: Yanoff M, Duker JS Ophthalmology, 3rd edn. Philadelphia, PA: Mosby, 2008.

Fig. 59.1, 131.1, IX.1A, 219.2: Canale ST, Beaty JH (eds) Campbell's operative orthopaedics, 11th edn. Philadelphia, PA: Mosby, 2007.

Fig. 59.2: Guggisberg D, Hadj-Rabia S, Viney C, et al. Skin markers of occult spinal dysraphism. Arch Dermatol 2004;140:1109–15.

Fig. 60.2: Courtney AM, Treadaway K, Remington G, Frohman E. Multiple sclerosis. Med Clin N Am 2009;93:451–76.

Fig. 62.2: Frontera WR, Silver JK, Rizzo TD. Essentials of physical medicine and rehabilitation, 2nd edn. Philadelphia, PA: Saunders, 2008.

Fig. 63.1, 116.1, 118.1, 120.1, V.1, 129.2, 154.2, 230.1, 246.1: Firestein GS, Budd RC, Harris ED, Jr. et al. Kelley's textbook of rheumatology, 8th edn. Philadelphia, PA: Saunders, 2008.

Fig. 66.2, 132.3: Currie G, Douglas G. Flesh and bones of medicine. Edinburgh: Elsevier, 2011.

Fig. 70.2, 129.1, 150.1, 155.1, 159.3, 178.1, 184.2, 190.1, 191.2, 217.1, 250.2: Habif TP. Clinical dermatology, 5th edn. Philadelphia, PA: Mosby, 2009.

Fig. 72.1: Schöllhammer M, von Rothenburg T, Schmid G, Köster O, Peters S. A red tongue and an unsteady gait: MRI in subacute combined degeneration of the spinal cord. Eur J Radiol Extra 2005;54:77–81.

Fig. 82.1: Lakshmi M, Glastonbury CM. Imaging of the cerebellopontine angle. Neuroimaging Clin North Am 2009;19:393–406

Fig. 95.1: Ling H, Lees AJ. How can neuroimaging help in the diagnosis of movement disorders? Neuroimaging Clin North Am 2010;20:111–23.

Fig. 98.3: Goldhaber SZ Lancet 2004;363:1295–305.

Fig. 106.1: Mason RJ, Broaddus VC, Murray JF, Nadel JA. Murray & Nadel's textbook of respiratory medicine, 4th edn. Philadelphia, PA: Saunders, 2005.

Fig. IV.1: Bosmann M, Schreiner O, Galle PR. Coexistence of Cullen's and Grey Turner's signs in acute pancreatitis. Am J Med 2009;122:333–4.

Fig. 115.1: Forbes A Misiewicz JJ, Compton CC. (eds) Atlas of clinical gastroenterology, 3rd edn. Oxford: Mosby, 2005.

Fig. 119.1: Hoffbrand AV, Pettite JE. Color atlas of clinical hematology, 3rd edn. London: Mosby, 2000.

Fig. 119.2: Hoffman R, Benz E, Shattil S, Furie B, Cohen H. Hematology: basic principles and practice, 5th edn. Philadelphia, PA: Churchill Livingstone, 2008.

Fig. 123.1: Bhangu AA, Keighley MRB. Flesh and bones of surgery. Edinburgh: Elsevier, 2007.

Fig. 126.1: His ED. The leukemias of mature lymphocytes. Hematol/Oncol Clin North Am 2009;23:843–71.

Fig. 127.2: Canoso JJ. Rheumatology in primary care, Philadelphia, PA: Saunders, 1997.

Fig. 128.1 Kelley WN Harris ED, Ruddy S, et al. (eds) Textbook of rheumatology, 5th edn, vol. 1. Philadelphia, PA: Saunders, 1997.

Fig. 149.2: Charles C, Clements P, Furst DE. Systemic sclerosis: hypothesis-driven treatment strategies. Lancet 2006;367:1683–91.

Fig. 131.2 Grainger RG, Allison D. Grainger & Allison's diagnostic radiology, a textbook of medical imaging, 4th edn. Edinburgh: Churchill Livingstone, 2001.

Fig. 132.2, 238.1: Roberts JR, Hedges JR. Clinical procedures in emergency medicine, 5th edn. Philadelphia, PA: Saunders, 2009.

Fig. 134.1, 134.2: Rogers LC, Bevilacqua NJ. The diagnosis of Charcot foot. Clin Podiatr Med Surg 2008;25:43–51.

Fig. 136.1, 139.1: Kronenberg HM, Melmed S, Polonsky KS, Larsen PR. Williams textbook of endocrinology, 11th edn. Philadelphia, PA: Saunders, 2008.

Fig. 137.1: Larsen PR, Kronenberg HM, Melmed S. Williams textbook of endocrinology, 10th edn. Philadelphia, PA: Saunders, 2003.

Fig. 137.2: Kanski JJ. Systemic diseases and the eye: signs and differential diagnosis. London: Mosby, 2001.

Fig. 138.1: Seidel HM, Ball JW, Dains JE, Benedict GW. Mosby's guide to physical examination, 5th edn. Philadelphia, PA: Mosby, 2004.

Fig. 140.1: Zimmermann MB, Jooste PL, Pandav C. Iodine deficiency disorders. Lancet 2008;372:1251–62.

Fig. 141.1: Burnside JW, McGlynn TJ. Physical Diagnosis, 17th edn. Baltimore, Williams & Wilkins, 1987.)

Fig. 156.1, 202.2, 216.1, 221.1, 231.1: Forbes CD, Jackson WF. Color atlas and text of clinical medicine, 3rd edn. London: Mosby, 2003.

Fig. 157.1: DeLee JC, Drez D, Jr, Miller MD. DeLee and Drez's orthopaedic sports medicine, 3rd edn. Philadelphia, PA: Saunders, 2009.

Fig. 162.1: Klippel JH, Dieppe PA (eds) Rheumatology, 2nd edn. London: Mosby, 1998.

Fig. 162.2: Powers DB. Systemic lupus erythematosus and discoid lupus erythematosus. Oral Maxillofac Surg Clin North Am 2008;20:661–2.

Fig. 163.1: Abeloff MD, Armitage JO, Niederhuber JE et al. Abeloff's clinical oncology, 4th edn. Edinburgh: Churchill Livingstone, 2008.

Fig. 165.1: Townsend CM, Jr, Beauchamp RD, Evers BM, Mattox KL. Sabiston textbook of surgery, 18th edn. Philadelphia, PA: Saunders, 2007.

Fig. 166.2: Mitani F, Mukai K, Miyamoto H. Polycystic ovary syndrome. Lancet 2007;370:685–97.

Fig. 167.2, 167.3: Moore RL, Devere TS. Epidermal manifestations of internal malignancy. Dermatol Clin 2008;26:17–29.

Fig. 173.1, 175.1: Durrington P. Dyslipidaemia. Lancet 2003;362:717–31.

Fig. 181.1: Winship IM, Dudding TE. Lessons from the skin: cutaneous features of familial cancer. Lancet Oncol 2008;9:462–72.

Fig. 182.2: Ennis O, Feroz A, Stephenson BM, Allison MC. Para-ileostomy pyoderma gangrenosum. Lancet 2001;358: 533.

Fig. 186.1, 201.3, 220.1: Kumar P, Clark M. Clinical medicine 6th edn. Edinburgh: Saunders, 2005.

Fig. 187.1: Kumar V, Abbas AK, Fausto N, Aster J. Robbins and Cotran pathologic basis of disease, 8th (professional) edn. Philadelphia, PA: Saunders, 2009.

Fig. 196.1: Rakel D. Textbook of family medicine, 7th edn. Philadelphia, PA: Saunders, 2007.

Fig. 202.1, 209.2: Wong T, Mitchell P. The eye in hypertension. Lancet 2007;369:425–35.

Fig. 206.1: Bindu PS, Kovoor JME, Christopher R. Teaching neuro. Neurology 2010;74:e14.

Fig. 208.1: Mandell GL, Bennett JE, Dolin R. Mandell, Douglas, and Bennett's Principles and Practice of Infectious Diseases, 7th edn. Edinburgh: Churchill Livingstone, 2009.

Fig. 214.2, 214.3: Coleman HR, Chan C-C, Ferris FL, Chew EY. Age-related macular degeneration. Lancet 2008;372:1835–45.

Fig. 215.1: Andersson DK, Svardsudd K. Long-term glycemic control relates to mortality in type 2 diabetes. Diabetes Care 1995;18:1534–43.

Fig. 215.2: Auerbach PS. Wilderness medicine, 5th edn. St Louis, PA: Mosby, 2007.

Fig. 218.1, 218.2: Marrie TJ, Brown N. Clubbing of the digits. Am J Med 2007;120:940–1.

Fig. 222.1 Leow CK, Lau WY. Sister Joseph's nodule. Can J Surg 1997;40:167.

Fig. 223.1: Sohn N, Korelitz BI, Weinstein MA. Anorectal Crohn's disease. Surg Clin North Am 2010;90:45–68.

Figure sources

Fig. 223.2: Marrero F, Qadeer MA, Lashner BA. Severe complications of inflammatory bowel disease. Med Clin North Am 2008;92: 671–86.

Fig. 224.1 Feldman M, Shiller R (eds) Gastroenterology and hepatology: the comprehensive visual reference. New York: Churchill Livingstone, 1997.

Fig. 229.1: Ralston SH, Langston AL, Reid IR. Pathogenesis and management of Paget's disease of bone. Lancet 2008;372:155–63.

Fig. 245.1: Rayman MP. The importance of selenium to human health. Lancet 2000;356:333–35.

Fig. 231.2: Walsh TD. Palliative medicine. Philadelphia, PA: Saunders, 2008.

Fig. 235.1: Song D, Maher CO. Spinal disorders associated with skeletal dysplasias and syndromes. Neurosurg Clin North Am 2007;18: 499–514.

Fig. 236.2: Davidson MA. Primary care for children and adolescents with Down syndrome. Pediatr Clin North Am 2008;55:1099–111.

Fig. 237.1: Pribitkin EA, Ezzat WH. Classification and treatment of the saddle nose deformity. Otolaryngolc Clin North Am 2009;42:437–61.

Fig. 239.1: Roche-Nagle G. Am J Surg 2009;197: e64–5.

Fig. 240.1: Yanoff M, Fine BS. Ocular pathology, 5th edn. St Louis, MO: Mosby, 2002.

Fig. 247.1: Hochberg MC, Silman AJ, Smolen JS, et al. (eds) Rheumatology, 3rd edn. St Louis, MO: Mosby, 2003.

Fig. 248.1: Levi B, Rees R. Diagnosis and management of pressure ulcers. Clin Plastic Surg 2007;34:735–48.

Fig. 250.1 Lerman MA, Laudenbach J, Marty FM. Management of oral infections in cancer patients. Dental Clin North Am 2008;52:129–53.

Contents

Contents

Respiratory system
History and examination of the chest 351

Abdomen
History and examination of the abdomen 415

Contents

Contents

Cardiovascular system
History and examination of the cardiovascular system

HISTORY

- Chest pain: exertional, at rest (when angina present, comment on the Canadian Cardiovascular Angina class, p. 59)
- Shortness of breath: exertional, at rest (when dyspnoea is present, comment on the New York Heart Association class, p. 3), paroxysmal nocturnal dyspnoea
- Palpitations (p. 50)
- Dizziness, presyncope, syncope
- Swelling of feet.

EXAMINATION OF THE CARDIOVASCULAR SYSTEM

1. Introduce yourself: 'I am Dr/Mr/Ms [???] May I examine your heart?'
2. Ensure adequate exposure of the precordium: 'Would you take your top off, please?' However, be sensitive of the feelings of female patients.
3. Get the patient to sit at 45 degrees: use pillows to support the neck.
4. Inspection: comment on the patient's decubitus (whether he or she is comfortable at rest or obviously short of breath); comment on malar flush (seen in mitral stenosis).
5. Examine the pulse: rate (count for 15 s), rhythm, character, volume; lift the arm to feel for the collapsing pulse. Feel the other radial pulse simultaneously.
6. Comment on the scar at antecubital fossa (cardiac catheterization scars).
7. Look at the tongue for pallor, central cyanosis.
8. Look at the eye for pallor, Argyll Robertson pupil.
9. Examine the jugular venous pulse: comment on the waveform and height from the sternal angle. Check the abdominojugular reflux.
10. Comment on any carotid pulsations (Corrigan's sign of aortic regurgitation).
11. Examine the precordium: comment on surgical scars (midline sternotomy scars; thoracotomy scars for mitral valvotomy may be missed under the female breast).
12. Feel the apex beat: position and character.
13. Feel for left parasternal heave and thrills at the apex and on either side of the sternum.
14. Listen to the heart, beginning from the apex: take care to palpate the right carotid pulse simultaneously so that the examiner notices that you are timing the various cardiac events:
    - Always comment on the first and second heart sounds; mention any additional heart sounds (Fig. I.1); listen to the heart murmurs and *be prepared to draw what your hear.*
    - If you do not hear the mid-diastolic murmur of mitral stenosis, make sure you listen to the apex in the left lateral position with the bell of the stethoscope.

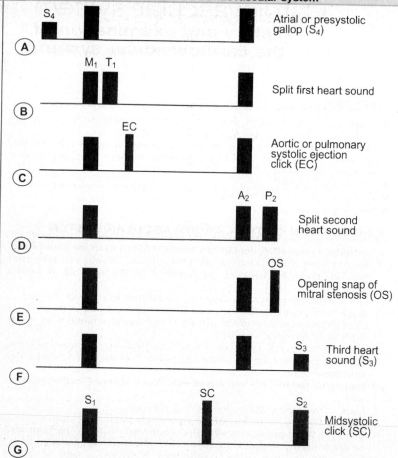

Fig. I.1 Timing of the different heart sounds and added sounds.

- If you hear a murmur at the apex, ensure that you get the patient to breathe in and out: the examiner will be observing whether or not you are listening for the variation in intensity with respiration.
- If you hear a pansystolic murmur, listen at the axilla (mitral regurgitant murmurs are conducted to the axilla).

Note: Be prepared to discuss approach of systolic and diastolic murmurs (see below).

15. Using the diaphragm of your stethoscope listen at the apex, below the sternum, along the left sternal edge, the second right intercostal space and the neck (for ejection systolic murmur of aortic stenosis, aortic sclerosis).

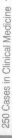

16. Request the patient to sit forward and listen with the diaphragm along the left sternal edge in the 3rd intercostal area with the patient's breath held in expiration for early diastolic murmur of aortic regurgitation.
17. Tell the examiner that you would like to do the following:
    - Listen to lung bases for signs of cardiac failure
    - Check for sacral and leg oedema
    - Examine the liver (tender liver of cardiac failure), splenomegaly (endocarditis)
    - Check blood pressure (BP)
    - Check the peripheral pulses and also check for radiofemoral delay.

ASSESSING MURMURS

● **Systolic murmur** What is the effect on the murmur of inspiration?
(a) Increases with inspiration (right sided):
   - Ejection or regurgitant?
   - If ejection, is there an ejection sound?
   - If no ejection sound, is S_2 fixed or not fixed?
(b) No increase with inspiration (left sided):
   - Is it ejection, regurgitant or uncertain?
   - For each what is the effect of the Valsalva manoeuvre or squatting?

● **Diastolic mumur** What is the effect on the murmur of inspiration?
(a) Increases with inspiration (right sided):
   - Assess quality of mumur and location
   - Is there pulmonary regurgitation.
(b) No increase with inspiration (left sided):
   - Assess quality of mumur (high or low pitched) and location.

CLASSIFYING SEVERITY OF HEART FAILURE

The severity of heart failure is classified by the New York Heart Association (NYHA) classification, which grades symptoms and gives estimated mortality.

NYHA class	Symptoms	Estimated 1-year mortality
I	Mild: no limitation of physical activity	5–10
II	Mild to moderate: slight limitation of physical activity, comfortable at rest but dyspnoea and fatigue on ordinary physical activity	15–30
III	Moderate: marked limitation of physical activity, comfortable at rest but dyspnoea and fatigue on less than ordinary physical activity	15–30
IV	Severe: symptoms at rest	50–60

Further reading

Bruns DLA: A general theory of the causes of murmurs in the cardiovascular system, *Am J Med* 27:360, 1959.

René Theophile Hyacinthe Laennec invented the stethoscope in 1816 and reported his early experience with auscultation in a two-volume book published 3 years later: Laennec RTH (1821) A Treatise on the Diseases of the Chest. London: T and G Underwood (translated by and with a preface and notes by John Forbes).

British physician Sir John Forbes (1787–1861) is best remembered for popularizing the stethoscope among English-speaking doctors. Forbes was born in Banff in the northeast of Scotland. He studied at Marischal College, Aberdeen, before he went to Edinburgh where he received his medical education. Forbes translated Laennec's monograph in English in 1821 and published his own book on the subject in 1824 (Forbes J (1824) Original Cases with Dissections and Observations Illustrating the Use of the Stethoscope and Percussion in the Diagnosis of the Diseases of the Chest. London: T and G Underwood). The latter included a brief biographical sketch of the Austrian physician Leopald Auenbrugger and the first English translation of his essay (which was in Latin) on percussion. It also contained a summary of Parisian physician Victor Collin's recent manual on cardiac physical diagnosis.

1 MITRAL STENOSIS

INSTRUCTION

This patient developed shortness of breath and orthopnoea during pregnancy, please examine.

This 55-year-old patient has atrial fibrillation, please do the relevant clinical examination.

SALIENT FEATURES

History

- Symptoms of left-sided heart failure: exertional dyspnoea, orthopnoea, paroxysmal dyspnoea.
- Less frequent symptoms: haemoptysis, hoarseness of voice, symptoms of right-sided failure (these symptoms are somewhat more specific for mitral stenosis).
- Obtain a history of rheumatic fever in childhood.

Examination

- Pulse is regular or irregularly irregular (from atrial fibrillation).
- Jugular venous pressure (JVP) may be raised.
- Malar flush.
- Tapping apex beat in the 5th intercostal space just medial to midclavicular line.
- Left parasternal heave (indicating right ventricular enlargement).
- Loud first heart sound.
- Opening snap (OS; often difficult to hear; a high-pitched sound that can vary from 0.04 to 0.10 s after the second sound (S) and is heard best at the apex with the patient in the lateral decubitus position).
- Rumbling, low-pitched, mid-diastolic murmur, best heard in the left lateral position on expiration. In sinus rhythm there may be presystolic accentuation of the murmur. If you are not sure about the murmur, tell the examiner that you want the patient to perform sit-ups or hopping on one foot to increase the heart rate. This will increase the flow across the mitral valve and the murmur is better heard.
- Pulmonary component of second sound (P) is loud.

Notes

1. Remember the signs of pulmonary hypertension include loud P_2, right ventricular lift, elevated neck veins, ascites and oedema. This is an ominous sign of the disease progression because pulmonary hypertension increases the risk associated with surgery (Br Heart J 1975;37:74–8).
2. In patients with valvular lesions, a candidate would be expected to comment on rhythm, the presence of heart failure and signs of pulmonary hypertension.
3. In atrial septal defect, large flow murmurs across the tricuspid valve can cause mid-diastolic murmurs. The presence of wide, fixed splitting of second sound, absence of loud first heart sound, and an opening snap and incomplete right bundle branch block should indicate the correct diagnosis. However, about 4% of the patients with atrial septal

defect have mitral stenosis, a combination called Lutembacher syndrome.

DIAGNOSIS

This patient has mitral stenosis (lesion), which is almost always caused by rheumatic heart disease (aetiology), and has atrial fibrillation, pulmonary hypertension and congestive cardiac failure (functional status).

QUESTIONS

What is the commonest cause of mitral stenosis?
Rheumatic heart disease.

What is the pathology of mitral stenosis?
The main features are leaflet thickening, nodularity and commissural fusion, all of which result in narrowing of the valve to the shape of a fish mouth.

What is the natural history of mitral stenosis?
- From the occurrence of rheumatic fever to the onset of symptoms, there is a long latent period of 20 to 40 years in Europe and North America.
- Moreover, there is a further period of about 10 years before symptoms become disabling.
- The 10-year survival of untreated patients is 50% to 60%, depending on symptoms at presentation:
  - When the patient is asymptomatic or minimally symptomatic the survival is >80% at 10 years with 60% of patients having no progression of symptoms.
  - Once significant limiting symptoms occur, the 10-year survival rate (is poor) 0–15%.
  - When there is severe pulmonary hypertension, mean survival drops to <3 years.
- Mortality of untreated patients is caused by:
  - progressive heart failure in 60% to 70%
  - systemic embolism in 20% to 30%
  - pulmonary embolism in 10%
  - infection in 1% to 5%.

What is the mechanism of tapping apex beat?
It is from an accentuated first heart sound.

What does the opening snap indicate?
The opening snap is caused by the opening of the stenosed mitral valve and indicates that the leaflets are pliable. The opening snap is usually accompanied by a loud first heart sound. It is absent when the valve is diffusely calcified. When only the tips of the leaflets are calcified, the opening snap persists.

What is the mechanism of a loud first heart sound?
The loud first heart sound occurs when the valve leaflets are mobile. The valve is open during diastole and is suddenly slammed shut by ventricular contraction in systole.

What is the mechanism of presystolic accentuation of the murmur?

In sinus rhythm it is caused by the atrial systole, which increases flow across the stenotic valve from the left atrium to the left ventricle (LV); this causes accentuation of the loudness of the murmur. This may also be seen in atrial fibrillation and is explained by the turbulent flow caused by the mitral valve starting to close with the onset of ventricular systole. This occurs before the first heart sound and gives the impression of falling in late diastole. It is, however, caused by the start of ventricular systole.

What are the complications?

- Left atrial enlargement and atrial fibrillation
- Systemic embolization, usually cerebral hemispheres
- Pulmonary hypertension
- Tricuspid regurgitation
- Right heart failure.

How does one determine clinically the severity of the stenosis?

- The narrower the distance between the second sound and the opening snap, the greater the severity. The converse is not true. (**Note**: This time interval between the second sound and opening snap is said to be inversely related to the left atrial pressure.)
- The longer the duration of the diastolic murmur, the greater the severity. Note that in tight mitral stenosis the murmur may be less prominent or inaudible and the findings may be primarily those of pulmonary hypertension.

ADVANCED-LEVEL QUESTIONS

What are the investigations you would do?

- *ECG* shows broad bifid P wave (P mitrale); atrial fibrillation in advanced disease, left atrial enlargement, right ventricular hypertrophy (Fig. 1.1).
- *Chest radiography* (Fig. 1.2) shows:
  - congested upper lobe veins
  - double silhouette from enlarged left atrium
  - straightening of the left border of the heart caused by prominent pulmonary conus and filling of the pulmonary bay by the enlarged left atrium
  - Kerley B lines (horizontal lines in the regions of the costophrenic angles)
  - uncommonly the left bronchus may be horizontal as a result of an enlarged left atrium
  - mottling caused by secondary pulmonary haemosiderosis.
- *Echocardiography:* two-dimensional and Doppler echocardiography is the diagnostic tool of choice for assessing the severity of mitral stenosis and for judging the applicability of balloon mitral valvotomy (N Engl J Med 1997;337:32–41):
  - can identify restricted diastolic opening of the mitral valve leaflets caused by 'doming' of the anterior leaflet and immobility of the posterior leaflet
  - allows assessment of the mitral valve apparatus and left atrial enlargement

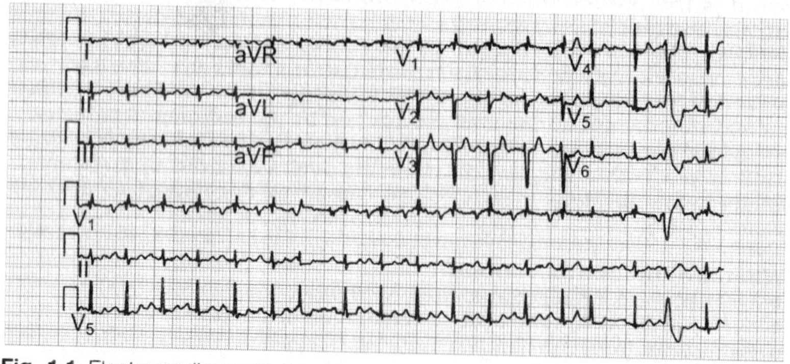

Fig. 1.1 Electrocardiography in severe mitral stenosis, showing right ventricular hypertrophy and left atrial enlargement.

- can usually permit an accurate planimetric calculation of the valve area (Am J Cardiol 1979;43:560–8)
- can also assess the severity of stenosis by measuring the decay of the transvalvular gradient or the 'pressure half-time', an empirical measurement (Br Heart J 1978;40:131–40)
- can accurately and reproducibly measure the mean transmitral gradient, using continuous wave Doppler signal across the mitral valve with the modified Bernoulli equation
- can determine the mitral valve area non-invasively from Doppler echocardiography with either diastolic half-time method or continuity equation; the continuity equation should be used when the area derived from the half-time does not correlate with the means transmitral gradient
- enables the estimation of the pulmonary artery systolic pressure from the tricuspid regurgitation velocity signal with Doppler and assess severity of concomitant mitral or aortic regurgitation.
- A *transoesophageal echocardiography* is not required unless a question about diagnosis remains after transthoracic echocardiography. It is also useful to exclude thrombus in the left atrial appendage before balloon valvotomy or cardioversion.
- *Cardiac catheterization:*
  - shows raised right heart pressures and an end-diastolic gradient from pulmonary artery wedge pressure (or left atrium if trans-septal puncture done to the LV)
  - (left and right heart catheterization) is indicated when percutaneous mitral balloon valvotomy is being considered
  - is indicated when there is a discrepancy between Doppler-derived haemodynamics and the clinical status of a symptomatic patient.
- *Coronary angiography* may be required in selected patients who need intervention.
- *Exercise haemodynamics* should be performed when the symptoms are out of proportion to the calculated mitral valve gradient area.

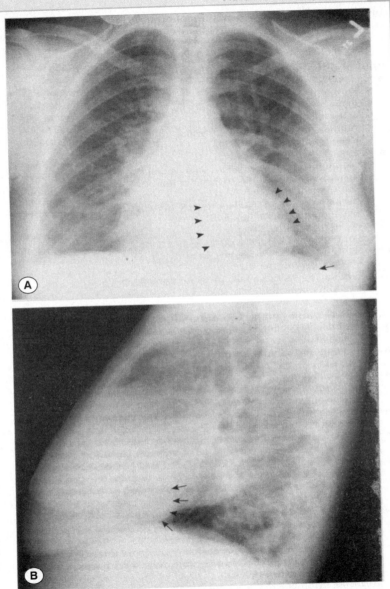

Fig. 1.2 Chest radiographs in severe mitral stenosis. (A) Posteroanterior view shows enlargement of the left atrium (arrowheads), prominence of the hilar vessels, and pulmonary venous redistribution. Transverse angle of the apex suggests right ventricular enlargement (arrow). (B) Lateral view confirms this, with filling in of the retrosternal airspace. Note also severe left atrial enlargement (arrows). (With permission from Zipes DP et al. 2007.)

What is the normal cross-sectional area of the mitral valve?
It ranges from 4 to 6 cm^2 and turbulence of the flow occurs when this area is <2 cm^2.

What are the features of severity of mitral stenosis?
- *Mild mitral stenosis:*
  - Symptoms: usually absent
  - Signs: S_2–OS >120 ms, normal P_2
  - Valve area (cm^2): >1.5
  - Pulmonary artery systolic pressure (mmHg): <30
  - Mean gradient (mmHg): <5.
- *Moderate mitral stenosis:*
  - Symptoms: New York Heart Association (NYHA) class II–III
  - Signs: S_2–OS 80–100 ms, normal or loud P_2
  - Valve area (cm^2): 1.0–1.5
  - Pulmonary artery systolic pressure (mmHg): 30–50
  - Mean gradient (mmHg): 5–10.
- *Severe or 'tight' mitral stenosis:*
  - Symptoms: NYHA class II–IV
  - Signs: RV lift, S_2–OS <80 ms, loud P_2
  - Valve area (cm^2): <1.0
  - Pulmonary artery systolic pressure (mmHg): >50
  - Mean gradient (mmHg): >10.

How would you manage the patient?
- Asymptomatic patient in sinus rhythm: prophylaxis against infective endocarditis only.
- Mild symptoms: diuretics to reduce left atrial pressure and, therefore, symptoms.
- Atrial fibrillation:
  - Rate control (digitalis, beta-blocker or calcium channel blocker)
  - Anticoagulants (Eur Heart J 1988;9:291–4).
- Anticoagulation should also be considered in patients with left atrial dimensions ≥55 mm.
- Moderate to severe symptoms or pulmonary hypertension is beginning to develop: mechanical relief of valve stenosis, including balloon valvotomy (N Engl J Med 1994;331:961–7, Br Heart J 1988;60:299–308) (percutaneous mitral balloon valvuloplasty is usually the procedure of choice when there is a non-calcified pliable valve) or surgery.

What are the indications for surgery?
- Patients with severe symptoms of pulmonary congestion and significant mitral stenosis (mitral valve area ≤1.5 cm^2).
- Patients with pulmonary hypertension (pulmonary artery systolic pressure >50 mmHg at rest or 60 mmHg with exercise) or haemoptysis even if minimally symptomatic.
- Recurrent thromboembolic events despite therapeutic anticoagulation.

Which surgical procedures are used to treat mitral stenosis?
- Closed commissurotomy:
  - Closed mitral valvotomy involves the use of mechanical dilators, inserted through the apex of the LV. It is complicated by mitral regurgitation, systemic embolization and restenosis.

- Balloon valvuloplasty (a form of closed commissurotomy) is a percutaneous trans-septal balloon mitral valvotomy (or valvuloplasty). Remember percutaneous balloon dilatation of the mitral valve is a useful option in patients who are unable to undergo cardiac surgery, as in late pregnancy or when the patient is too ill (severe respiratory disease, non-mitral cardiac disease, multiorgan failure).
- Open commissurotomy requires cardiopulmonary bypass and allows surgical repair of the valve under direct vision resulting in more effective and safer valvotomy than the closed procedure.
- Valve replacement entails risks including thromboembolism, endocarditis and primary valve failure.

What factors determine the success of balloon valvuloplasty?
- Good mobility of the valves
- Little calcification
- Minimal subvalvular disease
- Mild mitral regurgitation.

What are the indications for mitral valve replacement?
Patients who are not good candidates for percutaneous balloon valvotomy or mitral valve repair who have:
- moderate to severe mitral stenosis and NYHA class III–IV
- severe mitral stenosis (mitral valve area <1 cm^2) and severe pulmonary hypertension (pulmonary artery systolic pressure >60 mmHg).

In which trimester do pregnant patients with mitral stenosis usually become symptomatic?
Patients usually become symptomatic in the second trimester of pregnancy, when blood volume increases significantly and increases pulmonary pressures. As the blood volume diminishes late in third trimester, the symptoms might slightly improve.

Mention some rarer causes of mitral stenosis
- Calcification of mitral annulus and leaflets
- Rheumatoid arthritis
- Systemic lupus erythematosus (SLE)
- Malignant carcinoid
- Congenital stenosis.

Which conditions simulate mitral stenosis?
- Left atrial myxoma
- Ball valve thrombus in the left atrium
- Cor triatriatum (a rare congenital heart condition where a thin membrane across the left atrium obstructs pulmonary venous flow).

Have you heard of Ortner syndrome?
It refers to the hoarseness of voice caused by left vocal cord paralysis associated with enlarged left atrium in mitral stenosis.

What are the haemodynamic changes in mitral stenosis?
Depends on the severity of mitral stenosis and includes increase in left atrial pressure, increase in pulmonary arterial pressure and in severe cases decreased cardiac output.

N. Ortner (1865–1935), Professor of Medicine, Vienna, described the syndrome in 1897. He believed in laboratory research and its application to bedside clinical work and he said that the clinician's motto ought to be 'übers laboratorium dauernd zur Klinik' (translated: 'always via the laboratory to the clinic').

PJ Kerley (1900–1978), British radiologist.

Paul Wood was a cardiologist at the Hammersmith and National Heart Hospitals. His clinical skills are legendary and he had a profound influence on British cardiology.

Elliott Cutler, in 1923 in Boston, USA, was the first to attempt surgical treatment of mitral stenosis by inserting a knife through the apex of the LV and blindly cutting the valve at right angles to its natural orifice.

Henry Souttar, in 1925, relieved mitral stenosis with a finger inserted through the atrial appendage.

In 1948, four surgeons working independently performed successful valvotomies: Horace Smithy, Charles Bailey, Dwight Harken and Russell Brock.

In 1984, Kanji Inoue from Japan and in 1985, James E Lock, contemporary Professor of Pediatric Cardiology, Harvard Medical School, and colleagues introduced balloon valvuloplasty for mitral stenosis.

2   MITRAL REGURGITATION

INSTRUCTION

Examine this patient's heart.

SALIENT FEATURES

History

- Asymptomatic or mild symptoms: often
- Shortness of breath (from pulmonary congestion)
- Fatigue (from low cardiac output)
- Palpitation (from atrial fibrillation or LV dysfunction)
- Fluid retention (in late-stage disease)
- Obtain a history of myocardial infarction, rheumatic fever, connective tissue disorder, infective endocarditis.

Examination

- Peripheral pulse may be normal or jerky (i.e. rapid upstroke with a short duration).
- Apex beat will be displaced downwards and outwards and will be forceful in character.
- First heart sound will be soft.
- Third heart sound is common (left ventricular gallop sound).
- Pansystolic murmur (Hope murmur) (Fig. 2.1) conducted to the axilla, best detected with the diaphragm and on expiration. (**Note:** It is important to be sure that there is no associated tricuspid regurgitation.)

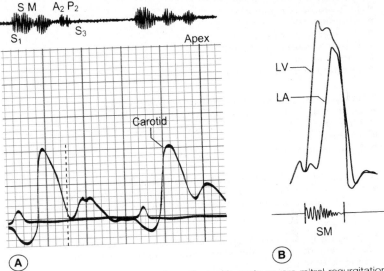

(A)

(B)

Fig. 2.1 (A) Phonocardiogram of a patient with acute severe mitral regurgitation showing a decrescendo early systolic murmur and diastolic filling sound (S_3). (B) Pressure waveforms showing an abrupt rise in LA pressure and attenuation of the LV–LA pressure gradient, resulting in the duration and configuration of the murmur.

- Loud pulmonary second sound and left parasternal heave when there is associated pulmonary hypertension.

Note: When mitral regurgitation is caused by left ventricular dilatation and diminished cardiac contractility, the systolic murmur may be mid, late or pansystolic. Other causes of short systolic murmurs at the apex include mitral valve prolapse, papillary muscle dysfunction and aortic stenosis. In calcific aortic stenosis of the elderly, the murmur may be more prominent in the apex and may be confused with mitral regurgitation. In such instances try to listen to the murmur after a pause with premature beat or listen to the beat after a pause with atrial fibrillation. The murmur of aortic stenosis becomes louder, whereas that of mitral regurgitation shows little change.

DIAGNOSIS

This patient has mitral regurgitation (lesion) as evidenced by grade III/VI pansystolic murmur, which is probably caused by ischaemic or rheumatic heart disease (aetiology), and is in cardiac failure as evidenced by bibasal crackles (functional status). The patient is in NYHA class III heart failure.

QUESTIONS

What are causes of chronic mitral regurgitation?
- Infective endocarditis
- Mitral valve prolapse

- Rheumatic heart disease
- Left ventricular dilatation
- Coronary artery disease
- Annular calcification
- Papillary muscle dysfunction
- Cardiomyopathy
- Connective tissue disorders.

What are causes of acute mitral regurgitation?

- Acute myocardial infarction (rupture of the papillary muscle)
- Endocarditis (from perforation of the mitral valve leaflet or the chordae)
- Trauma
- Myxomatous degeneration of the valve.

How would you investigate this patient?

- *ECG:* look for broad bifid P waves (P mitrale), left ventricular hypertrophy, atrial fibrillation. When coronary artery disease is the cause, there is often evidence of inferior or posterior wall myocardial infarction.
- *Radiography* can assess pulmonary congestion, large heart, left atrial enlargement and pulmonary artery enlargement (if severe and long-standing).
- *Echocardiography* determines the anatomy of the mitral valve apparatus, left atrial and left ventricular size and function (typical features include large left atrium, large LV, increased fractional shortening, regurgitant jet on colour Doppler, leaflet prolapse, floppy valve or flail leaflet). The echocardiogram provides baselines estimation of LV and left atrial volume, an estimation of left ventricular ejection fraction, and approximation of the severity of regurgitation. It can be helpful to determine the anatomic cause of mitral regurgitation. In the presence of even mild tricuspid regurgitation, an estimate of pulmonary artery pressure can be obtained.
- *Transoesophageal echocardiogram* is useful when transthoracic echocardiography provides non-diagnostic images. It may give better visualization of mitral valve prolapse. It is useful intraoperatively to establish the anatomic basis for mitral regurgitation and to guide repair.
- *Cardiac catheterization* is useful to determine coexistent coronary artery or aortic valve disease. Large 'v' waves are seen in the wedge tracing. Left ventriculogram and haemodynamic measurements are indicated when non-invasive tests are inconclusive regarding the severity of mitral regurgitation, LV function, or the need for surgery.

How would you differentiate between mitral regurgitation and tricuspid regurgitation?

	Mitral regurgitation	**Tricuspid regurgitation**
Pulse	Jerky or normal	Normal
Jugular venous pressure	Prominent 'v' wave	
Palpation	Left ventricular heave	Left parasternal heave

	Mitral regurgitation	Tricuspid regurgitation
Auscultation	Pansystolic murmur	Pansystolic murmur
	Intensity increases with expiration	Intensity increases with inspiration
	Radiates to the axilla	
Other signs	Hepatic pulsations	

Why may these patients have a jerky pulse?

Because of reduced systolic ejection time, secondary to a large volume of blood regurgitating into the left atrium.

When does the murmur of mitral regurgitation radiate to the neck (i.e. base of the heart)?

Rarely, in involvement of the posterior mitral leaflet or from ruptured chordae tendinae, the regurgitant jet strikes the left atrial wall adjacent to the aortic root and the murmur radiates to the base of the heart; therefore, it may be confused with the murmur of aortic stenosis.

How do you grade systolic murmurs?

Levine's grading of systolic murmurs (Ann Intern Med 1933;6:1371):

1: Murmur is so faint that it is heard only with special effort
2: Murmur is faint but readily detected
3: Murmur is prominent but not loud
4: Murmur is loud
5: Murmur is very loud
6: Murmur is loud enough to be heard with the stethoscope just removed from contact with the chest wall.

What are the causes of pansystolic murmur over the precordium?

- Mitral regurgitation
- Tricuspid regurgitation
- Ventricular septal defect (this generally radiates to the right of the sternum).

ADVANCED-LEVEL QUESTION

Which congenital cardiac conditions can be associated with mitral valve regurgitation?

- Ostium primum atrial septal defect (as a result of cleft mitral valve)
- Partial atrioventricular canal
- Corrected transposition of the great arteries.

What are the mechanisms of mitral regurgitation?

Mechanisms are grossly classified as:

- *functional* (mitral valve is structurally normal and disease results from valve deformation caused by ventricular remodelling), e.g. cardiomyopathy, myocarditis
- *organic* (intrinsic valve lesions), e.g. endocarditis, annular calcification, rheumatic heart disease, ruptured papillary muscle.

They can be subclassified by leaflet movement (Carpentier's classification):

- Type I (normal valve movement, such as annular dilatation or leaflet perforation), e.g. endocarditis

- Type II (excessive movement), e.g. ruptured papillary muscle
- Type III (restrictive movement:
  - IIIa: diastolic restriction, e.g. in rheumatic disease
  - IIIb: systolic restriction, e.g. in functional disease such as cardiomyopathy.

How would you determine the severity of the lesion?

- The larger the LV on clinical examination, the greater the severity.
- A third heart sound suggests that the disease is severe.
- Colour Doppler ultrasonography quantifies the severity of the regurgitant jet, usually into three grades. However echocardiography provides only a semiquantitative estimate of the severity of regurgitation. Left ventriculography performed during cardiac catheterization provides an additional but also imperfect estimate of the severity of mitral regurgitation.
- Prognosis is worsened if the right ventricular function is reduced and patients with a right ventricular ejection fraction of <30% are particularly at high risk (Circulation 1986;73:900-12).

How would you quantify the severity of the lesion?

Mild mitral regurgitation:
- Qualitative:
  - Angiographic grade: 1+
  - Doppler vena contracta width (cm): <0.3
  - Colour Doppler jet area: small central jet (<4 cm^2 or <20% left atria area).
- Quantitative (cath or echo):
  - Regurgitation volume (ml/beat): <30
  - Regurgitation fraction (%): <30
  - Regurgitant orifice area (cm^2): <0.20.

Moderate mitral regurgitation:
- Qualitative:
  - Angiographic grade: 2+
  - Doppler vena contracta width (cm): 0.3-0.69 cm
  - Colour Doppler jet area: signs of mitral regurgitation greater than mild but no criteria for severe mitral regurgitation.
- Quantitative (cath or echo):
  - Regurgitation volume (ml/beat): 30-59
  - Regurgitation fraction (%): 30-49
  - Regurgitant orifice area (cm^2): 0.2-0.39.

Severe mitral regurgitation:
- Qualitative:
  - Angiographic grade: 3-4+
  - Doppler vena contracta width (cm): >0.7
  - Colour Doppler jet area: large central jet (>40% left atria area) or with wall impinging jet of any size, swirling in LA, vena contracta width >0.7 quantitative (cath or echo)
  - Regurgitation volume (ml/beat): ≥60
  - Regurgitation fraction (%):≥50
  - Regurgitant orifice area (cm^2): ≥0.40.
- Additional criteria:
  - Left atrial size: enlarged
  - Left ventricular size: enlarged.

What is the significance of third heart sounds in mitral regurgitation?

The prevalence of third heart sounds increases with the severity of mitral regurgitation. However, in patients with mitral regurgitation, the third heart sound is caused by rapid ventricular filling and does not necessarily reflect left ventricular systolic dysfunction or increased filling pressure since in this situation the third heart sound is caused by rapid filling of the LV by the large volume of blood stored in the left atrium in diastole.

How would you follow an asymptomatic patient with mitral regurgitation?

- **Mild regurgitation**
  - Asymptomatic patients with no evidence of left ventricular enlargement or dysfunction or pulmonary hypertension may be followed up on an annual basis with instructions to alert the physician if symptoms develop in the interim period.
  - Annual echocardiography is unnecessary unless there is clinical evidence that the mitral regurgitation has worsened.

- **Moderate regurgitation**
  - Clinical evaluations should be performed annually.
  - Echocardiography is not necessary more than once a year.

- **Severe regurgitation**
  - Asymptomatic patients should be followed up every 6 to 12 months with a history, physical examination and echocardiography to assess symptoms or transition to asymptomatic LV dysfunction. (Most patients develop symptoms before developing LV dysfunction.)
  - Serial chest radiographs and ECGs are of less value but may be helpful in selected patients.
  - Exercise stress testing may be used to add objective evidence of symptoms and changes in exercise tolerance. Exercise testing may be helpful when a good history of the patient's exercise capacity cannot be obtained.

What is the medical management of such patients?

- Asymptomatic patients: antibiotic prophylaxis for endocarditis
- When atrial fibrillation develops: digitalis to slow ventricular response
- Heart failure: diuretics and inotropes, but major consideration should be given to surgery.

What are the indications for surgery in this patient?

- Moderate to severe symptoms despite medical therapy (NYHA functional class III or IV), provided that left ventricular function is adequate.
- Patients with minimal or no symptoms should be followed up every 6 months by echocardiographic or radionuclide assessment of left ventricular size and systolic function. When the ejection fraction falls to 60% (Circulation 1994;90:830–7), or when left ventricular end systolic dimension is greater than 45 mm (J Am Coll Cardiol 1984;3:235–42), mitral valve repair or replacement should be considered even in the absence of symptoms.

Remember that:

- valve repair improves outcome compared with valve replacement and reduces mortality of patient with severe organic mitral regurgitation by about 70%

- ischaemic mitral regurgitation carries the worse prognosis: operative mortality is 10 to 20% and long-term survival is substantially lower than with non-ischaemic mitral regurgitation (J Thorac Cardiovasc Surg 1986;91:379–88, Ann Thorac Surg 1994;58:668–75).

When is successful valve repair less likely?

It is less likely when the aetiology is ischaemic, infectious or rheumatic, when there is significant calcification, or when the prolapse is bileaflet or anterior.

What do you know about mitral regurgitation caused by flail leaflet?

In patients with mitral regurgitation caused by flail leaflet, the lesion usually results in high degrees of regurgitation (J Am Coll Cardiol 1990;16:232–9). In Western countries, flail leaflet is the most frequent cause of mitral regurgitation requiring surgical correction (Mayo Clinic Proc 1987;62:22–34, Eur Heart J 1991;12(suppl B):2–4). When treated medically, mitral regurgitation caused by flail leaflet is associated with excess mortality and high morbidity. Surgery is almost unavoidable within 10 years after the diagnosis and appears to be associated with an improved prognosis, suggesting that surgery should be considered early in the course of the disease (N Engl J Med 1996;335:1417–23).

What is the natural history of chronic mitral regurgitation?

Progression of the mitral regurgitation is variable and is determined by progression of lesions or mitral annulus size.

Samuel A Levine was Professor of Cardiology at Harvard Medical School and Peter Bent Brigham Hospital in Boston.

James Hope (1801–1841) was an English physician who worked at St George's Hospital, London, and wrote a book in 1831 entitled Diseases of the Heart and Great Vessels.

3 MIXED MITRAL VALVE DISEASE

INSTRUCTION

Listen to this patient's heart.

SALIENT FEATURES

- The patient will have signs of both mitral stenosis and regurgitation.
- The candidate will be expected to indicate the dominant lesion (see below).

Proceed as follows:

- Look carefully for surgical scars of mitral valvotomy in all patients (scars under the left breast in female patients are often missed). Patients with previous valvotomy may have regurgitation and restenosis.

	Dominant mitral stenosis	**Dominant mitral regurgitation**
Apex beat	Tapping, not displaced	Heaving and displaced
First heart sound	Loud	Soft
Third heart sound	Absent	Present

A third heart sound in mitral regurgitation indicates that any associated mitral stenosis is insignificant.

Note: There may be patients who do not have clear-cut signs such as a loud first heart sound with a displaced apex; in such cases you must say that it is difficult to ascertain clinically the dominant lesion and that cardiac catheterization should resolve the issue.

DIAGNOSIS

This patient has mitral stenosis with mitral regurgitation (lesion), with the dominant lesion being stenosis caused by rheumatic heart disease (aetiology), and is in cardiac failure (functional status).

QUESTIONS

What is the cause of mitral stenosis with regurgitation?
Mixed mitral valve disease is usually caused by chronic rheumatic heart disease.

Which valves are most often affected by rheumatic heart?
The approximate frequencies are:
- mitral valve disease, 80%
- aortic valve, 50%
- combined mitral and aortic valve lesion, 20%
- tricuspid valve, 10%
- pulmonary valve, <1%.

What is the significance of a diastolic rumble in mitral regurgitation?
It signifies the presence of coexistent mitral stenosis. In the absence of mitral stenosis, it suggests that there is high diastolic transmitral flow and severe mitral regurgitation. Inhalation of amyl nitrate increases both the duration and intensity of the diastolic murmur caused by mitral stenosis, whereas it decreases them if the diastolic rumble is solely caused by mitral regurgitation. Also the presence of an opening snap suggests mitral stenosis as the cause of the diastolic rumble.

In patients with mitral regurgitation and a diastolic rumble, what does the presence of a giant left atrium indicate?
It indicates that there is no significant mitral stenosis.

What is the significance of multiple small calcified nodules on chest radiograph in this patient?
It indicates long-standing elevation of pulmonary venous pressure (Fig. 3.1).

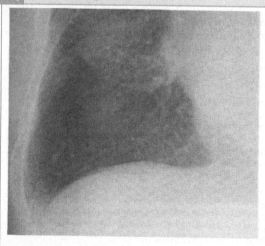

Fig. 3.1 Mixed mitral valve disease, showing multiple small calcified nodules. (With permission from Adam et al. 2008.)

4   AORTIC REGURGITATION

INSTRUCTION

Examine this patient's cardiovascular system.
Examine this patient's heart.

SALIENT FEATURES

History

- Asymptomatic (but may have normal or depressed left ventricular function)
- Dyspnoea and fatigue (from left ventricular impairment and low cardiac output initially on exertion)
- Symptoms of left ventricular failure in later stages
- Angina pectoris is less common than in aortic stenosis; usually indicates coronary artery disease.

Examination

Pulse

- Collapsing pulse (large volume, rapid fall with low diastolic pressure)
- Visible carotid pulsation in neck (dancing carotids or Corrigan's sign)
- Capillary pulsation in fingernails (Quincke's sign)
- A booming sound heard over femorals ('pistol-shot' femorals or Traube's sign)
- To and fro systolic and diastolic murmur produced by compression of femorals by stethoscope (Duroziez's sign or murmur).

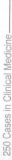

Heart
- Heart sounds are usually normal.
- Apex beat will be displaced outwards and forceful may be seen and/or felt.
- Third heart sound is heard (in early systole with bicuspid aortic valve).
- Early diastolic, high-pitched murmur is heard at the left sternal edge with the diaphragm; if not readily apparent, it is important to sit the patient forward and auscultate with the patient's breath held at the end of expiration (Fig. 4.1). When the ascending aorta is dilated and displaced to the right, the murmur may be heard along the right sternal border as well.
- An ejection systolic murmur may be heard at the base of the heart in severe aortic regurgitation (without aortic stenosis). This murmur may be as loud as grade 5 or 6, and underlying organic stenosis can be ruled out only by investigations.
- Ejection click suggests underlying bicuspid aortic valve.
- Mid-diastolic murmur of Austin–Flint may be heard at apex. It is typically low pitched, similar to the murmur of mitral stenosis but without preceding opening snap.
- Loud pulmonary component of second sound (suggests pulmonary hypertension).

General examination
- Head nodding in time with the heart beat (de Musset's sign) may be present.
- Visible carotid pulsation may be obvious in the neck: dancing carotids or Corrigan's sign.
- Blood pressure indicates wide pulse pressure.

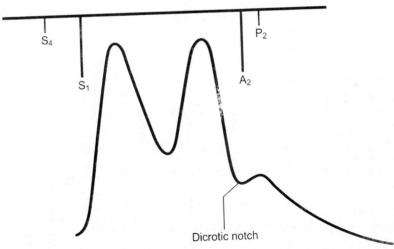

Fig. 4.1 Carotid pulse waveform and heart sound in severe aortic regurgitation: bifid pulse with two systolic peaks.

- Look for systolic pulsations of the uvula (Muller's sign).
- Check pupils for Argyll Robertson pupil of syphilis.
- Look for stigmata of Marfan syndrome: high-arched palate, arm span greater than height.
- Check joints for ankylosing spondylitis and rheumatoid arthritis.

DIAGNOSIS

This patient has pure aortic regurgitation (lesion), which is caused by associated ankylosing spondylitis (aetiology), and is in cardiac failure (functional status).

QUESTIONS

Mention a few causes of chronic aortic regurgitation:
- Rheumatic fever
- Hypertension (accentuated tambour quality of second sound)
- Atherosclerosis
- Bacterial endocarditis
- Idiopathic dilatation of the aortic root and annulus
- Syphilis
- Marfan syndrome
- Rheumatoid arthritis
- Cystic medial necrosis
- Seronegative arthritis (ankylosing spondylitis, Reiter syndrome)
- Bicuspid aortic valve.

How would you investigate a patient with aortic regurgitation?
- *Chest radiograph* is usually normal in mild aortic regurgitation; possibly valvular calcification, cardiomegaly.
- *ECG* (Fig. 4.2) typically shows features of left ventricular hypertrophy and strain (increased QRS amplitude and ST/T wave changes in

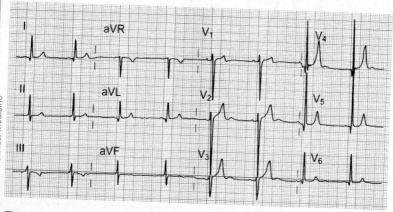

Fig. 4.2 Left ventricular hypertrophy with prominent positive anterior T waves.

precordial leads) and left atrial hypertrophy (wide P wave in lead II and biphasic P in lead V_1).

- *Echocardiogram* is indicated to confirm the diagnosis of aortic regurgitation, determine aetiology, assess valve morphology, acquire a semi-quantitative estimate of severity of regurgitation, assess LV dimension, mass and systolic function, assess aortic size, in estimating the degree of pulmonary hypertension (when tricuspid regurgitation is present), and in determining whether there is rapid equilibration of aortic and LV diastolic pressure. Doppler is the best method for detecting aortic regurgitation.
- *Exercise testing* in severe aortic regurgitation, when sedentary or where there are equivocal symptoms is useful to assess functional capacity, symptomatic responses and haemodynamic effects of exercise.
- *Radionuclide angiogram* is useful in asymptomatic patients with poor-quality echocardiographic images.
- *Cardiac catheterization* is necessary when coronary artery disease is suspected (e.g. in patients >40 years) and when severity of aortic regurgitation is doubted; injection of contrast into aortic root gives information on degree of regurgitation and state of aortic root (presence of dilatation, dissection, root abscesses).
- MRI or spiral CT can assess of aortic root size.

ADVANCED-LEVEL QUESTIONS

What is the prevalence of aortic regurgitation in the elderly?
According to the Helsinki Ageing Study, 13% of persons aged 75–86 years have moderate to severe aortic regurgitation (J Am Coll Cardiol 1993;21:1220–5).

What is the natural history of chronic aortic regurgitation?
- Asymptomatic patients with normal LV systolic function:
  - Progression to symptoms and/or LV dysfunction <6%/year
  - Progression to asymptomatic lv dysfunction <3.5%/year
  - Sudden death <0.2%/year.
- Asymptomatic patients with LV systolic dysfunction:
  - Progression to symptoms >25%/year.
- Symptomatic patients:
  - Mortality rate >10%/year.

What are the clinical signs of severity?
- Wide pulse pressure
- Soft second heart sound
- The duration of the decrescendo diastolic murmur
- Presence of the left ventricular third heart sound
- Austin Flint murmur
- Signs of left ventricular failure.

What do you know of Hill's sign?
Hill's sign is the presence of higher systolic pressure in the leg than in the arm and is said to be an indicator of the severity of aortic regurgitation: in mild aortic regurgitation the difference is <20 mmHg, in moderate regurgitation it is 20–40 mmHg and in severe regurgitation it is >60 mmHg.

Do characteristics of the early diastolic murmur correlate with severity?

Yes. In mild aortic regurgitation the murmur is short but, as the severity of the regurgitation increases, the murmur becomes longer and louder. In very severe regurgitation the murmur may extend throughout diastole.

What is an Austin Flint murmur?

It is an apical, low-pitched, diastolic murmur caused by vibration of the anterior mitral cusp in the regurgitant jet; it is heard at the apex.

Mention a few causes of acute aortic regurgitation

- Infective endocarditis
- Aortic dissection
- Trauma
- Failure of prosthetic valve
- Rupture of sinus of Valsalva.

What do you know about the natural history of asymptomatic aortic regurgitation?

About 4% of patients develop symptoms, left ventricular dysfunction or both every year.

What do you understand by the term cor bovinum?

In chronic aortic regurgitation, there is slow and progressive left ventricular dilatation and hypertrophy in an attempt to normalize wall stress. The heart may, therefore, become larger and heavier than in any other form of chronic heart disease, which is cor bovinum (bovine or ox heart).

How do you determine the severity of aortic regurgitation

Mild aortic regurgitation:
- Qualitative:
  - Angiographic grade: 1+
  - Colour Doppler jet width: central jet width <25% of LV outflow tract (LVOT)
  - Doppler vena contracta width (cm): <0.3.
- Quantitative:
  - Regurgitant volume (ml/beat): <30
  - Regurgitant fraction (%): <30
  - Regurgitant orifice area (cm^2): 0.10.

Moderate aortic regurgitation:
- Qualitative:
  - Angiographic grade: 2+
  - Colour Doppler jet width: central jet width >25% but <65% LVOT
  - Doppler vena contracta width (cm): 0.3–0.6.
- Quantitative:
  - Regurgitant volume (ml/beat): 30–59
  - Regurgitant fraction (%): 30–49
  - Regurgitant orifice area (cm^2): 0.1–0.29.

Severe aortic regurgitation:
- Qualitative:
  - Angiographic grade: 3–4+
  - Colour Doppler jet width: central jet width >65% LVOT
  - Doppler vena contracta width (cm): >0.6 cm.

- Quantitative:
  - Regurgitant volume (ml/beat): ≥ 60
  - Regurgitant fraction (%): ≥50
  - Regurgitant orifice area (cm²): ≥0.30.
- Additional essential criteria:
  - LV size increased.

What is the role of vasodilators in aortic regurgitation?

- Long-term vasodilator therapy with nifedipine reduces or delays the need for aortic valve replacement in asymptomatic patients with severe aortic regurgitation (N Engl J Med 1994;331:689). Patients in whom left ventricular dysfunction developed when treated with nifedipine respond favourably to valve replacement in terms of both survival and normalization of ejection fraction.
- Long-term treatment of patients with severe aortic regurgitation who have symptoms and/or LV dysfunction who are considered poor candidates for surgery because of other factors.
- Long-term vasodilator therapy should not be recommended for patients with left ventricular dysfunction.
- Patients with subnormal left ventricular ejection fractions should be considered candidates for aortic valve replacement rather than vasodilator therapy, since valve replacement remains the more definitive therapy to reduce volume overload.
- Vasodilator therapy is not recommended for asymptomatic patients with mild aortic regurgitation and normal LV function in the absence of systemic hypertension, as these patients have an excellent outcome with no therapy.
- The goal of vasodilator therapy is to reduce systolic BP. However, it is rarely possible to reduce systolic BP to normal because of increased LV stroke volume, and hence drug dosage should not be increased excessively in an attempt to achieve this goal. The benefit of vasodilator therapy in patients with normal BP and/or normal LV cavity size is not unknown and hence is not recommended (Circulation 1998;98:1949–84).
- A systematic review of vasodilators concluded that vasodilators inconsistently improve haemodynamic and structural parameters in asymptomatic patients with chronic aortic insufficiency. In addition, the impact of vasodilators on clinical outcomes is largely uncertain and requires further study (Am Heart J 2007;153:4542–61).

How is aortic regurgitation treated?

Aortic regurgitation is usually treated surgically. The timing of surgery is important and depends on severity of symptoms and extent of left ventricular dysfunction (Circulation 1998;98:1949–84). Valve replacement should be performed as soon as possible after the onset of ventricular dysfunction. Indications for surgery include:

- symptoms of heart failure and diminished left ventricular function (an ejection fraction of <50% but >20–30%)
- concomitant angina and severe aortic regurgitation
- a reduction in exercise ejection fraction (as estimated with radionuclide ventriculography and exercise testing) of 5% or more is considered by some an indication for surgery, even in the absence of symptoms

- an end-systolic dimension of 55 mm has been suggested by several investigators to represent the limit of surgically reversible dilatation of the LV, so aortic valve replacement is performed before this is exceeded; others have challenged the validity of this limit, as postoperative reduction in chamber size remains variable.
- when aortic root dilatation reaches or exceeds 50 mm by echocardiography, aortic valve replacement and aortic root reconstruction are indicated in patients with disease of the proximal aorta and aortic regurgitation of any severity (Circulation 1998;98:1949–84).

Notes
- In the young, mechanical prostheses are used as the valves are more durable.
- Tissue valves are prone to calcification and degeneration. In the elderly and in those for whom anticoagulants are contraindicated, tissue valves are preferred.

How would you follow-up a patient with aortic regurgitation?
- Asymptomatic patients with mild aortic regurgitation, little or no LV dilatation, and normal systolic LV function may be followed on an annual basis with the advice to alert the physician if symptoms develop between appointments (Circulation 1998;98:1949–84).
- Asymptomatic patients with normal systolic function but severe aortic regurgitation and significant LV dilatation should be followed up at least every 6 months, preferably with an echocardiogram (Circulation 1998;98:1949–84).
- Asymptomatic patients with normal systolic function but severe aortic regurgitation and with more severe LV dilatation (end-diastolic dimension >70 mm or end-systolic dimension >50 mm) have a 10–20% risk of developing symptoms and hence should have serial echocardiograms every 4 months (Circulation 1998;98:1949–84).
- Patients who have had valve replacement should also be seen regularly and monitored for signs of failure of the aortic valve prosthesis (particularly in patients with biological valves) and endocarditis (Circulation 1998;98:1949–84).

Alfred de Musset was a French poet whose nodding movements were described by his brother in a biography. When told of this, Alfred put his thumb and forefinger on his neck and the head stopped bobbing.

Austin Flint (1812–1886) was one of the founders of Buffalo Medical College, New York, and reported the murmur in two patients with aortic regurgitation, confirmed by postmortem. He also held chairs at New Orleans, Chicago, Louisville and New York.

HI Quincke (1842–1922) was a German physician who described angioneurotic oedema and benign intracranial hypertension.

PI Duroziez (1826–1897), a French physician, was widely acclaimed for his articles on mitral stenosis.

L Traube (1818–1876), a German physician, was the first to describe pulsus bigeminus.

Antonio Maria Valsalva (1666–1723) was an Italian anatomist and surgeon who discovered the labyrinth and developed the Valsalva manoeuvre to remove foreign bodies from the ear.

5 AORTIC STENOSIS

INSTRUCTION

Examine this patient's heart.

SALIENT FEATURES

History

- Asymptomatic (many patients do not have symptoms)
- Fatigue
- Angina (in ~70% of adults; average survival after onset of angina is 5 years)
- Syncope (in 25% of patients, during or immediately after exercise; average survival after onset of syncope is 3 years)
- Dyspnoea: common presenting symptom (suggests left ventricular dysfunction; heart failure reduces life expectancy to <2 years).

Examination

Pulse

- Low volume pulse, with a delayed upstroke (pulsus parvus et tardus). This is caused by a reduction in systolic pressure and a gradual decline in diastolic pressure.
- Normal pulse in mild aortic stenosis when the gradient is <50 mmHg.
- Slow rise with diminished 'volume', sometimes with notch on the upstroke ('anacrotic'): indicating severe aortic stenosis with associated aortic regurgitation, double pulse may be felt ('bisferious') (Fig. 5.1).

Heart

- Apex beat is heaving in nature but is not displaced. (A displaced apex beat indicates left ventricular dilatation and severe disease.)

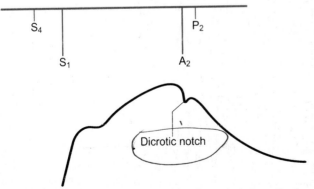

Fig. 5.1 Carotid pulse waveforms and heart sounds in aortic stenosis. Anacrotic pulse with slow upstroke and peak near S_2.

- Palpable systolic vibrations over the primary aortic area, with the patient in the sitting position during full expiration (often correlates with a gradient of >40 mmHg)
- Systolic thrill over the aortic area and the carotids
- Soft second heart sound
- Ejection click heard 0.1 s after first heart sound, along the left sternal border (indicates valvular stenosis). An ejection sound that moves with respiration is not aortic in origin (Fig. 5.2)
- An atrial (S4) sound may be heard
- Ejection systolic murmur at the base of the heart conducted to the carotids and the right clavicle (Fig. 5.2). (Listen carefully for an early diastolic murmur as mild aortic regurgitation often accompanies aortic stenosis. Remember Valsalva decreases duration of murmur of aortic stenosis and increases the murmur of hypertrophic cardiomyopathy
- Third heart sound: in patients with aortic stenosis, third heart sounds are uncommon but usually indicate the presence of systolic dysfunction and raised filling pressures.

General examination

- Check the BP, keeping in mind that the pulse pressure is low in moderate to severe stenosis.

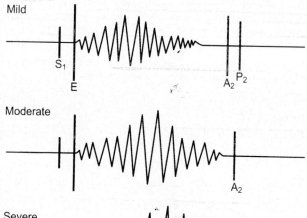

Mild

S₁

E

A₂ P₂

Moderate

A₂

Severe

A

P₂ A₂

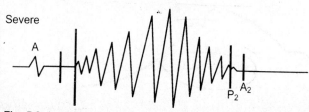

Fig. 5.2 Auscultatory and phonocardiographic signs in bicuspid aortic stenosis.

DIAGNOSIS

This patient has pure aortic stenosis (lesion), which may have a rheumatic aetiology or be from a bicuspid aortic valve (aetiology) he has severe aortic stenosis as he gives a history of recurrent syncope (functional status).

QUESTIONS

How would you differentiate aortic stenosis from aortic sclerosis?

Aortic sclerosis is seen in the elderly; the pulse is normal volume, the apex beat is not shifted and the murmur is localized.

Mention some causes of aortic stenosis

- <60 years: rheumatic, congenital
- 60–75 years: calcified bicuspid aortic valve, especially in men
- >75 years: degenerative calcification.

What does the second heart sound tell us in this condition?

- A soft second heart sound indicates valvular stenosis (except in calcific stenosis of the elderly, where the margins of the leaflets usually maintain their mobility).
- A single second heart sound may be seen when there is fibrosis and fusion of the valve leaflets.
- Reversed splitting of the second sound indicates mechanical or electrical prolongation of ventricular systole. *severe AS*
- A perfectly normal second heart sound (i.e. normal splitting with A$_2$ of normal intensity) is strong evidence against the presence of critical aortic stenosis.

What do you understand by the term ejection systolic murmur?

It is a crescendo–decrescendo murmur that begins after the first heart sound (or after the ejection click when present), peaks in mid or late systole and ends before the second heart sound. This peak is delayed with increasing severity of aortic stenosis.

ADVANCED-LEVEL QUESTIONS

Does the loudness of the murmur reflect the severity of the aortic stenosis?

No, the loudness of the murmur is related more to the cardiac output and the systolic turbulence surrounding the valve than to the severity of the stenosis. Thus, a loud murmur may be associated with trivial stenosis and, in severe heart failure, it may be soft because of decreased flow across the valve from the diminished cardiac output.

What are other causes of ejection systolic murmur at the base of the heart?

- Pulmonary stenosis
- Hypertrophic obstructive cardiomyopathy
- Supravalvular aortic stenosis.

What is the prevalence of aortic stenosis in the elderly?

According to the Helsinki Ageing Study, almost 3% of the individuals aged between 75 and 86 years have critical aortic stenosis (J Am Coll Cardiol 1993;21:1220–25).

$< 1 cm \rightarrow 1.5 cm \rightarrow > 1.5 cm$

What is the mechanism of syncope in aortic stenosis?

- The LV is suddenly unable to contract (transient electromechanical dissociation) against the stenosed valve
- Cardiac arrhythmias (bradycardia, ventricular tachycardia or fibrillation)
- Marked peripheral vasodilatation without a concomitant increase in cardiac output, particularly after exercise.

What investigations would you do?

Note: The degree of aortic stenosis is graded as mild (valve area >1.5 cm^2), moderate (>1.0 to 1.5 cm^2) or severe (≥1.0 cm^2).

- ECG usually shows left ventricular hypertrophy, ST–T changes, possibly left axis deviation, later left atrial hypertrophy (negative P waves in V$_1$), conduction abnormalities from calcification of conducting tissues (first-degree heart block, left bundle branch block).
- *Chest radiograph* may show cardiac enlargement, post-stenotic dilatation of aorta (a bicuspid valve should be suspected if the proximal aorta is greatly enlarged), calcification of aortic valve (particularly in older patients) (Fig. 5.3).
- *Echocardiography* is useful in:
  - the diagnosis and assessment of severity of aortic stenosis as it can estimates valve gradient; a normal valve appearance excludes significant aortic stenosis in adults
  - helping to define the level of obstruction (i.e. valvar, supravalvar, subvalvar)
  - identifying calcified valves
  - assessing left ventricular size, function and/or haemodynamics
  - re-evaluating patients with known aortic stenosis with changing symptoms and signs
  - re-evaluating asymptomatic patients with severe aortic stenosis
  - assessing patients with known aortic stenosis during pregnancy.
- *Exercise testing* in adults with aortic stenosis has been discouraged largely because of safety; it should not be performed in symptomatic patients as it may be fatal; in asymptomatic patients an abnormal haemodynamic response (e.g. hypotension) is sufficient to consider aortic valve replacement. In selected patients it may be useful to provide a basis for advice about physical activity.
- *Cardiac catheterization* is done to assess the coronary circulation and to confirm or clarify the diagnosis. When the echocardiogram is inadequate, cardiac haemodynamics using both left- and right-heart catheterization is indicated and requires:
  - measurement of transvalvular flow
  - determination of transvalvular pressure gradient
  - calculation of the effective valve area.

What are the complications of aortic stenosis?

- Left ventricular failure indicates poor prognosis unless the valve is replaced.
- Sudden death occurs in 10–20% of adults and 1% of children. It has been rarely documented to occur without prior symptoms. It is an uncommon event: probably <1% per year.
- Arrhythmias and conduction abnormalities include ventricular arrhythmias (more common than supraventricular arrhythmias) and heart block (may occur because of calcification of conducting tissues).

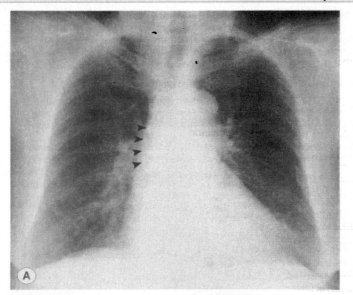

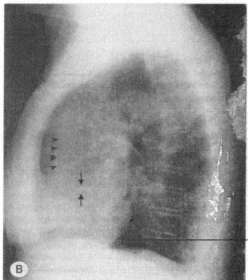

Normal LV contour

Fig. 5.3 Chest radiographs in severe aortic stenosis. (A) Frontal view shows prominent aortic root to the right of the midline (arrowheads). (B) Lateral view demonstrates calcification of the aortic valve leaflets (arrows), suggestive of a bicuspid valve. There is a prominent, mildly dilated aortic root (arrowheads). (With permission from Zipes DP et al. 2007.)

- Systemic embolization is caused by disintegration of the aortic valve apparatus or by concomitant aortic atheroma.
- Infective endocarditis (in 10% of cases) should be considered when these patients present with unexplained illness.
- Haemolytic anaemia.

What are the clinical signs of severity of aortic stenosis?
- Narrow pulse pressure
- Soft second sound
- Narrow or reverse split second sound
- Systolic thrill and heaving apex beat
- Fourth heart sound
- Cardiac failure.

How is the severity of aortic stenosis determined?
Mild aortic stenosis:
- Jet velocity (m/s): <3
- Mean gradient (mmHg): <25
- Valve area (cm^2): >1.5.

Moderate aortic stenosis:
- Jet velocity (m/s): 3.0–4.0
- Mean gradient (mmHg): 25–40
- Valve area (cm^2): 1.0–1.5.

Severe aortic stenosis:
- Jet velocity (m/s): >4.0
- Mean gradient (mmHg): >40
- Valve area (cm^2): <1.0
- Valve area index (cm^2/m^2): 0.6.

How would you manage this patient?
- If the patient is asymptomatic and the valvular gradient is ≤50 mmHg, then observation. Surgery is not recommended in asymptomatic patients.
- Valve replacement in the following circumstances:
  - The patient is *symptomatic* or the valvular gradient is >50 mmHg. Surgery is mandatory in symptomatic patients.
  - It should be considered in asymptomatic patients objectively with severe aortic stenosis (peak-to-peak gradient >50 mmHg) particularly when any one or more of the following features is present: left ventricular systolic dysfunction, abnormal response to exercise (e.g. hypotension), ventricular tachycardia, marked excessive left ventricular hypertrophy (≥15 mm) and valve area <0.6 cm^2.
  - In asymptomatic patients with moderate aortic stenosis it is generally acceptable to perform valve replacement in those who are undergoing mitral valve or aortic root surgery or coronary artery bypass surgery.
  - Severe aortic stenosis with low mean systolic aortic valve gradient (≤30 mmHg) and severe LV dysfunction (Circulation 2000;101: 1940–6).
  - The valve area is <0.8 cm^2 (normal area 2.5–3.0 cm^2). Patients with severe aortic stenosis should have valve replacement early to avoid deterioration.
  - Patients with severe aortic stenosis, with or without symptoms, who are undergoing coronary artery bypass surgery, surgery on the aorta

or other heart valves should undergo aortic valve replacement at the time of their surgery.

- Often, patients require coronary artery bypass grafts during aortic valve replacement.
- Balloon valvuloplasty should be limited to moribund patients requiring emergency intervention or those with a very poor life expectancy from other pathology. In one study, although in-hospital mortality rates were similar to those following conventional surgical replacement, there were more deaths in the valvuloplasty group in the subsequent follow-up period (J Am Coll Cardiol 1992;20:796–801).

If a young person presents with signs and symptoms of aortic stenosis but the aortic valve is normal on echocardiography which condition would you suspect?
Supravalvular or subvalvular aortic stenosis.

What is the genetics of supravalvular stenosis?
- Studies suggest that mutation in the gene for elastin causes supraval-vular stenosis (Cell 1993;73:159).
- In Williams syndrome (also known as Williams–Beurens syndrome) there is a microdeletion in chromosome 7.

If this patient had bleeding per rectum what unusual cause would come to mind?
Angiodysplasia of the colon (Radiology 1974;113:11).

If the patient was icteric and had haemolytic anaemia, what would the mechanism be?
Microangiopathic haemolysis has been described in severe calcified aortic stenosis, manifesting with anaemia and icterus (Semin Hematol 1969;6:133).

What is the relationship between skin and gastrointestinal tract bleeding and aortic stenosis?
Skin and gastrointestinal (GI) tract bleeding is caused by an acquired defect in von Willebrand factor; aortic valve replacement restores the normal structure of von Willebrand factor and thus restores normal hae-mostasis. Von Willebrand factor abnormalities are directly related to the severity of aortic stenosis and are improved by valve replacement in the absence of mismatch between patient and prosthesis. Von Willebrand factor normally circulates as very large, homologous multimers com-posed of 250 kDa subunits. In aortic stenosis, von Willebrand factor is subjected to high fluid shear stress as it passes through the stenotic valve, which renders the multimers susceptible to cleavage by ADAMTS 13 (a plasma metalloprotease that acts on von Willebrand factor pre-ferentially under conditions of high fluid shear stress). A deficit in large, haemostatically effective multimers is the result (N Engl J Med 2003;349:343–9).

What do you understand by 'Gallavardin phenomenon'?
The high-frequency components of the ejection systolic murmur may radiate to the apex. This can then falsely suggests mitral regurgitation. This is known as the Gallavardin phenomenon (Lyons Med 1925;135:523).

What do you know about the Ross operation?

Ross operation (or pulmonary autograft aortic root replacement) involves translocation of the pulmonary valve to the aortic position with subsequent replacement of the pulmonary valve with either a homograft or heterograft valved conduit.

> Williams syndrome is characterized by elfin facies, supravalvular aortic stenosis and hypercalcaemia (JCP Williams, New Zealand physician).

---

6   MIXED AORTIC VALVE LESION

INSTRUCTION

Examine this patient's heart.
Examine this patient's cardiovascular system.
Examine this patient's pulse.

SALIENT FEATURES

- Pulse may be bisferious, small volume or large volume depending on the dominant lesion
- There is a displaced apex beat (remember a small LV is inconsistent with chronic severe aortic regurgitation)
- Early diastolic murmur of aortic regurgitation (Fig. 6.1)
- Ejection systolic murmur of aortic stenosis
- Proceed by telling the examiner that you would like to check the BP, in particular to determine the pulse pressure (systolic minus diastolic pressure).

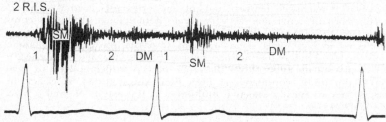

Fig. 6.1 Phonocardiogram of the murmurs present in a patient with valvar aortic stenosis and regurgitation. Note the diamond-shaped systolic murmur peaking in early to midsystole and the high-frequency, lower-intensity murmur throughout diastole. 2 R.I.S., second right intercostal space; SM, systolic murmur; DM, diastolic murmur; 1, first heart sound, 2, second heart sound.

DIAGNOSIS

This patient has mixed aortic stenosis with aortic regurgitation (lesion) caused by rheumatic heart disease (aetiology). He has a dominant stenosis and is in cardiac failure (functional status).

Note

In dominant aortic stenosis:
- Pulse volume is small
- BP is normal and pulse pressure is narrow.

In dominant aortic regurgitation:
- Pulse is collapsing.
- Pulse pressure is wide.

QUESTIONS

What are common causes of mixed aortic lesions?
- Rheumatic heart disease
- Bicuspid aortic valve
- Degenerative disease.

What is the pathophysiology of mixed aortic valve disease?
- In mixed aortic valve disease, one lesion usually predominates over the other and the pathophysiology resembles that of the pure dominant lesion. When aortic stenosis predominates, the pathophysiology and, therefore, the management resembles that of pure aortic stenosis (J Am Coll Cardiol 1998;32:1486–588). The LV in these patients develops concentric hypertrophy rather than dilatation. The timing of aortic valve replacement (like pure aortic stenosis) depends on symptoms (Circulation 1998;98:1949–84).
- When aortic regurgitation is more than mild and the aortic stenosis is predominant, the concentrically hypertrophied and non-compliant LV is on the steeper portion of the diastolic pressure–volume curve, resulting in pulmonary congestion. Therefore, although neither lesion by itself is severe enough to merit surgery, both together produce substantial haemodynamic compromise requiring surgery (Circulation 1998;98:1949–84).
- When the aortic regurgitation is severe and the aortic stenosis is mild, the high total stroke volume caused by extensive regurgitation may produce a substantial transvalvular gradient. Because the transvalvular gradient varies with the square of the transvalvular flow (Am Heart J 1951;41:1–29), a high gradient in predominant regurgitation may be predicted primarily on excess transvalvular flow rather than on a severely compromised orifice area (Circulation 1998;98:1949–84).

In mixed aortic valve disease is cardiac catheterization more accurate than Doppler echocardiography to measure valve area?

Aortic valve area would be measured inaccurately at the time of cardiac catheterization in mixed aortic valve lesions if the cardiac output is measured by either the Fick or the thermodilution method as both these methods usually underestimate total valve flow. The valve area can be measured more accurately using Doppler echocardiography (by continuity equation) in mixed aortic stenosis and aortic regurgitation. However, the confusing nature of mixed valve disease makes cardiac catheterization necessary to obtain additional haemodynamic information in most patients (including coronary anatomy) (Circulation 1998;98:1949–84).

How would you manage such a patient?

- Surgical correction of disease that produces more than mild symptoms
- When the aortic stenosis is dominant, surgery in the presence of even mild symptoms
- When the aortic regurgitation is dominant, surgery can be delayed until symptoms develop or asymptomatic LV dysfunction become apparent on echocardiography.

7 MIXED MITRAL AND AORTIC VALVE DISEASE

INSTRUCTION

Examine this patient's precordium.
Examine this patient's cardiovascular system.
Examine this patient's heart.

SALIENT FEATURES

- Pulse may be small volume (from either dominant aortic stenosis or mitral stenosis), regular or irregularly irregular
- Apex beat may be displaced
- Left parasternal heave
- Mid-diastolic murmur of mitral stenosis
- Pansystolic murmur of mitral regurgitation
- Ejection systolic murmur of aortic stenosis at the base of the heart
- Early diastolic murmur of aortic regurgitation heard with the patient sitting forward on end expiration.

Note

- If the apex beat is not displaced in such mixed lesions, then mitral stenosis is the dominant lesion. (However, if the mitral stenosis developed earlier it can mask the signs of a significant stenosis.)
- In aortic stenosis, the murmur of mitral stenosis may be diminished or absent. The presence of the following features should alert the clinician to a coexisting mitral stenosis because they are not commonly associated with isolated aortic stenosis:
  - Atrial fibrillation
  - Absence of left ventricular hypertrophy in patients with left heart failure
  - Female sex
  - Giant-sized left atrium
  - Calcification of the mitral valve
  - Absence of aortic valve calcification in the symptomatic patient.

Combined mitral stenosis and aortic stenosis

- Severe mitral stenosis and low cardiac output may mask moderate to severe aortic stenosis. A history of angina, syncope or ECG evidence of left ventricular hypertrophy or calcification of the aortic valve on the chest radiograph suggests the presence of aortic stenosis (Circulation 1998;98:1949–84).

- The murmur of aortic stenosis is occasionally better heard at the apex than at the base, particularly in the elderly (Gallavardin phenomenon). When this occurs in younger individuals with a coexisting mitral stenosis, the murmur of aortic stenosis may be mistaken for mitral regurgitation (Circulation 1998;98:1949–84).

- In patients with significant aortic stenosis and mitral stenosis, the physical findings of aortic stenosis generally dominate and those of mitral stenosis may be missed, whereas the symptoms are usually those of mitral stenosis. 'Combination stenosis' is almost always caused by rheumatic heart disease (Circulation 1998;98:1949–84).

Combined mitral stenosis and aortic regurgitation

The combination of severe mitral stenosis and severe aortic regurgitation may present with confusing pathophysiology and often leads to misdiagnosis. Mitral stenosis restricts left ventricular filling and thus diminishing the impact of the aortic regurgitation on left ventricular volume (J Am Coll Cardiol 1984;3:703–11). Consequently, even severe aortic regurgitation may fail to cause a hyperdynamic circulation and the typical signs of aortic regurgitation will be absent during physical examination (Circulation 1998;98:1949–84).

Combined mitral and aortic regurgitation

Both lesions cause left ventricular dilatation, but aortic regurgitation causes systolic hypertension and mild left ventricular thickness. Treatment depends on the dominant lesion and to treat primarily that lesion.

Combined aortic stenosis and mitral regurgitation

Aetiology includes rheumatic heart disease, congenital aortic stenosis with mitral valve prolapse in young patients and degenerative aortic stenosis and mitral regurgitation in the elderly. When severe, aortic stenosis will worsen the degree of mitral regurgitation. Also, mitral regurgitation may cause difficulty in assessing the severity of aortic stenosis because of reduced forward flow. Mitral regurgitation will also enhance LV ejection performance, thereby masking the early development of LV systolic dysfunction caused by aortic stenosis (J Am Coll Cardiol 1998;32:1486–588).

- Treatment
- In patients with severe aortic stenosis and severe mitral regurgitation with symptoms, LV dysfunction or pulmonary hypertension: combined aortic and mitral valve replacement or mitral valve repair.
- In patients with severe aortic stenosis and milder degrees of mitral regurgitation: the severity of mitral regurgitation may improve with isolated aortic valve replacement, particularly when there is normal mitral valve morphology.
- In patients with mild to moderate aortic stenosis and severe mitral regurgitation in whom surgery on mitral valve is indicated because of symptoms of LV dysfunction or pulmonary hypertension: preoperative assessment of the severity of aortic stenosis may be difficult because of reduced forward stroke volume. If the mean aortic valve gradient is ≥30 mmHg, aortic valve replacement should be performed. In patients with less severe gradients, intraoperative transesophageal

echocardiography and visual assessment by the surgeon may be necessary to determine the need for aortic valve replacement (Circulation 1998;98:1949–84).

DIAGNOSIS

This patient has mixed mitral valve and aortic valve disease (lesion) of rheumatic aetiology with a dominant mitral regurgitation, as evidenced by the hyperdynamic circulation. The patient is in cardiac failure (functional status).

QUESTIONS

Mention a few causes of combined aortic and mitral valve disease
- Rheumatic valvular disease
- Infective endocarditis
- Collagen degenerative disorder, e.g. Marfan syndrome
- Calcific changes in the aortic and mitral valve apparatus.

What are the indications for surgery?
- NYHA class III status
- NYHA class II status where there is volume overload of the LV, e.g. in severe aortic regurgitation with moderate mitral valve disease or severe mitral regurgitation with moderate aortic stenosis and regurgitation.

8 HYPERTENSION

INSTRUCTION

This patient has hypertension; would you like to examine her?

SALIENT FEATURES

History

- Chest pain or shortness of breath
- Intermittent claudication
- Headaches or visual disturbances (in accelerated or severe hypertension)
- Family history of hypertension
- Ask about hypertension during pregnancy
- Ask about medications.

Examination

Look for aetiology:
- Comment on Cushingoid facies if present
- Look for radiofemoral delay of coarctation of aorta
- Examine BP in both upper arms (the arm with the higher BP is used for serial follow-up of patients)
- Listen for renal artery bruit of renal artery stenosis and feel for polycystic kidneys.

Look for target organ damage (heart, kidney, nervous system, eyes:
- Palpate the apex for left ventricular hypertrophy
- Look for signs of cardiac failure
- Examine the fundus for changes of hypertensive retinopathy (see Case 238)
- Tell the examiner that you would like to check urine for protein (renal failure) and sugar (associated diabetes): increases risk of cardiovascular disease.

DIAGNOSIS

This patient has retinopathy (lesion) caused by hypertension, which is probably renovascular (aetiology) as evidenced by the renal artery bruit. She probably has damage to other target organs (functional status).

QUESTIONS

How would you record the BP?

Use a device whose accuracy has been validated and one that has been recently calibrated.

Patient should be seated with the arm at the level of the heart. The BP cuff should be appropriate for the size of the arm and the cuff should be deflated at 2 mm/s and the diastolic BP is measured to the nearest 2 mmHg. Diastolic BP is recorded as disappearance of the sounds (phase V).

At least two recordings of BP should be made during at least two subsequent clinic visits where BP is assessed under the best conditions available.

What are the causes of BP discrepancy between the arms or between the arms and legs?

- Coarctation of aorta (p. 117)
- Patent ductus arteriosus (p. 108)
- Dissecting aortic aneurysm
- Arterial occlusion or stenosis of any cause
- Supravalvular aortic stenosis (see p. 34)
- Thoracic outlet syndrome.

How would you investigate a patient with hypertension in outpatients?

In patients without established cardiovascular disease, assess cardiovascular risk. Investigation should aim to identify diabetes, evidence of hypertensive damage to the heart and kidneys, and secondary causes of hypertension such as kidney disease:

- Full blood count (FBC)
- Urine for sugar, albumin and specific gravity
- Urea, electrolytes and serum creatinine
- Fasting lipids, fasting blood sugar, serum uric acid
- Serum total cholesterol to high density lipoprotein (HDL) cholesterol ratio.
- ECG
- Chest radiograph
- 24-h urine collection to measure vanillyl mandelic acid.

What are the indications for ambulatory blood pressure recording?

- When clinic BP shows unusual variability (it allows detection of patients who are truly hypertensive but office BP measurements are normal – the patients with 'masked' hypertension).
- Hypertension is resistant to drug treatment with three or more agents.
- When symptoms suggest that the patient may have hypotension.
- To exclude 'white-coat hypertension'.

What are causes of hypertension?

- Unknown or idiopathic (in 90% of cases)
- Renal: glomerulonephritis, diabetic nephropathy, renal artery stenosis, pyelonephritis
- Endocrine: Cushing syndrome, steroid therapy, phaeochromocytoma
- Others: coarctation of aorta, contraceptives, toxaemia of pregnancy.

What special investigations would you do to screen for an underlying cause?

- Renal digital subtraction angiography
- Urinary catecholamines: 24-h collection of at least three samples (phaeochromocytoma)
- Overnight dexamethasone suppression test

What are the NICE guidelines for initiating hypertensive agents?

- **Aim** The aim for drug therapy in hypertension is to reduce risk of cardiovascular disease (myocardial infarction, stroke, and heart failure) and mortality:
  - sustained systolic BP ≥160 mmHg or sustained diastolic BP ≥100 mmHg
  - patients at raised cardiovascular risk (10-year risk of cardiovascular disease of ≥20%, existing cardiovascular disease or target organ damage) with persistent BP >140/90 mmHg.

- **Initial therapy** The first choice for initial therapy should be:
  - lifestyle measures which should be offered initially and continually
  - either a calcium channel blocker or a thiazide-type diuretic in hypertensive patients aged ≥55 years or black patients of any age, the first choice for initial therapy. (Black patients are considered to be those of African or Caribbean descent, not mixed-race, Asian or Chinese.)
  - an angiotensin-converting enzyme (ACE) inhibitor (or an angiotensin-II receptor antagonist if an ACE inhibitor is not tolerated) in hypertensive patients ≤55 years.

What are the NICE recommendations for follow up of a patient with well controlled blood pressure?

- Annual review of care to monitor BP, provide patients with support and discuss their lifestyle, symptoms and medication.
- Patients may become motivated to make lifestyle changes and want to stop using antihypertensive drugs. If at low cardiovascular risk and with well-controlled BP, these patients should be offered a trial reduction or withdrawal of therapy with appropriate lifestyle guidance and ongoing review.

What the optimal treatment targets?

The optimal treatment targets are systolic BP ≤140 mmHg and diastolic BP ≤85 mmHg. The minimal acceptable level of control is 150/90 mmHg (BMJ 1999;319:630–5).

Why is there increased emphasis on management of systolic blood pressure in those over the age of 50 years?

Although typically guidelines recommend a 'threshold' BP for targets (e.g. in 2002 guidelines classify persons with systolic BP of 120–139 mmHg or diastolic BP of 80–89 mmHg as prehypertensive), it is well recognized that the risk is a continuum: for every 20 mmHg increase in systolic BP >115 mmHg, the risk of heart and stroke disease death doubles in patients over the age of 40 and 50 years, respectively. Even a 2–5 mmHg decrease in systolic BP results in significant improvement in mortality.

How would you manage a patient with mild hypertension?

Lifestyle measures:
- Diet: weight reduction in obese patients, low cholesterol diets for associated hyperlipidaemia, salt restriction (2–3 g sodium/day), increased consumption of fruit and vegetables
- Regular physical exercise that should be predominantly dynamic (for example brisk walking) rather than isometric (weight lifting).
- Limit alcohol consumption (<14 units per week for women and <21 units/week for men)
- Stop smoking.

Why are beta-blockers no longer recommended as first-line agents in the management of hypertension?

- Beta-blockers are no longer routinely recommended as first-line agents in hypertension because of an increased long-term risk of diabetes, particularly when used with diuretics.
- The CAFE study (Circulation 2006; 113:1213–25) showed that beta-blocker-based treatment was significantly less effective than regimens based on calcium channel blockers at lowering aortic systolic BP and pulse pressure despite identical brachial BP in both treatment groups (pseudo-hypertensive effects).
- In head-to-head clinical trials, beta-blockers were usually less effective than comparator antihypertensive medications at reducing major cardiovascular events, in particular stroke. Atenolol was the beta-blocker used in most of these studies and, in the absence of substantial data on other agents, it is unclear whether this conclusion applies to all beta-blockers. It has been proposed that, in the case of atenolol, insufficient duration of action leaves night-time BP untreated, which is one reason for its lack of efficacy.

However, when hypertension is accompanied by coronary artery disease, congestive heart failure, increased sympathetic activity, and arrhythmia, beta-blocker therapy could be beneficial.

What is the role of alpha-blocker-based regimens in the control of blood pressure?

The Antihypertensive and Lipid Lowering Treatment to Prevent Heart Attack (ALLHAT) trial showed that an alpha-blocker-based regimen is less effective than a diuretic-based regimen in preventing heart failure (JAMA 2000;283:1967–75). Additionally, there was a marginally significant excess of stroke in the alpha-blocker group. Although poorer BP control might account for the higher risk of stroke, it does not entirely explain the two-fold greater risk of heart failure.

What is role of calcium channel blockers in the treatment of hypertension?

- In the SYST-EUR study, nitrendipine showed a reduction in the risk of stroke in isolated systolic hypertension when compared to diuretics (Lancet 1997;350:757–64).
- In the Swedish Trial in Old Patients with Hypertension-2 (STOP-2) study, there was some evidence that the risks of myocardial infarction and of heart failure were greater with calcium antagonist-based therapy than with ACE inhibitor-based therapy, but there were no clear differences between either of these regimens and a third based on diuretics and beta-blockers (Lancet 1999;354:1751–56). In this study 34–39% of patients withdrew from the three treatment regimens.
- The International Nifedipine GITS Study: Intervention as a Goal in Hypertension Treatment (INSIGHT) trial compared long-acting nifedipine with a diuretic (hydrochlorthizide and amiloride combination) and found that the calcium channel antagonist was as effective as diuretics in preventing overall cardiovascular or cerebrovascular complications (Lancet 2000;356:366–72). There was a marginally significant excess of heart failure with nifedipine-based treatment. Fatal myocardial infarctions were more common in the nifedipine group. There was an 8% excess withdrawal of drug in the nifedipine group because of peripheral oedema, whereas serious adverse events were more frequent in the diuretic group.
- In the Nordic Diltiazem Study (NORDIL) from Sweden, ditliazem was compared with diuretics, beta-blockers or both (Lancet 2000;356;359–65). This study found that diltiazem was as effective as treatment based on diuretics, beta-blockers or both in preventing the primary end-point of all stroke, myocardial infarction and other cardiovascular death. There was a marginally significant lower risk of stroke in the diltiazem group despite a lesser reduction in BP. In this study, 23% of the patients withdrew from the diltiazem-based group and 7% withdrew from diuretic-based and beta-blocker-based therapy.

What is role of ACE inhibitors in hypertension?

- In the HOPE (Heart Outcomes Prevention Evaluation) study, the use of ramipril was associated with reductions of stroke, coronary artery disease and heart failure in both hypertensive and non-hypertensive groups when compared with placebo (N Eng J Med 2000;342:145–53).
- In the Captopril Prevention Project (CAPPP), the risk of stroke was slightly greater with ACE inhibitor-based therapy than with diuretic-based or beta-blocker-based therapy but the higher baseline and follow-up BP among patients assigned the ACE inhibitor regimen may largely or entirely account for the excess risk of stroke (Lancet 1998;353:611–16).

What are the indications for specialist referral?

- Hypertensive emergency: malignant hypertension, impending complications.
- To investigate possible aetiology when evaluation suggests this possibility.
- To evaluate therapeutic problems or failures.
- Special circumstances: unusually variable BP, possible white-coat hypertension, pregnancy (BMJ 1999;319:630–5).

What do you understand by resistant hypertension?

Resistant or refractory hypertension is defined as BP persistently greater than target (i.e. >140/90 mmHg for most patients and >130/80 mmHg in those with diabetes or renal disease) despite therapy with three different antihypertensive medication classes including a diuretic. True resistant hypertension can occur in volume overload, use of contraindicated drugs or exogenous substances and with some associated conditions (e.g. smoking, obesity, pain, excessive alcohol intake). Resistant hypertension can occur secondary to Conn's adenoma, sleep apnoea, chronic kidney disease.

'I have also been treating the high cholesterol and then I stopped the medicine because I got my cholesterol down low. And, I had in the past, a little [blood pressure] problem, which I treated and then I got it down...'
(Former US President Clinton, awaiting coronary bypass surgery, calls into Larry King Live from his hospital bed; posted 3 September 2004).

---

9 ATRIAL FIBRILLATION

INSTRUCTION

Examine this patient's pulse.

SALIENT FEATURES

History

- Palpitations
- Pre-syncope, dizziness
- Fatigue
- Dyspnoea
- Asymptomatic and atrial fibrillation (AF) is discovered incidentally
- History of ischaemic heart disease, hypertension, valvular heart disease, rheumatic heart disease, chronic obstructive airway disease (COPD), congenital heart disease (atrial septal defect, ventricular septal defect), thyrotoxicosis (p. 506)
- History of consumption of caffeine, digitalis, theophylline.

Examination

- Irregularly irregular pulse (patients are often digitalized and in slow AF)
- Look for:
  - malar flush (mitral stenosis)
  - mitral valvotomy scar
  - warm hands, goitre, pretibial myxoedema (thyrotoxicosis).
- Elevated JVP without 'a' waves
- Varying intensity of first heart sound (the intensity is inversely related to the previous RR cycle length; a longer cycle length produces a softer first heart sound)

- Pulse deficit, which is the difference between the rate of the apex and the pulse rate (because of varying stroke volumes resulting from varying periods of diastolic filling, not all ventricular beats produce a palpable peripheral pulse). The pulse deficit is greater when the ventricular rate is high
- If you are not sure tell the examiner that you would like to differentiate from ventricular ectopics by asking the patient to exercise: after exercise, ventricular ectopics diminish in frequency whereas there is no change in the rhythm of AF
- Look for the underlying cause:
  - Examine the heart for mitral valvular lesion
  - Check the BP for hypertension
  - Ask the patient for history of ischaemic heart disease
  - Check the patient's thyroid status for thyrotoxicosis.
- Calculate the $CHAD^2$ score (see below) to determine the eligibility for anticoagulation.

DIAGNOSIS

This patient has fast atrial fibrillation (lesion), which is commonly caused by ischaemic heart disease (aetiology). The patient is short of breath, indicating that he may be in cardiac failure (functional status).

QUESTIONS

What are the components of the CHADS2 score?

Annual risk of stroke (adjusted stroke rate per 100 patient-years) in patients with AF is stratified by a score based on:

C, recent congestive heart failure

H, hypertension

A, age ≥75 years

D, diabetes

S, history of stroke or transient ischaemic attack (TIA).

The CHADS2 score is calculated by adding one point for each of the first four risk factors and two points for a history of previous stroke or TIA (JAMA 2001;285:2864–70). Patients with a CHADS score ≥2 and patients with rheumatic mitral stenosis should be managed with adjusted-dose warfarin to achieve an international normalized ratio (INR) of 2 to 3. At this intensity of anticoagulation, the annual risk of intracerebral haemorrhage is low: between 0.1% and 0.6%. For patients with a CHADS score of 1, anticoagulation with either aspirin or warfarin is reasonable. Patients with AF and no risk factors do not need anticoagulation. Opinion is divided about anticoagulation for those at intermediate risk (CHADS2 score 2 where stroke rate is 3–5% per year). Adjusted-dose oral anticoagulation is highly efficacious for prevention of all stroke (both ischaemic and haemorrhagic), with a risk reduction of 61% (95% confidence interval (CI), 47–71) versus placebo in randomized clinical trials. Aspirin offers only modest protection against stroke, a stroke reduction of 19% (95% CI, 2–34) (Ann Intern Med 1999;131:492–501).

What are the components of the bleeding risk index?

Scoring system for estimating risk of major bleeding related to warfarin (the bleeding risk index; J Gen Intern Med 2005;20:1008–13) gives points for the risk factors:

- Age >65 years: 1 point
- History of stroke: 1 point
- History of GI bleeding: 1 point
- Any, or several combined, of the following: 1 point:
  - Diabetes mellitus
  - Recent myocardial infarction
  - Packed cell volume <30%
  - Serum creatinine >1.5 mg/l.

The annual risk of stroke (based on points accrued) is then:

- low (0 points): 0.8%
- intermediate (1–2 points): 2.5%
- high (3–4 points): 10.6%

What are the common causes of atrial fibrillation?

- Mitral valvular disease in the young and middle aged
- Ischaemic heart disease or hypertension in the elderly
- Thyrotoxicosis (AF may be the only clinical feature in the elderly)
- Constrictive pericarditis
- Chronic pulmonary disease.

Mention common sites of systemic embolization

Brain, leg, kidney, superior mesenteric artery, coronary artery and spleen.

At the bedside how would you differentiate atrial fibrillation from multiple ventricular ectopics?

If the patient is not in heart failure, exercise the patient: ventricular ectopics after exercise tend to diminish in frequency whereas there is no change in the rhythm of AF.

How would you investigate this patient?

- *ECG* shows absent P waves. Fibrillatory or 'f' waves are present at a rate that may vary between 350 and 600 beats/min and the 'f' waves vary in shape, amplitude and intervals. The RR interval is irregularly irregular. Narrow QRS complex with varying RR interval (irregular unless there is an underlying ventricular conduction defect). It should be differentiated from sinus arrhythmia (Figs 9.1 and 9.2).
- *Echocardiogram* (transthoracic and transoesophageal) is useful to determine left atrial size and left ventricular systolic function, and to exclude underlying valvular heart disease and intracardiac thromboemboli. Transoesophageal echocardiography prior to cardioversion.
- *Test of thyroid function* to exclude thyrotoxicosis.
- *Exercise treadmill* will identify AF precipitated by exercise.
- *Holter monitor* is useful in paroxysmal AF to determine whether it was triggered by another arrhythmia, such as when a premature atrial complex during a rapid paroxysmal atrial tachycardia may cause the immediate onset of AF.

ADVANCED-LEVEL QUESTIONS

Mention a few causes of irregularly irregular pulse

- AF
- Multiple ventricular ectopics
- Atrial flutter with varying block (Fig. 9.1)
- Complete heart block (there is associated bradycardia).

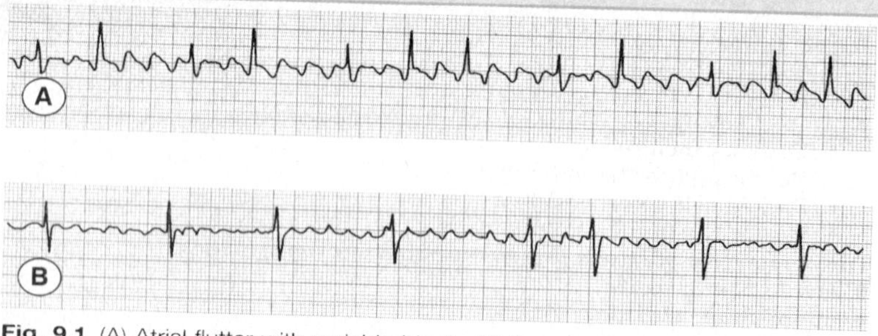

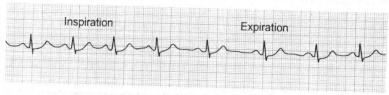

Fig. 9.1 (A) Atrial flutter with variable block. (B) Coarse atrial fibrillation. The ventricular rate is completely erratic and the atrial waves are not identical from segment to segment (as they are with atrial flutter).

Fig. 9.2 Respiratory sinus arrhythmia: normally, heart rate increases slightly with inspiration and decreases slightly with expiration.

In which congenital disorders is atrial fibrillation common?
● Atrial septal defect
● Ebstein's anomaly.

What is the clinical classification of atrial fibrillation?
1. Recent onset or first detected: first diagnosed episode (sometimes an incidental diagnosis and precise duration is not known); may or may not recur.
2. Recurrent: when a patient has had two or more episodes:
   • Paroxysmal AF: when the arrhythmia terminates spontaneously
   • Persistent AF: when sustained beyond 7 days.
3. Permanent: cardioversion has failed or restoration of sinus rhythm is no longer considered possible; or established. (The definition of permanent AF is often arbitrary.) The duration of AF refers both to individual episodes and to how long the patient has been affected by the arrhythmia. Thus, a patient with paroxysmal AF may have episodes that last seconds to hours occurring repeatedly for years.
4. Secondary AF that occurs following acute myocardial infarction, hyperthyroidism, cardiac surgery, pericarditis, myocarditis, pulmonary embolism, pneumonia, or other acute pulmonary disease.
5. Lone AF occurs in the absence of cardiopulmonary disease or a history of hypertension and before the age of 60 years. Such patients have a low risk of stroke (0.5% per year).

Notes
● Termination with pharmacological therapy or direct-current cardioversion does not change the designation.

- First-detected AF may be either paroxysmal or persistent.
- The category of persistent AF also includes long-standing AF (e.g. greater than 1 year), usually leading to permanent AF, in which cardioversion has failed or has not been attempted.
- These categories are not mutually exclusive in a particular patient, who may have several episodes of paroxysmal AF and occasional persistent AF, or the reverse. Regarding paroxysmal and persistent AF, it is practical to categorize a given patient by the most frequent presentation.

How would you treat a patient with atrial fibrillation?
- The 4C approach:
  - Control the rate
  - CHAD2 score and anti-coagulate
  - Cause: look for a cause
  - Correct the rhythm: cardioversion (electrical or chemical) or AF ablation.
- Attempt to restore slow ventricular rate:
  - In the hypertensive patient, use calcium antagonists (verapamil, diltiazem)
  - In thyroid disease use a beta-blocker (e.g. propranolol)
  - In ischaemic heart disease, use a beta-blocker or diltiazem, verapamil
  - In heart failure, use digoxin or verapamil
  - In hypertrophic cardiomyopathy, use a beta-blocker or calcium antagonists
  - In those who are intolerant or do not respond to drugs, radiofrequency catheter ablation of the atrioventricular node (with a cardiac pacemaker) may provide symptomatic relief but it does not change the risk of systemic emboli or the need for anticoagulation (N Engl J Med 1999;340:534)
  - In paroxysmal AF when the ectopic foci is in the pulmonary veins, radiofrequency ablation of the pulmonary veins has been shown to be effective.
- Attempt to restore sinus rhythm by cardioversion if the following conditions apply:
  - Left atrial size by echocardiogram is <4.5 cm (left atrial size >4.5 cm is not associated with long-term maintenance of sinus rhythm)
  - Duration of the arrhythmia (acute AF is likely to remain in sinus rhythm)
  - Drugs used to restore sinus rhythm include propafenone, flecainide, amiodarone, dofetilide and ibutilide.
- Anticoagulation with warfarin is advised for certain patients:
  - Undergoing cardioversion (electrical or drug)
  - With underlying mitral valve disease
  - In left ventricular failure
  - With cardiomyopathy
  - Above the age of 60 years.

What is the role of oral anticoagulants in chronic atrial fibrillation?
- Non-rheumatic AF is an important risk factor for stroke (AF raises the risk of ischaemic stroke by a factor of four to five, primarily as a result of cardioembolism of a fibrin-rich thrombus), even though it is recognized that only 80% of strokes in such patients are caused by embolism from the heart. All patients with non-rheumatic AF should receive

warfarin for anticoagulation unless there are contraindications (Br J Hosp Med 1993;50:452–7).

- Oral anticoagulation is highly efficacious for prevention of all stroke (both ischaemic and haemorrhagic), with a risk reduction of 62% (95% CI, 48–72) versus placebo identified in a meta-analysis of five large randomized trials. This reduction was similar for both primary and secondary prevention and for both disabling and non-disabling strokes. By on-treatment analysis (excluding patients not undergoing oral anticoagulation at the time of stroke), the preventive efficacy of oral anticoagulation exceeded 80%.

- Aspirin offers only modest protection against stroke for patients with AF. Meta-analysis of the five randomized trials showed a stroke reduction of 19% (95% CI, 2–34).

- The Atrial Fibrillation Clopidogrel Trial with Irbesartan for Prevention of Vascular Events (ACTIVE) investigators reported that the combination of clopidogrel and aspirin significantly reduced the rate of major vascular events in certain patients with AF (in those not eligible for vitamin K-antagonist therapy such as warfarin), driven primarily by fewer strokes, when compared with aspirin alone (N Engl J Med 2009;360:2066–78). One disabling or fatal stroke would be prevented for approximately 200 patients treated for 1 year with clopidogrel added to aspirin. One extra major bleeding episode and one extra intracranial haemorrhage would occur for approximately 143 and 500 patients, respectively, treated for 1 year with clopidogrel added to aspirin. The same investigators in a separate study found that vitamin K-antagonist therapy was more efficacious than clopidogrel plus aspirin in patients at high risk for stroke.

- The Randomized Evaluation of Long-Term Anticoagulation Therapy (RE-LY) reported that dabigatran, a direct oral thrombin inhibitor, given at a dose of 110 mg was associated with rates of stroke and systemic embolism that were similar to those associated with warfarin, as well as lower rates of major haemorrhage (N Engl J Med 2009;361:1139). The number needed to treat to prevent one (non-haemorrhagic) stroke with dabigatran (150 mg twice daily) was 357.

- Dabigatran etexilate, after conversion to its active form by a serum esterase that is independent of cytochrome P450, competitively inhibits thrombin. Therefore, dabigatran should be less susceptible to dietary and drug interactions and to genetic polymorphisms that affect warfarin. Furthermore, neither anticoagulation monitoring nor dose adjustments are necessary with dabigatran. P-glycoprotein inhibitors, including verapamil, amiodarone and especially quinidine, raise dabigatran serum concentrations considerably. The long-term hepatic risks of dabigatran are unclear but in the short term it was similar to warfarin (ximelagatran, an earlier direct thrombin inhibitor, appeared to be similar to warfarin with respect to efficacy and safety but was found to be hepatotoxic). Dabigatran is excreted by the kidney and has a half-life of 12 to 17 h. In a separate study, dabigatran was also found to be comparable to warfarin in the management of deep venous thromboembolism (N Engl J Med 2009;361:2342).

- Rivaroxaban is a direct factor Xa inhibitor which has been shown to prevent strokes in the ROCKET AF (Rivaroxaban Once Daily Oral Direct Factor Xa Inhibition Compared with Vitamin K Antagonism for

Prevention of Stroke and Embolism Trial in Atrial Fibrillation) trial (N Engl J Med 2011).

What is the role of surgery in the treatment of atrial fibrillation?

- The Maze procedure involves multiple incisions in the atria to prevent re-entrant loops (Clin Cardiol 1991;14:827–34). This procedure is highly effective in preventing AF, with only 1 patient out of 65 suffering a clinical recurrence of the arrhythmia 3 or more months after the procedure. Although the long-term outcome is not known, it remains a promising procedure when AF is not controlled by medical therapy or in those complicated by recurrent thromboembolism.
- The 'corridor' procedure effectively isolates both the left and right atrium, leaving a strip of myocardium connecting the sinus node to the atrioventricular node. This procedure does not prevent AF but isolates the fibrillating atria. Although a 70% 'cure' rate is reported, sequential atrioventricular contraction is not restored (with the consequent haemodynamic effects), and there is a risk of thromboembolism.

What do you know about holiday heart syndrome?

It is the occurrence of supraventricular arrhythmias, usually AF and atrial flutter, following an acute alcoholic binge in chronic alcoholics. These are usually transient.

Rhythm control versus rate control for atrial fibrillation and heart failure

Mention newer antiarrhythmic drugs for AF:

- Vernakalant, a new atrial selective agent, is effective for rapid cardioversion of recent onset AF
- Dronedarone, a derivative of amiodarone, is more effective than placebo in maintaining sinus rhythm and reducing admission to hospital but increased mortality in patients with heart failure (the results from a study comparing dronedarone with amiodarone are expected soon).

It was James Mackenzie (1853–1925), a Scottish general practitioner working in Burnley, England, utilizing an ink polygraph to record and label JVP, who would pioneer the deciphering of normal and abnormal cardiac rhythms. His key observation that the jugular 'a' wave disappeared in a patient who went from a normal to an irregular rhythm provided the first insight into the mechanism of AF.

In 1909, Lewis in England and Rothberger and Winterberg in Vienna, taking advantage of Einthoven's newly developed string galvanometer, were the first to establish electrocardiographically that auricular fibrillation was the cause of pulsus irregularis perpetuus.

In 1924, Willem Einthoven (1860–1927) of Leyden University, the Netherlands, was awarded the Nobel Prize for his discovery of the mechanism of electrocardiography (Am J Cardiol 1994;73:384–9).

Dr Neil Dewhurst, President of the Royal College of Physicians of Edinburgh (RCPE), is a Consultant Cardiologist and General Physician at Perth Royal Infirmary and an Honorary Senior Lecturer in Medicine at the University of Dundee. He is a highly regarded physician with over 30 years of experience gained in District and Teaching Hospitals in Scotland and England. His clinical interests include arrhythmogenesis and presentations of heart disease in young adults.

250 Cases in Clinical Medicine

10 PALPITATIONS

INSTRUCTION

This patient has palpitations: would you like to ask her a few questions?

SALIENT FEATURES

History

- How old are you? Supraventricular tachycardias (SVT), particularly ones that use a bypass tract (atrioventricular re-entry tachycardia) may be experienced in earlier life. Atrial fibrillation, flutter, atrial tachycardia and ventricular tachycardia (VT) tend to occur later in life associated with structural heart disease.
- Are the palpitations regular or irregular? Patients should be asked to tap out the rhythm or choose from cadences tapped by the clinician. (Rapid regular rhythms suggest SVT or VT whereas rapid, irregular rhythms suggest atrial fibrillation, atrial flutter or tachycardia with varying block.)
- Is the onset abrupt (paroxysmal tachyarrhythmias)?
- How frequent are the palpitations?
- Do you have palpitations at work? (More likely to be a cardiac arrhythmia.)
- Do the palpitations start on sleeping or on termination of exercise? (Both these are states of increased vagal tone suggesting vagally mediated atrial fibrillation or certain subtypes of long-QT syndrome.)
- What is the duration of each episode? (palpitations lasting <5 min makes the diagnosis of cardiac arrhythmia slightly less likely) (JAMA 2009;302:2135–43).
- Is there accompanying pounding sensation in the neck? (The presence of regular rapid pounding sensation in the neck or visible neck pulsations increases the likelihood of atrioventricular nodal re-entry tachycardia when contraction of the atria against closed atrioventricular valves produces increased right atrial pressures and reflux of blood into the inferior vena cava.)
- Is each episode followed by polyuria? (Seen in supraventricular tachycardia.)
- Is there any relation to exercise? (For example, polymorphic VT in long-QT syndrome.)
- What happens on standing? (Postural hypotension, atrioventricular nodal tachycardia.)
- Are there any precipitating factors such as coffee, tea, alcohol or medications such as thyroid extract, ephedrine, aminophylline, monoamino oxidase inhibitors?
- Are there any associated symptoms such as chest pain or shortness of breath?
- Associated shirt flapping, which is defined as visible movements of patients' clothes during the episode (described with both atrioventricular node re-entry tachycardia and atrioventricular re-entry tachycardia).
- Is there associated syncope? (Dizziness, or syncope accompanying palpitations should prompt a search for ventricular tachycardia.)

- Are the palpitations associated with anxiety or panic attacks? (Anxiety or panic can result in palpitations; a known history of panic disorder makes diagnosis of cardiac arrhythmia slightly less likely.)
- Is there a family history of palpitations, especially history of atrial fibrillation or a diagnosis of arrhythmogenic right ventricular cardiomyopathy?

Note: Palpitations are a common complaint in up to 16% of outpatients. They are non-specific and in only 15% of patients do they correlate with cardiac arrhythmia.

Examination

- Check the pulse for arrhythmia.
- JVP is distended in heart failure and 'frog' sign in atrioventricular node re-entry tachycardia (Lancet 1993;341:1254–8). The presence of cannon A waves suggests associated atrioventricular dissociation such as VT.
- Auscultate the heart for murmurs (mitral valve prolapse, valvular heart disease, harsh systolic murmur of hypertrophic cardiomyopathy), split second heart sound (atrial fibrillation).
- Look for signs of atrial fibrillation.
- Although palpitations may not be present at rest, when the ventricular response is slow, a brisk walk down the corridor may result in palpitations.
- Tell the examiner that you would like to examine the ECG for:
  - presence of Q waves typical of old myocardial infarction, prompting a search for non-sustained VT.
  - left ventricular hypertrophy with left atrial enlargement (as suggested by notched P wave in lead II or terminal P wave force in lead V_1 more negative than 0.04 s) as this is a likely substrate for atrial fibrillation
  - short PR interval and delta waves, which suggests ventricular pre-excitation and substrate for SVT (Wolff–Parkinson–White syndrome)
  - marked left ventricular hypertrophy with deep septal Q waves in I, L and V_4 through V_6, suggests hypertrophic cardiomyopathy
  - prolonged QT interval and abnormal T wave morphology, which may suggest the presence of long-QT syndrome
  - bradycardias and complete heart block since they may be associated with ventricular premature depolarizations, long QT syndrome and torsade de pointes (Fig. 10.1)
  - abnormal morphology of a ventricular ectopic may suggest that one of the two types of idiopathic VT is present
  - Brugada syndrome (Fig. 10.2).

DIAGNOSIS

This patient has palpitations (lesion) accompanied by polyuria, indicating a supraventricular tachycardia (aetiology).

QUESTIONS

What are the causes?
- Extrasystole
- Tachycardia or bradycardia

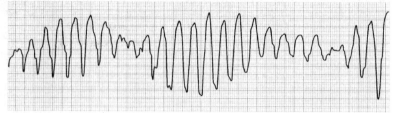

Fig. 10.1 Torsades de pointes, with polymorphic QRS morphology.

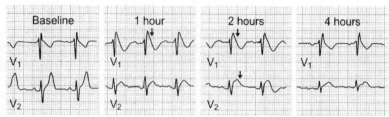

Fig. 10.2 Brugada syndrome. Typical repolarization changes (arrows) elicited by a single oral dose of 400 mg flecainide.

- Drugs (see above)
- Other: thyrotoxicosis, hypoglycaemia, unaccustomed exertion, phaeochromocytoma, fever
- Anxiety state (also known as da Costa syndrome or cardiac neurosis).

How would you investigate a patient suspected of having a disorder of cardiac rhythm?

- *12-lead ECG* (look for evidence of a rhythm disturbance and pre-excitation syndrome)
- *Continuous ambulatory (Holter) echocardiography* (many patients with palpitations may have stable sinus rhythm)
- *Exercise ECG* particularly in those whose palpitations occur on exercise or are provoked by cardiac ischaemia
- *Loop monitors* have the highest diagnostic yield (34–84%) for diagnosing arrhythmia.

JM da Costa (1833–1900) was Professor of Medicine at Jefferson Medical College, Philadelphia.

11 SLOW PULSE RATE

INSTRUCTION

Examine this patient's pulse.

SALIENT FEATURES

History

- Drug history: beta-blockers, digoxin, verapamil
- Ask whether the patient is an athlete
- Symptoms, which are usually non-specific (e.g. dizziness, fatigue, weakness, heart failure)
- History of recent myocardial infarction
- Ask if the bradycardia is episodic? If so, ask about precipitating factors and associated symptoms or signs
- Ask regarding nocturnal bradycardia (a feature of obstructive sleep apnoea).

Examination

Pulse

- Pulse rate <60 beats/min (N Engl J Med 2000;342:703–9)
- Pulse rate may be either regular or irregular
- If the pulse is irregular: get the patient to stand and then count the pulse rate (in complete heart block there is no increase in rate)
- Look at the JVP for cannon 'a' waves
- Auscultate the heart for cannon first heart sound
- Look for signs of hypothyroidism particularly in the elderly.

DIAGNOSIS

This patient has a complete heart block (lesion) probably caused by ischaemic heart disease (aetiology) and is disabled by syncopal attacks (functional status).

QUESTIONS

What are the causes of bradycardia?

- Physical fitness in athletes
- Idiopathic degeneration (aging)
- Acute myocardial infarction
- Drugs (beta-blockers, digitalis, calcium channel blockers)
- Hypothyroidism
- Obstructive jaundice
- Increased intracranial pressure
- Hypothermia
- Hyperkalaemia.

ADVANCED-LEVEL QUESTIONS

How would you investigate this patient?

- ECG:
  - 12-lead assessment to confirm bradycardia

- 24–48 h ambulatory recording in patients with frequent or continuous symptoms
- Exercise or ambulatory monitoring for chronotropic incompetence.
- Tilt-table testing when neurocardiogenic syncope is suspected.

What are the indications for temporary cardiac pacing in bradyarrhythmias?

- Symptomatic second-or third-degree heart block caused by transient drug intoxication or electrolyte disturbance (Fig. 11.1A,B)
- Complete heart block, Mobitz II (Fig. 11.1D) or bifascicular (Fig. 11.2) in the setting of an acute myocardial infarct
- Symptomatic sinus bradycardia, atrial fibrillation with slow ventricular response.

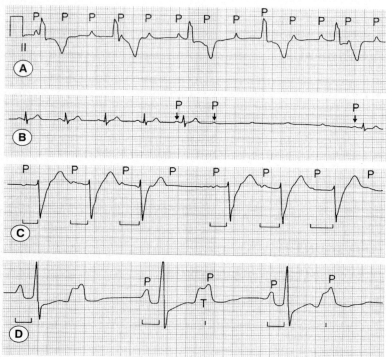

Fig. 11.1 ECG showing heart block. (A) Complete atrioventricular (AV) block: P waves bear no relationship to the QRS complexes, which are regular and wide. (B) Intermittent complete heart block: sinus rhythm with normal PR intervals and normal QRS complexes followed by sudden absence of AV conduction. (C) Mobitz I second-degree heart block with progressive lengthening of the PR interval and eventual failure of the P wave to generate a QRS complex. (D) Mobitz type II second-degree heart block, with failure to produce a QRS complex on every second P wave.

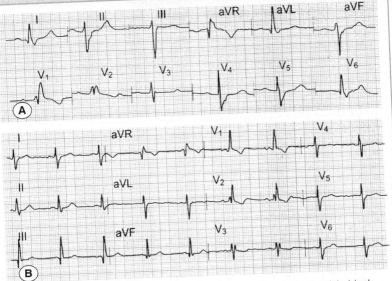

Fig. 11.2 Bifascicular right bundle branch block (A) Left anterior fascicle block.
(B) Left posterior fascicle block.

What are the indications for permanent pacing in bradyarrhythmias?
- Symptomatic congenital heart block
- Symptomatic sinus bradycardia
- Symptomatic second- or third-degree heart block.

Which drug would you use to treat sinus bradycardia seen in the setting of an acute myocardial infarction?
Intravenous atropine.

What do you understand by the term chronotropic incompetence?
Failure to reach a heart rate that is 85% of the age-predicted maximum (220 – age in years) at peak exercise, the failure to achieve a heart rate of 100 beats/min or a maximal heart rate >2SD below that in a control population (N Eng J Med 2000;342:703–9).

What you know about Stokes–Adams syndrome?
It refers to syncope or fits occurring during complete heart block.

W Stokes (1804–1878), Regius Professor of Medicine in Dublin, graduated from Edinburgh.
R Adams (1791–1875), Professor of Surgery in Dublin, was an authority on gout and arthritis.

12 GALLOP RHYTHM

INSTRUCTION

Listen to the precordium.
Examine this patient's heart.

SALIENT FEATURES

History

- Dyspnoea
- Determine NYHA class
- Paroxysmal nocturnal dyspnoea
- Swelling of the feet.

Examination

- Presence of an abnormal third or fourth heart sound (Fig. 12.1) with tachycardia. (The presence of a normal third or fourth heart sound does not connote a gallop rhythm unless there is associated tachycardia.)
- Auscultate with the bell as third and fourth heart sounds are low pitched
- Gallop rhythm as a result of third heart sound seems to sound like 'Kentucky', whereas that because of the fourth heart sound sounds like 'Tennessee'.

Notes

- A left ventricular third heart sound is best heard at the apex, whereas the right ventricular third heart sound is best heard along the left sternal border.
- The left ventricular third heart sound is heard over the left ventricular impulse, especially when the impulse is brought closer to the chest wall by placing the patient in a partial left lateral decubitus position.
- In emphysematous patients, the gallop is better heard when listening over the xiphoid or epigastric area.

DIAGNOSIS

This patient has gallop rhythm (lesion), which indicates that he is in cardiac failure (functional status).

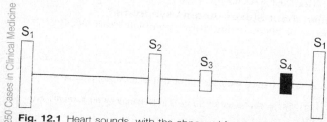

Fig. 12.1 Heart sounds, with the abnormal fourth sound.

QUESTIONS

What is the expression used when both the third and fourth heart sounds are heard with tachycardia?
This is known as the summation gallop. It can sometimes be confused for a diastolic rumbling murmur.

ADVANCED-LEVEL QUESTIONS

What is the mechanism of production of the third heart sound?
It is caused by rapid ventricular filling in early diastole.

What is the mechanism of production of the fourth heart sound?
It is caused by vigorous contraction of the atria (atrial systole) and is hence heard towards the end of diastole.

How do you differentiate between the fourth heart sound, a split first heart sound and an ejection click?
The fourth heart sound is not heard when pressure is applied on the chest piece of the stethoscope, but pressure does not eliminate the ejection sound or the splitting of the first heart sound.

What are the causes of a third heart sound?
- Physiological: in normal children and young adults
- Pathological:
  - Heart failure (third heart sound gallop is relatively specific for elevated left ventricular end-diastolic pressure and left ventricular dysfunction)
  - Left ventricular dilatation without failure: mitral regurgitation, ventricular septal defect, patent ductus arteriosus
  - Right ventricular third heart sound in right ventricular failure, tricuspid regurgitation.

What are the implications of a third heart sound in patients with valvular heart disease?
- In patients with mitral regurgitation, they are common but do not necessarily reflect ventricular systolic dysfunction or increased filling pressure (N Engl J Med 1992;327:458–62).
- In patients with aortic stenosis, third heart sounds are uncommon but usually indicate the presence of systolic dysfunction and raised filling pressure.

What is the significance of third heart sound in heart failure?
N Engl J Med 2001;345:574–581

What are the causes of a fourth heart sound?
- Normal: in the elderly
- Pathological:
  - Acute myocardial infarction
  - Aortic stenosis (the presence of a fourth heart sound in individuals <40 years indicates significant obstruction)
  - Hypertension (it is a constant finding in hypertension)
  - Hypertrophic cardiomyopathy
  - Pulmonary stenosis.

Note: The fourth heart sound does not denote heart failure, unlike the third heart sound gallop.

Potain credited Jean Baptiste Bouillaud (1786–1881), Professor of Medicine in Paris, as being the first person to describe gallop rhythm (Jean Baptiste Bouillaud. Proc R Soc Med 1931;24:1253–1931).

Pierre Carl Edouard Potain (1825–1901), Parisian physician, was the first to distinguish between various types of gallop in a short account titled Théorie du Bruit de Gallop, in 1885.

13 ANGINA PECTORIS

INSTRUCTION

This patient is suspected to have angina pectoris. Would you like to ask her a few questions and perform a relevant examination, to confirm these suspicions?

SALIENT FEATURES

History

- Have you ever had any pain or discomfort in the chest?
- How would you describe the chest discomfort (heavy, burning, tightness, stabbing, pressure)?
- Do you get this on walking at ordinary pace on the level or does it come when you walk uphill or hurry?
- When you get the pain/discomfort, do you stop, slow down or continue at the same pace?
- Does the pain/discomfort go away when you stand still? (It is typically relieved by rest or glyceryl trinitrate within 10 min.)
- Where do you get this pain? (Because angina is a visceral sensation, it is poorly localized and, therefore, patients rarely point to the location of their discomfort with one finger.)
- Does it radiate elsewhere (e.g. arms, jaw, epigastrium)?
- Does food or cold weather bring on the pain?
- Ask about risk factors such as smoking, diabetes, hypertension, family history of ischaemic heart disease.
- Ask about past medical history of coronary artery disease.

Examination

Typically no signs are manifest, but patients should be examined for evidence of the following:
- Hypertension (p. 38)
- Hyperlipidaemia (p. 616)
- Diabetes (p. 749)
- Left ventricular outflow obstruction (aortic stenosis, hypertrophic cardiomyopathy)
- Previous myocardial infarction (MI) (p. 64)

DIAGNOSIS

This patient has angina pectoris (lesion), which is caused by atherosclerotic coronary artery disease (aetiology). She is in Canadian Cardiovascular Society functional class II (functional status).

QUESTIONS

How is angina graded by the Canadian Cardiovascular Society?

There are four functional classes:

- I: angina occurs only with strenuous or rapid or prolonged exertion
- II: slight limitation of ordinary activity (e.g. climbing more than one flight of ordinary stairs at a normal pace and in normal conditions)
- III: marked limitation of ordinary activity (e.g. climbing more than one flight in normal conditions)
- IV: inability to carry out any physical activity without discomfort — anginal syndrome may be present at rest.

How would you investigate a patient with angina pectoris?

- Haemoglobin: anaemia aggravates angina
- *Rest ECG* to detect left ventricular hypertrophy, prior Q-wave MI or ST-T changes
- *Rest echocardiogram* is carried out only when there is clinical suspicion of aortic stenosis or hypertrophic cardiomyopathy
- *Exercise ECG* can precipitate symptoms, document workload at onset and record any associated ECG abnormality (≥1 mm of horizontal or downsloping ST-segment depression or elevation for ≥60 to 80 ms after the end of the QRS complex) or arrhythmia (Fig. 13.1)
- *Exercise myocardial perfusion imaging or exercise echocardiography* is used in patients where considerations of functional significance of lesions or myocardial viability are important or who have one of the following baseline ECG abnormalities:
  - Left bundle branch block
  - >1 mm of rest ST depression
  - Electronically paced ventricular rhythm and in patients with prior revascularization (percutaneous transluminal coronary angioplasty (PTCA) or coronary artery bypass graft (CABG))

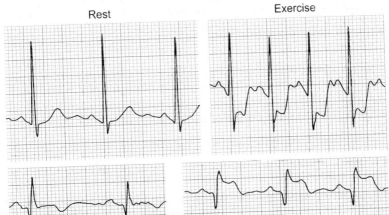

Fig. 13.1 Exercise ECG test.

- *Coronary angiography:* provides detailed anatomical information about site and severity of luminal narrowing caused by coronary atherosclerosis and less-common non-atherosclerotic causes such as coronary artery spasm, coronary anomaly, primary coronary artery dissection and radiation-induced coronary vasculopathy.

How would you treat a patient with chronic stable angina pectoris?

Treatment is remembered with the mnemonic ABCDE (Circulation 1999;99:2829–48).

A: aspirin, antianginal therapy and ACE inhibitor therapy. Aspirin has been shown to reduce the incidence of non-fatal MI and the overall incidence of cardiac events, although overall death rate and the incidence of fatal MI were similar to those obtained with placebo in the Swedish Angina Pectoris Aspirin Trial (SAPAT) study. Ramipril up to 10 mg once a day should be offered to all patients in view of the new HOPE trial. Antianginal therapy includes nitrates, ranalozine and nicorandril.

B: beta-blocker and blood pressure

C: cigarette smoking and cholesterol (clopidogrel)

D: diet and diabetes

E: education and exercise.

What other treatments are there?

- **Percutaneous transluminal coronary angioplasty (with or without coronary stent)**
- Complementary to drug treatment and surgery; no improvement in survival.
- Best results are achieved in discrete single-vessel coronary artery disease.
- The restenosis rate is ~30% at 6 months; for balloon angioplasty with stenting, restenosis is lower, ~20%.
- The ACME (Angioplasty Compared to Medicine) study showed that PTCA can offer better symptomatic relief than medical therapy in patients with single-vessel coronary artery disease, but is a much more expensive procedure and is associated with complications (including emergency and elective coronary bypass and second PTCA).
- The RITA (Randomized Intervention Treatment of Angina) study compared PTCA with CABG and found that both procedures have similar prognostic implications with risk of death or myocardial infarction similar in the two groups, but more patients in the PTCA group required a second revascularization procedure and more antianginal therapy.

- **Coronary artery bypass grafting**
- This has prognostic value in patients with left main-stem coronary stenosis or three-vessel coronary artery disease and impaired left ventricular function.
- The risk of surgery is related to the degree of impairment of left ventricular function.

- **Neurostimulation** Stimulation of the spinal cord region that receives the cardiac nerve fibres has been shown to ease angina and improve functional status.

- **External enhanced counterpulsation** Can improve angina and exercise capacity, with effects that can persist for up to 2 years. It uses three sets of pneumatic cuffs wrapped around the lower extremities to achieve a haemodynamic effect similar to an intra-aortic balloon pump. Usually patients undergo this therapy every day for 6 weeks. The mechanism of improvement is unknown.

ADVANCED-LEVEL QUESTIONS

What is the mechanism of angina pectoris?

It is commonly caused by increased myocardial oxygen demand triggered by physical activity, but it can also be caused by transient decreases in oxygen delivery as a result of coronary vasospasm. Unstable angina is caused by non-occlusive intracoronary thrombi.

What is the prognosis of patients with angina?

- Progression to unstable angina, MI or death within 1 year occurs in 14% of patients with newly diagnosed angina pectoris.
- Mortality at CABG with normal ventricular function is 1%.

What is the significance and the mechanism of postprandial angina?

The presence of postprandial angina indicates severe coronary artery disease; one mechanism is 'intramyocardial steal' with blood being distributed from the stenotic territories to the normal territories (Circulation 1998;97;1144–49). It is caused by the carbohydrate content of the meal (Am J Cardiol 1997;79:1397–1400) and can be ameliorated by prior treatment with octreotide (Circulation 1996;94:I-730), which prevents postprandial vasodilatation of the superior mesenteric artery.

How would you follow a patient with stable angina in your clinic?

Successfully treated chronic stable angina pectoris should have a follow-up evaluation every 4–12 months. During the first year of therapy, evaluations every 4–6 months are recommended. After this, annual evaluations are recommended provided the patient is stable and reliable enough to call or make an appointment when anginal symptoms become worse or other symptoms occur. Patients who are co-managed by their general practitioner and cardiologist may alternate these visits (Circulation 1999; 99:2829–48).

The ACC/AHA give 'Five questions' that must be answered regularly during the follow-up of the patient who is receiving treatment for chronic stable angina (Circulation 1999;99:2829–48):

1. Has the patient decreased the level of physical activity since the last visit?
2. Have the patient's anginal symptoms increased in frequency and become more severe since the last visit? If the symptoms have worsened or the patient has decreased physical activity to avoid precipitating angina, then he or she should be evaluated and treated according to either the unstable angina or chronic stable angina guidelines, as appropriate.
3. How well is the patient tolerating therapy?
4. How successful has the patient been in reducing modifiable risk factors and improving knowledge about ischaemic heart disease?

5. Has the patient developed any new comorbid illnesses or has the severity or treatment of known comorbid illnesses worsened the patient's angina?

What changes in resting 12-lead ECG are consistent with coronary artery disease and suggest ischaemia or previous infarction?

- Pathological Q waves in particular
- Left bundle branch block
- ST segment and T wave abnormalities (e.g. flattening or inversion).

In people without confirmed coronary artery disease in whom stable angina cannot be diagnosed or excluded based solely on clinical assessment alone, how would you manage the patient?

In such patients first the likelihood of coronary artery disease is estimated from a consideration of their age, the clinical assessment and the resting 12-lead ECG. Further diagnostic testing is then done as follows:

- Estimated likelihood 10–29%: CT calcium score as the first-line diagnostic investigation indicates:
  - 0: consider other causes of chest pain
  - 1–400: offer 64-slice (or above) CT coronary angiography
  - >400: offer invasive coronary angiography; if this is not clinically appropriate or acceptable to the person and revascularization is not being considered, offer non-invasive functional imaging.
- Estimated likelihood 30–60%: functional imaging as the first-line diagnostic investigation.
- Estimated likelihood 61–90%: invasive coronary angiography as the first-line diagnostic investigation may be considered.

What is Prinzmetal's angina?

It is angina occurring at rest, unpredictably and associated with transient ST segment elevation on the ECG. Coronary vasospasm is the cause often in the presence of atherosclerosis.

How is exercise testing useful in determining the prognosis of chest pain?

A study at Duke University used exercise testing to determine high- and low-risk subsets in patients with chest pain suggestive of ischaemic heart disease:

- *Low-risk subset:* subjects who could complete 9 min of exercise using the Bruce protocol without evidence of ischaemic ST segment changes and achieve a maximal sinus heart rate in excess of 160 beats/min. These were found to have a 1-year survival rate of 99% and a 4-year survival rate of 93%. This means that cardiac catheterization and CABG can be deferred.
- *High-risk subset:* those who were forced to stop exercising in stages I or II (under 6 min); survival rate was 85% at 1 year and 63% at 4 years.

What do you understand by significant coronary artery disease?

Significant coronary artery disease found during invasive coronary angiography is ≥70% diameter stenosis of at least one major epicardial artery segment or ≥50% diameter stenosis in the left main coronary artery.

- *Factors intensifying ischaemia*: these factors allow less-severe lesions (e.g. ≥50%) to produce angina:
  - Large mass of ischaemic myocardium: proximally located lesions
  - Longer lesion length
  - Reduced oxygen delivery: anaemia, coronary spasm
  - Increased oxygen demand: tachycardia, left ventricular hypertrophy.
- *Factors reducing ischaemia*: these factors may render severe lesions (≥70%) asymptomatic:
  - Well developed collateral supply
  - Small mass of ischaemic myocardium: distally located lesions, old infarction in the territory of coronary supply.

What the indications for CABG in stable angina?

ACC/AHA guidelines 2004 (Circulation 2004;110:e340–437):

1. Recommended in patients with:
   - significant left main coronary artery stenosis
   - left main coronary artery disease: ≥70% of stenosis of proximal left anterior descending artery and proximal left circumflex artery
   - three-vessel disease
   - two-vessel disease with significant proximal left anterior descending stenosis and left ventricular ejection fraction <50% or demonstrable ischaemia on non-invasive testing.
2. Beneficial in patients with:
   - one- or two-vessel disease without significant proximal left anterior descending stenosis but with a large area of viable myocardium and high-risk criteria on non-invasive testing
   - developed disabling angina despite maximal non-invasive therapy, when surgery can be performed with acceptable risk (if angina is not typical, objective evidence of ischaemia should be obtained).

What do you understand by the term syndrome X?

- Syndrome X, or microvascular angina, is the presence of classic angina and ST depression on exercise stress testing and a normal coronary angiogram in the absence of any other demonstrable cardiac abnormalities.
- Reaven syndrome or 'endocrine' syndrome X is the association of insulin resistance, hypertension, and increased very low density lipoprotein (VLDL) and decreased HDL cholesterol concentrations in the plasma.

Coronary artery bypass grafting was introduced by RG Favaloro in 1969 while he was at the Cleveland Clinic, USA (J Thorac Cardiovasc Surg 1969;58:178–85).

Balloon angioplasty was introduced by Arthur Gruntzig, a Swiss cardiologist, in 1977 (Lancet 1978;i: 263).

14 ACUTE MYOCARDIAL INFARCTION

INSTRUCTION

This patient has had a myocardial infarction 2 days ago; would you like to take a short history and examine him?

SALIENT FEATURES

History
- Age
- Post-infarct angina
- Shortness of breath
- Palpitations
- Dizziness or syncope
- Family history of cardiovascular disease, hyperlipidaemia, gout
- Smoking
- Past history of diabetes mellitus, hypertension, stroke, myocardial infarction (MI), intermittent claudication and hyperlipidaemia
- History of oral contraceptives in young women
- Prior use of aspirin particularly in the previous 7 days
- Previous history of coronary stenosis (>50%).

Examination
- Hands: nicotine staining of fingers
- Pulse: check pulse rate (keeping in mind heart block and tachycardia), rhythm (keeping in mind atrial fibrillation, ventricular arrhythmias)
- Check blood pressure
- JVP may be raised in cardiac failure or right ventricular infarction
- Eyes: look for arcus senilis, xanthelasma
- Cardiac apex: look for double apical impulse (ventricular aneurysm)
- Auscultate for fourth heart sound, pericardial rub, pansystolic murmur of papillary muscle dysfunction (or ventricular septal defect)
- Examine:
  - chest for crackles and pleural effusion
  - abdomen for tender liver of cardiac failure
  - legs for deep venous thrombosis and peripheral pulses.
- Tell the examiner that you would like to:
  - check the ECG for ST segment changes (Fig. 14.1)
  - know whether serum cardiac markers were elevated (be prepared to compute the TIMI (thrombolysis in myocardial infarction) risk score if asked, see below).

DIAGNOSIS

This patient with myocardial infarction (aetiology) has papillary muscle dysfunction (lesion) and is in Killip class II cardiac failure (functional status).

Be prepared to discuss the 'number needed to treat' (NNT) for each therapy:

Table 14.1: NNT+to treat in acute MI.

Treatment	NNT	Time Period	Continue Post-MI
Nitrates	333	Short term	Sublingual PRN
Beta blocker	33	16 months	Indefinitely
Aspirin	38	15 months	Indefinitely
ACE inhibitors	17	2.5 years	Indefinitely
Fibrinolytics	53	35 days	No
Heparin	200	Short term	No
Aldosterone inhibitor	44	16 months	Selected patients
Statin	38	2 years	Indefinitely
Thienopyridines	43	30 days	Unknown
Primary PCI	25	Long term	No

†The Number Needed to Treat (NNT) is the number of patients you need to treat to prevent one additional bad outcome (death, stroke, etc.). For example, if a drug has an NNT of 6, it means you have to treat 6 patients with the drug to prevent one additional bad outcome. The ideal NNT is 1, where everyone improves with treatment and no-one improves with control. The higher the NNT, the less effective is the treatment.

QUESTIONS

What is Levine's sign?
In acute myocardial infarction the patient often describes the pain by illustrating a clenched fist.

What are the major risk factors for an acute myocardial infarction?
- Smoking
- Dyslipidaemia
- Diabetes
- Hypertension
- Family history of premature coronary artery disease.

What is the clinical classification of myocardial infarction?
Type 1: spontaneous MI related to ischaemia caused by a primary coronary event such as plaque erosion and/or rupture, fissuring or dissection.
Type 2: MI secondary to ischaemia caused by either increased oxygen demand or decreased supply, such as coronary spasm, coronary embolism, anaemia, arrhythmias, hypertension or hypotension.

What are the diagnostic criteria for acute MI?
Any two of the following three:
- Ischaemic symptoms including chest pain
- ECG changes (Fig. 14.1)
- Elevated serum cardiac markers particularly troponin.

250 Cases in Clinical Medicine

(A) ST segment elevation (⟹ injury)

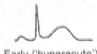

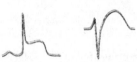

Early ('hyperacute') stage

Coved ('frowny') ST segment elevation (acute injury pattern)

(B) T wave inversion (⟹ ishaemia)

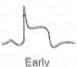

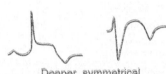

Early

Deeper, symmetrical inversion (ischaemia)

(C) Development of Q waves

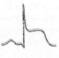

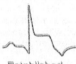

Early   Established   QS complex

(D) Reciprocal ST segment depression

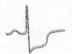

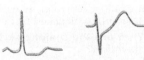

Mirror image ST depression

Subtler reciprocal ST segment depression

Fig. 14.1 Principal electrocardiographic indicators of acute infarction.

Mention some causes of elevated troponin not the result of acute coronary syndrome

- Myocarditis
- Heart failure
- Thromboembolism.

Describe the Killip (or Killip–Kimball) classification

The Killip classification is used to characterize heart failure following MI (Am J Cardiol 1967;20:457–64):

Killip I: absent third heart sound and absence of crackles

Killip II: third heart sound or crackles in <50% of lung fields

Killip III: crackles in greater than 50% of lung fields
Killip IV: cardiogenic shock.

What are the three main types of acute coronary syndrome

- Unstable angina
- Non ST elevation MI (NSTEMI)
- ST elevation MI (STEMI).

How would you use the ECG to localize STEMI?

- *Anterior or anteroseptal:* The QS complexes in leads V_1 and V_2 indicate anteroseptal infarction. A characteristic notching of the QS complex, often seen with infarcts, is present in lead V_2. The septum is supplied with blood by the left anterior descending coronary artery. Septal infarction generally suggests this artery or one of its branches is occluded, whereas a strictly anterior infarct generally results from occlusion of the left anterior descending coronary artery.
- *Anterolateral:* ST segment elevation in leads I, L, and V_1 to V_6 with Q waves in V_1 to V_4. (Fig. 14.1B,C)
- *Posterior:* tall R waves in leads V_1 and V_2. In most cases of posterior infarctions, the infarct extends either to the lateral wall of the LV (resulting in characteristic changes in lead V_6) or to the inferior wall of that ventricle (resulting in characteristic changes in leads II, III and aVF). Because of the overlap between inferior and posterior infarctions, the more general term inferoposterior is used when the ECG shows changes consistent with either inferior or posterior infarction.
- *Inferior:* ST elevations in leads II, III, and aVF and the reciprocal ST depressions in leads I and aVL. Inferior wall infarction is generally caused by occlusion of the right coronary artery. Less commonly, it occurs because of a left circumflex coronary obstruction.
- *Right ventricular infarction:* Q waves and ST segment elevations in leads II, III and aVF are accompanied by ST elevations in the right precordial leads.

This classification is not absolute, and infarct types often overlap.

How would you manage a patient with acute MI?

- In A&E, a patient with chest pain should have a quick clinical examination and an ECG done within 10 min of arrival to hospital.
- Aspirin: chewable non-coated 160–325 mg should be administered immediately and then 160–325 mg daily. In the ISIS-2 and ISIS-3 trials, 160 mg dosage was effective whereas a 325 mg dose was used successfully in GISSI-2. An initial large dose of aspirin of 325 mg orally or 160 mg chewable aspirin is preferred because lower doses may still allow significant thromboxane activity and may take a few days.
- Pain relief: immediate relief of pain should be a top priority because severe pain can result in autonomic disturbances that can result in sudden death.
- Reperfusion strategies: either thrombolysis or primary PTCA should be performed within 30 min of the patient's arrival in hospital.
- Beta-blockers: patient should receive beta-blockers when there are no contraindications within 12 h of onset of infarction, irrespective of administration of concomitant thrombolytic therapy or performance of primary angioplasty.

- ACE inhibitors: should be administered within the first 24 h of a suspected acute STEMI in ≥2 anterior precordial leads or with clinical heart failure in the absence of hypotension (systolic BP <100 mmHg) and known contraindications to use of ACE inhibitors.

What are the complications of myocardial infarction?

- Extension of infarct and post-infarct ischaemia
- Rhythm disorders: tachycardia, bradycardia, ventricular ectopics, ventricular fibrillation, atrial fibrillation and tachycardia
- Heart failure: acute pulmonary oedema
- Circulatory failure: cardiogenic shock
- Infarction of papillary muscle: mitral regurgitation and acute pulmonary oedema
- Rupture of interventricular septum
- Left ventricular aneurysm
- Mural thrombus
- Thromboembolism, cerebral or peripheral
- Venous thrombosis
- Pericarditis
- Dressler syndrome: characterized by persistent pyrexia, pericarditis, pleurisy (first described in 1956 when Dressler recognized that chest pain following MI is not caused by coronary artery insufficiency).

What is a silent myocardial infarct?

A painless infarct, common in diabetics and the elderly (particulary women); it may present with complications of myocardial infarction.

How is short-term risk determined in acute coronary syndromes?

The TIMI risk score can be used for unstable angina/NSTEMI and for STEMI.

- **Unstable angina/NSTEMI** The TIMI risk score for NSTEMI is one method of evaluating short-term (14-day) risk for death and non-fatal MI in patients presenting with unstable angina and NSTEMI. The TIMI trial risk score for death or myocardial infarction at 14 days assigns a value of 0 when a factor is absent and 1 when a factor is present. The score utilizes seven independent risk factors:
- Age >65 years
- >3 risk factors for coronary artery disease
- Documented coronary artery disease at catheterization
- ST deviation >0.5 mm
- >2 episodes of angina in last 24 h
- Aspirin within prior 7 days
- Elevated cardiac markers.

Use of this scoring system was able to risk-stratify patients across a 10-fold gradient of risk, from 4.7% to 40.9% (p <0.001). The TIMI risk score predicts outcome and response to therapy.

Outcome:

0–2: low risk (8% rate of recurrent MI or death)
3–4: intermediate risk
6–7: high risk (~31% rate of recurrent MI or death).

Response to therapy: patients with higher TIMI risk scores had significant reductions in events when treated with enoxaparin than when treated with unfractionated heparin, treated with a glycoprotein IIb/IIIa antagonist inhibitor compared with placebo, and with invasive compared with conservative strategy.

● **STEMI:** In the TIMI scoring system for STEMI (1 through 14 points), risk rises progressively with higher scores and is maximal for a composite score >8. A score >6 identifies a segment of the population (12%) that has double the mean 30-day mortality risk of the total population. However, this scoring system should not substitute for clinical judgment in individual cases. For example, patients with inferior STEMI, who might be considered to have a low risk of mortality (and for whom many physicians have questioned the benefits of thrombolysis), might actually be in a much higher mortality risk subgroup if their inferior infarction is associated with ST segment elevation in the lateral precordial leads indicating right ventricular infarction, or precordial ST segment depression.

● **The Global Registry for Acute Coronary Events (GRACE) system** This is another risk score for prediction of death and myocardial infarction that incorporates renal dysfunction.

What are TIMI grades?

Grades (0–3) determined in the thrombolysis in myocardial infarction trial (TIMI) measure coronary blood flow and luminal narrowing:

0: no flow of contrast beyond the point of occlusion
1: penetration with minimal perfusion (contrast fails to opacify the entire coronary bed distal to the stenosis for the duration of investigation)
2: partial perfusion (contrast opacifies the entire distal coronary artery, but the rate of entry or clearance or both is slower in the previously blocked artery than in nearby normally perfused vessels
3: complete perfusion (contrast filling and clearance are as rapid in the previously blocked vessel as in normally perfused vessels).

Which thrombolytic agents are available?

● Streptokinase: for non-anterior MI
● Tenecteplase: for anterior MI, previous streptokinase use, systolic BP <100 mmHg, new left bundle branch block; can be given by paramedics and administered as a bolus
● Alteplase (rt-PA): in younger patients with anterior MI; given within 6 h of symptoms in accelerated manner and followed by heparin
● Reteplase: given in two intravenous boluses 2 h apart.

What is the relation between thrombolysis and onset of symptoms?

Thrombolytic therapy reduces mortality and limits infarct size. The shorter the interval between the onset of symptoms and the initiation of thrombolysis, the greater is the survival. The greatest benefit occurs if the treatment is initiated within the first 3 h, when a 50% or greater reduction in mortality rate can be achieved. The magnitude of benefit declines rapidly thereafter, but a 10% mortality reduction can be achieved up to 12 h after the onset of pain.

Duration from symptom onset to therapy initation	Lives saved per 1000 treated
<60 min	65
2–3 h	27
4–6 h	25
7–12 h	8

What is the benefit of late administration of thrombolytic therapy?

ISIS-2 (Lancet 1988;ii:349–60) showed benefit for up to 24 h (after onset of symptoms) with thrombolysis, but more recent studies — the LATE (Late Assessment of Thrombolytic Therapy) and EMERAS (Estudio Multicentrico Estreptoquinasa Republicas de America del Sur) — have shown no benefit for treatment given beyond 12 h.

What is the role of heparin with thrombolysis?

In the ISIS-3 (Lancet 1992;339:753–70) and GISSI-2 (Lancet 1990;336:65–75) studies, heparin therapy was not beneficial with streptokinase or anistreplase, and it is believed that it may even be harmful. The GUSTO trial showed that early intravenous heparin with tPA results in a further reduction in the mortality rate compared with that found with a combination of heparin and streptokinase.

What is the role of prehospital thrombolysis?

Two studies — the GREAT (Grampian Region Early Administration of Thrombolysis) and EMIP (European Myocardial Infarction Project) — showed that a single bolus dose of anistreplase reduced the total mortality rate. These results suggest that early thrombolysis has greater benefit, and hence the importance in many hospitals for 'door to needle time'.

What is the role of primary angioplasty in acute infarction?

● Angioplasty results in both lower mortality rates and reduction in the incidence of recurrent ischaemic events. Also angioplasty is associated with lower enzyme rise, better left ventricular function and less reinfarction. Angioplasty led to shorter hospital stay, fewer re-admissions and lower follow-up costs. However, the major limitation of this approach is the access to both facilities and personnel to carry out the procedure.

● Angioplasty should be considered in patients who have recognized contraindication to thrombolysis (even if this means transferring the patient) or who are considered high risk and present with their infarction to a hospital where angioplasty can be performed. Patients who have received thrombolysis and who seem on clinical grounds (reduction in maximal ST segment elevation by 50% and resolution of chest pain) not to have reperfused at 90 min review should be seriously considered for rescue angioplasty, again even if this means transferring the patient.

● Patients who do not receive reperfusion therapy should be treated immediately with fondaparinux.

Why is the Asian population in Britain susceptible to premature myocardial infarction?

Premature ischaemic heart disease in migrants from the Indian subcontinent is associated with insulin resistance. The site of this defective insulin action has been localized to the skeletal muscle by means of positron emission tomography (PET) (Circulation 1995;92(suppl I):16).

What do you know about right ventricular infarction?

Right ventricular infarction presents with retrosternal chest discomfort, nausea, vomiting and diaphoresis, unlike left ventricular infarction, which presents with dyspnoea. On examination in right ventricular infarction, there is a raised JVP with no evidence of pulmonary congestion; the patient often has a low cardiac output with hypotension. The patient typically presents with ST elevation in the inferior leads (II, III and aVF) and in one or more right-sided lead, particularly V_4R. The cornerstones of therapy include restoration of infarct artery patency, intravascular volume expansion and inotropic support.

What do you know about the open-infarct related coronary artery hypothesis?

This hypothesis holds that early reperfusion of the infarct-related coronary artery results in myocardial salvage, which preserves left ventricular function and is responsible for improved survival. Patients with complete occlusion of the coronary artery (TIMI grade 0) 90 min following thrombolysis had a 30-day mortality of 8.4%, whereas mortality was 4% in patients with TIMI grade 3 flow (complete perfusion).

What is the role of glycoprotein IIb/IIIa antagonists as adjuncts to thrombolytic therapy in acute myocardial infarction?

After thrombolytic therapy for acute MI, full anterograde perfusion (TIMI grade 3 flow) occurs in only 29–54% of patients at 90 min, while reocclusion occurs in at least 12%, with increased morbidity and mortality. Thrombolytic therapy may itself be prothrombotic by releasing clot-bound thrombin, which in turn stimulates platelet activation. Preclinical and early clinical trials have suggested that glycoprotein IIb/IIIa receptor blockers (which prevent fibrinogen binding to platelets) used as adjuncts to thrombolytic therapy may improve early patency and reduce the incidence of reocclusion. Though there are as yet no data showing a reduction in mortality from such use of these blockers, a large randomized trial has recently confirmed the early findings on patency and suggests that adjunct treatment with glycoprotein IIb/IIIa receptor blockers may hold promise for better management of acute MI – the results from the GUSTO-AMI phase III trial using abciximab with reduced dose reteplase are awaited.

What are the indications for drug-eluting stents?

According to NICE guidelines (issued in Oct 2003) drug-eluting stent should be used if the person has symptoms of angina and the artery is <3 mm across, or the narrowed part (the 'lesion') is >15 mm. When more than one artery is narrowed, the interventional cardiologist should make the decision on which type of stent to use for each artery separately. (Note that the Taxus stent elutes paxlitaxel to inhibit cell division; the Cypher stent elutes sirolimus (previously known as rapamycin), an immunosuppressive agent that reduces inflammation).

What do you know about risk stratification after myocardial infarction?

● Risk stratification before hospital discharge is an important aspect of management and determines whether coronary angiography is indicated. The first step is to determine whether the clinical variables indicating a relatively high risk for future cardiac events are present:

- Patients who have recurrent ischaemia at rest or with mild activity, who have had evidence of congestive heart failure or who are known to have an ejection fraction <40% and in whom there are no contraindications for revascularization should undergo cardiac catheterization and coronary angiography. Revascularization should then be carried out if the coronary anatomy is suitable and there are no contra-indications.

- Patients who have had episode of ventricular fibrillation or sustained ventricular tachycardia >48 h after acute MI should be considered for electrophysiologic study or amiodarone therapy, or both.

- In patients with non-STEMI or unstable angina who appear on clinical grounds to be candidates for coronary revascularization, coronary vascularization should be performed. Revascularization may then be carried out if the coronary anatomy is appropriate.

- Patients without these clinical indicators of high risk should undergo an assessment of left ventricular function (echocardiogram or radionuclide angiogram and submaximal stress) before hospital discharge:
  - If the test is negative the patient may return for a symptom limited exercise test at 3 to 6 weeks. If that too is negative they can remain on medical therapy and risk factor reduction.
  - If the resting ejection fraction is <40% or if the stress is markedly abnormal (>2 mm ST segment depression, hypotension at peak exercise or low working capacity) then coronary angiography should be carried out if there are no contraindications to revascularization.

- In patients in whom the ECG is not interpretable because of resting ST–T wave abnormalities, digitalis therapy or left bundle branch block, rest and exercise radionuclide myocardial perfusion scintigraphy (with thallium or sestamibi) or rest and exercise echocardiography should be performed. Patients who cannot exercise should undergo pharmacologic stress imaging study such as adenosine or dipyridamole myocardial perfusion scintigraphy or echocardiography with dobutamine or dipyridamole stress. A marked abnormality in any of these tests or a resting ejection fraction <40%, measured by echocardiography or a radionuclide technique, should be followed by coronary angiography.

How is non-invasive testing used to risk stratify patients?

Risk stratification based on non-invasive testing (J Am Coll Cardiol 1999;33:2092–197) comprises:

High risk (>3% annual mortality rate):

- Severe resting LV dysfunction (LV ejection fraction <35%)
- High-risk treadmill score (score ≥–11)
- Severe exercise LV dysfunction (exercise LV ejection fraction <35%)
- Stress-induced large perfusion defect (particularly if anterior)
- Stress-induced multiple perfusion defects of moderate size
- Large, fixed perfusion defect with LV dilation or increased lung uptake (thallium-201)
- Stress-induced moderate perfusion defect with LV dilation or increased lung uptake (thallium-201)

- Echocardiographic wall motion abnormality (involving >2 segments) developing at a low dose of dobutamine (%10 mg/min per kg) or at a low heart rate (<120 beats/min)
- Stress echocardiographic evidence of extensive ischaemia.

Intermediate risk (1–3% annual mortality rate):
- Mild/moderate resting LV dysfunction (LV ejection fraction 35–49%)
- Intermediate-risk treadmill score (−11 to <5)
- Stress-induced moderate perfusion defect without LV dilation or increased lung intake (thallium-201)
- Limited stress echocardiographic ischaemia with a wall motion abnormality only at higher doses of dobutamine involving >2 segments.

Low risk (<1% annual mortality rate):
- Low-risk treadmill score (≥5)
- Normal or small myocardial perfusion defect at rest or with stress
- Normal stress echocardiographic wall motion or no change of limited resting wall motion abnormalities during stress.

What advice would you give this patient on discharge?

Secondary prevention of myocardial infarction (BMJ 1998;316:838–42) as follows:
- Smoking cessation: it should be emphasized to the patient that within 2 years of discontinuing smoking, the risk of a non-fatal recurrent MI falls to the level observed in a patient who has never smoked.
- Lipid profile: a lipid profile should be obtained in all patients with acute MI. Since cholesterol may fall after 24 to 48 h, it is important these measurements be obtained on admission; otherwise a 6-week wait is necessary for cholesterol to reach pre-MI levels. It is desirable to fractionate the cholesterol, and patients with LDL cholesterol >3.37 mmol/l should be treated with lipid lowering agents (p. 616).
- Cardiac rehabilitation: all discharged patients should be referred for outpatient cardiac rehabilitation. Patients should be encouraged to increase activity gradually over 1–2 months.
- Risk factors: diabetes (target HbA1C <6) and hypertension (target BP <130/85 mmHg) should be aggressively controlled.
- Aspirin: led to a 12% reduction in death, a 31% reduction in re-infarction and a 42% reduction in non-fatal stroke in a study of 19791 patients who had myocardial infarctions reviewed by the Antiplatelet Therapy Trialists. Low to medium doses (75–325 mg/day) seems to be as effective as high doses (1200 mg/day).
- Beta-blockers: several controlled trials in >35000 survivors of MI have shown the benefit of long-term treatment with beta-blockers in reducing the incidence of recurrent MI, sudden death and all cause mortality. Beta-blockers reduce myocardial workload and oxygen consumption by reducing the heart rate, BP and contractility, and they increase the threshold for ventricular fibrillation. The beneficial effect of beta-blockers seems to be a class effect, but those with agonist activity do not show a beneficial effect on mortality, and their use cannot be recommended at present.
- ACE inhibitors: low-dose ramipril should be considered in all patients with uncomplicated MI (N Engl J Med 2000;342:145–53). Treatment with full dose ACE inhibitors is recommended for an indefinite period in all patients with congestive heart failure, an ejection fraction <40% or a large regional wall motion abnormality.

Eugene Braunwald (b. 1929) was consecutively Chair and Professor of Medicine in San Diego and Harvard Medical School, Boston. His research interests included heart failure, factors influencing cardiac contraction and hypertrophic cardiomyopathy and he was responsible for the idea that late patency of an occluded artery can lead to clinical benefit. His wife, Nina H Starr Braunwald, was a cardiothoracic surgeon who made important contributions to heart valve replacement.

Thomas Killip described Killips class in 1967.

Professor Jaspal Kooner, is Professor of Clinical Cardiology at Imperial College, Consultant Cardiologist at Hammersmith and Ealing Hospitals. His research includes gene identification of coronary artery disease.

15   JUGULAR VENOUS PULSE

INSTRUCTION

Examine this patient's neck.
Examine this patient's cardiovascular system.

SALIENT FEATURES

History

- Shortness of breath
- Symptoms of right heart failure (leg oedema, ascites).

Examination

- The JVP is measured ..... cm above the angle of Louis (manubriosternal angle). Remember that the distance between the angle of Louis and the mid-right atrium can be varied and the JVP may be measured as high as at the level of the ear lobes.
- Comment on the waveform (timing it with the carotid pulse):
  - 'v' waves of tricuspid regurgitation
  - Cannon waves of heart block
  - Absent 'a' waves in atrial fibrillation (irregular carotid pulse)
  - Large 'a' waves of pulmonary hypertension, pulmonary stenosis, tricuspid stenosis.
- Check the hepatojugular reflex.
- Tell the examiner that you would like to look for other signs of heart failure:
  - Basal crackles and pleural effusion
  - Dependent oedema (ankle and sacral oedema)
  - Tender hepatomegaly.

DIAGNOSIS

This patient has raised jugular venous pulse with 'v' waves (lesion) caused by tricuspid regurgitation (see Case 19) and is in heart failure (functional status).

QUESTIONS

What are the causes of a raised jugular venous pulse?
- Congestive cardiac failure (N Engl J Med 2001;345:574–81)
- Cor pulmonale
- Tricuspid regurgitation (prominent 'v' waves)
- Tricuspid stenosis (prominent 'a' waves)
- Complete heart block (cannon waves)
- Non-pulsatile neck veins seen in superior venal caval obstruction (p. 796).

How do you differentiate jugular venous pulsations from carotid artery pulsations?
Unlike the arterial pulse, the venous pulse has a definite upper level which falls during inspiration and changes with posture. The venous pulse is seen to have a dominant inward motion, towards the midline (the 'y' descent), whereas the arterial pulse exhibits a dominant outward wave. The venous pulse is better seen than felt, whereas the arterial pulse is readily felt by very slight pressure of the clinician's finger.

What do you know about the hepatojugular reflux?
A positive hepatojugular (abdominojugular) reflux is a feature of left ventricular systolic failure with secondary pulmonary hypertension. It is elicited by upper abdominal compression for ~10 s and an abnormal response is one where there is an increase followed by an abrupt fall. The hepatojugular manoeuvre is often useful in eliciting venous pulsations when not readily visible.

ADVANCED-LEVEL QUESTIONS

What do you know about the waveforms in the jugular pulse?
There are two outward moving waves ('a' and 'v' wave) and two inward moving waves (the 'x' and 'y' descent) (Fig 15.1):
- The 'a' wave is caused by atrial contraction and is presystolic. It can be identified by simultaneous auscultation of the heart and the examination of the jugular venous pulse. The 'a' wave occurs at about the first heart sound.
- The 'c' wave is caused by closure of the tricuspid valve and is not readily visible.
- The 'v' wave is caused by venous return to the right heart (not from ventricular contraction) and occurs nearer to the second heart sound.
- The 'x' descent is caused by atrial relaxation (sometimes referred to as systolic collapse).
- The 'y' descent is produced by opening of the tricuspid valve and rapid inflow of blood into the RV.

What is Kussmaul's sign?
Normally there is an inspiratory decrease in JVP. In constrictive pericarditis, there is an inspiratory increase in JVP. Kussmaul's sign is also seen in severe right heart failure regardless of aetiology. It is caused by the inability of the heart to accept the increase in right ventricular volume without a marked increase in the filling pressure.

What is the prognostic value of raised JVP in heart failure?
Raised JVP and third heart sounds are associated with adverse outcomes, including subsequent hospitalization for heart failure, progression of heart failure as defined by death from pump failure and by the composite

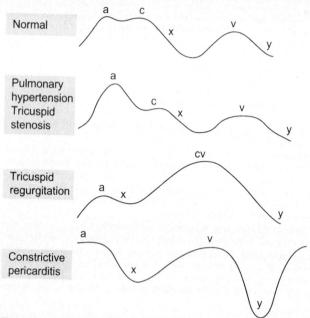

Fig. 15.1 Normal jugular venous pulse.

end-point of death or hospitalization for heart failure, and death from all causes (N Engl J Med 2001;345:574–81).

What is the mechanism of anaemia in heart failure?

The aetiology and pathophysiology of anaemia in heart failure is also multifactorial and is caused by a complex interaction between cardiac function, renal dysfunction, neurohormonal and inflammatory responses, haemodilution, iron deficiency, impaired ability to utilize available iron stores, bone marrow suppression caused by cytokines (e.g. tumour necrosis factor α (TNF-α), interleukin-1, interleukin-6 (IL-6) and C-reactive protein), blunted bone marrow responsiveness to erythropoietin, impaired iron mobilization and effects of medications. Aspirin and ACE inhibitors contribute to the anaemia potentially through the actions of haematopoiesis inhibitor N-acetyl-seryl-aspartyl-lysyl-proline. IL-6 stimulates the production of hepcidin in the hepatic cells, which blocks absorption of iron in duodenum and downregulates ferroprotein expression; this, in turn, prevents release of iron from total body stores. TNF-α (and IL-6) inhibits erythropoietin production in the kidney by activating the GATA-binding protein GATA2 and nuclear factor-κB and it also inhibits proliferation of bone marrow erythroid progenitor cells.

Adolf Kussmaul (1822–1902) was Professor of Medicine successively at Heidelberg, Enlargen, Freiburg and Strasbourg, and coined the term polyarteritis nodosa (Berl Klin Wochnschr 1873;10:433). Kussmaul breathing is deep sighing respiration seen when the arterial pH is low.

In 1867, Potain described the waveforms of the internal jugular vein.

In 1902, James Mackenzie championed that the jugular venous pulse is an essential part of the cardiovascular physical examination.

In 1928, Carl Wiggers wrote that the jugular venous pulse might have utility in the interpretation of dynamic events in the heart.

In 1956, Paul Wood wrote, 'Precise analysis of the cervical venous pulse and measurement of the height of each individual wave with reference to the sternal angle is not only possible at the bedside but highly desirable'.

16   CONGESTIVE CARDIAC FAILURE

INSTRUCTION

Examine this patient's cardiovascular system.

SALIENT FEATURES

History

- Dyspnoea on exertion
- Past history of hypertension, ischaemic heart disease or cardiomyopathy

Examination

- Signs of fluid retention: raised JVP, lung crepitations, pitting leg oedema, tender hepatomegaly
- Signs of impaired perfusion: cold clammy skin, low BP
- Signs of ventricular dysfunction: displaced left ventricular apex, right ventricular heave, third or fourth heart sound, functional mitral or tricuspid regurgitation, tachycardia
- Look for the aetiology:
  - Valvular disease
  - Atherosclerotic vascular disease
  - Severe hypertension
  - Severe anaemia or volume overload, e.g. arteriovenous shunt
  - Pathological arrhythmia
  - Evidence of generalized myopathy or poisoning.

DIAGNOSIS

This patient has congestive cardiac failure caused by hypertension and is severely limited with NYHA class 4 dyspnoea.

Be prepared to discuss mortality in heart failure depending on the NYHA functional class (see p. 3).

How would you investigate this patient?

- *Chest radiography* (Fig. 16.1). Presence of pulmonary oedema on chest radiograph suggests that left ventricular end-diastolic pressure is 25 mmHg (normal ~7 mmHg).

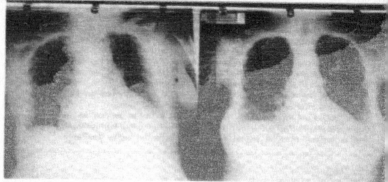

Fig. 16.1 Radiograph of person with heart failure before (left) and after treatment (right). (With permission from Krum 2009.)

- *ECG* to look for underlying cause, e.g. ischaemia or infarction, left ventricular hypertrophy, arrhythmia, other causes of pathological Q waves. Monitoring with 24-Holter can identify ventricular arrhythmias.
- *Echocardiogram* detects valvular disease and determines whether LV function is globally impaired (e.g. idiopathic dilated cardiomyopathy) or whether there is segmental wall motion abnormalities (e.g. in ischaemic heart disease). Ejection fraction can be estimated and usually treatment is initiated when ejection fraction is ≤40. Doppler echocardiography allows determination of diastolic dysfunction.
- *Exercise testing* is useful to identify ischaemic heart disease.
- *Cardiopulmonary exercise testing* is useful to determine functional capacity before cardiac rehabilitation and to determine eligibility for cardiac transplantation.
- *Blood tests* can identify associated disease: renal, liver and electrolyte disturbances (common); metabolic causes (e.g. haemochromatosis, hypocalcaemic cardiomyopathy, thyroid heart disease, anaemia, heavy metal poisoning), amyloid (serum electrophoresis, rectal biopsy), sarcoid (serum ACE).
- *Coronary angiography* is used to identify ischaemic heart disease.
- *Ventricular biopsy* for specific myocarditis, especially viral, and to exclude infiltrative diseases such as cardiac sarcoidosis and amyloidosis.
- *Radionuclide ventriculography or echocardiography* to quantitate severity of systolic dysfunction (ejection fraction).

What is the pharmacologic treatment of left ventricular systolic dysfunction?

- Diuretics for symptomatic patients to maintain appropriate fluid balance
- For patients with systolic dysfunction (ejection fraction <40%) who have no contraindications:
  - ACE inhibitors for all patients
  - Beta-blockers for all patients except those who are haemodynamically unstable or who are intolerant

- Spironolactone for patients with rest dyspnoea or with a history of rest dyspnoea
- Digoxin both for patients who remain symptomatic despite diuretics, ACE inhibitors and beta-blockers and for patients with rest dyspnoea or who have a history of rest dyspnoea.

ADVANCED-LEVEL QUESTIONS

What drugs should be avoided in heart failure?

- Antiarrhythmic drugs
- Non-dihydropyridine calcium antagonists, e.g. verapamil, diltiazem in patients with systolic chronic heart failure
- Tricyclic antidepressants
- Non-steroidal anti-inflammatory drugs (NSAIDs)
- Cyclo-oxygenase 2 inhibitors
- Corticosteroids
- Doxorubicin and trastuzamab
- Thiazolidinediones.

What is diastolic dysfunction?

It is excessive stiffness of the heart resulting in an inability of the heart to fill properly (Eur Heart J 1998;19:990–1003). This is in contrast to systolic dysfunction, where contractility is impaired. Patients have clinical features of left heart failure but normal systolic function by echocardiography or radionuclide ventriculography. It is a feature of hypertrophic cardiomyopathy, severe left ventricular hypertrophy (e.g. aortic stenosis or hypertension) and restrictive cardiomyopathy (e.g. amyloidosis). Treatment is directed towards the underlying cause.

What is the role of devices in heart failure?

Three types of device have been found to effective in treatment of systolic heart failure:

- Atrial-synchronized biventricular pacing (also called cardiac resynchronization therapy); ventricular dyssynchrony is currently defined as a QRS duration of at least 120 ms on the 12 lead ECG.
- Implantable cardioverter defibrillators: a 23–31% reduction in all-cause mortality is attributable to diminished risk for sudden cardiac death in patients randomly allocated an implantable cardioverter defibrillator and best medical treatment versus those assigned best medical care alone.
- Left ventricular assist devices may be considered in three situations:
  - For individuals listed for transplantation but who need support before a suitable donor heart becomes available
  - As a bridge to recovery in people with potentially reversible forms of heart failure, such as myocarditis or postpartum cardiomyopathy
  - As 'destination therapy' for patients not judged candidates for transplantation.

What are the indications for heart transplantation?

When patients are refractory to treatment, both medical and surgical (such as valve replacement), and are in NYHA class IV, then they are unlikely to survive for 1 year and should be considered for heart transplantation. The survival rate is about 69% at 5 years, although most patients have one episode of rejection and 25% have multiple episodes. They are also prone to accelerated coronary atherosclerosis.

In 1967 Christiaan Barnard, a South African surgeon, was the first to perform cardiac transplantation in humans.

Sir Magdi Yacoub, contemporary professor of cardiology at University of London and Royal Brompton Hospital and Harefield Hospital is Egyptian-born surgeon who performed several pioneering cardiac surgeries.

Professor Shoumo Bhattacharya is Professor of Cardiovascular Medicine at Oxford. He is Fellow of Green Templeton College and his research interest includes cardiac development, congenital heart disease and myocardial homeostasis. His clinical interest is chemotherapy induced cardiomyopathy.

17 INFECTIVE ENDOCARDITIS

INSTRUCTION

This patient is suspected to have endocarditis; would you like to examine him?

SALIENT FEATURES

History

- Fever, malaise, anorexia, weight loss, rigors: non-specific symptoms of inflammation
- Progressive heart failure: caused by valve destruction (can be dramatic)
- Stroke, pulseless limb, renal infarct, pulmonary infarct: caused by embolization of vegetations
- Arthralgia, loin pain: caused by immune-complex deposition
- Obtain a history of recent dental procedures
- History of valvular heart disease, history of IV drug abuse

Examination

- Look for the following signs:
  - Anaemia
  - Clubbing (seen in 20% of the cases)
  - Splinter haemorrhages in the nails (vasculitic phenomenon; probably caused by embolic phenomena in the nail bed) (Fig. 17.1)
  - Osler's nodes (vasculitic phenomenon): tender, erythematous, pea-sized nodules seen in the pulp of the fingers caused by inflammation around the site of the infected emboli lodged in distal arterioles (Fig. 17.2)
  - Janeway lesions (vasculitic phenomenon): flat, non-tender red spots found on the palms and soles; they blanch on pressure)
  - Petechiae: conjunctiva, palate and skin
  - Digital infarcts
  - Maculopapular rash.
- Record the temperature.
- Listen to the heart for murmurs and look for signs of cardiac failure.
- Examine the fundus for Roth's spots (vasculitic phenomena).
- Examine the abdomen for splenomegaly.

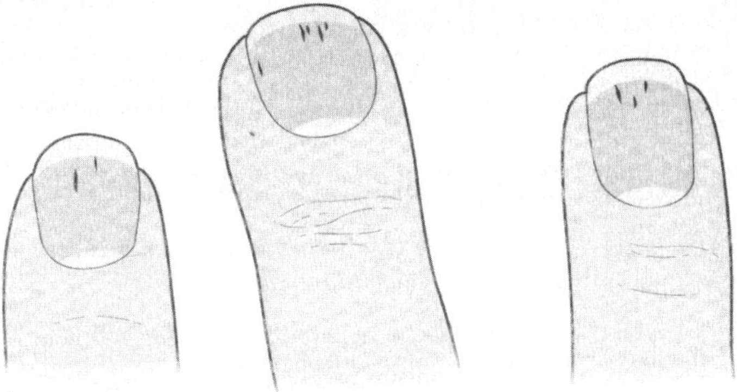

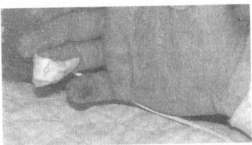

Fig. 17.1 Splinter haemorrhages: parallel streaks in the distal third of the finger.

Fig. 17.2 Osler's nodes. (With permission from Goldman L, Ausiello DA 2007.)

- Look for embolic phenomena: stroke, viscera or occlusion of peripheral arteries.
- Test urine for microscopic haematuria (vasculitic phenomena).
- Remember that ostium secundum atrial septal defects almost never have infective endocarditis.

DIAGNOSIS

This patient has Janeway lesions and Roth's spots (lesions), confirming infective endocarditis, and is in severe heart failure (functional status).

QUESTIONS

How would you investigate such a patient?

- Test the urine for microscopic haematuria.
- Take a FBC to show normocytic, normochromic anaemia and raised white cell count.
- Test for raised erythrocyte sedimentation rate (ESR).
- Blood culture: take three samples from different sites in 24 h. It is the most important test for diagnosing endocarditis and cultures are negative in >50% of cases of fungal aetiology.

- Transthoracic echocardiography may show vegetations. A negative study does not rule out endocarditis as vegetations <3–4 mm in size cannot be detected. Furthermore, all the leaflets of the aortic, tricuspid and pulmonary valves may not be visualized in every patient. Transoesophageal echocardiography is usually indicated in infective endocarditis.

What are the major categories of infective endocarditis?

Infective endocarditis can be classified as:
- native-valve infective endocarditis
- prosthetic-valve infective endocarditis
- infective endocarditis in intravenous drug users
- nosocomial infective endocarditis.

These four categories allow delineation of clinical conditions and help in predicting the likely microbial organisms involved.

What do you know about the pathogenesis of this condition?

1. The primary event is bacterial adherence to damaged valves. This occurs within minutes during transient bacteraemia and involves valve tissue and bacterial factors.
2. The second step involves persistence and growth of bacteria within the cardiac lesions, usually associated with local extension and tissue damage.
3. Third step is the dissemination of septic emboli to kidney, spleen and brain

What are the major manifestations of bacterial endocarditis?

- Manifestations of a systemic infection: fever, weight loss, pallor, splenomegaly.
- Manifestations of vasculitic phenomenon: cardiac failure, changing murmurs, petechiae, Roth's spots, Osler's nodes, Janeway lesions, splinter haemorrhages, stroke, infarction of viscera, mycotic aneurysm.
- Manifestations of immunological reactions: arthralgia, finger clubbing, uraemia.

Note: Mnemonic to remember Duke's criteria for bacterial endocarditis, BE FEVER:

Major:

B, blood culture positive at least twice, 12 h part
E, endocardial involvement from echocardiogram.

Minor:

F, fever
E, evidence from microbiology
V, vascular findings
E, evidence from immunology
R, risk factors/predisposing factors, e.g.drug abuse, valvular diseases.

Name the common organisms found in infective endocarditis?

Streptococcus viridans, Staphylococcus aureus, Streptococcus faecalis, fungi.

How would you treat a patient suspected to have endocarditis?

Until the bacteriology results are available, with intravenous benzylpenicillin and gentamicin.

ADVANCED-LEVEL QUESTIONS

Mention a few prognostic factors

- Heart failure
- Non-streptococcal endocarditis, especially *S. aureus*, fungal endocarditis
- Infection of prosthetic valve
- Elderly patients
- Valve ring or myocardial abscess.

Mention a few conditions that can simulate clinical manifestations of infective endocarditis

- Atrial myxoma
- Non-bacterial endocarditis
- Systemic lupus erythematosus
- Sickle cell disease.

What do you know of prosthetic valve endocarditis?

About 3% of patients will develop prosthetic valve endocarditis by the end of the first year of valve replacement; thereafter, the incidence is lower. Prosthetic valve endocarditis is classified into two groups.

- *Early:* occurring within 2 months of surgery. It develops as a result of intraoperative contamination of the prosthetic valve or as a consequence of a postoperative nosocomial infection, such as sternotomy infection, postoperative pneumonia, urinary tract infection or intravenous catheter-related insertion. The clinical features may be masked by the ordinary events in the postoperative course or by another infection. Cutaneous signs are not common.
- *Late:* develops >2 months after valve surgery. It can occur after transient bacteraemia as in minor skin or upper respiratory tract infections or following dental or urinary manipulations. The non-cardiac manifestations resemble those of native valve infective endocarditis.

Although this classification is convenient, the high prevalence of *S. epidermidis* and diphtheroids among patients suggests that this division is not absolute.

What are the complications of infective endocarditis?

- Congestive heart failure: may develop acutely or insidiously; it portends a grave prognosis
- Conduction disturbances caused by abscesses in ventricular septum
- Valve destruction: acute regurgitation, pulmonary oedema, heart failure
- Embolism: occurs in 22–50% of cases, leading to infarction in any vascular bed, including lungs, coronary arteries, spleen, bowel, renal (flank pain and haematuria) and extremities
- Local extension of infection: purulent pericarditis, aortic root abscess (may cause sinus Valsalva fistula), myocardial abscess (conduction disturbance)
- Septic emboli to vaso vasorum: may lead to mycotic aneurysms anywhere on vascular tree; most worrying in cerebral vessels, resulting in cerebral haemorrhage
- Distal infection (metastatic): caused by septic emboli, e.g. brain abscess, cerebritis
- Candidal endocarditis: may be manifest by fungal endophthalmitis

- Glomerulonephritis: there are two types of renal lesion in subacute bacterial endocarditis (SBE), a diffuse proliferative glomerulonephritis and a focal embolic glomerulonephritis. This is associated with low complement levels and immune complexes.

What are the indications for surgery?
- Positive blood cultures or relapse after several days of the best available antibiotic therapy indicates the need for valve replacement
- Drainage of myocardial or valve ring abscesses
- Patients with aortic valve endocarditis who develop second- or third-degree heart block
- Prosthetic valve replacement for non-streptococcal endocarditis, valve dysfunction, valve dehiscence or myocardial invasion
- Development of a new aneurysm of the sinus of Valsalva
- Fungal endocarditis.

What do you understand by the term marantic endocarditis?
Marantic or Libman–Sacks endocarditis is seen in SLE and is a postmortem diagnosis. It is rarely clinically significant.

What are MSCRAMMs?
MSCRAMMs (microbial surface component reacting with adhesive matrix molecules) are surface adhesives on microbial pathogens that promote attachment to damaged valves and vegetations. These include fibrinogen-binding protein (also called clumping factor) and fibronectin-binding proteins in *S. aureus*, protein M in streptococci; these proteins act as surface adhesions, platelet-activating factors and exopolysaccharides.

What are the recommendations for prophylaxis?
According to NICE guidelines (March 2008).

Prophylaxis should be considered in those at increased risk of developing infective endocarditis including those with:
- acquired valvular heart disease with stenosis or regurgitation
- valve replacement
- structural congenital heart disease, including surgically corrected or palliated structural conditions, but excluding isolated atrial septal defect, fully repaired ventricular septal defect or fully repaired patent ductus arteriosus, and closure devices that are judged to be endothelialized
- previous infective endocarditis
- hypertrophic cardiomyopathy.

Sir William Osler (1849–1919) was successively a Professor of Medicine in Montreal, Pennsylvania, Baltimore and Oxford. He was reputed to be a brilliant clinician and educationist.

M Roth (1839–1914), Professor of Pathology in Basel, Switzerland.

EG Janeway (1841–1911) followed Austin Flint as Professor of Medicine at Bellevue Hospital, New York.

E Libman (1872–1946), US physician.

B Sacks (1873–1939), US physician who wrote on Hindu medicine.

18 PROSTHETIC HEART VALVES

INSTRUCTION

Listen to this patient's heart.

SALIENT FEATURES

- *Mitral* valve prostheses can be recognized by their site, metallic first heart sound, normal second heart sound and metallic opening snap. Systolic murmurs are often also present and it is important to note that this does *not* indicate valve malfunction. Diastolic flow murmurs may be heard normally over the disc valves.
- *Aortic* valve prostheses may be recognized by their site, normal first heart sound and metallic second heart sound.
- Both *mitral and aortic* valves may be replaced and both the first and second heart sounds will be metallic. The presence of a systolic murmur does not indicate valve dysfunction. However, the presence of an early diastolic murmur indicates a malfunctioning aortic valve.

Note

- Comment on the midsternal vertical thoracotomy scar and state whether or not the metallic valve sounds are audible to the unaided ear (they are most often audible). Some mechanical valves cause so many clicks that it may not be possible to determine which valve has been replaced solely by auscultation. Porcine and cadaveric heterografts do not cause metallic clicking or plopping sounds.

DIAGNOSIS

This patient has both first and second heart sounds with a metallic quality, indicating that both mitral and aortic valves are artificial valves (lesion) and the patient is not in heart failure (functional status).

QUESTIONS

What are the different kinds of valves?

- Mechanical valves
- The Starr–Edwards valve is a caged ball device (Fig. 18.1C) and, because blood flows around the ball, there is a high incidence of haemolysis. This valve was introduced in 1960. The silastic ball is specially cured to prevent lipid accumulation (which can result in ball variance). The struts of the modern Starr–Edwards prosthesis are not covered with cloth.
- The Medtronic–Hall is a tilting disc valve (Fig. 18.1A) made of pyrolytic carbon. The disk tilts to an opening of 75 degrees for aortic prostheses and 70 degrees for mitral prostheses.
- The Bjork–Shiley pivoted single-tilting disc valve has laminar flow and hence a lower incidence of haemolysis. It was introduced in 1969. In the current model the entire ring and struts are machined from one piece (i.e. there are no welds). This is referred to as the 'monostrut valve'.
- The St Jude valve is a double-tilting disc valve (bileaflet valve) (Fig. 18.1B). Other examples of bileaflet prostheses include Carbomedics and Duromedics valve.

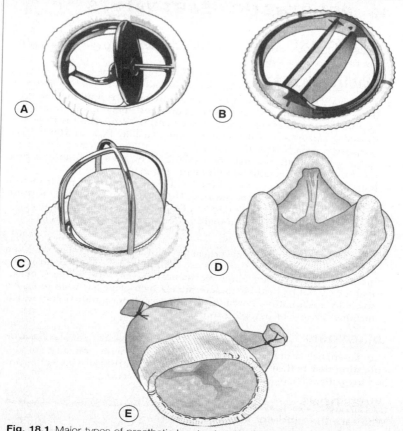

Fig. 18.1 Major types of prosthetic heart valve. (A) Tilting disc; (B) bileaflet; (C) ball; (D) stented bioprosthesis; (E) stentless bioprosthesis.

- **Xenografts**
- Porcine valves (Fig. 18.1E; Carpentier–Edwards, Hancock Modified Orifice, C/E Duraflex, Medtronic Intact).
- Pericardial valves mounted on a frame (Mitroflow, Carpentier–Edwards pericardial, Ionescu–Shiley, Hancock). A design flaw predisposed the Ionescu–Shiley valve to sudden rupture of the cusps. Currently, the Baxter pericardial valve is being used but its long-term durability remains to be ascertained.

- **Homografts**
- These are cadaveric aortic or pulmonary valves. Homografts are considered the valve of first choice in a young patient requiring aortic valve replacement. They are useful in replacing infected aortic valves as they are more resistant to re-infection than other prosthetic valves.

What are the complications of prosthetic valves?

- Thromboembolism
- Valve dysfunction, including valve leakage, valve dehiscence and valve obstruction caused by thrombosis and clogging. Perivalvular leak is always abnormal. 'Built-in' transvalvular leakage should be <10 ml per beat. The loss of expected valve sounds is an important sign of mechanical valve thrombosis
- Bleeding (such as upper GI haemorrhage) caused by anticoagulants
- Haemolysis at valve, causing anaemia
- Endocarditis, which carries a mortality rate of up to 60%; patients should be urgently referred to a tertiary cardiothoracic centre (p. 80)
- Structural dysfunction: fracture, poppet escape, cuspal tear, calcification
- Non-structural dysfunction: paravalvular leak, suture/tissue entrapment, noise.

Notes

- All patients with prosthetic valve should have an echocardiogram performed 2 to 3 months after surgery to establish baseline values.
- When prosthetic valve dysfunction is suspected, transoesophageal echocardiogram is the procedure of choice but findings may be somewhat limited by acoustic shadowing and reverberations from prosthetic material.

What are causes of anaemia in a patient with a prosthetic valve?

- Bleeding caused by anticoagulants
- Haemolytic anaemia
- Secondary to bacterial endocarditis.

What are the advantages of a porcine heart valve?

There is no need for chronic anticoagulation and hence it is safe in women of childbearing age and in the elderly.

What are the complications of a porcine heart valve?

- Degeneration with time
- Calcification.

Note: Increasingly warfarin is recommended for valves in the mitral position for first 3 postoperative months to allow complete endothelialization of the new valve.

ADVANCED-LEVEL QUESTIONS

What are the indications for valve replacement?

- Mitral stenosis (p. 5)
- Mitral regurgitation (p. 12)
- Aortic regurgitation (p. 20)
- Aortic stenosis (p. 27).

What kind of valve would you use to replace the mitral valve?

Mechanical prosthesis. However, patients in whom the risk posed by anticoagulants is unacceptably high may receive a bioprosthesis, but at the increased risk of further operation at a later date.

What kind of valve would you use to replace the aortic valve?

Mechanical valves in younger patients in whom the risk of porcine valve failure is higher and for whom durability of the valve is of paramount importance. Porcine valves may be considered for elderly

250 Cases in Clinical Medicine

patients whose life expectancy may not exceed that of the prosthesis used.

Why are mechanical valves increasingly preferred over bioprosthetic valves?

Two randomized controlled trials have shown a lower rate of reoperation with mechanical prostheses than with porcine prostheses, and a smaller increased risk of anticoagulant-related bleeding.

What do you know about the convexo-concave model for the Bjork–Shiley prosthesis?

This was a modification of the previously reliable design that resulted in the strut retaining the tilting disc becoming liable to fracture several years after implantation, causing fatality. All Bjork–Shiley valves manufactured after 1975 have a radioopaque ring marker in the edge of a tilting disc. This ring marker is missing if the strut is fractured. The disc may be spotted in the peripheral circulation. About two-thirds of the patients with strut fracture die acutely. The risk of strut fracture is 7 per 10 000 per year, but the risk of another mitral valve replacement exceeds this. This risk is greatest in patients with a large-size mitral prosthesis (31 and 33 mm) and a weld date between 1 January 1981 and 30 July 1982.

Is there any difference between the lifespan of a porcine mitral prosthesis and a porcine aortic prosthesis?

Porcine mitral bioprostheses usually fail after about 7 years whereas those in the aortic position fail in about 10 years owing to degeneration of the valve leaflets. In younger patients, these prostheses tend to degenerate more rapidly.

Which patients should receive a bioprosthetic valve?

- Those unable to take anticoagulants and those not expected to live longer than the predicted lifespan of the prosthesis.
- Patients over the age of 70 years who require an aortic valve replacement as the rate of degeneration is relatively slow in these patients.

In a woman of childbearing age, which kind of valve, bioprosthetic or mechanical, do you prefer?

Until recently, bioprosthetic valves were advocated in women of child-bearing age to avoid the risks of warfarin on the fetus. More recently, it has been found that the risk of fetal abnormalities is very low in pregnant women receiving warfarin, although there is an increased risk of spontaneous abortion. Also there appears to be an accelerated risk of bioprosthetic valve degeneration during pregnancy. Therefore, the risks of spontaneous abortion have to be weighed against the operative mortality rate of 10% during reoperation following valve failure. Increasingly it is believed that a mechanical prosthesis should be used if valve replacement is needed (Br Heart J 1994;71:196–201).

If a patient with atrial fibrillation requires a prosthetic mitral valve, which kind of valve would you prefer?

A mechanical valve, as these patients need warfarin treatment for atrial fibrillation.

What is the role of percutaneous valve replacements?

Currently the role of transcatheter valve-in-valve implantation seems to be best suited for failed bioprosthetic valves (Circulation 2010;121:1848–57). Aortic, pulmonary, mitral and tricuspid tissue valves are amenable to this approach. Currently, the percutaneous valves are not suited for replacement of native valves because the variation in the shape of the annulus makes positioning of the symmetrical sewing ring of transcatheter valves (which are deployed by expansion of a balloon) suboptimal (increasing the incidence of paravalvular leaks and valve regurgitation). However, it may increasingly be used for aortic valve disease as better and better prosthetic valves are developed.

The first aortic valve replacement (caged ball device) was performed by Dr Dwight Harken in March 1960 at Peter Bent Brigham Hospital in Boston. Shortly thereafter, Dr Nina Braunwald, at the National Institutes for Health, USA, performed a total mitral valve replacement with an artificial flexible leaflet valve.

A Starr and ML Edwards, both US physicians.

---

19 TRICUSPID REGURGITATION

INSTRUCTION

Examine this patient's heart.
Examine this patient's cardiovascular system.

SALIENT FEATURES

History

- Intravenous drug abuse
- Trauma to the chest
- Rheumatic fever
- COPD.

Examination

- Peripheral cyanosis
- Large 'v' waves in the jugular venous pulse (Fig. 19.1)
- Left parasternal heave
- Palpable or loud P2
- Pansystolic murmur at the left lower sternal border, which increases in inspiration (Carvallo's sign)
- Right ventricular third heart sound may be present
- Atrial fibrillation may be present
- Proceed by looking for:
  - mid-diastolic murmur of mitral stenosis
  - systolic pulsations of an enlarged liver
  - ascites and ankle oedema.

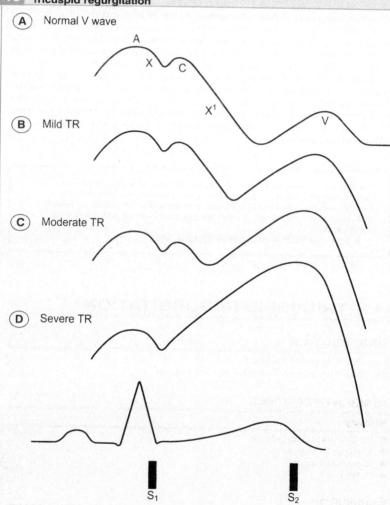

Fig. 19.1 Jugular venous pulse in tricuspid regurgitation (TR). The jugular venous pulse wave normally drops during ventricular systole. As TR becomes more severe, the CV wave becomes more obvious.

DIAGNOSIS

This patient has tricuspid regurgitation (lesion) secondary to chronic lung disease and cor pulmonale (aetiology of the lesion) and is in cardiac failure (functional status).

QUESTIONS

What are the causes of tricuspid regurgitation?
- Functional:
  - Pulmonary hypertension
  - Congestive cardiac failure.
- Rheumatic (associated with mitral and/or aortic valve disease)
- Right heart endocarditis as in drug addicts
- Uncommon: carcinoid syndrome, Ebstein's anomaly, endomyocardial fibrosis, infarction of right ventricular papillary muscles, tricuspid valve prolapse, blunt trauma to the heart.

How would you treat organic tricuspid regurgitation?
Surgically with:
- valve plication or annuloplasty
- valve replacement.

How is tricuspid regurgitation quantified?
On echocardiography it is quantified by colour Doppler imaging into:
- *mild:* flow disturbance in systole localize to the area adjacent to the vale closure plane (jet area <5 cm^2)
- *moderate:* fills between 5 and 10 cm^2 of the right atrium
- *severe:* fills >10 cm^2 of the enlarged right atrium.

> JMR Carvallo, Mexican cardiologist who worked in Mexico City (Rivero-Carvallo JM (1946) Signo para el diagnostico de las insuficiencias tricuspideas. Arch Inst Cardiol Mex 16:531).

20 MITRAL VALVE PROLAPSE

INSTRUCTION
Examine this patient's heart.

SALIENT FEATURES

History
- Palpitations associated with mild tachyarrhythmias
- Increased adrenergic symptoms
- Chest pain
- Anxiety or fatigue.

Examination
- Midsystolic click followed by late or midsystolic murmur
- Look for features of Marfan syndrome (high arched palate, arm span greater than height).

Notes
- Squatting will bring the midsystolic click closer to the second heart sound and decrease the duration of the murmur.

- A Valsalva manoeuvre and standing have the opposite effect.
- The midsystolic murmur begins after the first heart sound; the late systolic murmurs begin after the first heart sound but continue to or through the second heart sound (S_2). Both types of murmur may have a crescendo–decrescendo configuration

DIAGNOSIS

This patient has mitral valve prolapse (lesion) and a long pansystolic murmur, indicating significant mitral regurgitation, which will require prophylaxis for infective endocarditis (functional status).

QUESTIONS

What are eponyms for mitral valve prolapse?
Barlow syndrome (Br Heart J 1968;30:203), click–murmur syndrome, floppy mitral valve.

What is the prevalence in the normal population?
The new awareness that the mitral valve is saddle shaped rather than a planar valve has resulted in new echocardiographic definition for mitral valve prolapse as one or both mitral leaflets exhibit at least 2 mm displacement superior to the long-axis annular plane (a line connecting the annular hinge points), with or without leaflet thickening (Fig. 20.1). With this new description, the prevalence of prolapse is estimated at 2–3%, and is equally distributed between men and women.

What are the complications of mitral valve prolapse?
- Severe mitral regurgitation
- Arrhythmias: ventricular premature contractions, ventricular tachycardia, paroxysmal supraventricular tachycardia
- Atypical chest pain
- Transient ischaemic attacks, embolism
- Infective endocarditis in those with mitral regurgitation
- Sudden death.

Mention a few associated conditions
- Marfan syndrome
- Chronic rheumatic heart disease
- Ischaemic heart disease
- Cardiomyopathies
- 20% of patients with atrial septal defects — secundum type'
- Ehlers–Danlos syndrome
- Psoriatic arthritis
- Ebstein's anomaly
- SLE.

How would you manage such patients?
- Reassure the asymptomatic patient
- Relief of atypical chest pain with analgesics or beta-blockers (empiric treatment)
- Aspirin or anticoagulants in those with transient ischaemic attacks
- Antiarrhythmics in those with frequent tachyarrhythmias or ventricular premature contractions
- Prophylaxis for infective endocarditis (see Case 17)
- Consider surgery in those with severe mitral regurgitation.

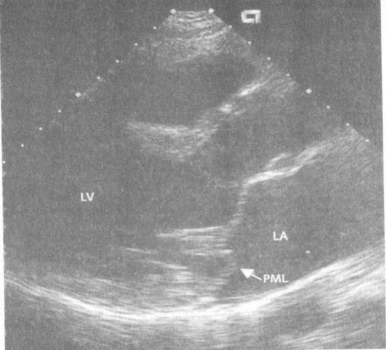

Fig. 20.1 Transthoracic echocardiographic image in parasternal long-axis view, showing posterior mitral leaflet (PML) bowing backward and prolapsing into left atrium during systole. (With permission from Hayek E et al. 2005.)

ADVANCED-LEVEL QUESTIONS

What is the mechanism of click in the mitral valve prolapse?
Clicks result from sudden tensing of the mitral valve apparatus as the leaflets prolapse into the left atrium during systole

What do you know about Carpentier's nomenclature of the mitral valve?
Anatomically, the posterior and anterior leaflets of the mitral valve each may be divided into three sections:
- Three posterior leaflet scallops: the lateral (P1), middle (P2), and medial (P3)
- Three anterior segments: lateral (A1), middle (A2) and medial (A3).

Which segments of the mitral valve commonly prolapse?
- Most cases of prolapse involve the posterior middle scallop (easily identified on long-axis echocardiographic images)
- Lateral scallop prolapse (not clearly seen on long-axis images; this aspect is best seen in the apical four-chamber view).

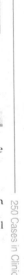

Notes

- Superior leaflet displacement in a four-chamber view should not be judged diagnostic of prolapse. Therefore, transthoracic echocardiography can confirm the diagnosis of prolapse but may not be able to exclude lateral scallop prolapsed without taking into account several planes of imaging. Transoesophageal echocardiography is, consequently, very effective in identifying prolapsing segments.

> John Barlow, South African Professor of Cardiology.
> The term mitral valve prolapse was introduced in 1966 by Criley et al. (Br Heart J 1966;28:488–96) and has been frequently used as a synonym for 'billowing mitral leaflet', which was used by Barlow et al. (Br Heart J 1968;30:203–18) to describe the same condition.
> The French surgeon Carpentier suggested that the term prolapse should be reserved to indicate that the free edge of the leaflet protrudes beyond the mitral annulus level during systole (J Thorac Cardiovasc Surg 1983;86:323–37), whereas the term billowing should be used when the leaflet body bulges into the left atrium, overriding the mitral annulus plane and usually maintaining the free edge of the leaflets on the ventricular side (Am J Cardiol 1985;55:501–2), although the two conditions may coexist.

21 VENTRICULAR SEPTAL DEFECT

INSTRUCTION

Listen to this patient's heart.

SALIENT FEATURES

History

- Small defects are usually asymptomatic
- Large defects with shunts: repeated respiratory tract infections, debilitating dyspnoea and exercise intolerance
- Symptoms of infective endocarditis or past history of endocarditis
- Symptoms of Eisenmenger syndrome (p. 122).

Examination

- There is a normal pulse.
- There are normal findings on palpation (there may be either left or right ventricular enlargement).
- With substantial left-to-right shunting and little or no pulmonary hypertension, the left ventricular impulse is dynamic and laterally displaced, and the right ventricular impulse may not be felt. The murmur of a moderate or large defect is pansystolic, loudest at the lower left sternal border, and usually accompanied by a palpable thrill.
- A short mid-diastolic apical rumble (caused by increased flow through the mitral valve) may be heard.

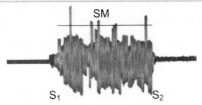

Fig. 21.1 Phonocardiogram showing the holosystolic murmur of isolated ventricular septal defect.

- A decrescendo diastolic murmur of aortic regurgitation may be present if the ventricular septal defect (VSD) undermines the aortic valve annulus.
- Small, muscular VSDs may produce high-frequency systolic ejection murmurs that terminate before the end of systole (when the defect is occluded by contracting heart muscle) (Fig. 21.1).
- If pulmonary hypertension develops, a right ventricular heave and a pulsation over the pulmonary trunk may be palpated. The pansystolic murmur and thrill diminish and eventually disappear as flow through the defect decreases, and a murmur of pulmonary regurgitation (Graham Steell's murmur) may appear. Finally, cyanosis and clubbing are present.
- The second sound may be normal when the defect is small; A_2 is obscured by the pansystolic murmur of large defects. A single second sound indicates that the ventricular pressures are equal and a loud P indicates pulmonary hypertension.
- Look for signs of cardiac failure.

Note: VSD is the most common congenital cardiac anomaly, occurring in 2 per 1000 births. It is a feature of Down syndrome (p. 806).

DIAGNOSIS

This patient has a ventricular septal defect (lesion) of congenital origin (aetiology) and has pulmonary hypertension (functional status).

QUESTIONS

Is the loudness of the murmur related to the size of the defect?
No; in fact, very small defects (maladie de Roger) cause loud murmurs (Bull Acad Med, 1879;VIII:1074–94).

What are causes of a ventricular septal defect?
- Congenital
- Rupture of the interventricular septum as a complication of myocardial infarction.

Where is the defect usually situated?
In the membranous portion of the interventricular septum.

Can such defects close spontaneously?
Spontaneous closure usually occurs in a small defect, during early childhood in about 50% of the patients.

What are complications of a ventricular septal defect?

- Congestive cardiac failure
- Right ventricular outflow tract obstruction (muscular infundibular obstruction develops in about of 5% of VSDs)
- Aortic regurgitation
- Infective endocarditis
- Pulmonary hypertension and reversal of shunt (Eisenmenger complex).

How would you investigate this patient?

- *ECG and chest radiography* provide insight into the magnitude of the haemodynamic impairment: with a small ventricular septal defect, both ECG and chest radiograph are normal:
  - With a large defect, there is ECG evidence of left atrial and ventricular enlargement, and left ventricular enlargement and 'shunt vascularity' is evident on the chest radiograph (Fig. 21.2).
  - If pulmonary hypertension occurs, the QRS axis shifts to the right, and right atrial and ventricular enlargement are noted on the ECG; the chest radiograph shows marked enlargement of the proximal pulmonary arteries, rapid tapering of the peripheral pulmonary arteries, and oligaemic lung fields.
- *Doppler echocardiography* can identify the presence and location of the ventricular septal defect, and Doppler colour-flow mapping can identify the magnitude and direction of shunting.
- Magnetic resonance imaging (MRI).
- *Cardiac catheterization and angiography* can confirm the presence and location of the ventricular septal defect, as well as determine the magnitude of shunting and the pulmonary vascular resistance.

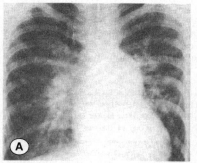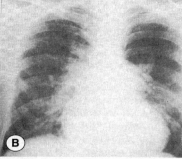

Fig. 21.2 (A) Radiograph of a moderately restrictive perimembranous ventricular septal defect with left-to-right shunt. Pulmonary arterial vascularity is increased, the pulmonary trunk and its proximal branches are markedly dilated, and a moderately enlarged convex LV occupies the apex. (B) Radiograph of a non-restrictive perimembranous ventricular septal defect and a bidirectional shunt. Pulmonary arterial vascularity is increased, the pulmonary trunk and its proximal branches are markedly dilated, an enlarged convex LV occupies the apex, and a prominent right atrium forms the right lower cardiac border. (With permission from Perloff 2003.)

ADVANCED-LEVEL QUESTIONS

What types of ventricular septal defect do you know?

- The supracristal type (above the crista supraventricularis, a muscular ridge that separates the main portion of the right ventricular cavity from the infundibular or outflow portion) is a high defect just below the pulmonary valve and the right coronary cusp of the aortic valve. The latter may not be adequately supported, resulting in aortic regurgitation. In Fallot's tetralogy, this defect is associated with a rightward shift of the interventricular septum, and in double-outlet LV with subaortic stenosis the supracristal defect is associated with a leftward shift of the septum.
- The infracristal defect, which may be in either the upper membranous portion of the interventricular septum or the lower muscular part (<5% of the defects):
  - Small defects (maladie de Roger)
  - Swiss cheese appearance (multiple small defects)
  - Large defects
  - Gerbode defect (defect opening into the right atrium) (Ann Surg 1958;148:433).

Mention other cardiac lesions that may be associated with a ventricular septal defect

- Conditions in which VSD is an essential part of the syndrome:
  - Fallot's tetralogy
  - Truncus arteriosus
  - Double-outlet RV
  - Atrioventricular canal defects.
- Conditions frequently associated with a VSD but not an essential part of the syndrome:
  - Patent ductus arteriosus
  - Pulmonary stenosis
  - Secundum atrial septal defects
  - Coarctation of aorta
  - Tricuspid atresia
  - Transposition of the great arteries
  - Pulmonary atresia.

What is the effect of pregnancy in women with a ventricular septal defect?

- Small defects should present with no problems.
- Moderate-sized defects and moderate pulmonary hypertension are at the risk of developing acute right ventricular failure and rapidly worsening pulmonary hypertension in pregnancy.
- Pregnancy should be avoided in pulmonary hypertension and pregnancy.

What is the management of patients with a ventricular septal defect?

- The natural history of ventricular septal defect depends on:
  - the size of the defect
  - the pulmonary vascular resistance.
- Adults with small defects and normal pulmonary arterial pressure are usually asymptomatic, and pulmonary vascular disease is unlikely to develop. Such patients do not require surgical closure of their defect,

but they are at risk for infective endocarditis and should, therefore, receive antibiotic prophylaxis.

- Patients with large VSDs who survive to adulthood usually have left ventricular failure or pulmonary hypertension with associated right ventricular failure. Surgical closure of such defects is recommended, if the magnitude of pulmonary vascular obstructive disease is not prohibitive. Once the ratio of pulmonary to systemic vascular resistance exceeds 0.7, the risk associated with surgery is excessive.

Which patients merit surgical attention?

Usually, in an adult, VSD is small enough to be safely ignored, or the patient has Eisenmenger syndrome. However, there are exceptions to this and these patients may benefit from surgery:

- Recurrent endocarditis
- Development of aortic regurgitation caused by prolapse of the right coronary cusp through the septal defect
- Progressive left ventricular dilatation caused by volume overload imposed by the shunt (pulmonary to systemic ratio is 3:1)
- When the defect is caused by an acute rupture of the ventricular septum.

Note: If the VSD is large enough to cause heart failure or pulmonary hypertension, it usually manifests in the first few years of life.

Henri Roger (1809–1891), a French paediatrician, described maladie de Roger in 1879 in a paper entitled 'Clinical researches on the congenital communication of the two sides of the hearts, but failure of occlusion of the interventricular septum': 'A developmental defect of the heart occurs from which cyanosis does not ensue in spite of the fact that a communication exists between the cavities of the two ventricles and in spite of the fact that admixture of venous blood and arterial blood occurs. This congenital defect, which is even compatible with a long life, is a simple one. It comprises a defect in the interventricular septum'.

---

22   ATRIAL SEPTAL DEFECT

INSTRUCTION

Examine this patient's heart.
Listen to her heart.

SALIENT FEATURES

History

- **Ostium secundum defect (anatomically in the region of the fossa ovalis)**
- Asymptomatic particularly small defects with minimal left to right shunting; moderate or large defects often have no symptoms until third or fourth decades despite substantial left-to-right shunting (characterized by a ratio of pulmonary to systemic flow of 1.5 or more)
- Fatigue
- Dyspnoea

- Palpitations indicating atrial arrhythmias
- Productive cough indicating recurrent pulmonary infections
- Symptoms of paradoxical emboli
- Right heart failure.

- **Ostium primum defect (anatomically in the lower part of the atrial septum)**
- Patients may develop symptoms and heart failure in childhood
- Failure to thrive
- Chest infections
- Poor development
- In adults in addition to the same symptoms as for secundum defect, the following occur:
  - Syncope: indicating heart block
  - Symptoms suggesting endocarditis.

Examination

- Diffuse or normal apical impulse
- Left parasternal heave
- Ejection systolic flow murmur in the left second and third intercostal space
- Wide, fixed, split second heart sound (occasionally a slight movement of P occurs) that does not vary with respiration (Fig. 22.1)
- Infrequently, a mid-diastolic murmur may be heard in the tricuspid area (indicating a large left-to-right shunt)
- Proceed by looking for signs of:
  - pulmonary hypertension (Eisenmenger syndrome)
  - congenital defects of the thumb (Holt–Oram syndrome).

Note: Atrial secundum defect is often confused with pulmonary stenosis (P is soft, delayed and moves with respiration).

DIAGNOSIS

This patient has an atrial septal defect (ASD) (lesion) that is congenital in origin (aetiology); she is not in cardiac failure and there is no reversal of shunt (functional status).

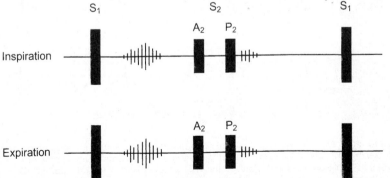

Fig. 22.1 Auscultatory findings resulting from an atrial septal defect. S_1, first heart sound; A_2, aortic valve closure; P_2; pulmonic valve closure.

ADVANCED-LEVEL QUESTIONS

What are the types of atrial septal defect

- *Ostium secundum defect* accounts for 70% of the cases. The defect is in the middle portion of the atrial septum and is usually 2–4 cm in diameter (incomplete right bundle branch block pattern, QRS axis rightward) (Fig. 22.2A,B).
- *Sinus venosus type* is a defect in the septum just below the entrance of the superior vena cava into the right atrium (leftward P wave axis so that P waves are inverted in at least one inferior lead) (Fig. 22.2C).
- *Ostium primum type* is a defect in the lower part of the septum and clefts may occur in the mitral and tricuspid valves (QRS axis leftward). A junctional or low atrial rhythm (inverted P waves in the inferior leads) occurs with sinus venosus defects.

What do you understand by the term patent foramen ovale?

In the fetus, the right and left atria communicate with each other through an oblique valvular opening, which is called the foramen ovale. The foramen ovale persists throughout fetal life. After birth, the left atrium receives blood from the lungs and the pressure in this chamber becomes greater than that in the right atrium; this causes the closure of the foramen ovale.

What is the importance of patent foramen ovale?

The prevalence of patent foramen ovale is significantly higher in patients with stroke (N Engl J Med 1988;318:1148–52).

What is Holt–Oram syndrome?

This is an ostium secundum ASD with a hypoplastic thumb and an accessory phalanx. In addition, the thumb lies in the same plane as the other digits (Br Heart J 1960; 22:236). The inheritance is autosomal dominant and

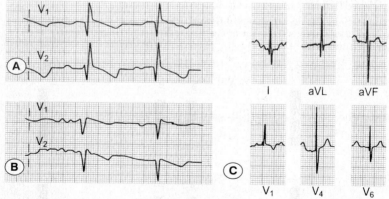

Fig. 22.2 Electrocardiography in atrial septal defect. (A,B) Ostium secundum defect right precordial leads V₁ and V₂ illustrate two variants of an incomplete right bundle branch block pattern, the rSrT pattern (A) and the rSr' pattern (B). (C) Ostium primum type: endocardial cushion defect with the QRS axis is leftward counterclockwise and superior.

is associated with mutations in chromosome 12q2 (N Engl J Med 1994;330:885–91).

At what age does the reversal of shunt occur?
Usually after the end of the second decade.

What is the mechanism of fixed split second sound?
In normal individuals, on inspiration there is a widening of the split between the two components of the second sound caused by a delay in closure of the pulmonary valve. In ASD, the effect of respiration is eliminated because of communication between the left and right sides of the heart.

In which conditions is an abnormally widely split second sound present?
- ASD, ventricular septal defect (VSD), pulmonary regurgitation (caused by increased right ventricular volume)
- Pulmonary stenosis (caused by increased right ventricular pressure)
- Right bundle branch block (caused by right ventricular conduction delay)
- Mitral regurgitation, VSD (caused by premature left ventricular emptying).

What is Lutembacher syndrome?
ASD with an acquired rheumatic mitral stenosis (Arch Mal Coeur 1916;9:237).

What is Fallot's triology?
ASD, pulmonary stenosis and right ventricular enlargement.

How would you investigate a patient with atrial septal defect?
- *ECG:*
  - Often has right axis deviation and incomplete right bundle branch block (Fig. 22.2A,B)
  - In ostium primum defects left axis deviation also occurs (Fig. 22.2C)
  - In sinus venosus defects, a junctional or low atrial rhythm (inverted P waves in inferior leads) occurs.
- *Chest radiography:*
  - Prominent pulmonary arteries (large pulmonary conus)
  - A peripheral pulmonary vascular pattern of 'shunt vascularity' (in which the small pulmonary arteries are especially well visualized in the periphery of both lungs)
  - Small aortic knob
  - Enlarged RV and right atrium
  - 'Uilar dance' on fluoroscopy.
- *Echocardiography:*
  - Transthoracic echocardiography visualizes ostium secundum and primum defects but usually does not identify sinus venosus defects
  - Sensitivity can be enhanced by injecting microbubbles in the peripheral vein after which the movement across the defect can be seen
  - Transoesophageal and Doppler colour-flow echocardiography is useful in detecting and determining the location of atrial septal defects and also in identifying anomalous venous drainage and sinus venosus defects.

- MRI
- *Cardiac catheterization* is often unnecessary in diagnosis but is useful in determining the magnitude and direction of shunting and to determine the severity and reversibility of pulmonary hypertension

What are the complications of atrial septal defect?

- Atrial arrhythmias: atrial fibrillation is most common. Atrial fibrillation is often accompanied by the appearance of tricuspid regurgitation. Patients are usually in normal sinus rhythm in the first three decades of life, after which atrial arrhythmias including atrial fibrillation and supraventricular tachycardia may appear
- Pulmonary hypertension with the development of right ventricular disease
- Eisenmenger syndrome with reversal of shunt
- Paradoxical embolus
- Infective endocarditis in patients with ostium primum defects only
- Recurrent pulmonary infections.

How is pregnancy tolerated in a women with an atrial septal defect?

Pregnancy is usually well tolerated in uncomplicated atrial septal defects. However, when complicated by significant pulmonary hypertension, there is increased maternal and fetal morbidity and mortality and hence pregnancy should be avoided in Eisenmenger syndrome. Rapidly progressive pulmonary vascular disease may develop during pregnancy and, therefore, routine closure of atrial septal defect is recommended before pregnancy.

How would you manage an uncomplicated atrial septal defect?

- When detected in early childhood, surgical closure is recommended between the age of 5 and 10 years to prevent the late onset of either right ventricular failure, atrial arrhythmias or right heart failure.
- In adults, small ASDs can be left alone, although many believe all ASDs must be closed. Those operated on before the age of 25 years have an excellent prognosis and one may anticipate normal long-term survival, but older patients require regular supervision. In a recent study, surgical repair of atrial septal defects in middle-aged and elderly patients was found to improve longevity and reduce functional limitation caused by heart failure and was, therefore, superior to medical treatment. However, the risk of atrial arrhythmias, especially fibrillation and flutter, and the attendant risk of thromboembolic events were not reduced by closure of the defect.
- Left-to-right shunt saturations of 1.5:1 or more require surgical closure to prevent right ventricular dysfunction.
- Other indications for surgery include evidence of pulmonary vascular reactivity when challenged with pulmonary vasodilators or a lung biopsy with pulmonary arterial changes being potentially reversible.
- A history of a cryptogenic cerebrovascular event in the presence of a small ASD with right-to-left shunting is also recommended for closure.
- Closure in adults results in a reduction in right ventricular size and improves symptoms.

More recently, ASDs are being occluded by transcatheter button or 'clamshell devices', particularly when the ASD is under 35 mm in diameter and in patients who have a sufficient (>5 mm) rim of surrounding atrial tissue present. Percutaneous closure of secundum ASD is safe (periprocedural morbidity <10%, periprocedural mortality 0%), highly effective (procedural success >95%) and durable. Periprocedural and long-term morbidity and mortality are particularly low in patients whose defect is closed when patients are under <25 years of age. Even in older individuals, however, closure is recommended to reduce morbidity and mortality. During long-term follow-up after successful closure, atrial tachyarrhythmias may become manifest. The next generation of percutaneous devices would be biodegradable devices

Is prophylaxis against infective endocarditis recommended in atrial septal defect?

Prophylaxis against infective endocarditis is not recommended for patients with atrial septal defects (repaired or unrepaired) unless a concomitant valvular abnormality (e.g. mitral valve cleft or prolapse) is present.

What do you know about the embryology of atrial septal defect?

There are seven septa involved in the partitioning of the heart: three form passively (i.e. when an area of tissue forms a septum because of the rapid growth of contiguous tissue) and these include septum secundum at the atrial septum, the muscular portion of the ventricular septum and the aorticopulmonary septum. The actively formed portions of the septums of the heart include the septum of the atrioventricular canal, the conal septum and the truncal septum. The atrial septum begins as a passively formed septum; however, active growth from the endocardial cushions completes the septum.

What do you know about ostium primum defects?

They are associated with endocardial cushion defects often resulting in cleft mitral valve (usually anterior leaflet) causing mitral regurgitation. The ECG shows right bundle branch block and left axis deviation (Fig. 22.2C). Treatment is surgical closure with repair of cleft mitral valve, which generally involves simple interrupted suture repair of the cleft or the addition of a mitral annuloplasty for annular reduction and stabilization.

Leonardo da Vinci's description in 1513 of a 'perforating channel' in the atrial septum is believed to be the first recorded account of a congenital malformation of the human heart.

Rene Lutembacher, a French physician, described the Lutembacher syndrome in 1916.

Mary Holt, cardiologist, King's College Hospital, London.

Samuel Oram, cardiologist, King's College Hospital, London.

---

23 HYPERTROPHIC CARDIOMYOPATHY

INSTRUCTION

Examine this patient's cardiovascular system.

SALIENT FEATURES

History

- Patients may be asymptomatic
- Severe cardiac failure (in infants)

- Premature unexpected death: may be presenting symptom in children or young adults
- Dyspnoea on exertion: in ~50% of patients
- Chest pain: in ~50%; may be exertional or occur at rest
- Syncope (in 15–25%)
- Dizziness and palpitations
- Obtain a family history of the following:
  - Similar cardiomyopathy
  - Sudden death.

Examination

- Carotid pulse is bifid (Fig. 23.1)
- 'a' wave in the JVP (see Case 15)
- *Double apical impulse* (left ventricular heave with a prominent presystolic pulse caused by atrial contraction)
- Pansystolic murmur at the apex caused by mitral regurgitation
- Ejection systolic murmur along the left sternal border (across the outflow tract obstruction); accentuated by standing and Valsalva manoeuvre and softer on squatting (squatting increases LV cavity size and reduces outflow tract obstruction). Remember the Valsalva manoeuvre decreases the duration of murmur of aortic stenosis and increases the murmur of hypertrophic cardiomyopathy
- Fourth heart sound.

DIAGNOSIS

This patient has hypertrophic cardiomyopathy (aetiology) as evidenced by a double apical impulse and ejection systolic murmur along the left sternal border, which is heard better on standing (lesion); the patient is in cardiac failure.

ADVANCED-LEVEL QUESTIONS

How would you investigate this patient?

- *Echocardiogram* is useful for assessing LV structure and function, gradients (Fig. 23.2), valvular regurgitation, and atrial dimensions. Doppler echocardiography shows characteristic high-velocity late peaking or

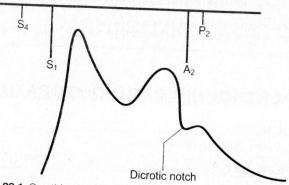

Fig. 23.1 Carotid pulse is bifid pulse with two systolic peaks. The second peak (tidal or reflected wave) is of lower amplitude than the initial percussion wave.

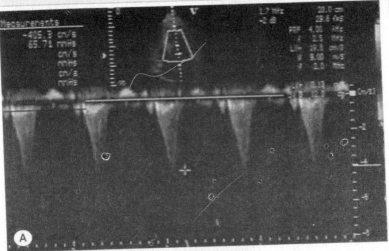

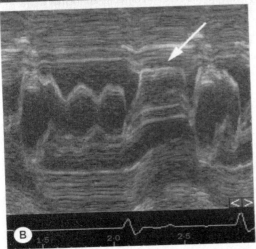

Fig. 23.2 Echocardiology. (A) Continuous wave Doppler in dynamic left ventricular outflow tract obstruction. Note characteristic dagger-shaped velocity envelope. (B) M-mode shows the protracted contact between the anterior mitral valve leaflet and the interventricular septum in systole (arrow). (With permission from Elliott P, McKenna WJ 2004.)

dagger-shaped spectral waveform (Fig. 23.2A). Characteristic findings include systolic anterior motion of mitral valve (SAM), asymmetric hypertrophy (ASH) and mitral regurgitation.

- *ECG* may be normal (in about 5% of patients) or show abnormalities including left ventricular hypertrophy, atrial fibrillation, left axis deviation, right bundle branch block and myocardial disarray (e.g. ST–T

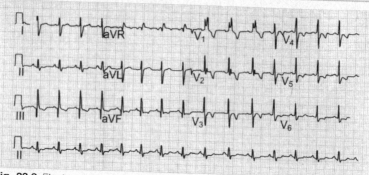

Fig. 23.3 Electrocardiographic patterns in hypertrophic cardiomyopathy. A 12-lead tracing, in concentric left ventricular hypertrophy, with T wave inversion extending from V_1 to V_5, and deep Q waves in leads III and aVF.

wave changes, intraventricular conduction defects, abnormal Q waves); bizarre or abnormal findings in young patients should raise suspicion of hypertrophic cardiomyopathy, (especially if family members also affected) (Fig. 23.3).

- *Chest radiograph* may be normal or show evidence of left or right atrial or left ventricular enlargement.
- *Treadmill exercise test* is performed when patients have angina (ST segment changes of >2 mm documented in 25% associated with symptoms of angina).
- *48-hour Holter monitoring* identifies established atrial fibrillation (in about 10% of patients), paroxysmal supraventricular arrhythmias (in 30%), non-sustained ventricular tachycardia (in 25%) and ventricular tachycardia (in 25%); ventricular tachycardia is invariably asymptomatic during Holter monitoring but is a most useful risk marker of sudden death in adults; sustained supraventricular arrhythmias often symptomatic and predispose to thromboembolic complications.
- *Endomyocardial biopsy* possibly necessary to exclude specific heart muscle disorder (amyloid, sarcoid) but has no role in diagnosis because of patchy nature of myofibrillar disarray.
- *Cardiac MRI* shows patchy areas of hyperenhancement, the extent of which is greatest in patients with risk markers for sudden cardiac death and in those in whom progressive remodelling of the LV can be seen. The predominant site of hypertrophy is usually the 1-o'clock position in the short-axis view at the confluence of anterior septum and anterior wall
- *Left heart catheterization* is rarely needed to make the diagnosis. In the presence of left ventricular outflow obstruction, the LV-to-aortic late-peaking gradient is seen with characteristic aortic pressure tracing showing a rapid rise and fall followed by a plateau — the 'spike and dome' pattern.

What are the complications of hypertrophic cardiomyopathy?
- Sudden death
- Atrial fibrillation
- Infective endocarditis
- Systemic embolization.

How would you manage such a patient?

- Relief of symptoms
- Improvement of ventricular function using beta-blocker (propranolol up to 640 mg/day), verapamil, amiodarone and diuretics (N Engl J Med 1997;336:775)
- Prevention of infective endocarditis
- Dual-chamber pacing or DDD pacing is considered by some as the initial procedure in symptomatic patients resistant to treatment with drugs. DDD pacing causes depolarization from the right ventricular apex, resulting in altered motion of the interventricular septum and diminished subaortic gradient
- Implantable-cardiac defibrillators to prevent sudden death
- Prevention of arrhythmias and sudden death by administration of amiodarone (Br Heart J 1985;53:412–16)
- Septal ablation with alcohol or surgery — such as myotomy or myectomy — relieves symptoms but does not alter the natural history of the disease. Mitral valve replacement may be done simultaneously for severe mitral regurgitation
- Counselling of sufferers and relatives is essential and they should be encouraged to contact the Hypertrophic Cardiomyopathy Association
- Cardioversion in patients with atrial fibrillation
- Digoxin and vasodilators should be avoided as they worsen outflow obstruction.

What is the most characteristic pathophysiological abnormality in hypertrophic cardiomyopathy?

Diastolic dysfunction.

Which condition has the most common association with hypertrophic cardiomyopathy?

Friedreich's ataxia.

What do you know about the genetics of hypertrophic cardiomyopathy?

Hypertrophic cardiomyopathy is an autosomal dominant heart muscle disorder. Mutations in the gene encoding contractile proteins cause disease in 50–60% of patients. At least nine individual genes have been identified. Mutations in the gene for β-heavy chain myosin is associated with left ventricular outflow obstruction; mutations affecting troponin T are associated with rather modest left ventricular wall thickening; mutations affecting myosin-binding protein C are associated with onset in late adult life. Also mutations leading to arginine as the new amino acid have a worse prognosis than ones substituting with leucine.

What do you know about the Brockenbrough–Braunwald–Morrow sign?

Diminished pulse pressure in post-extrasystolic beat occurs in hypertrophic cardiomyopathy/aortic stenosis.

What do you know about the epidemiology of this condition?

- The male to female ratio is equal, although the disease tends to affect younger men and older women.
- In children and adolescents, myocardial hypertrophy often occurs during growth spurts (a negative diagnosis made before adolescent growth does not exclude the condition and re-assessment at a later age is important).

- Myocardial hypertrophy does not ordinarily progress after adolescent growth is completed.
- Sudden death can occur at any age (from childhood over to 90 years), and in subjects who have been asymptomatic all their life. The annual mortality from sudden death is 3 to 5% in adults and at least 6% in children and young adults.
- First-degree relatives of affected patients have a 50% chance of carrying the disease gene; they should be investigated by ECG and two-dimensional echocardiogram. Genetic counselling is therefore important.

What are the risk predictors of sudden death?

	Criteria	Comment
History	Exertional or recurrent syncope and presyncope	Risk greatest in children
	Family history of sudden death, known malignant genotype	Risk related to family size and number of members with sudden cardiac death
Diagnostic evaluation	Severe left ventricular hypertropy	Risk increases with increase in wall thickness
	Non-sustained ventricular tachycardia	Higher predictive value in children and those with syncope
	Abnormal haemodynamic response to exercise (failure to augment systolic BP by at least 20 mmHg)	Less applicable to those >40 years

The pathology of hypertrophic cardiomyopathy was first described by two French pathologists in the mid 19th century and by a German pathologist in the early 20th century. The simultaneous reports of Sir Russel Brock, thoracic surgeon at Guy's and Brompton Hospitals (Guy's Hosp Rep 1957;106:221–38), and of Teare (Br Heart J 1958;20:1) brought this to modern medical attention.

24 PATENT DUCTUS ARTERIOSUS

INSTRUCTION

Examine this patient's heart.
Examine this patient's cardiovascular system.

SALIENT FEATURES

History

- Asymptomatic
- Bronchitis or dyspnoea on exertion in severe cases
- Take a maternal history of rubella, particularly in the first trimester

- Determine whether the patient was a premature baby or had a low birth weight. Remember the frequency of patent ductus arteriosus (PDA) in infants weighing 501–1500 g is 31% (Pediatrics 1993;91:540–5)
- Determine whether the patient was born in a place located at a high altitude.

Examination

- Collapsing pulse (caused by an aortic diastolic run-off)
- Heaving apex beat
- Systolic and/or diastolic thrill in the left second interspace
- Loud, continuous 'machinery' murmur, i.e. pansystolic and extending into early diastole — known as Gibson murmur — is heard along the left upper sternal border and outer border of the clavicle. The murmur begins after the first heart sound, peaks with the second sound, and trails off in diastole (Edinb Med 1890;8:1) (Fig. 24.1)
- The second sound is not heard.

DIAGNOSIS

This patient has a patent ductus arteriosus (lesion) which is probably congenital in origin (aetiology); the patient is not in heart failure (functional status).

QUESTIONS

Mention a few causes of a collapsing pulse

- Hyperdynamic circulation caused by:
  - aortic regurgitation
  - thyrotoxicosis
  - severe anaemia
  - Paget's disease
  - complete heart block.

ADVANCED-LEVEL QUESTIONS

Mention a few causes of continuous murmurs

- Venous hum
- Mitral regurgitation murmur with aortic regurgitant murmur
- Ventricular septal defect with aortic regurgitation
- Pulmonary arteriovenous fistula
- Rupture of the sinus of Valsalva

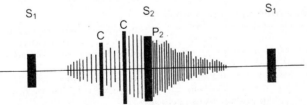

S_1 S_2 S_1

C C P_2

Fig. 24.1 The machinery murmur of patent ductus arteriosus is typically maximally loud at the time of the second heart sound (S_2); clicking noises (C) in systole contribute to the machinery sound.

- Coronary arteriovenous fistula
- Arteriovenous anastomosis of intercostal vessels following a fractured rib.

What happens to the continuous murmur of patent ductus arteriosus in pulmonary hypertension?

First the diastolic murmur, then the systolic murmur, becomes softer and shorter, and P increases in intensity.

How would you investigate this patient?

- *ECG* may be normal or shows left ventricular hypertrophy.
- *Chest radiograph* may be normal, or there may be left ventricular and left atrial enlargement. The chest film shows pulmonary plethora, proximal pulmonary arterial dilatation and a prominent ascending aorta. The ductus arteriosus may be visualized as an opacity at the confluence of the descending aorta and the aortic knob. If pulmonary hypertension develops, right ventricular hypertrophy is noted.
- *Echocardiography* can usuually visualize the ductus arteriosus. Doppler studies demonstrate continuous flow in the pulmonary trunk.
- *Cardiac catheterization* is useful to determine the presence and severity of the shunt and determines pulmonary vascular resistance. Angiography defines its anatomy.
- *Cardiac MRI.*

Mention a few associated lesions

- Ventricular septal defect
- Pulmonary stenosis
- Coarctation of aorta.

What are complications?

- Congestive cardiac failure is the commonest complication.
- Infective endocarditis or endarteritis (involves the pulmonary side of the ductus arteriosus or the pulmonary artery opposite the duct orifice, from which septic pulmonary emboli may arise).
- Pulmonary hypertension and reversal of shunt (causes differential cyanosis and clubbing, i.e. toes—*not* fingers—are clubbed and cyanosed).
- Substantial left-to-right shunting through the ductus in infants may increase the risk of intraventricular haemorrhage, necrotizing enterocolitis, bronchopulmonary dysplasia and death.
- The ductus may become aneurysmal and calcified, which may lead to its rupture

Remember: One-third of patients with a PDA that is not surgically repaired die of heart failure, pulmonary hypertension or endarteritis by the age of 40 years, and two-thirds die by the age of 60 years.

How would you manage such patients?

- Within 1–3 weeks of birth: administer a prostaglandin E synthesis inhibitor such as indometacin or ibuprofen. Ibuprofen is as effective as indometacin but is associated with a lower incidence of renal toxic effects (N Engl J Med 2000;343:674–81).
- PDA can be closed percutaneously by two types of device: coils (e.g. Gianturco-Grifka Vascular Occlusion Device, Nit-Occlud PDA occluder) or occluders (e.g. Amplatzer PDA occluder).
- Surgery is required in children or adults with large shunts: ligation or division of the PDA.

Notes
- Because of the risk of endarteritis associated with unrepaired PDA (estimated at 0.45% annually after the second decade of life) and the low risk associated with ligation (mortality of <0.5%), it is recommended that even a small PDA be ligated surgically or occluded with a percutaneously placed closure device.
- Once severe pulmonary vascular obstructive disease develops, surgical ligation or percutaneous closure is contraindicated.

Which congenital cardiac lesions are dependent on a patent ductus arteriosus?
- Hypoplastic left heart syndrome
- Complex coarctations of aorta
- Critical congenital aortic stenosis.

Collapsing pulse is also called Corrigan's pulse after Sir Dominic J Corrigan (1802–1880), a Dublin-born physician who graduated from Edinburgh.
RE Gross was the first to report surgical closure of the PDA in 1939.

---

25 PULMONARY STENOSIS

INSTRUCTION

Examine this patient's heart.

SALIENT FEATURES

History

- Patients may be asymptomatic.
- Ask if there is a history of maternal rubella.
- Dyspnoea on exertion or fatigability may occur (when the stenosis is severe), less often, patients may have retrosternal chest pain or syncope with exertion. Eventually, right ventricular failure may develop, with resultant peripheral oedema and abdominal swelling.
- Cyanosis and clubbing (if the foramen ovale is patent, shunting of blood from the right to the left atrium may occur).

Remember: The presence or absence of symptoms, their severity and the prognosis are influenced by the severity of stenosis, the right ventricular systolic function and the competence of the tricuspid valve.

Examination

- Round plump facies
- Normal pulse
- Prominent 'a' wave in the JVP
- Left parasternal heave
- Ejection click, which *decreases* on inspiration (this is the only right sided sound that decreases with inspiration) (valvular stenosis) (Br Heart J 1951;13:519)

- Soft P_2, with a wide split second sound
- Ejection systolic murmur in the left upper sternal border, best heard on inspiration. The murmur radiates to the left shoulder and left lung posteriorly. The more severe the stenosis, the longer is the murmur, obscuring the second aortic sound A_2
- Then proceed by looking for central cyanosis and clubbing (Fallot's tetralogy).

DIAGNOSIS

This patient has pulmonary stenosis (lesion), which is a congenital anomaly (aetiology) and the patient is severely limited by her symptoms (functional status).

QUESTIONS

What is the underlying cause of pulmonary stenosis?
- Congenital (commonest cause)
- Carcinoid tumour of the small bowel

ADVANCED-LEVEL QUESTIONS

What is the normal valve area of the pulmonary valve?
The area of the pulmonary valve orifice in a normal adult is about 2.0 cm^2/ m^2 body surface area, and there is no systolic pressure gradient across the valve.

How is the severity of pulmonary valve stenosis determined?
Mild: valve area larger than 1.0 cm^2/m^2, transvalvular gradient <50 mmHg or peak right ventricular systolic pressure <75 mmHg.

Moderate: valve area 0.5–1.0 cm^2/m^2, transvalvular gradient 50–80 mmHg or right ventricular systolic pressure 75–100 mmHg.

Severe: valve area <0.5 cm^2/m^2, transvalvular gradient >80 mmHg or right ventricular systolic pressure >100 mmHg.

How would you investigate this patient?
- *Electrocardiogram* shows right-axis deviation and right ventricular hypertrophy (Fig. 25.1).
- *Chest radiograph* shows a normal aortic knuckle whereas the pulmonary conus is either normal or enlarged (caused by post-stenotic dilatation of the main pulmonary artery) and the pulmonary vascular markings are diminished. The cardiac silhouette is usually normal in size or may be enlarged (when the patient has right ventricular failure or tricuspid regurgitation) (Fig. 25.2).
- *Echocardiography* can visualize the site of obstruction in most patients, but right ventricular hypertrophy and paradoxical septal motion during systole are evident. Doppler flow studies accurately assesses the severity of stenosis so that cardiac catheterization and angiography are usually unnecessary.

What are the complications of this condition?
- Cardiac failure
- Infective endocarditis: blood cultures are rarely positive; the emboli are entirely in the pulmonary circulation and not systemic.

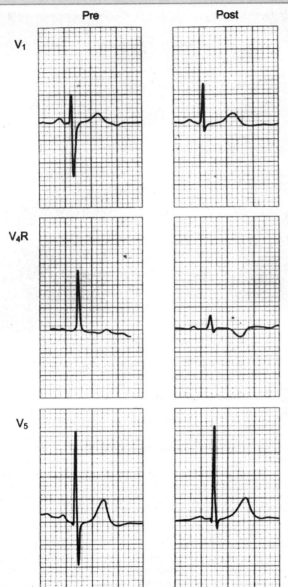

Fig. 25.1 Electrocardiogram in severe valvar pulmonary stenosis showing prehypertrophy before dilation and after QRS axis shift, and regression of hypertrophy after gradient reduction.

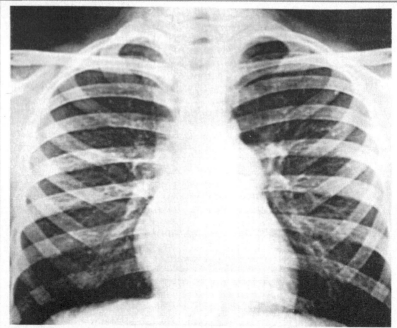

Fig. 25.2 Roentgenogram in valvular pulmonary stenosis with a normal aortic root. The heart size is within normal limits, but there is poststenotic dilatation of the pulmonary artery (usually the left branch). (With permission from Kliegman et al. 2007.)

- **What are the types of pulmonary stenosis?**
- Valvular
- Subvalvular: infundibular and subinfundibular
- Supravalvular.

Do you know of any eponymous syndromes linked to pulmonary stenosis?

- *Noonan syndrome:* short stature, ptosis, downward slanting eyes, wide-spaced eyes (hypertelorism), low-set ears, webbed neck, mental retardation and low posterior hairline. About two-thirds of patients with Noonan syndrome have pulmonary stenosis caused by valve dysplasia.
- *Watson syndrome:* café-au-lait spots, mental retardation and pulmonary stenosis.
- *Williams syndrome:* infantile hypercalcaemia, elfin facies and mental retardation, in addition to supravalvular pulmonary stenosis. Subvalvular pulmonary stenosis, which is caused by the narrowing of the right ventricular infundibulum or subinfundibulum, usually occurs in association with a ventricular septal defect.

How would you manage a patient with pulmonary stenosis?

Pulmonary balloon valvuloplasty should be considered when the peak systolic gradient >50 mmHg in symptomatic patients with domed pulmonary valve or mean pulmonary valve gradient >40 mm Hg, when right ventricular hypertrophy is present or when the peak gradient is >60 mmHg or mean >40 mm Hg in a patient who is asymptomatic.

- *Mild valvular pulmonary stenosis:* patients are usually asymptomatic and survival is excellent (with 94% still alive 20 years after diagnosis); therefore surgical correction is not required.
- *Moderate pulmonary stenosis* has an excellent prognosis with either medical or interventional therapy. Interventional therapy is usually recommended since most patients with moderate pulmonary stenosis eventually have symptoms requiring such therapy. Valve replacement is required if the leaflets are dysplastic or calcified or if marked regurgitation is present.
- *Severe stenosis:* relieve the the stenosis since only 40% of such patients do not require any intervention by 10 years after diagnosis.

Note: It is important that patients with mild valvular stenosis who are undergoing elective dental or surgical procedures should receive antibiotic prophylaxis against infective endocarditis.

What is the role of balloon valvuloplasty in pulmonary stenosis?

Relief of valvular stenosis can be accomplished easily and safely with percutaneous balloon valvuloplasty (Am J Cardiol 1990;65:775) and a delay in intervention offers no advantage. Balloon valvuloplasty, the procedure of choice, is usually successful, provided the valve is mobile and pliant; its long-term results are excellent. The secondary hypertrophic subpulmonary stenosis that may occur with valvular stenosis usually regresses after successful intervention. In a series of 100 patients, balloon dilatation resulted in a significant reduction in the transvalvular gradient, which was maintained at the 12-month follow-up (Int J Cardiol 1988;21:335–342).

What is Erb's point?

The third left intercostal space adjacent to the sternum is Erb's point, and the murmur of infundibular pulmonary stenosis is best heard in this space and in the left fourth intercostal space.

26   DEXTROCARDIA

INSTRUCTION

Examine this patient's precordium.
Listen to this patient's heart.

SALIENT FEATURES

History

- Asymptomatic
- Obtain history of cough with purulent expectoration (bronchiectasis) and sinusitis.

Examination

- Apex beat is absent on the left side and present on the right.
- Heart sounds are better heard on the right side of the chest.
- Ascertain whether the liver dullness is present on the right or left side.

- Examine the chest for bronchiectasis.
- Proceed by telling the examiner that you would like to perform the following checks:
  - Chest radiograph (looking for right-sided gastric bubble; (Fig. 26.1)
  - ECG (inversion of all complexes in lead I; Fig. 26.2).

Notes

- Dextrocardia without evidence of situs inversus is usually associated with cardiac malformation. It may occur with cardiac malformation in Turner syndrome.
- Situs solitus means normal position.

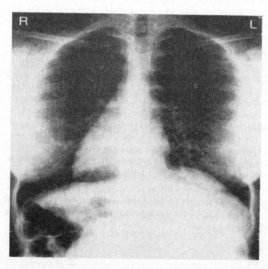

Fig. 26.1 Situs inversus. The heart, stomach, and liver are all in reversed positions (check that the right and left markers are placed correctly). (With permission from Mettler 2004.)

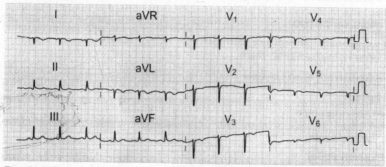

Fig. 26.2 Dextrocardia. Negative QRS wave on lead I and negative P, QRS and T waves on leads I and aVL. Isoelectric aVR. Negative QRS and T waves in all the precordial leads.

DIAGNOSIS

This patient has dextrocardia (lesion) of congenital aetiology.

ADVANCED-LEVEL QUESTIONS

What is Kartagener syndrome?

A type of immotile cilia syndrome in which there is dextrocardia or situs inversus, bronchiectasis and dysplasia of the frontal sinuses (Beitr Klin Tuberk 1933;83:489; N Engl J Med 1953;248:730).

Which other abnormality has been associated with dextrocardia?

Asplenia (blood smear may show Heinz bodies, Howell–Jolly bodies) (Br Heart J 1975;37:840).

What do you understand by the term situs inversus?

Right-sided cardiac apex, right stomach, right-sided descending aorta. The right atrium is on the left. The left lung has three lobes and the right lung has two.

What do you understand by the term dextroversion?

Right-sided cardiac apex, left-sided stomach and left-sided descending aorta.

What do you understand by the term levoversion?

Left-sided apex, right-sided stomach and right descending aorta.

M Kartagener (b. 1897), a Swiss physician, described this condition in 1933.

---

27   COARCTATION OF AORTA

INSTRUCTION

Examine this patient's cardiovascular system.

SALIENT FEATURES

History

- Asymptomatic usually
- Symptoms are usually those of hypertension: headache, epistaxis, dizziness, and palpitations
- Claudication (caused by diminished blood flow the legs)
- Occasionally, diminished blood
- Patients sometimes seek medical attention because they have symptoms of heart failure or aortic dissection. Women with coarctation are at particularly high risk for aortic dissection during pregnancy.

Examination

- The upper torso is better developed than the lower part (as the lower body has chronic low systolic blood pressure compared to the upper part).

- The systolic arterial pressure is higher in the arms than in the legs, but the diastolic pressures are similar; therefore, a widened pulse pressure is present in the arms. (**Note**: This condition results in hypertension in the arms. Less commonly, the coarctation is immediately proximal to the left subclavian artery, in which case a difference in arterial pressure is noted between the arms.)
- Radial pulse on the left side may be less prominent.
- The femoral arterial pulses are weak and delayed (simultaneous palpation of the brachial and femoral arteries using the thumbs is the most convenient method of comparing pulsations in the upper and lower limbs).
- A systolic thrill may be palpable in the suprasternal notch.
- Heaving apex caused by left ventricular enlargement.
- A systolic ejection click (caused by a bicuspid aortic valve which occurs in 50% of cases) is frequently present, and the second heart sound is accentuated.
- A harsh systolic ejection murmur may be identified along the left sternal border and in the back, particularly over the coarctation.
- Scapular collaterals are visible (listen over these collaterals for murmur).
- A systolic murmur, caused by flow through collateral vessels, may be heard in the back.
- In about 30% of patients with aortic coarctation, a systolic murmur indicating an associated bicuspid aortic valve is audible at the base.
- Look for:
  - Turner syndrome (female, webbing of the neck, increased carrying angle)
  - berry aneurysms (extraocular movements impaired caused by third cranial nerve involvement).

DIAGNOSIS

This patient has coarctation of the aorta (lesion) with left ventricular failure (functional status).

ADVANCED-LEVEL QUESTIONS

What are the types of aortic coarctation?

- Common:
- Infantile or preductal where the aorta between the left subclavian artery and patent ductus arteriosus is narrowed. It manifests in infancy with heart failure. Associated lesions include patent ductus arteriosus, aortic arch anomalies, transposition of the great arteries, ventricular septal defect.
- *Adult type:* the coarctation in the descending aorta is juxtaductal or slightly postductal. It may be associated with biscuspid aortic valve or patent ductus arteriosus. It commonly presents between the ages of 15 and 30 years.

- Rare:
- Localized juxtaductal coarctation
- Coarctation of the ascending thoracic aorta
- Coarctation of the distal descending thoracic aorta
- Coarctation of the abdominal aorta

- Pseudocoarctation is of no haemodynamic significance and is a 'kinked' appearance of the aorta in the juxtaductal region without stenosis.

Is aortic coarctation commoner in men or women?

This condition is two to five times as frequent in men and boys as in women and girls.

What conditions are associated with coarctation of aorta?

It may occur in conjunction with gonadal dysgenesis (e.g. Turner syndrome), bicuspid aortic valve, ventricular septal defect, patent ductus arteriosus, mitral stenosis or regurgitation or aneurysms of the circle of Willis.

At what age does the condition manifest?

It is particularly likely to produce significant symptoms in early infancy (presenting as cardiac failure) or between the ages of 20 and 30 years.

How would you investigate this patient?

- *Electrocardiogram* usually shows left ventricular hypertrophy (Fig. 27.1).
- *Chest radiograph* shows symmetric rib notching. The coarctation may be visualized as the characteristic '3' sign on a chest radiograph (Fig. 27.2). The upper bulge is formed by dilatation of the left subclavian artery high on the left mediastinal border; the sharp indentation is the site of the coarctation and the lower bulge is called the poststenotic dilatation of the aorta.
- *Echocardiography* may visualize the coarctation; Doppler examination makes possible an estimate of the transcoarctation pressure gradient.
- *Computed tomography (CT), MRI and contrast aortography* are useful to determine the precise anatomy regarding the location and length of the coarctation; in addition, aortography permits the visualization of the collateral circulation.

What do you understand by the term pseudocoarctation?

It refers to buckling or kinking of the aortic arch without the presence of a significant gradient.

What causes rib notching?

Collateral flow through dilated, tortuous and pulsatile posterior intercostal arteries typically causes notching on the undersurfaces of the posterior portions of the ribs. The anterior parts of the ribs are spared because the anterior intercostal arteries do not run in the costal grooves. Notching is seldom found above the third or below the ninth rib and rarely appears before the age of 6 years.

Mention a few conditions in which rib notching is seen

- Coarctation of aorta
- Pulmonary oligaemia
- Blalock–Taussig shunt
- Subclavian artery obstruction
- Superior vena caval syndrome
- Neurofibromatosis
- Arteriovenous malformations of the lung or chest wall.

What are the complications of aortic coarctation?

- Severe hypertension and resulting complications:
  - Stroke
  - Premature coronary artery disease
  - Left ventricular failure (two-thirds of patients >40 years who have uncorrected aortic coarctation have symptoms of heart failure)
  - Rupture of aorta.

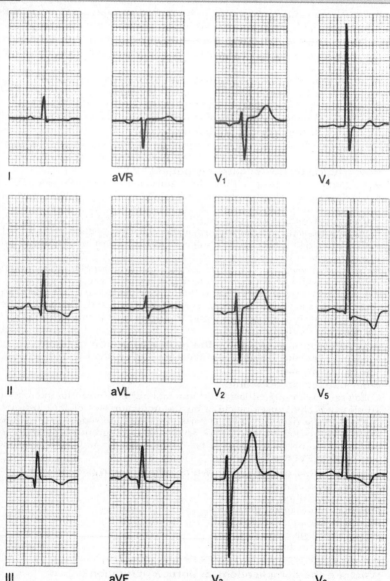

Fig. 27.1 Electrocardiogram usually shows left ventricular hypertrophy.

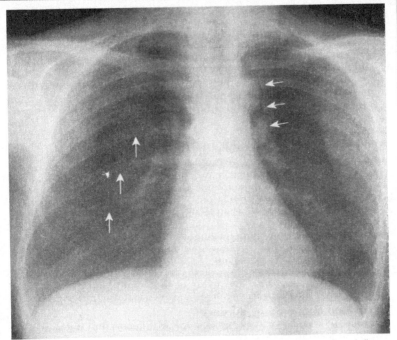

Fig. 27.2 Chest radiograph shows the 'number 3' sign (short arrows) and rib notching (long arrows) is seen on the inferior portion of the posterior ribs (ribs 3 to 9). (With permission from Carey WD 2009.)

- Infective endocarditis endarteritis (at the site of the coarctation or on a congenitally bicuspid aortic valve).
- Intracranial haemorrhage (combination of hypertension and ruptured berry aneurysm).
- Death occurs in 75% by the age of 50, and 90% by the age of 60 (Br Heart J 1970;32:633–40).

What are the fundal findings in coarctation of aorta?

Hypertension caused by coarctation of aorta causes retinal arteries to be tortuous with frequent 'U' turns; curiously, the classical signs of hypertensive retinopathy are rarely seen (see Fig. 202.1).

What are the indications for treatment of coarctation?

- Proximal hypertension
- A withdrawal gradient greater than 20 mmHg at angiography
- An echo peak gradient of >20 mmHg in the absence of extensive collaterals or <20 mmHg in their presence.

What is the treatment of such patients?

- Balloon dilatation with stent insertion in patients with native coarctation and recoarctation can be done with good immediate and medium-term results in adolescents and adults and should probably be the procedure of choice when the anatomy is suitable and expert skills are available.

- When the anatomy is not suitable (i.e. long tunnel-like stenosis) surgical resection and end-to-end anastomosis may be needed, although a tubular graft may be required if the narrowed segment is too long. After surgical repair of isolated aortic coarctation, the obstruction is usually relieved with minimum mortality (<2%). However, mortality is increased for reoperation (5–15%).

What are the postoperative complications?
- Recurrent coarctation
- Persistent hypertension
- Possible sequelae of a bicuspid aortic valve.

What happens to the hypertension after surgery?
Despite surgery, some patients may continue to have residual or recurrent hypertension and will require monitoring for hypertension and premature coronary artery disease (Circulation 1989;80:840–5). The incidence of persistent or recurrent hypertension, is influenced by the patient's age at the time of surgery:

- Among patients who undergo surgery during childhood, 90% are normotensive 5 years later, 50% are normotensive 20 years later, and 25% are normotensive 25 years later.
- Among those who undergo surgery after the age of 40 years, half have persistent hypertension, and many of those with a normal resting BP after successful repair have a hypertensive response to exercise.

Is survival improved by surgery?
Survival after repair of aortic coarctation is influenced by the age of the patient at the time of surgery:

- Repair during childhood: 89% of patients are alive 15 years later and 83% are alive 25 years later
- Repair between ages of 20 and 40 years: 25-year survival is 75%
- Repair in patients >40 years: the 15-year survival is only 50%.

28 EISENMENGER SYNDROME

INSTRUCTION

Examine this patient's heart.
Examine this patient's cardiovascular system.

SALIENT FEATURES

History

- Symptoms may not appear until early late childhood or early adulthood
- Cyanosis (appears as right-to-left shunting develop)
- Dyspnoea on exercise and impaired exercise tolerance
- Palpitations (common and usually caused by atrial fibrillation or flutter)
- Angina of effort
- Haemoptysis (may occur as a result of pulmonary infarction, or rupture of dilated pulmonary arteries or aorticopulmonary vessels)

- Syncope (owing to inadequate cardiac output or, less commonly, an arrhythmia)
- Symptoms of hyperviscosity including visual disturbances, fatigue, headache, dizziness and paraesthesia
- Symptoms of heart failure are uncommon until the disease is in advanced stages.

Examination

- Clubbing of fingers and central cyanosis
- An 'a' waves in the JVP, 'v' wave if tricuspid regurgitation is also present
- Left parasternal heave and palpable P_2
- Loud P_2, pulmonary ejection click, early diastolic murmur of pulmonary regurgitation (Graham Steell murmur)
- Loud pansystolic murmur of tricuspid regurgitation
- Listen carefully to the second sound. The clinical findings from the underlying defect are as follows:
  - Ventricular septal defect (VSD): single second sound
  - Atrial septal defect (ASD): fixed, wide split second sound
  - Patent ductus arteriosus (PDA): reverse split of second sound and differential cyanosis where lower-limb cyanosis is marked.

DIAGNOSIS

This patient has Eisenmenger syndrome with a shunt at the ventricular level (lesion) that is congenital in origin (aetiology), and severe pulmonary hypertension (functional status).

QUESTIONS

What do you understand by the term Eisenmenger syndrome?
Pulmonary hypertension with a reversed or bidirectional shunt. It matters very little where the shunt happens to be (e.g. VSD, ASD, PDA, persistent truncus arteriosus, single ventricle or common atrioventricular canal).

ADVANCED-LEVEL QUESTIONS

What do you understand by the term Eisenmenger complex?
Eisenmenger complex is a VSD with a right-to-left shunt in the absence of pulmonary stenosis. The onset of Eisenmenger syndrome is often heralded by a softening of the murmur, a decrease in the left heart size and in increase in the second pulmonic sound.

Mention some cyanotic heart diseases of infancy
- Tetralogy of Fallot
- Transposition of the great vessels
- Tricuspid regurgitation
- Total anomalous pulmonary venous connection.

What is the age of onset of Eisenmenger syndrome?
In the case of PDA and VSD, about 80% occur in infancy, whereas in the case of ASD over 90% occur in adult life.

What factors worsen deteriorate pulmonary hypertension in these patients?

- Pregnancy
- Dehydration or acute vasodilation (e.g. sauna, hot tub)
- Increased fluid volume
- Worsened renal or hepatic function
- Chronic environmental hypoxia
- Increased left-sided filling pressure:
  - Left ventricular diastolic dysfunction
  - Obstructive congenital lesion
  - Myocardial restriction
  - Systemic hypertension with increased left ventricular afterload.
- Erythrocytosis and increased blood viscosity; anaemia
- Hypercoagulability: thrombosis
- Acute infection
- Arrhythmias.

(See Clin Chest Med 2007;28:243–53.)

What are the complications of Eisenmenger syndrome?

- Haemoptysis
- Erythrocytosis
- Right ventricular failure
- Cerebrovascular accidents (as a result of paradoxical embolization, venous thrombosis of cerebral vessels or intracranial haemorrhage)
- Sudden death
- Brain abscess
- Bleeding and thrombosis (patients at increased risks for both as a consequence of an abnormal haemostasis secondary to chronic arterial desaturation)
- Paradoxical embolization
- Infective endocarditis
- Hyperuricaemia
- Recurrent haemoptysis.

How would you investigate this patient?

- *Electrocardiogram* shows right ventricular hypertrophy; atrial arrhythmias particularly in those with underlying ASD.
- *Chest radiograph* shows conspicuous dilatation of the pulmonary artery (Fig. 28.1) with narrowed 'pruned' peripheral vessels (caused by pulmonary hypertension); slight to moderate enlargement of the heart (predominantly RV) may be seen in ASD whereas the size of the heart is normal in VSD or PDA.
- *Echocardiography* provides evidence of right ventricular overload and pulmonary hypertension; the underlying cardiac defect can be visualized, although shunting may be difficult to demonstrate by colour Doppler imaging because of low velocity jet; contrast echocardiography permits localization of shunt.
- *Cardiac catheterization* determine the extent and severity of pulmonary vascular disease and accurately quantify the magnitude of the intracardiac shunting; assessment of reversibility of shunting is done using pulmonary vasodilators (e.g. oxygen, inhaled nitrous oxide, intravenous adenosine or epoprostenol).

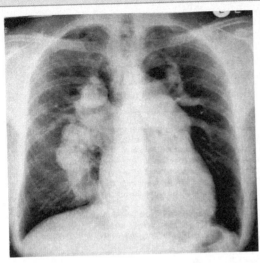

Fig. 28.1 Chest radiograph demonstrating gross dilatation of the main, left and right pulmonary arteries in a patient with Eisenmenger ASD. (With permission from Adam et al. 2008.)

What is the prognosis in these patients?

- Survival is 80% 10 years after diagnosis, 77% at 15 years, and 42% at 25 years.
- Death is usually sudden; other causes include heart failure, haemoptysis, brain abscess or stroke.
- Poor prognostic factors include syncope, clinically evident right ventricular systolic dysfunction, low cardiac output and severe hypoxaemia.

Is pregnancy safe in this patient?

Pregnancy is associated with a high incidence of early spontaneous abortion and rarely results in the birth of a healthy child. Mortality of the mother is high (30–60%) in those with underlying VSD, particularly in late pregnancy and postpartum period. Pregnancy is, therefore, contraindicated and if occurs is best terminated at an early stage. If pregnancy proceeds to term, a vaginal delivery is the preferred route with careful management of hydration, arrhythmias and hypoxaemia. Epidural anaesthesia is preferred over general anaesthesia in complicated cases.

What treatment is available for Eisenmenger syndrome?

- Phlebotomy done cautiously in symptomatic hyperviscosity due to secondary erythrocytosis when the haematocrit >0.65 (but not due to dehydration). Always replace fluid intravenously following phlebotomy
- Long-term intravenous epoprostenol (Circulation 1999;99:1858–65; Ann Intern Med 1999;130:740–3)
- Uncontrolled studies suggest that prostacyclin analogues and phosphodiesterase 5 inhibitors (e.g. sildenafil) may have benefits in advanced pulmonary vascular disease

- In a randomized, controlled trial of bosentan versus placebo, bosentan showed a significant improvement in exercise capacity based on 6-minute walk distance, with serious safety concerns (Circulation 2006;114:48–54)
- Combined heart–lung transplantation (limited success and hence patients should be carefully selected).

Victor Eisenmenger was a German physician who described this condition in an infant in 1897. His patient had cyanosis since infancy and a fairly good quality of life until he succumbed at the age of 32 years. The patient was active until the age of 29 years when he developed right heart failure and died 3 years later following a massive haemoptysis. Post-mortem revealed a large VSD (2.5 cm) with both the LV and RV with equally thick walls. The pulmonary arteries revealed atheroma with multiple thrombi leading to pulmonary infarctions.

Paul Wood at the Brompton Hospital in 1958 published a study of 127 patients and was the first to suggest that Eisenmenger reaction occurred with defects other than the ventricular level (BMJ 1958;2:701, 709).

---

29 FALLOT'S TETRALOGY

INSTRUCTION

Examine this patient's heart.

SALIENT FEATURES

History

- Syncope (in 20% of cases)
- Squatting
- Shortness of breath
- Decrease in exercise tolerance
- Growth retardation.

Examination

- Clubbing
- Central cyanosis
- Left parasternal heave with normal left ventricular impulse
- Second sound is single (absent second pulmonic sound)
- Ejection systolic murmur heard in the pulmonary area
- Signs indicating Blalock–Taussig shunt:
  - The left radial pulse is not as prominent as the right
  - The arm on the side of the anastomosis (usually the left) may be smaller than the other arm
  - Blood pressure is difficult to obtain because of the narrow pulse pressure in the arm supplied by the collateral vessels
  - Thoracotomy scar.

DIAGNOSIS

This patient has Fallot's tetralogy with a Blalock–Taussig shunt and is mildly cyanosed, indicating a right to left shunt (functional status).

QUESTIONS

What are the constituents of Fallot's tetralogy?
- Ventricular septal defect with a right-to-left shunt
- Pulmonary stenosis (infundibular or valvular)
- Right ventricular hypertrophy
- Dextroposition of the aorta with it overriding the ventricular septal defect.

What are the complications of Fallot's tetralogy?
- Cyanotic and syncopal spells
- Cerebral abscess (in 10% of cases)
- Endocarditis (in 10% of cases)
- Strokes: thrombotic secondary to erythrocytosis and hyperviscosity
- Paradoxical emboli.

ADVANCED-LEVEL QUESTIONS

What anomalies may occur in association with tetralogy of Fallot?
- Right aortic arch in 25% of patients
- Atrial septal defect in 10% (so-called pentalogy of Fallot)
- Coronary arterial anomalies in 10%.

What do you understand by a Blalock–Taussig shunt?
It is the anastomosis of the left subclavian artery to the left pulmonary artery with the intention to increase pulmonary blood flow.

Why is a Blalock–Taussig shunt seen less frequently in adults in the recent past?
With ready availability of cardiopulmonary bypass, such patients have total correction of their anomalies at an early age.

What is the survival of Fallot's Tetralogy?
The rate of survival in uncorrected patients (Am J Cardiol 1978;42:458–66) is:
66% at 1 year of age
40% at 3 years
11% at 20 years
6% at 30 years
3% at 40 years.
The rate of survival 32 years after surgery in one series was 86% among patients with repaired tetralogy and 96% in an age-matched control population (N Engl J Med 1993;329:593–5); the difference reflected the increased risk of sudden death.

What do you know about the embryological development of Fallot's tetralogy?
It arises from the anterior displacement of the conal septum, which leads to unequal partitioning of the conus at the expense of the right ventricular infundibulum and results in the obstruction of the right ventricular outflow tract and failure to close the intraventricular foramen.

What do you know regarding the relation between congenital heart disease and embryology of heart development?

In order of embryologic development, the steps embryogenesis include:

1. Looping, laterality and single-ventricle defects (e.g. double-inlet LV, situs inversus totalis)
2. Conotruncal defects (e.g. tetralogy of Fallot, double-outlet RV)
3. Atrioventricular canal defects (e.g. endocardial cushion defect, common atrioventricular canal defect)
4. Right ventricular outflow tract obstruction (e.g. pulmonary valve atresia or stenosis, Ebstein's anomaly)
5. Left ventricular outflow tract obstruction (e.g. aortic valve atresia or stenosis, hypoplastic left heart)
6. Septal defects (e.g. ventricular septal defect, atrial septal defect)
7. Total or partial anomalous pulmonary venous return.

What is the treatment for Fallot's tetralogy?

- Total correction under the age of 1 year when there is no need for an outflow transannular patch. A second-stage total correction can be performed when the child is over the age of 2 years. The mortality associated with surgery is <3% in children and 2.5 to 8.5% in adults.
- Blalock–Taussig shunting is performed nowadays only if the anatomy is unfavourable for a total correction.
- Modified Blalock–Taussig shunting is the interposition of a tubular graft between the subclavian and pulmonary arteries.
- The Waterston shunt involves anastomosis of the back of the ascending aorta to the pulmonary artery. It is used when surgery is required in a child younger than 3 months, because the subclavian artery is too small for a good Blalock–Taussig shunt.
- The Potts shunt involves anastomosis of the descending aorta to the back of the pulmonary artery (JAMA 1946;132:627).
- The Glenn operation involves anastomosis of the superior vena cava to the right pulmonary artery. The bidirectional Glenn procedure involves anastomosis of the superior vena cava to both pulmonary arteries.
- Pulmonary balloon valvuloplasty is sometimes used as an alternative for surgery.

What cardiac lesions favour an initial shunt?

- Anomalous coronary artery
- Single pulmonary artery
- Hypoplastic pulmonary arteries
- Single pulmonary artery.

What is Fallot's triology?

Atrial septal defect, pulmonary stenosis and right ventricular hypertrophy.

What is Fallot's pentalogy?

Fallot's tetralogy with associated atrial septal defect.

What conditions are associated with Fallot's tetralogy?

- Right-sided aortic arch (in 30% of cases)
- Double aortic arch
- Left-sided superior vena cava (in 10% of cases)
- Hypoplasia of the pulmonary arteries
- Atrial septal defect.

Mention the common congenital heart diseases

Ventricular septal defect, atrial septal defect of the secundum type, patent ductus arteriosus and Fallot's tetralogy are the common congenital heart diseases, in order of frequency.

What are the findings from investigations?

● Chest radiography:
● Boot-shaped heart (Fig. 29.1)
● Enlarged RV
● Decreased pulmonary vasculature
● Right-sided aortic arch (in 30% of cases).

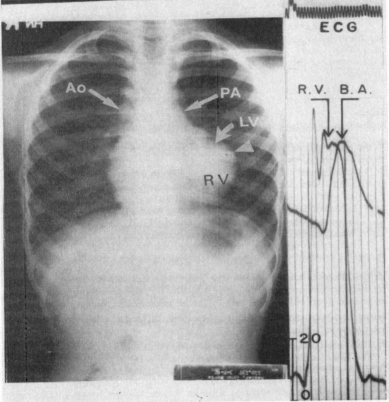

Fig. 29.1 Radiograph in classic cyanotic Fallot's tetralogy. The left ventricle (LV) is small and underfilled and lies superior to a relatively horizontal ventricular septum and an elevated interventricular sulcus (arrowhead) inferior to which lies the concentrically hypertrophied apex forming right ventricle (RV). The ascending aorta (Ao) is prominent, the main pulmonary artery segment (PA) is concave, and the lungs are oligaemic. (With permission from Perloff 2003.)

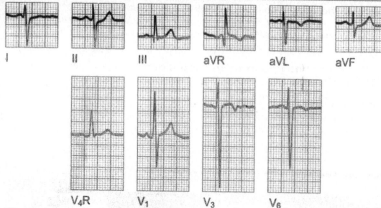

Fig. 29.2 Electrocardiogram in tetralogy of Fallot, with tall R waves in the right precordium, deep S waves in V_6, and positive T waves in V4R and V_1 characteristic of right ventricular hypertrophy.

ECG
Right axis deviation right ventricular hypertrophy (Fig. 29.2).

What are the arrhythmias detected with Holter monitoring with repaired tetralogy of Fallot?
- Ventricular arrhythmias can be detected in 40–50% of such patients and are most likely to occur in those who:
  - are older at the time of surgical repair
  - have moderate or severe pulmonary regurgitation
  - have systolic and diastolic left ventricular dysfunction
  - have prolonged cardiopulmonary bypass
  - have prolongation of the QRS interval (to >180 ms).
- Atrial fibrillation or flutter, which may cause considerable morbidity

What do you know about the Taussig–Bing syndrome?
In this condition, the aorta arises from the RV; the pulmonary trunk overrides both ventricles at the site of an interventricular septal defect.

What are long-term complications in patients with repaired tetralogy of Fallot?
- Pulmonary regurgitation may develop as a result of surgical repair of the right ventricular outflow tract).
- Enlargement of the RV occurs, resulting in RV dysfunction, and repair or replacement of the pulmonary valve may be required.
- An aneurysm may form at the site where the RV outflow tract was repaired.
- Residual or recurrent obstruction of the RV outflow tract, requiring repeated surgery.
- Residual ventricular septal defects in approximately 10–20% of patients with repaired tetralogy of Fallot; such patients may require repeated surgery if the defects are of sufficient size.

- Right bundle branch block is common after repair of tetralogy of Fallot, but complete heart block is rare.
- Aortic root dilatation resulting in aortic regurgitation, usually mild.

Further reading

Apitz C, Webb GD, Reddington AN: Tetralogy of Fallot, *Lancet* 374:1469–1471, 2009.

Etienne-Louis Arthur Fallot (1850–1911), Professor of Hygiene and Legal Medicine in Marseilles, published his 'Contribution to the pathologic anatomy of morbus coeruleus cardiac cyanosis' in 1888.

The tetralogy was first described by Niels Stensen, Professor of Anatomy in Copenhagen, in 1672 but the term tetralogy of Fallot is attributed to Canadian Maude Abbott in 1924. (Fallot A. Contribution à l'anatomie pathologique de la maladie bleue (cyanose cardiaque). Marseille Med 1888;25:418–20).

Helen Brook Taussig (1898–1986) is the founder of American paediatric cardiology. She collaborated with Alfred Blalock (1899–1964), a vascular surgeon, in the development of palliative surgery for Fallot's tetralogy (JAMA 1945;128:189).

---

30 ABSENT RADIAL PULSE

INSTRUCTION

Examine this patient's pulses.

SALIENT FEATURES

History

- Past history of insertion of an arterial line for blood gases or arterial pressure
- Systemic symptoms in the past (Takayasu's arteritis)
- Past history of cardiac surgery (Blalock–Taussig shunt)
- Cervical rib.

Examination

- Left radial pulse is weaker than the right.
- Examine all other pulses (including carotid, brachial, femoral, popliteal, posterior tibial and dorsalis pedis pulses).
- Check the BP in both the upper limbs (differences in BP between both arms of >10 mmHg systolic or 5 mmHg diastolic are abnormal).

DIAGNOSIS

This patient has an absent radial pulse (lesion) that is caused by a previous Blalock–Taussig shunt.

QUESTIONS

In which conditions may the pulse rate in one arm differ from that in the other?

Usually, slowing of the pulse on one side occurs distal to the aneurysmal sac. Therefore, an aneurysm of the transverse or descending aortic arch causes a retardation of the left radial pulse. Also the artery feels smaller and is more easily compressed than usual. An aneurysm of the ascending aorta or common carotid artery may result in similar changes in the right radial pulse.

What are the causes of absent radial pulse?

- Aberrant radial artery or congenital anomaly (check the brachials and BP)
- Tied off at surgery or previous surgical cut-down
- Catheterization of the brachial artery with poor technique
- Following a radial artery line for monitoring of blood gases or arterial pressure
- Subclavian artery stenosis
- Blalock–Taussig shunt on that side (shunt from subclavian to pulmonary artery)
- Embolism into the radial artery (usually caused by atrial fibrillation)
- Takayasu's arteritis (rare).

What are the causes of differences in blood pressure between arms or betweens the arms and legs?

- Occlusion or stenosis of the artery of any cause
- Coarctation of the aorta
- Dissecting aortic aneurysm
- Patent ductus arteriosus
- Supravalvular aortic stenosis
- Thoracic outlet syndrome.

ADVANCED-LEVEL QUESTIONS

What is Adson's test?

The clinician palpates the radial pulse and abducts the arm slightly (Fig. 30.1). The clinician asks the patient to hyperextend the neck and turn it to the affected side and inhale deeply. Adson's test is positive if the patient reports paraesthesias or if the pulse fades away. Diminution or obliteration of the pulse probably is caused by compression of the axillary artery by the anterior scalene muscle. The patient should turn the head to the opposite side (reverse Adson's test) to test compressive effect of the middle scalene.

What do you know about Takayasu's arteritis?

It tends to affect young women and most of the cases have been from Japan. Prodromal systemic symptoms include fever, night sweats, anorexia, weight loss, malaise, fatigue, arthralgia and pleuritic pain. It predominantly involves the aorta and is of three types: type I (Shimizu–Sano),

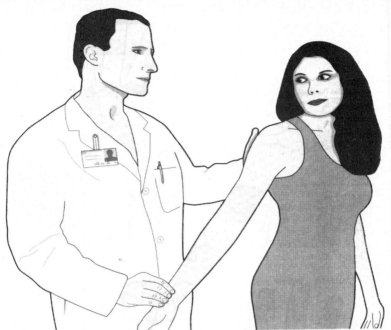

Fig. 30.1 Adson's test. Hold patient's arm in slight abduction while palpating the radial pulse. Ask the patient to extend the neck and rotate toward the affected side. Adson's test is positive if the patient reports paresthesias or if the pulse fades away.

which involves primarily the aortic arch and brachiocephalic vessels; type II (Kimoto), which affects the thoracoabdominal aorta and particularly the renal arteries; and type III (Inada), which has features of types I and III. Types I and III may be complicated by aortic regurgitation.

What is the Allen test?

The Allen test is used to determine patency of radial or ulnar artery (Fig. 30.2). To perform an Allen test, both the radial and the ulnar artery should be occluded while the atient elevates the hand and makes fist. The patient extends the fingers and blanching of the hand is seen. When the radial artery alone is released, and colour of hand returns to normal. An abnormal test result occurs when the colour of the hand does not return within 5–10 s. In thrombosis of the ulnar artery, the hand remains blanched when this artery alone is released. Allen's test can be used before puncturing the radial artery for cannulation as it is important to identify a competent ulnar artery should injury to the radial artery occur.

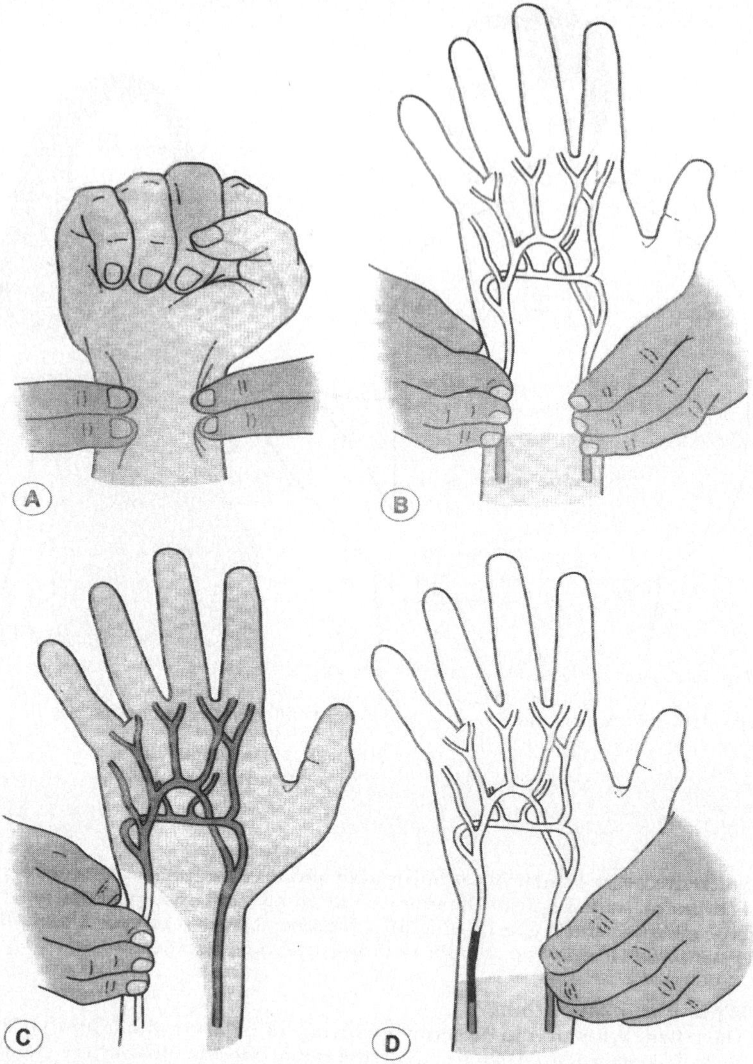

Fig. 30.2 Allen test for patency of radial and ulnar arteries. Blanching can be seen with both arteries occluded (B); releasing the radial artery alone returns the hand colour to normal (C). If the ulnar artery alone is released, the hand remains blanched if there is thrombosis of the ulnar artery.

M. Takayasu (1860–1938), Japanese ophthalmologist.

31 CONSTRICTIVE PERICARDITIS

INSTRUCTION

Examine this patient's cardiovascular system.

SALIENT FEATURES

History

- Dyspnoea
- Fatigue
- Ankle or abdominal swelling
- Nausea, vomiting, dizziness and cough.

Examination

- The patient may appear cachectic.
- Pulse may be regular or irregularly irregular (one-third have atrial fibrillation).
- Prominent 'x' and 'y' descents in the JVP and the level of the jugular venous pulse may rise with inspiration (Kussmaul's sign; Fig. 31.1).
- Apex beat is not palpable and there may be apical systolic retraction (Broadbent sign).
- Early diastolic pericardial knock along the left sternal border, which may be accentuated by inspiration.
- Lungs are clear but there may be pleural effusion.
- Markedly distended abdomen with hepatomegaly and ascites.
- Pitting leg oedema.

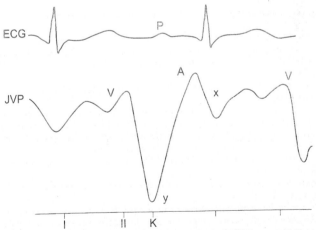

Fig. 31.1 Abnormal jugular venous waveform (JVP) in constrictive pericarditis with a prominent 'y' descent. Note the timing of the pericardial knock (K) relative to S$_2$. The abrupt rise in pressure after the nadir of the 'y' descent is caused by the rapid rise in venous pressure with ventricular filling.

DIAGNOSIS

This patient has constrictive pericarditis (lesion) caused by radiation therapy for previous Hodgkin's disease (aetiology) and is now limited by dyspnoea and marked ascites (functional status).

QUESTIONS

Mention some causes of constrictive pericarditis

- Tuberculosis (TB; <15% of patients)
- Connective tissue disorder
- Neoplastic infiltration
- Radiation therapy (often years earlier)
- Post-purulent pericarditis
- Haemopericardium after surgery (rare)
- Chronic renal failure.

ADVANCED-LEVEL QUESTIONS

What is the mechanism for pericardial knock?

It is caused by the abrupt halting of rapid ventricular filling.

Mention the differential diagnosis of the early diastolic sound

- Loud P_2 (p. 146)
- S_4 gallop (p. 56)
- Opening snap (mitral stenosis)
- Pericardial sound
- Tumour plop (atrial myxoma).

What is Beck's triad?

The presence of low arterial BP, high venous pressure and absent apex in cardiac tamponade is known as Beck's triad.

How would you investigate a patient with constrictive pericarditis?

- *Chest radiograph* typically shows normal heart size and pericardial calcification (note the combination of pulsus paradoxus, pericardial knock and pericardial calcification favour the diagnosis of constrictive pericarditis) (Fig. 31.2).
- *ECG* shows low voltage complexes, non-specific T wave flattening or atrial fibrillation.
- *Echocardiogram* shows myocardial thickness is normal and may reveal thickened pericardium; normal ventricular dimensions with enlarged atria and good systolic and poor diastolic dysfunction. Doppler shows increased right ventricular systolic and decreased left ventricular systolic velocity with inspiration, expiratory augmentation of hepatic-vein diastolic flow reversal.
- *CT or MRI* shows normal myocardial thickness usually and pericardial thickening and calcification.
- *Cardiac catheterization* typically shows identical left and right ventricular filling pressures and pulmonary artery systolic pressure usually <45 mmHg, with normal myocardial biopsy: haemodynamic tracings show rapid 'y' descent in atrial pressure and early dip in diastolic pressure, with pressure rise to plateau in mid or late diastole. Cardiac tamponade and constrictive pericarditis are basically similar in

restricting the filling of the heart and raising the systemic and pulmonary venous pressures. The venous pressure waveforms differ, however, reflecting a single wave of forward flow (during systole) in tamponade, compared with a biphasic pattern (a lesser wave in systole and a greater wave in early diastole) in constrictive conditions.

How would you treat a patient with constrictive pericarditis?
- Surgery is the only satisfactory treatment: complete surgical resection of the pericardium (myocardial inflammation or fibrosis may delay symptomatic response).
- Patients with tuberculous pericarditis should be pretreated for TB; if the diagnosis is confirmed after pericardial resection, full anti-tuberculous therapy should be continued for 6–12 months after resection.

What do you understand by the term effusive–constrictive pericarditis?
This is a clinical haemodynamic syndrome in which constriction of the heart by the visceral pericardium occurs in the presence of tense effusion in a free pericardial space. The hallmark is the persistence of elevated right atrial pressure after intrapericardial pressure has been reduced to normal levels by removal of pericardial fluid. Removing the pericardial fluid from a patient with effusive–constrictive pericarditis tends to change the venous waveform pattern from one more like that found in tamponade to one more like that associated with constriction.

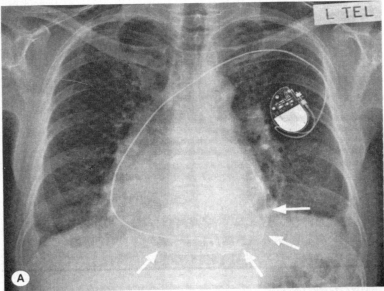

Fig. 31.2 Dense pericardial calcification demonstrated on chest radiograph (arrows). (With permission from Adam et al. 2008.)

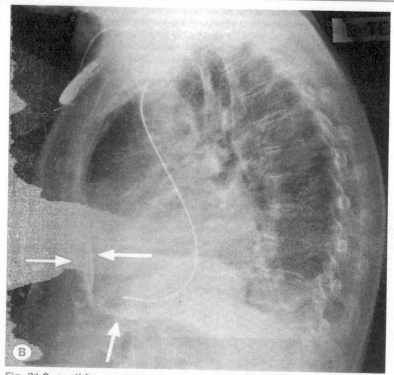

Fig. 31.2, cont'd

CS Beck (1894–1971), surgeon, Peter Bent Brigham Hospital in Boston.

W Broadbent (1868–1951), English physician who qualified from St Mary's Hospital Medical School, London. He described the Broadbent sign in constrictive pericarditis, which is an indrawing of the 11th and 12th left ribs with a narrowing and retraction of the intercostal space posteriorly; this occurs as a result of pericardial adhesions to the diaphragm.

32 PERMANENT CARDIAC PACEMAKER/IMPLANTABLE CARDIOVERTER-DEFIBRILLATOR

INSTRUCTION

Examine this patient's cardiovascular system.

SALIENT FEATURES

History

- Past history of syncope (Stokes–Adams attacks) and heart block
- Dizziness (pacemaker syndrome).

Examination

- Dropped beats caused by occasional ventricular ectopics
- Infraclavicular scar indicating pacemaker insertion
- Palpate the infraclavicular area gently to confirm the presence of a pacemaker.

Remember: electromagnetic interference during MRI or lithotripsy may transiently cause malfunction of pacemakers. Be prepared to discuss the anatomy of cardiac conduction system.

DIAGNOSIS

This patient has a permanent pacemaker (lesion) for previous heart block (aetiology), which is functioning adequately (functional status).

QUESTIONS

What are the indications for a permanent pacemaker?

- Symptomatic bradyarrhythmias: heart rate <40 beats/min or documented periods of asystole >30 s when awake. Symptoms include syncope, presyncope, confusion, seizures, or congestive heart failure and they must be clearly related to the bradycardia.
- Asymptomatic Mobitz type II atrioventricular block (N Engl J Med 1998;338:1147–48): you may asked to differentiate between Mobitz type I and II (see Fig. 11.1C,D).
- Complete heart block (see Fig. 11.1A,B).

ADVANCED-LEVEL QUESTIONS

What do you know about permanent pacemakers?

- They are connected to the heart by one or two electrodes and are powered by long-lasting (5–10 years) solid-state lithium batteries. Most pacemakers are designed to pace and sense the ventricles: called the VVI pacemakers because they pace the ventricle (V), sense the ventricle (V) and are inhibited (I) by the ventricular signal. They are inserted under local anaesthesia and fluoroscopic guidance, subcutaneously under the pectoral muscles.
- In symptomatic sinus tachycardia, an atrial pacemaker may sometimes be implanted (AAI).
- In sick sinus syndrome, a dual chamber pacemaker DDD (because it paces two or dual chambers, senses both (D) and reacts in two (D) ways, i.e. pacing in the same chamber is inhibited by spontaneous atrial and ventricular signals, and ventricular pacing is triggered by spontaneous atrial events) is implanted.
- Rate-responsive pacemakers measure activity, respiration, biochemical and electrical indicators, and change their pacing rate so that it is suitable for that level of exertion.

How soon after pacemaker insertion can a patient drive?

They may not drive until the pacemaker has been shown to be functioning correctly for at least 1 month after implantation. Patients must inform driving licensing authorities and the motor insurers.

Mention some expanded use of cardiac pacing

- Dual chamber pacing has been used to optimize cardiac output and minimize the outflow tract gradient in patients with hypertrophic obstructive cardiomyopathy.
- Dual chamber pacing is currently being utilized in dilated cardiomyopathy with heart failure and intraventricular conduction delay to optimize atrioventricular delay and improve cardiac output: cardiac resynchronization therapy.
- Dual-site atrial pacing to prevent atrial fibrillation is being evaluated.

What are the complications of pacemakers?

- Erosion through the skin caused by mechanical factors
- Infection
- Lead displacement or lead fracture (the most common site of pacing lead fracture is between the first rib and the clavicle)
- Pacemaker malfunction
- Electromagnetic interference
- Pain/ecchymoses at site of insertion
- Pneumothorax.

What are the potential sources of electromagnetic interference?

Electromagnetic interference can occur from heavy electric motors and arc welding. Devices such as airport security devices and ham radios cause single-beat inhibition but they should not cause significant clinical interference. Microwave ovens do not interfere with pacemakers. Cellular phones and anti-theft devices or electronic article surveillance equipment can potentially interfere with pacemakers (N Engl J Med 1997;336:1473–79,1518–19). Analogue phones are less likely to cause interference than phones based on digital technology. Patients should avoid carrying the cellular phones in a pocket directly over the pacemaker.

What is the pacemaker syndrome?

- It is seen in individuals with a single-chamber pacemaker who experience symptoms of low cardiac output (dizziness, etc.) when erect; it is attributed to the lack of atrial kick. Pacemaker syndrome results from haemodynamic changes following inappropriate use of ventricular pacing: it occurs when ventricular pacing is uncoupled from atrial contraction. It is most common when the VVI mode is used in patients with sinus rhythm, but it can occur in any pacing mode when atrioventricular synchrony is lost. Levels of atrial natriuretic factor are high in pacemaker syndrome.
- If pacemaker syndrome occurs in a patient with VVI pacemaker, the only definitive treatment is converting to a DDD. If the patient has occasional use of bradycardia then often symptoms may be ameliorated by programming the pacemaker to a lower limit and programming with

hysteresis 'on'. This allows the patient to stay in normal sinus rhythm for longer periods by minimizing the pacing.

If a patient with an implantable defibrillator requires a pacemaker would you put a separate device or replace it with a ICD with associated pacemaker function?

Placement of a separate pacemaker into a patient who has a defibrillator has the potential to cause serious pacemaker–defibrillator interactions. The most commonly implanted defibrillators have the additional ability to attempt termination of ventricular tachycardia with anti-tachycardia pacing. The obvious advantage of this feature is that an arrhythmia can be terminated painlessly without delivery of a shock. If anti-tachycardia pacing is unsuccessful then the device will administer a shock.

Mention some indications for implantable cardiac defibrillators

- Cardiac arrest as a result of ventricular tachyarrhythmia not the result of a reversible cause or transient cause (**remember**: patients who have cardiac arrest unrelated to acute myocardial infarction have approximately a 35% chance of recurrent ventricular arrhythmias within the first year)
- Spontaneous sustained ventricular tachycardia
- Syncope of undetermined origin with inducible sustained ventricular tachycardia on electrophysiologic study and when drug therapy is not effective or tolerated
- Non-sustained ventricular tachycardia with coronary artery disease and inducible ventricular tachycardia or electrophysiologic study that is not suppressible by class I antiarrhythmic drug.

What are the contraindications to patients with ICDs?

- MRI
- Lithotripsy is contraindicated if the pulse generator is in the field.

What are the indications for lead removal?

Mandatory:
- Life-threatening condition, leads must be removed
- Indications include septicaemia (endocarditis), migration (causing emboli, arrhythmia, or perforation)
- Device interference (i.e. abandoned ICD lead), and occlusion of all usable vessels.

Necessary:
- Great potential for morbidity or mortality, leads should be removed
- Indications include pocket infection, chronic draining sinus, erosion
- Potential device interference, venous thrombosis, and lead replacement (extract and reimplant via thrombosed vein).

Discretionary:
- Lead removal is optional
- Indications include pain, malignant disease, and replacement of leads abandoned for <3–4 years (not advisable to remove non-infected leads that have been implanted for >8–10 years).

(see Lancet 2004; 364:1701–19.)

33 PERICARDIAL RUB

INSTRUCTION

Listen to this patient's heart.

SALIENT FEATURES

History

- Precordial pain changing with posture (worse on lying down and relieved by sitting forward)
- Myocardial infarction
- Viral infection (coxsackie A and B viruses)
- Chronic renal failure
- Trauma
- TB.

Examination

- Scratching and grating sound heard best with the diaphragm at the left sternal border, with the patient leaning forward and the breath held in expiration.

Note: A pericardial rub does not occur in acute pericarditis and it is common for the rub to disappear when a pericardial effusion develops.

- Tell the examiner that you would like to do an ECG (Fig. 33.1), see a chest radiography (Fig. 33.2) and echocardiogram (Fig. 33.3).

DIAGNOSIS

This patient has a pericardial rub (lesion) caused by pericarditis secondary to uraemia (aetiology) and is not in pain (functional status).

QUESTIONS

What are the characteristic features of a pericardial friction rub?
It typically consists of three components:

- A presystolic rub during atrial contraction
- A ventricular systolic rub, which is almost always present and usually the loudest component
- A diastolic rub, which follows the second heart sound (during rapid ventricular filling).

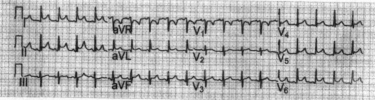

Fig. 33.1 Pericarditis with sinus tachycardia, diffuse, concave upward ST segment elevation, PR segment depression (lead II) and PR segment elevation (lead aVR).

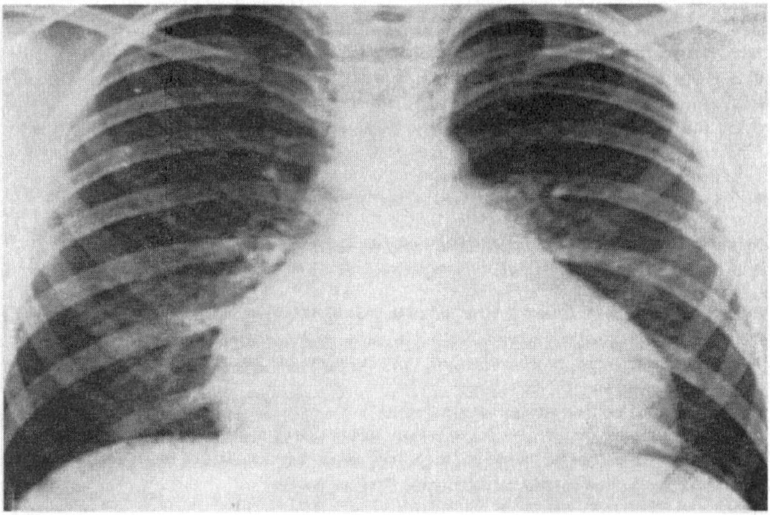

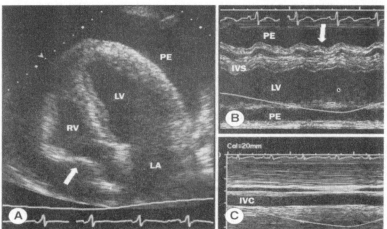

Fig. 33.2 Chest radiograph in acute non-specific pericarditis, showing cardiopericardial shadow caused by pericardial effusion. (With permission from Kliegman et al. 2007.)

Fig. 33.3 Echocardiographic images of large pericardial effusion (PE) with features of tamponade. (A) Apical four-chamber view showing large PE with diastolic right-atrial collapse (arrow). (B) M-mode image in parasternal long axis showing circumferential PE with diastolic collapse of RV free wall (arrow) during expiration. (C) M-mode image from subcostal window showing IVC plethora without inspiratory collapse. (With permission from Troughton et al. 2004.)

ADVANCED-LEVEL QUESTIONS

What are the characteristic electrocardiographic findings?

● ST elevation in most ECG leads with the concavity upwards.
● T wave inversion occurs after the ST segment returns to baseline (unlike in acute myocardial infarction where the ST segment is concave downwards like a cat's back and there is some amount of T wave inversion accompanying the ST elevation).
● PR-segment depression (caused by inflammation of the atrial wall).

How common is pericardial rub in constrictive pericarditis?

It is not heard in constrictive pericarditis.

What is the treatment for acute pericarditis?

● Pain relief (codeine) and NSAIDs (e.g. indometacin)
● Steroids should be considered only when the pain does not respond to a combination of NSAIDs
● Treatment of the underlying cause
● Treatment of pain: colchicine has been used to treat recurrent pain of pericarditis; rarely pericardiectomy may be required for pain even in the setting of no haemodynamic impairment.

What do you know about transient constrictive phase of acute pericarditis?

About 10% of the patients with acute pericarditis have a transient constrictive phase, which may last 2 to 3 months before it gradually resolves either spontaneously or with treatment with anti-inflammatory drugs. These patients usually have a moderate amount of pericardial effusion and as the effusion resolves, the pericardium remains thickened, inflamed and non-compliant, resulting in constrictive haemodynamics. Clinical features include shortness of breath, raised JVP, peripheral oedema and ascites. Constrictive haemodynamics can be documented by Doppler echocardiography and resolution of constrictive physiology can be serially followed by this technique.

What are the indications for drainage of pericardial fluid?

● Overt clinical tamponade, in those with suspicion of purulent pericarditis and in patients with idiopathic chronic large pericardial effusion.
● Tamponade, either unresolved or relapsing after pericardiocentesis, and persistent active illness 3 weeks after hospital admission.

Note: Pericardial drainage is not indicated in the initial management of patients with large pericardial effusions without clinical tamponade because of its low diagnostic yield and poor influence on the evolution of pericardial effusion. Even the presence of right chamber collapse (suggesting raised intrapericardial pressure) on echocardiography does not by itself warrant pericardial drainage because most of these patients do not evolve to overt tamponade.

What is Dressler syndrome?

It is characterized by persistent pyrexia, pericarditis and pleurisy. It was first described in 1956 when Dressler recognized that postmyocardial infarction chest pain is not caused by coronary artery insufficiency. It usually occurs 2–3 weeks after myocardial infarction and is considered to be of autoimmune aetiology; it responds to NSAIDs.

What do you know about postcardiotomy syndrome?

It occurs in about 5% of patients who have cardiac surgery and with symptoms of pericarditis from 3 weeks to 6 months after surgery. It is initially treated with NSAIDs, and with systemic steroids if refractory. Pericardiectomy is rarely required. It is said to be the result of autoimmune response and is most likely to be related to surgical trauma and irritation of blood products in the mediastinum and pericardium.

What are the functions of pericardium?

- The pericardium protects and lubricates the heart.
- It contributes to the diastolic coupling of the LVs and RVs: an effect that is important in cardiac tamponade and constrictive pericarditis.

W Dressler (1890–1969), US physician educated in Vienna. He worked at the Manimoides Hospital, Brooklyn, New York.

34 PRIMARY PULMONARY HYPERTENSION

INSTRUCTION

Listen to this patient's heart.

SALIENT FEATURES

History

- Dyspnoea (60–89%)
- Fatigue (19–73%)
- Syncope, near syncope or dizziness (13–88%)
- Oedema (3–37%)
- Palpitations (5–33%)
- Determine whether the patient is on oral contraceptives, fenfluramine or aminorex (N Engl J Med 1996;335:609–16).
- Determine whether the patient has habitually consumed plant products from *Crotalaria* species (particularly if from the Caribbean).
- Determine whether there is a family history: the chromosome locus 2q31-q32 has been identified in one familial cohort of primary pulmonary hypertension (Circulation 1997;95:2603–6).
- Determine whether the patient is positive for the human immunodeficiency virus (HIV) (HIV-associated pulmonary hypertension is associated with poor prognosis).

Examination

- Young woman
- Loud pulmonary second sound
- Early diastolic murmur of pulmonary regurgitation best heard on inspiration (Graham Steell murmur)
- Examine the chest for chronic lung disease

- Tell the examiner that you would like to:
  - Investigate for a tight or occult mitral stenosis
  - Perform a ventilation–perfusion (V/Q) scan to exclude pulmonary emboli.

DIAGNOSIS

This patient has pulmonary hypertension (lesion) and should be investigated for an underlying cause; she is in cardiac failure (functional status) and belongs to WHO class III (see below).

QUESTIONS

What are the signs of pulmonary hypertension?

- Large 'a' waves in JVP
- Left parasternal heave
- Loud or palpable P_2
- Ejection click in the pulmonary area
- Early diastolic murmur (Graham Steell murmur) caused by pulmonary regurgitation.

ADVANCED-LEVEL QUESTIONS

What is clinical classification of pulmonary hypertension that guides therapy?

National Pulmonary Hypertension Centres of the UK and Ireland Physicians Committee classification (Thorax 2008 63(suppl ii):1–41):

- Pulmonary arterial hypertension: disease-targeted therapies (but caution in venoocclusive disease)
- Pulmonary hypertension with left heart disease: medical, interventional and surgical therapies for chronic heart failure, coronary artery disease, valve disease and pericardial disease
- Pulmonary hypertension associated with lung diseases and/or hypoxaemia: therapy to treat the primary lung disorder, oxygen, disease-targeted therapies when pulmonary hypertension out of proportion to lung disease
- Pulmonary hypertension caused by chronic thrombotic and/or embolic disease: pulmonary endarterectomy (PEA) for proximal disease; disease-targeted therapies for distal disease, significant residual post-PEA pulmonary hypertension or late redevelopment of symptomatic pulmonary hypertension post-PEA
- Miscellaneous: specific to individual diseases.

How would you investigate such a patient?

- Blood investigations include routine haematology and biochemistry, thyroid function, thrombophilia screen in chronic thromboembolic pulmonary hypertension; autoimmune screen (for anti-centromere antibody, anti-SCL70, U1-ribonucleoprotein (U1RNP), anti-phospholipid antibodies, hepatitis serology, serum ACE, HIV.
- Urine for human chorionic gonadotrophin.
- Chest radiograph shows enlarged main pulmonary arteries with reduced peripheral branches, enlargement of the RV.
- Pulmonary function testing includes arterial blood-gas study, 6 min walk test and nocturnal oxygen saturation monitoring.
- ECG will show right ventricular and right atrial hypertrophy.

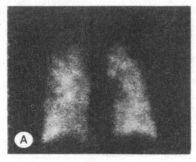 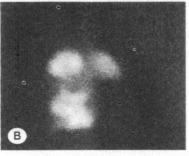

IPAH   PTE

Fig. 34.1 Perfusion–ventilation lung scans in pulmonary hypertension. (A) In idiopathic pulmonary hypertension, there is a mottled distribution in a non-segmental, non-anatomical manner. (B) In pulmonary hypertension caused by a pulmonary thromboembolism there are area-specific defects suggestive of obstructed blood flow. (With permission from Zipes DP et al. 2007.)

- Ventilation–perfusion scan can exclude pulmonary emboli (Fig. 34.1).
- Echocardiography with right heart catheterization and pulmonary angiography.

What are the measurements made during right heart catheterization in such a patient?
National Pulmonary Hypertension Centres of the UK and Ireland Physicians Committee recommendations (Thorax 2008 63(suppl ii): 1–41):
A. Pressure measurements should be made in the following places:
   1. Systemic artery
   2. Pulmonary capillary wedge (or left ventricular end diastolic pressure if not obtainable)
   3. Pulmonary artery
   4. RV
   5. Right atrium
   6. Left atrium (if entered via a patent foramen ovale or atrial septal defect).
B. Blood samples for oximetry should be taken from:
   1. Systemic artery
   2. Left atrium
   3. Pulmonary artery (take 3 saturations and average results).
C. Derived variables to be calculated:
   1. Cardiac output and index
   2. Pulmonary and systemic vascular resistances.

What are the imaging procedures to be considered in such a patient?
The National Pulmonary Hypertension Centres of the UK and Ireland Physicians Committee recommendations (Thorax 2008 63(suppl ii): 1–41):
- *Chest radiography* to looking for increase in cardiac chambers, increased pulmonary artery size, hypoperfused areas of lung and evidence of parenchymal lung disease.

- *High-resolution CT* of lungs to look for parenchymal lung disease, mosaic perfusion (a sign of pulmonary vascular embolism or thrombosis but for which there are other causes such as air trapping) and features of pulmonary venous hypertension.
- *CT pulmonary angiography* to look for enlargement of pulmonary arteries, filling defects and webs in the arteries. Detects enlarged bronchial circulation.
- *Ventilation–perfusion scanning* is more sensitive for chronic pulmonary thromboembolism than CT pulmonary angiography but is not helpful when there is underlying parenchymal lung disease.
- *Selective pulmonary angiography* by direct injection of the pulmonary arteries (Fig. 34.2): gold standard for delineating chronic pulmonary thromboembolism to define the location and extent of disease. It may be superseded by MR angiography or multislice CT.
- *Echocardiography* is the screening tool of choice as it detects cardiac disease (congenital, myocardial, valvular, intracavity clot or tumour, pericardial). Use of contrast may be helpful to identify shunts.
- *Cardiac MRI* is a good tool for imaging the RV and is helpful in delineating congenital heart defects, and the pulmonary circulation by angiography.
- Abdominal ultrasound is used for investigation of liver disease and suspected portal hypertension.

What are the pathological features of primary pulmonary hypertension?

They are those of plexogenic pulmonary arteriopathy (which also occurs in post-tricuspid left-to-right atrial shunts such as ventricular septal defect or patent ductus arteriosus, and collagen vascular diseases), characterized by medial hypertrophy and concentric intimal fibrosis of the pulmonary arteries with complex plexiform lesions. Others have no plexiform lesions or concentric intimal fibrosis but rather have recanalized thrombotic small pulmonary arteries, which are said to be caused by small thrombi or recurrent emboli. The least common histological pattern is veno-occlusive disease.

What are the theories for the cause of primary pulmonary hypertension?

- Excess endothelial production of the vasoconstrictor thromboxane relative to dilator prostaglandins such as prostaglandin I_2 (prostacyclin)
- Excess endothelin-1 levels relative to nitric oxide. Inhaled nitric oxide and endothelin-1 antagonists reduce pulmonary hypertension
- Excessive thrombosis in situ caused by increased platelet activation, plasminogen activator inhibitor levels and decreased thrombomodulin
- Increased sertonin levels
- Inhibition or down regulation of potassium (Kv) channels in pulmonary artery smooth muscle cells and platelets
- Activation of elastase and matrix metalloprotease, which enhances production of mitogens
- Monoclonal proliferation of endothelial cells.

What is the prognosis in pulmonary hypertension?

Untreated prognosis is poor, with median survival of approximately 3 years from the time of diagnosis, with about one-third of patients

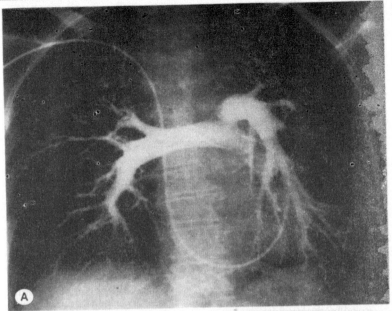

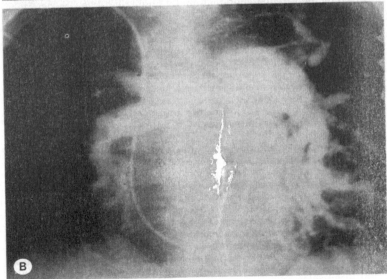

Fig. 34.2 Pulmonary angiograms. (A) Normal; (B) pulmonary arterial hypertension, with marked pruning of peripheral vasculature. (With permission from Albert et al. 2008.)

surviving for 5 years. Death usually occurs suddenly, presumably from arrhythmias or right ventricular infarction.

What are the predictors of survival?

These include indicators of severity of diseases as assessed by measurement of haemodynamic characteristics (mean pulmonary-artery pressure, right atrial pressure, cardiac index and mixed venous oxygen concentration), functional class, exercise tolerance (6-min walk test), anticoagulant therapy and the response to vasodilators. Most patients succumb to progressive right-sided failure, but sudden death accounts for approximately 7% of deaths.

What treatment is available for primary pulmonary hypertension?

- Diuretics: useful in reducing excessive preload in patients with right heart failure, particularly when hepatic congestion and ascites are present.
- Oral anticoagulants: warfarin is the anticoagulant of choice, in doses adjusted to achieve an international normalized ratio (INR) of approximately 2.0. Anticoagulants nearly double the 3-year survival rate (Circulation 1984;70:580–7).
- Calcium channel blockers (nifedipine, diltiazem): patients who respond to calcium channel blockers have a 5-year survival rate of 95% (N Engl J Med 1992;327:76–81).
- Intravenous epoprostenol (formerly prostacyclin): potent short-acting vasodilator and inhibitor of platelet aggregation that is natually produced by the vascular endothelium (N Engl J Med 1996;334:296–301, N Engl J Med 1998;338:273–7).
- Atrial septostomy: the creation of a right-to-left shunt by blade–balloon atrial septostomy has been reported to improve forward output and alleviate right-sided heart failure by providing blood with a low-resistance channel, thereby decompressing the right atrium and improving filling of the left side of the heart (Circulation 1995;91:2028–35).
- Lung transplantation and combined heart–lung transplantation: survival rates after the two procedures are similar. Even markedly depressed right ventricular function improves considerably with single- or double-lung transplantation.
- Other drugs:
  - UT-15, a prostaglandin I analogue, has shown to have sustained and favourable effects in patients when administered subcutaneously (Circulation 2000;102(suppl II):101).
  - Sitaxsentan, an oral selective endothelin A receptor blocker has been shown to produce sustained improvements in pulmonary artery pressure (Circulation 2000;102(suppl II):427).
- PPARγ-activating agents: data suggest that the genes involved in development of pulmonary hypertension are targets of the insulin-sensitizing transcription factor peroxisome proliferator-activated receptor γ (PPARγ), and that PPARγ activation could lead to their beneficial induction or repression and subsequent antiproliferative, anti-inflammatory, proapoptotic and direct vasodilatory effects in the vasculature. PPARγ acts downstream of bone morphogenetic protein receptor II (BMP-RII), which is the cell surface receptor that is mutated or dysfunctional in many forms of pulmonary hypertension. Insulin resistance may be

an environmental risk factor or disease modifier ('second hit'); it has, therefore, been suggested that PPARγ-activating agents might be beneficial in the future treatment of both insulin-resistant and insulin-sensitive PAH patients with or without BMP-RII mutations (Sci Transl Med 2009;1:12–14).

Graham Steell (1851–1942), assistant physician to the Manchester Royal Infirmary, described the murmur in a paper titled 'The murmur of high pressure in the pulmonary artery' (Med Chron (Manchester) 1888;9:182–8).

---

35 EBSTEIN'S ANOMALY

INSTRUCTION

Listen to this patient's heart. He was told he had an innocent murmur during a school medical examination many years ago but now has a large globular heart on chest radiography.

SALIENT FEATURES

History

- An incidental cardiac murmur
- Ask the patient about palpitations (paroxysmal supraventricular tachycardia)
- Symptoms of right-sided heart failure
- History of maternal lithium ingestion.

Examination

- Raised jugular venous pulse; the large 'v' of tricuspid regurgitation is absent because the giant right atrium absorbs most of the regurgitant volume
- Left parasternal heave
- Loud first heart sound produced by the sail-like anterior tricuspid leaflet
- Pansystolic murmur which increases on inspiration
- Hepatomegaly
- Proceed to:
  - ascertain whether the patient has exertional cyanosis or dyspnoea
  - exclude an atrial septal defect.

DIAGNOSIS

This patient has isolated tricuspid regurgitation (lesion) that is probably of congenital aetiology as there is no pulmonary hypertension. He has Ebstein's anomaly with cardiomegaly and cardiac failure (functional status).

ADVANCED-LEVEL QUESTIONS

What is the pathology in Ebstein's anomaly?

The tricuspid leaflets are abnormal and are displaced into the body of the RV. The septal leaflet is variably deficient or even absent. The posterior leaflet is also variably deficient and there is large 'sail-like' anterior leaflet, which is the hallmark of this condition. The anterior leaflet is rarely affected. The abnormally located tricuspid orifice produces a part of the RV lying between the atrioventricular ring and the origin of the valve, which is continuous with the right atrial chamber. This proximal segment is known as the 'atrialized' portion of the RV. Approximately 50% of the patients have either a patent foramen ovale or a secundum atrial septal defect, and 25% have one or more accessory atrioventricular conduction pathways. The anomaly is said to be associated with maternal lithium ingestion.

What are the mechanisms of cyanosis in these patients?

Right-to-left shunting at the atrial level, i.e. through a patent foramen ovale or atrial septal defect.

What are the poor predictors of outcome?

- The earlier the presentation higher the risk of mortality
- A large right atrium or cardiothoracic ratio >60%
- Severe right outflow tract abnormalities.

How would you investigate such a patient?

- *Chest radiography* (Fig. 35.1) shows the large right atrium with oligaemic lung fields.
- *ECG* shows right bundle branch block, prolonged PR interval, P pulmonale (indicating right atrial enlargement), large P waves (Himalayan P waves), type B Wolff–Parkinson–White syndrome (where the QRS complex is downward in lead V_1) (Fig. 35.2B). (**Note**: Wolff–Parkinson–White syndrome comprises a trial of short PR interval, delta wave and wide QRS complex.) Approximately 10% of patients with Ebstein's anomaly have the Wolff–Parkinson–White syndrome.
- *Echocardiography* characteristic findings include the abnormal positional relation between the tricuspid valve and mitral valve with septal displacement of the septal tricuspid leaflet.
- *Cardiac catheterization* has no place in classical cases as in the past it has been associated with serious morbidity and mortality.

What are the indications for surgery?

- Severe functional limitation
- A cardiothoracic ratio >60%
- An atrial communication and if the patient has cyanosis (caused by risk of stroke)
- Accessory pathway is present
- Severe tricuspid regurgitation.

How are such patients treated?

- Tricuspid valve replacement plus closure of atrial septal defect
- Tricuspid annuloplasty with plication of the atrialized portion of the RV.

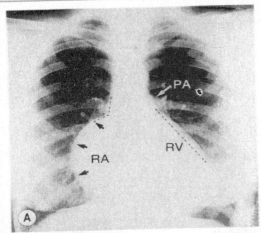

Fig. 35.1 Ebstein's anomaly. (A) A giant right atrium (RA) causes a shoulder along the right cardiac silhouette (arrows). A giant right ventricular (RV) outflow tract causes the left cardiac border to be straight; the pulmonary artery (PA) is very small. (B) The left atrium (LA) and left ventricle (LV) are essentially normal, but the RA and RV are filling in the retrosternal space (arrows). (With permission from Mettler 2004.)

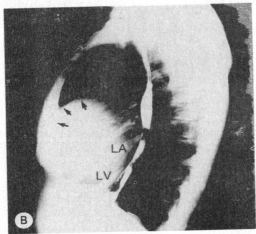

Wilhelm Ebstein (1836–1912), German physician who also described the Armanni–Ebstein nephropathy (where there is glycogen vacuolation in the proximal convoluted tubules)
    L Armanni (1839–1903) was an Italian pathologist.

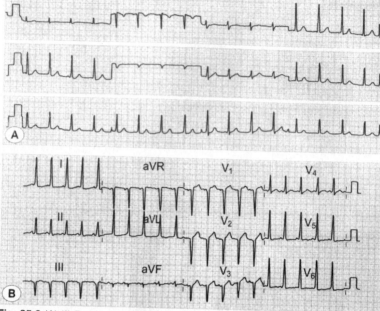

Fig. 35.2 Wolff–Parkinson–White syndrome. (A) Type A. The delta wave is recognized clearly in leads II, III, aVF, and V₁ through V₄. (B) Type B. The tracing also shows left ventricular hypertrophy. Tachycardia can be seen, which may be caused by a re-entry phenomenon.

Neurology
History and examination of the nervous system

HISTORY

- Note the mnemonic SHOVE:
  Syncope, speech defect, swallowing difficulty
  Headache
  Ocular disturbances: diplopia, field defects
  Vertigo
  Epilepsy: seizures.
- History pertaining to motor and sensory components of the cranial nerves and limbs (e.g. pain, paraesthesia, weakness, incoordination).

EXAMINATION OF THE CRANIAL NERVES

First cranial nerve

- Ask the patient, 'Have you noticed any change in your sense of smell recently?' 'Can you differentiate between the odour of tea, coffee and bananas?'
- If the examiner requires you to test the sense of smell, use an odour that can be readily identified, such as soap or clove oil. If the patient has frequent nasal troubles, the value of this examination is limited.

Second cranial nerve

- First check visual acuity with a pocket Snellen's chart and finger counting.
- Make sure that the patient is their spectacles should they use them, as one is not concerned with refractive errors.
- Check visual fields with a white hat pin (10 mm in diameter); your instructions to the patient should be clear and precise. Smaller hat pins (5 mm in diameter) are used for detecting small scotomata. Red hat pins, for reasons that are not clear, are useful in the detection of pregeniculate lesions and are, therefore, useful in compression of the optic nerve, optic chiasm or optic tract.
- Comment on the pupils (size, shape or inequality) and test their reaction to light (direct and indirect reaction) and to accommodation. The popular acronym PERRLA (pupils equal, round and reactive to light and accommodation) is a convenient description of normal pupillomotor function.
- Examine the fundus in a definite sequence: retina, retinal vessels, optic nerve and macula.

Third, fourth and sixth cranial nerves

Test eye movements:

- The Parks–Bielschowsky three-step test is used to determine which muscle is weak in a patient who has a vertical deviation because of a weakness in a single muscle:
  - Step 1: determine which eye is hypertropic; paralysis of the superior oblique is one cause of hypertropia

- Step 2: determine whether the hypertropia is greater in left or right gaze; hypertropia caused by superior oblique paralysis is greater on gaze to the contralateral side
- Step 3: determine whether the hypertropia is greater in left or right head tilt; hypertropia caused by superior oblique paralysis is greater in a head tilt to the ipsilateral side
- A further step 4 can confirms that the correct muscle has been identified and helps to rule out other causes of vertical deviation: determine whether the hypertrophia is worse in upgaze or downgaze.

- Remember to ask the patient if they see a double image: this is the most sensitive sign of defective eye movement and may be present even when there is no apparent weakness of extraocular muscle or an abnormality of gaze.
- *Saccadic movements* are tested by asking the patient to look voluntarily to the right and left and up and down. Note whether these movements are carried out rapidly to the extremes of gaze.
- *Pursuit movements* are examined by asking the patient to follow an object moved to the right and left and up and down.

Note whether these movements are carried out smoothly without interruption.

- Remember to comment on nystagmus: nystagmus is a repetitive drift of the eyeball away from the point of fixation, followed by a fast corrective movement towards it.
- Comment on ptosis if present (seen in third nerve palsy).

Fifth cranial nerve

- Test the masseters: 'Clench your teeth'; take care to palpate the muscles.
- Test the pterygoids: 'Open your mouth'; note the jaw deviates to the side of the lesion.
- Test corneal (not conjunctival) sensation by touching a wisp of cotton-wool to the cornea while the patient looks upward and away from the examiner.
- Test facial sensation: keep in mind that this nerve supplies not only the face but also the anterior half of the scalp. Impairment of sensation limited to the face only is usually psychogenic in origin.
- Test jaw jerk: ask the patient to have his or her mouth half open; place your thumb over the patient's chin and lightly tap on the thumb. A mild jaw jerk or absent jerk is seen in normal individuals. In upper motor neuron lesions above the cervical cord, the jaw will manifest a marked jerk with this procedure.

Seventh cranial nerve

Remember that the facial nerve is a motor nerve:
- Test the lower half of the face: 'Show me your teeth'. Note the nasiolabial fold, which often disappears in mild facial palsy.
- Test the upper half of the face: 'Screw your eyes tightly shut and don't let me open them'.
- Ask the patient to wrinkle his or her forehead and note the movement of the muscles of the forehead.

Note: Taste may be lost on the anterior two-thirds of the tongue, but this is not usually tested.

Eighth cranial nerve

- Test by bringing a watch from beyond auditory acuity into the zone of hearing.
- Occlude each external auditory meatus with your finger and whisper short phrases, asking the patient to repeat them.
- Perform Rinne's and Weber's tests (use a tuning fork with a frequency of 256 or 512 cycles/s). Normally air conduction is better than bone conduction:
  - Rinne's test: in obstructive deafness, bone conduction is better; in nerve deafness the normal relations are kept (i.e. air conduction is greater than bone conduction in the deaf ear)
  - Weber's test: if the base of the tuning fork is placed on the middle of the forehead of a person with an obstructive deafness, she will hear it better in the deaf ear; with a nerve deafness, the fork will be heard better in the normal ear.

Ninth and tenth cranial nerves

- Ask the patient 'Open your mouth and say "aah"'; observe the soft palate with a torch (the soft palate is pulled to the normal side on saying 'aah').
- Tell the examiner that you would like to check the gag reflex. An absence of gag reflex is significant only if it is unilateral.

Eleventh cranial nerves

- Ask the patient 'Shrug your shoulders'; try to push them down simultaneously (this tests the trapezii muscles).
- Test the sternomastoids by the patient's ability to resist lateral movement of the neck. Keep in mind that one rotates the head to the *right* by use of the *left* sternomastoid muscle.

Twelfth cranial nerve

- Ask the patient, 'Open your mouth'; comment on fasciculations of the tongue while in the mouth. Comment on wasting.
- Ask the patient, 'Stick out your tongue'; the tongue will deviates to the side of the lesion but a slight deviation of the tongue can be disregarded.

NEUROLOGICAL EXAMINATION OF THE UPPER LIMBS

1. Introduce yourself to the patient and ask him to take his top off so that both his arms are well exposed. If the patient is female, cover her breasts with suitable clothing so that she is decent.
2. Comment on wasting, tremor (p. 221), fasciculations.
3. Assess tone: 'Let your arms go loose and let me move them from you':
   - Flex and extend wrists passively: cogwheel rigidity is elicited by this method
   - Flex and extend at the elbows, pronate and supinate at the forearm: lead-pipe rigidity and clasp-knife spasticity is elicited by these methods.
4. Test power: 'I am going to test the strength of the muscles of your arms' Ask the patient the following, evaluating strength on a scale of 0 to 5:
   - 'Hold your arms stretched out in front of you and then close your eyes': observe for drift, action tremor

- 'Hold your arms outwards at your sides (like this) and keep them up; don't let me stop you': shoulder abduction, the chief movers are the deltoids C5. (**Note:** supraspinatus is responsible for the initiation of abduction and for the first 60 degrees of this movement but this method of testing only assesses the power of the deltoids)
- 'Push your arms in towards you and don't let me stop you': shoulder adduction, chief movers are the pectoral muscles, C6–C8
- 'Bend your elbows and pull me towards you; don't let me stop you': elbow flexion, chief mover is the biceps, C5
- 'Straighten your elbows and push me away; don't let me stop you': elbow extension, chief mover is the triceps, C7
- 'Clench your fist and cock your wrists up; don't let me stop you': wrist extension, chief mover is C7
- 'Now push the other way': wrist flexion, chief mover is C7 (Fig. II.1)
- 'Spread your fingers wide apart and don't let me push them together': finger abduction, chief movers are the dorsal interossei, T1 (ulnar nerve). (**Note:** Dorsal interossei abduct mnemonic, DAB.)
- 'Hold this piece of paper between your fingers and don't let me snatch it away': finger adduction, chief movers are the palmar interossei T1 (ulnar nerve). (**Note:** Palmar interossei adduct mnemonic, PAD)
- 'Hold your palms facing the ceiling and now point your thumb towards the ceiling; don't let me stop you': thumb abduction, chief mover is the abductor pollicis brevis, C8, T1 (median nerve)
- 'Grip these two fingers of mine tightly and don't let them go': flexion of fingers, chief movers are the long and short flexors of the fingers, C8.

Notes

- The median nerve supplies the lateral two lumbricals, opponens pollicis, abductor pollicis brevis, flexor pollicis brevis (mnemonic, LOAF).
- The ulnar nerve supplies all other small muscles of the hand.
- The lumbricals are responsible for flexion at the metacarpophalangeal joint when the interphalangeal joints are in extension.
- Power is graded from 0 to 5:
  0, absence of movement
  1, flicker of movement on voluntary contraction
  2, movement present when gravity is eliminated
  3, movement against gravity but not against resistance
  4, movement against resistance but not full strength
  5, normal power.

5. Test deep tendon reflexes: (Fig. II.1E):
   - Biceps jerk, C5, C6
   - Triceps, C7
   - Supinator, C5, C6.

Notes

- If the reflexes are absent, test after reinforcement: ask the patient to clench his or her teeth.
- Inversion of the supinator reflex. When the supinator jerk is elicited the normal response is a slight flexion of the fingers, contraction of the brachioradialis and flexion at the elbow joint. The jerk is said to be 'inverted' when finger flexion is the sole response, with contraction of

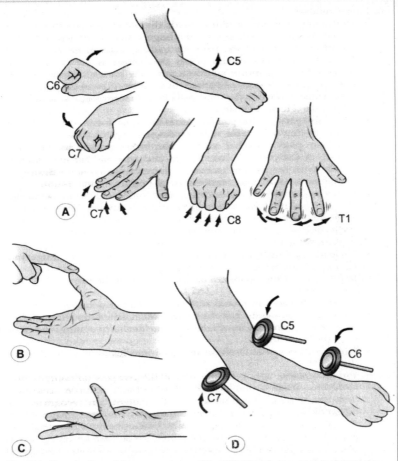

Fig. II.1 Examination of the upper extremities. (A) Muscle groups, designated by their respective nerve root innervation. These a e C5, elbow flexion; C6, wrist extension; C7, finger extension; C8, finger flexion and T1, finger abduction. (B,C) Motor innervation of muscles of the hand. (B) Thumb abduction tests median motor nerve function. (C) Little finger flexion at the metacarpophalangeal joint with simultaneous interphalangeal joint extension tests ulnar motor nerve function. (D) Stretch reflexes and nerve roots of origin.

the brachioradialis and elbow flexion being absent. There is associated absence of the biceps jerk and exaggeration of the triceps jerk.
- The inverted jerk indicates a lower motor neuron lesion at the fifth cervical level and an upper motor neuron lesion below this level. It could be caused by cervical spondylosis, trauma to the cervical cord, spinal cord tumours at this level and syringomyelia.

6. Finger reflexes:
   - Hoffman's sign: the examiner holds the patient's wrist in the horizontal pronated position with the fingers and wrists relaxed. Then the distal phalanx of the patient's middle finger is forcibly flexed. Normally no reflex occurs unless the patient is under emotional tension. In upper motor neuron lesions, the patient's thumb undergoes a quick flexion–adduction–opposition movement while the other fingers move in flexion–adduction. This response is labelled as a 'positive' Hoffman's sign.
   - Wartenberg's sign: the patient places his or her hand in partial supination resting on a table with the fingers slightly flexed. Then the examiner places his/her middle and index fingers on the volar surface of the patient's four fingers and taps his/her own fingers briskly with the tendon hammer. The response is one of flexion of the patient's four fingers and the distal phalanx of the thumb.
   - Mayer's sign: with the patient's thumb abducted and the hand relaxed, the proximal phalanx of the middle finger is forcibly flexed towards the palm. Normally the thumb adducts. In upper motor neuron lesions the thumb usually remains in the position of abduction.
7. Test coordination:
   - Finger–nose–finger test: 'Touch your nose with your index finger and now touch my finger'.
   - Rapid alternating movement of one hand over the other.
8. Test sensation:
   - Light touch: use cottonwool and check each dermatome.
   - Pinprick: demonstrate first the sharp end and then the blunt end on the sternum; then check each dermatome for sharp or blunt sensation with the eyes closed.
   - Joint position sense: check in the distal interphalangeal joint of the thumb.
   - Vibration sense: use a tuning fork of 128 cycles/s (although some authorities believe that a fork of 64 cycles/s is more accurate). First test on the sternum so that the patient can recognize the vibration and then check over the fingers, moving proximally if the vibration sense is absent distally. Pallaesthesia is the ability to perceive the presence of vibration when an oscillating tuning fork is placed over certain bony prominences. Loss of vibratory perception is referred to as pallanaesthesia.

Remember:
- joint sense and vibration sense are carried in the dorsal columns
- pain and temperature are carried in the lateral spinothalamic tracts
- light touch is carried in both the above tracts.

NEUROLOGICAL EXAMINATION OF THE LOWER LIMBS

1. Introduce yourself and then ensure that the lower limbs are well exposed. It is important to ensure that the patient is decent – cover the genital area with a towel or any suitable clothing.
2. Inspect for wasting, fasciculations (tap the muscles of the leg and thigh to elicit fasciculations if not seen).
3. Assess tone:
   - Ask the patient, 'Let your leg go loose and lax, and let me move it for you'; then passively flex and extend the leg at the knee and hip:

- Roll the extended leg, feeling for resistance
- Put your hand behind the knee and pull it upwards, observing the foot to check whether or not it flops
- If there is spasticity or increased tone, then test for ankle clonus and patellar clonus.
  - *Patellar clonus.* With the patient in the supine position, grasp the upper edge of the patella between the thumb and index finger and apply a quick constant pressure in a downward direction. Avoid prolonging this manoeuvre as it is often painful to the patient. In upper motor neuron lesions the patella may manifest a few jerks (unsustained clonus) or a constant jerking as long as the pressure is applied (sustained clonus).
  - *Ankle clonus.* Ensure that the patient's knee is semiflexed and the foot relaxed. The foot is suddenly pushed dorsally with moderate force and held there. In upper motor neuron lesions, the posterior muscles of the leg will enter into a persistent contraction.

4. Test power (begin at the hips): 'I am going to test the strength of the muscles of your legs'; then ask the patient to:
   - 'lift your leg straight up and keep it there; don't let me stop you': hip flexion, chief mover is iliopsoas L1, L2
   - 'push your leg downwards into your bed and don't let me stop you': hip extension, chief movers are glutei, L4, L5
   - 'push your thigh inwards against my hand': chief movers are adductors of the thigh, L2–4 (Fig. II.2A)
   - 'bend your knee and pull your heel towards you; don't let me stop you': knee flexion, chief movers are the hamstrings, L5, S1
   - 'straighten your knee and don't let me stop you': knee extension, chief movers are quadriceps, L3, L4
   - 'push your foot downwards against my hand': plantar flexion of the ankle, chief mover is the gastrocnemius, S1
   - 'move your foot up and don't let me stop you': dorsiflexion of the ankle, chief movers are the tibialis anterior and long extensors, L4, L5
   - 'push your foot inwards against my hand': inversion of the foot, chief movers are tibialis anterior and posterior, L4
   - 'push your foot outwards against my hand': eversion of the foot, chief movers are the peronei, S1
   - 'pull your toe upwards and don't let me stop you': extension of the great toe, chief mover is the extensor hallucis longus, L5.

5. Test the plantar response: (Fig. II.2B) 'I am going to tickle the bottom of your foot'; use an orange stick to stimulate the outer portion of the sole and then across the ball to the base of the big toe. Always describe the response as either downgoing or upgoing. Normally the response is downgoing (i.e. all the toes flex towards the plantar surface). Upgoing plantars or the Babinski response (Fig. II.2C) is a feature of upper motor neuron lesions where the four small toes fan and turn towards the sole while the big toe extends dorsally. There is associated slight flexion of the hip and knee. The contraction of the tensor fasciae lata is referred to as the Brissaud's reflex and is a part of the spinal defence reflex mechanism. Other responses to plantar stimulation include the quick avoidance response, the grasp reflex and the support reaction. Remember that if the feet are cold (when outside the bedclothes for long) the response may be equivocal.

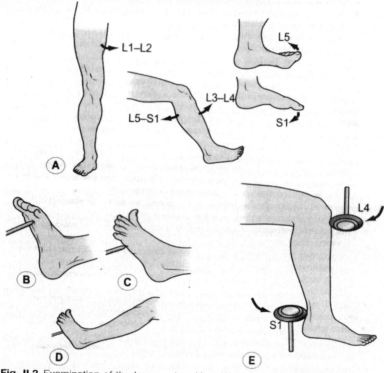

Fig. II.2 Examination of the lower extremities. (A) Muscle groups, designated by their respective nerve root innervation: L1–L2, hip abductors; L3–L4, knee extension; L5–S1, knee flexion; L5, great toe extension; S1, great toe flexion. (B) Plantar reflex. (C) Babinski sign. (D) Triple flexion response. (E) Stretch reflexes and nerve roots of origin.

6. Test deep tendon reflexes (Fig. II.2E):
   - Knee jerk, L4
   - Ankle jerk, S1. In the elderly, the plantar-strike technique is said to be more reliable than the tendon-striking method for eliciting ankle jerks. The plantar-strike technique of eliciting ankle jerks is as follows: the patient's legs are side by side and the foot is passively dorsiflexed; the reflex hammer strikes the examiner's own fingers, which are placed over the plantar surface.
   - When the reflexes are absent, reinforce by asking the patient to pull outwards his or her clasped hands (Jendrassik manoeuvre). Do not tie your hands into a knot while testing the left ankle jerk from the patient's right-hand side. Avoid jabbing the patient while eliciting reflexes.

Notes

- By convention, deep tendon reflexes are graded as follows:
  0, no response, abnormal
  1+, slight but definitely present response which may be normal or abnormal
  2+, brisk response, normal
  3+, very brisk response, which may be normal or abnormal
  4+, a tap elicits clonus, abnormal
- Asymmetry of reflexes suggests abnormality.
7. Test coordination:
   - Heel–shin test. Have the patient place the heel of one foot upon the knee of the opposite leg, and then move the heel downwards along the tibia. In a positive test, the patient has difficulty placing or holding the heel on the opposite knee or cannot keep the heel firmly on the tibia as the heel is moved downwards.
8. Test sensation. Avoid testing in a given rhythm where the patient can expect to be stimulated at a given time. Always compare sensory responses in different areas of the same side of the body, as well as the two sides of the body:
   - Light touch
   - Pinprick: test irregularly with the pin-point and pin-head, asking the patient whether the perceived sensation is sharp or blunt
   - Joint position sense: hold the lateral aspect of the patient's big toe (not the dorsum of the toe) while eliciting this and move the toe gently up and down; the examiner's fingers should not rub against the skin of the adjoining toe during this test and the joint should not be put in the extreme position of flexion during the test
   - Vibration sense.

Note: When there is weakness of the limbs, tell the examiner that you would like to check sensation in the sacral area.

9. Romberg's test: 'Please stand up with your legs together and now close your eyes'. Take care to protect the patient if he or she sways or tends to fall. A positive test result is shown by pronounced swaying of the trunk. Sometimes functional cases will sway without having a true Romberg. This may be proved by diverting the attention of the patient by instituting the finger–nose test at the same time as Romberg is being tested. In functional cases the 'rombergism' will usually disappear.
10. Check gait and, if the heel–shin test is affected, then test tandem walking (asking the patient to walk along a straight line with one heel in front of the other foot). *Candidates frequently forget to check the gait when asked to examine the legs.*
11. Special manoeuvres in suspected upper motor neuron lesions:
    - Rossalimo's sign: the undersurface of the patient's toes are tapped with the examiner's fingers to produce abrupt extension (dorsiflexion) of the toes. In normal individuals, there is no response, whereas in patients with upper motor neuron lesions all the toes respond with a quick plantar flexion.
    - In upper motor neuron lesions, the big toe will often dorsiflex (i.e. upgoing toe) when any of the following manoeuvres is conducted:
      - Gordon reflex: on applying pressure to the muscle of the calf
      - Oppenheim sign: on applying heavy pressure with the thumb and index finger to the shin, stroking downwards from below the knee down to the ankle

- Bing reflex: when the dorsum of the toe is pricked with a pin
- Schaefer reflex: pinching the Achilles tendon enough to cause pain
- Chaddock reflex: on stroking the lateral side of the foot, beginning below the malleolus and extending anteriorly along the dorsum of the foot to the base of the big toe
- Gonda reflex: grasping the small toes between the fingers, slowly and forcibly flex the toe and then suddenly release the toe.

APPROACH TO A MYOPATHIC PATIENT

There are six key questions (Neurology 2009;73:1592–7):
1. Does the patient have negative or positive signs and symptoms?
    - Negative: weakness, fatigue, atrophy
    - Positive: pain. crampls, contractures, stiffness, hypertrophy.
2. What is the timing of the weakness, pain or stiffness?
    - Constant or episodic
    - Monophasic or relapsing
    - Age at onset
    - Lifelong
    - Progressive or non-progressive.
3. What is the distribution of weakess?
    - Proxmial arms/legs
    - Distal arms/legs
    - Proximal and distal
    - Neck
    - Cranial: ocular, pharyngeal, facial, atrophy/hypertrophy.
4. Are there triggering events?
    - During or immediately after exercise
    - After brief or prolonged exercise
    - After exercise followed by rest
    - After carbohydrate meal
    - Relieved by exercise drugs/toxins
    - Temperature (internal/external).
5. Family history of myopathy?
6. Any associated medical conditions?
    - Rash
    - Baldness
    - Fever
    - By organ system.

HA Rinne (1819–1868), German ear, nose and throat physician.
  FE Weber-Liel (1832–1891), a German otologist.
  JJ Babinski (1857–1932), of Polish origin, graduated from the University of Paris with a thesis on multiple sclerosis. The Babinski response refers to upgoing plantars in upper motor neuron lesions. He described adiposogenitalis a year before Frolich.

36 BILATERAL SPASTIC PARALYSIS (SPASTIC PARAPLEGIA)

INSTRUCTION

Carry out a neurological examination of this patient's lower limbs.

SALIENT FEATURES

History

- Ask about onset, duration and course of symptoms
- Back pain: whether localized
- Ask about radicular pain
- Numbness and parasthesia particularly below the level of lesion
- Weakness: whether gradual or sudden
- Sphincter control and bladder sensation
- Functional status: wheelchair transfers, walking aids, orthotic shoes and whether house has been modified for the patient's disability
- Take a family history (hereditary spastic paraplegia)
- Take a history of birth anoxia (cerebral palsy)
- History of urinary infections, pressure sores and deep venous thromboses.

Examination

- Increased tone in both lower limbs
- Hyperreflexia
- Ankle clonus
- Weakness in both lower limbs
- Wasting
- Then proceed to:
  - Check the sensory level
  - Examine the spine (spinal tenderness or deformity).
- Tell the examiner that you would like to do the following:
  - Check sacral sensation
  - Examine the hands to rule out involvement of upper limbs
  - Check for cerebellar signs (multiple sclerosis, Friedreich's ataxia).
- Try to localize the level of lesion using the following:
  - Spasticity of the lower limb alone: lesion of thoracic cord (T2–L1)
  - Irregular spasticity of lower limbs with flaccid weakness of scattered muscles of lower limbs: lesion of lumbosacral enlargement (L2–S2)
  - Radicular pain: useful early in the disease, with time becomes diffuse and ceases to have localizing value
  - Superficial sensation: not good for localizing as the level of sensory loss may vary greatly in different individuals and in different types of lesions.

DIAGNOSIS

This patient has bilateral spastic paraparesis (lesion) at L1 spinal level caused by trauma (aetiology); it is complicated by bladder involvement (functional status).

QUESTIONS

What are the causes of spastic paraparesis?

Youth:

- Trauma
- Multiple sclerosis
- Friedreich's ataxia
- HIV.

Adults:

- Multiple sclerosis
- HIV (Neurology 1989;39:892)
- Trauma (motor vehicle or diving accident)
- Spinal cord tumour (meningioma, neuroma)
- Motor neuron disease
- Syringomyelia
- Subacute combined degeneration of the cord (associated peripheral neuropathy)
- Tabes dorsalis
- Transverse myelitis
- Familial spastic paraplegia.

Elderly:

- Osteoarthritis of the cervical spine
- Vitamin deficiency
- Metastatic carcinoma
- Anterior spinal artery thrombosis
- Atherosclerosis of spinal cord vasculature.

ADVANCED-LEVEL QUESTIONS

What intracranial cause for spastic paraparesis do you know?
Parasagittal falx meningioma.

What do you know about transverse myelitic syndrome?

- Causes include trauma, compression by bony changes or tumour, vascular disease.
- All the tracts of the spinal cord are involved.
- The chief clinical manifestation is spastic or flaccid paralysis.
- The lesion can be incomplete cord compression or total cord transection.

	Total cord transection	Incomplete cord compression
Paraplegia in flexion	+	+
Paralysis	Symmetrical	Asymmetrical
Flexor-withdrawal reflex	+ without return (withdrawal phase only	Associated with return to original position
Other	Vasomotor and sphincter changes	Variable area of anaesthesia that is not consistent with motor loss

What do you know about paraplegia-in-flexion?
Paraplegia-in-flexion is seen in partial transection of the cord where the limbs are involuntarily flexed at the hips and knees because the extensors

are more paralysed than the flexors. In complete transection of the spinal cord, the extrapyramidal tracts are also affected and hence no voluntary movement of the limb is possible, resulting in paraplegia-in-extension.

What investigations would you do?

- CBC for anaemia
- ESR for infection
- Serology: syphilis, vitamin B_{12}, prostate-specific antigen (PSA) and serum acid phosphatase; and serum protein electrophoresis
- MRI of the spine (Fig. 36.1)
- CT myelography, or plain CT
- CT of the head to exclude parasagittal meningiomas
- Check CSF (CSF) for oligoclonal bands.
- Serum vitamin B_{12} levels.

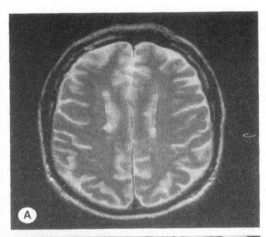

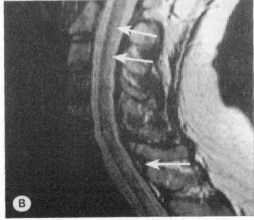

Fig. 36.1 T_2-weighted MRI of brain (A) and spinal cord (B) in progressive spastic paraplegia (lesions arrowed). (With permission from Compston et al. 2005.)

Where is the lesion in patients with spastic weakness of one leg?

The lesion may be localized to the spinal cord or the brain. Progression to involve the arm does not help to differentiate between the spinal cord or the brain. Similarly, spread to the opposite leg does not necessarily indicate that the lesion is the spinal cord. Full investigation would include radiography of the spine, CT and MRI with spinal angiography to exclude spinal dural arteriovenous fistula.

What do you know about hereditary spastic paraplegia?

This is an autosomal dominant condition, first described by Seeligmuller and Strumpell, in which spasticity is more striking than muscular weakness. The age of onset is variable and the condition has a relatively benign course. When the onset is in childhood, there may be shortening of the Achilles tendon, often requiring surgical lengthening. There is usually no sensory disturbance. An autosomal dominant form of hereditary spastic paraplegia is associated with mutations in the mitochondrial import chaperonin HSP60 (Am J Hum Genet 2002;70:1328–32). An autosomal recessive form of hereditary spastic paraplegia is the result of mutations in the gene *SPG7*, which encodes paraplegin, a mitochondrial protein similar to yeast metalloproteases (Cell 1998;93:973–83).

What do you know about tropical spastic paraplegia?

This is seen in Japan, the Caribbean and parts of western Africa and South America where women, more often than men, in their third and fourth decades have spastic paraparesis with neurogenic bladder. Viral infection with human T-lymphotrophic virus 1 has been implicated as a cause of this disorder.

How do you localize the lesion to the second and third lumbar root level?

- Muscular weakness: hip flexors and quadriceps
- Deep tendon reflexes affected: knee jerk
- Radicular pain/paraesthesia: anterior aspect of thigh, groin and testicle
- Superficial sensory deficit: anterior thigh.

How do you localize the lesion to the fourth lumbar root level?

- Muscular weakness: quadriceps, tibialis anterior and posterior
- Deep tendon reflexes affected: knee jerk
- Radicular pain/paraesthesia: anteromedial aspect of the leg
- Superficial sensory deficit: anteromedial aspect of the leg.

How do you localize the lesion to the fifth lumbar root level?

- Muscular weakness: hamstrings, peroneus longus, extensors of all the toes
- Deep tendon reflexes affected: none
- Radicular pain/paraesthesia: buttock, posterolateral thigh, anterolateral leg, dorsum of foot
- Superficial sensory deficit: dorsum of the foot and anterolateral aspect of the leg.

How do you localize the lesion to the first sacral root level?

- Muscular weakness: plantar flexors, extensor digitorum brevis, peroneus longus and hamstrings
- Deep tendon reflexes affected: ankle jerk

- Radicular pain/paraesthesia: buttock, back of thigh, calf and lateral border of the foot
- Superficial sensory deficit: lateral border of the foot.

How do you localize the lesion to the lower sacral root level?
- Muscular weakness: none
- Deep tendon reflexes affected: none (but anal reflex impaired)
- Radicular pain/paraesthesia: buttock and back of thigh
- Superficial sensory deficit: saddle and perianal areas.

What is the characteristic type of diplegia in cerebral palsy?
Diplegia associated with prematurity is a striking clinical entity—striking for the symmetry of neurological signs, for their distribution, for the relatively good intelligence of the patients and for the comparative absence of seizures; the disability is often purely motor without sensory deficits.

What surgical treatment is available for the management of spastic diplegia in cerebral palsy?
Dorsal rhizotomy may be beneficial in selected patients.

What are the clinical features of spinal cord compression from epidural metastasis?
The initial symptom is progressive axial pain, referred or radicular, which may last for days to months. Recumbency frequently aggravates the pain, unlike the pain of degenerative joint disease where it is relieved. Weakness, sensory loss and incontinence typically develop after the pain. Once a neurological deficit appears, it can evolve rapidly to paraplegia over a period of hours to days. In suspected cases, MRI of the spine must be done by the next day. About 50% of cases in adults arise from breast, lung or prostate cancer. Compression usually occurs in the setting of disseminated disease. It is at the thoracic level in 70% of cases, lumbar in 20% and cervical in 10%, and it ccurs at multiple, non-contiguous levels in less than half of the cases. The tumour usually occupies the anterior or anterolateral spinal canal. CSF findings are non-specific in metastatic epidural compression. The cell count is usually normal, but protein levels may be raised because the flow of CSF is impeded. Lumbar puncture has been known to worsen the neurological deficit, presumably caused by impaction of the cord.

37 HEMIPLEGIA

INSTRUCTION
Carry out a neurological examination of this patient.

SALIENT FEATURES

History
- Obtain history of headache, seizures and loss of consciousness (more common in subarachnoid haemorrhage or intracerebral bleeds than in cerebral infarction)
- History of speech defects, sensory loss and weakness of face and limbs

- Risk factors: hypertension, smoking, diabetes mellitus
- History of functional status: swallowing, mobility, pressure sores, independence in activities of daily living, visual difficulties (for visual field defects).

Examination

- Unilateral upper motor neuron seventh nerve palsy.
- The arm is held to the side, the elbow is flexed and the fingers and wrist are flexed on to the chest.
- The leg is extended at both the hip and knee, while the foot is plantar flexed and inverted.
- Weakness of the upper and lower limbs on the same side with upper motor neuron signs: increased tone, hyper-reflexia and upgoing plantar response.
- Hemiplegic weakness of the upper limbs affects the shoulder abductor, elbow extensors, wrist and finger extensors, and small hand muscles.
- Hemiplegic weakness of the lower limbs affects hip flexors, knee flexors and dorsiflexors and evertors of the foot.
- Do not forget sensory signs, in particular joint sensation which is important in rehabilitation.
- Proceed by examining for:
  - homonymous hemianopia and sensory inattention
  - Horners syndrome (p. 176): contralateral to hemiplegia suggests carotid dissection
  - carotid bruits
  - speech defects
  - atrial fibrillation with the pulse
  - murmurs from the heart.
- Tell the examiner that you would like to check the patient's BP and check the urine for sugar.

DIAGNOSIS

This patient has had a stroke causing a right or left hemiplegia (lesion), which can be the result of either a vascular event, such as thrombosis, embolism or haemorrhage, or a neoplasm of the brain (aetiology). This patient is limited by hemiplegia and hemianopia (functional status).

QUESTIONS

What are the causes of hemiplegia?

About 80% of all strokes are caused by cerebral infarction resulting from thrombotic or embolic occlusion of a cerebral artery (J Neurol Neurosurg Psych 1990;53:16–22). The remainder 20% are caused by either intra-cerebral or subarachnoid haemorrhage.

Elderly:

- Vascular event (thrombosis, embolism or haemorrhage)
- Tumour
- Subdural haematoma
- Syphilis.

Youth:

- Multiple sclerosis
- Tumour

- Trauma
- Embolism: look for underlying valvular heart disease and atrial fibrillation
- Connective tissue disorder
- Neurosyphilis
- Intracranial infection: look for underlying acquired immunodeficiency syndrome (AIDS), otitis media, cyanotic heart disease.

How would you manage such a patient?

- Early hospital admission preferably to a dedicated stroke unit, which has been shown to produce long-term reductions in death, dependency and need for institutional care (BMJ 1997;314:1151–9)
- Aspirin given within 48 h of ischaemic stroke reduces the risk of death and recurrent stroke. The International Stroke Trial (Lancet 1997;349:1569–81) and the Chinese Stroke Trial (Lancet 1997;349:1641–9), each involved 20 000 patients and found that aspirin was associated with about 10 fewer deaths or recurrent strokes, but with slightly more haemorrhagic strokes. The International Stroke Trial reported no benefit from subcutaneous heparin given with or without aspirin
- FBC, ESR
- Urine sugar
- ECG
- Chest radiography
- Echocardiography (looking for source of emboli), CT and carotid digital subtraction angiography (DSA) in selected patients
- Carotid Doppler: prior to endartrectomy, presurgical evaluation of saccular aneurysm
- MRI: diffusion-weighted sequences allow early detection. MRI has a much higher sensitivity than CT for acute ischaemic changes, especially in the posterior fossa and in the first hours after an ischaemic stroke
- Physiotherapy, speech therapy and occupational therapy
- Control of risk factors: hypertension, hyperlipidaemia and diabetes; stop smoking and oral contraceptives.

Discuss the importance of blood pressure reduction in a patient with acute ischemic stroke

Randomized clinical trials suggest that patients with acute ischemic stroke treated with antihypertensive agents may have an adverse clinical outcome and increased mortality (BMJ 1988;296:737–41, Cerebrovasc Dis 1994;4:204–10).

ADVANCED-LEVEL QUESTIONS

What are the measures used to determine the outcome after an acute stroke?

Some of the standard measures include:

- Barthel index: reliable and valid measure of the ability to perform activities of daily living such as eating, bathing, walking and using the toilet.
- Modified Rankin Scale: simplified overall assessment of function in which a score of 0 indicates the absence of symptoms and a score of 5 shows severe disability.
- Glasgow Outcome Scale: global assessment of function in which a score of 1 indicates good recovery, a score of 2 moderate disability, a score of 3 severe disability, a score of 4 survival but in a vegetative state, and a score of 5 death.

- NIH Stroke Scale: a serial measure of neurological deficit using a 42-point scale that quantifies neurological deficits in 11 categories. For example, a mild facial paralysis is given a score of 1 and complete right hemiplegia with aphasia, gaze deviation, visual field deficit, dysarthria and sensory loss is given a score of 25. Normal function without neurological deficit is scored as 0.

What is the role of thrombolysis in acute stroke?

Treatment with intravenous tissue plasminogen activator (tPA) when administered within 3 h after onset of the ischaemic event (and in the absence of any sign of brain injury on CT) improves clinical outcome at 3 months (N Engl J Med 1995;333:1581–7). The CT scan in these patients must be examined very carefully for evidence of hemispheric brain ischaemia, which may increase the risk of deterioration with or without cerebral haemorrhage, after thrombolytic treatment. An overview of previous trials found significant excesses of early and total deaths, and of symptomatic and fatal intracranial haemorrhages, after acute thrombolysis, but a significant reduction in death or dependency in patients randomized to treatment within 3 h of stroke onset (Lancet 1997;350:607–14). It remains unclear which patients are most likely to benefit or be harmed. Therapy with alteplase may be effective in patients who present 3–4.5 h after the onset of stroke symptoms

Note: If the examiner asks: 'If a patient presents to you 60 min after the onset of a left hemispheric stroke; how long do you have to initiate thrombolytic therapy?' The correct answer is 1 min, not 2 h! Time is neurons saved!

What is the role of anticoagulants in the immediate treatment of acute ischaemic stroke?

Anticoagulants (including unfractionated heparin, low-molecular-weight heparin or specific thrombin inhibitors) offer no short or long-term benefits in the immediate treatment of acute ischaemic stroke. Although the risks of deep venous thrombosis or pulmonary embolus are significantly reduced, these benefits are offset by a dose-dependent increased risk of intracranial or extracranial bleeding.

What are the important principles of rehabilitation after a stroke?

- Long-term use of aerobic training
- Exercises to enhance flexibility, balance and coordination
- Resistance exercises within daily activities.

What are the clinical features that would interest you for the rehabilitation of a stroke?

- Independence in activities of daily living: bathing, dressing, toileting, transferring, continence and feeding.
- Independence in more complex activities such as meal preparation, shopping, financial management, housekeeping, transportation, medication-taking and laundering.

What are key goals before and after discharge of a stroke patient?

- Before discharge the patient should be able to:
  - provide reliable yes and no responses to questions
  - express himself or herself in short phrases
  - use the unaffected hand effectively for self-care

- walk 50 m slowly with hands-on supervision (with the aid of a cane and/or ankle–foot orthosis).

Note: The patient would be expected to require some physical help for self-care.

- After discharge:
  - Physical, occupational and speech therapy with a focus on on training in skills needed to increase independence for activities of daily living both at home and in the community; successful learning of such personal skills may require 20 or more hours of practice
  - Formal training of caregivers
  - Depression should be identified and treated
  - Improvement in movement and language skills is possible with further practice at any time after stroke (because of the plasticity of neural pathways that remain intact).

(See N Engl J Med 2005;352:1677.)

What is the prognosis in a patient with acute ischaemic stroke?

About 25% of stroke patients are dead within a month, about 30% by 6 months and 50% by 1 year. Prognosis is worse when it is caused by intracerebral and subarachnoid haemorrhage, where the 1-month mortality is close to 50%. Of those who survive the acute event, about half will experience some disability after 6 months (J Neurol Neurosurg Psych 1987;50:177–82).

What is the significance of carotid artery stenosis?

Carotid artery stenosis is an important predisposing factor for cerebrovascular ischaemic events, the risk increasing with the severity of the stenosis and the presence of symptoms.

For *severe symptomatic stenosis* (>70% narrowing), carotid endarterectomy is recommended.

For *severe symptom-free stenosis*, optimal management has yet to be defined: one meta-analysis of trials showed only a small absolute benefit from surgery in reducing the odds of ipsilateral stroke (BMJ 1998;317:1477–80). Also 45% of strokes in patients with asymptomatic stenosis with 60–99% narrowing are attributable to lacunaes or cardioembolism (N Engl J Med 2000;342:1693–1700). Hence carotid endarterectomy cannot be routinely recommended.

For *mild to moderate symptomatic stenosis* (<70% narrowing), an antiplatelet agent such as aspirin is recommended. Persistent symptoms may necessitate use of other agents such as ticlopidine or clopidogrel, which reduce the relative risk for further ischaemic events slightly more than aspirin or anticoagulation with aspirin (CAPRIE trial, Lancet 1996;348:1329–39).

How would you manage a patient with a transient ischaemic attack?

- Advise to stop smoking
- Aspirin
- Duplex ultrasonography of the carotid vessels
- Carotid artery digital subtraction angiography
- MRI scan of the head. It has been argued that all patients with TIA should be scanned since permanent damage may be seen in the brain on MRI in about 25% of patients with TIAs. The best approach to such patients is using the ABCD scoring system:

- **Age** ≥60 years: 1 point
- **BP** elevation at first assessment (≥140/90 mmHg): 1 point
- **Clinical feature of TIA:** unilateral weakness: 2 points; speech impairment without weakness: 1 point
- **Duration of TIA:** 10–59 min: 1 point; ≥60 min: 2 points
- **Diabetes:** 1 point.

What do you understand by the term transient ischaemic attack?

An acute loss of focal cerebral or ocular function with symptoms lasting <24 h.

Why is it important to differentiate a carotid transient ischaemic attack from a vertebrobasilar attack?

Carotid TIAs may be amenable to surgery. Furthermore, a TIA in the anterior circulation is generally of more serious prognostic significance than a TIA in the posterior circulation.

What are the features of a carotid transient ischaemic attack?

Hemiparesis, aphasia or transient loss of vision in one eye only (amaurosis fugax).

What are the features of a vertebrobasilar transient ischaemic attack?

- Vertigo, dysphagia, ataxia and drop attacks (at least two of these should occur together)
- Bilateral or alternating weakness or sensory symptoms
- Sudden bilateral blindness in patients aged over 40 years.

What are the risk factors for stroke?

Hypertension, ischaemic heart disease, atrial fibrillation, peripheral vascular disease, diabetes, smoking, previous TIA, cervical bruit, hyperlipidaemia, raised haematocrit, oral contraceptive pill and cardiomyopathy.

Why is it important to treat transient ischaemic attacks?

Prospective studies have shown that within 5 years of a TIA:
- 1 in 6 patients will have suffered a stroke
- 1 in 4 patients will have died (from either stroke or heart disease).

What is the role of carotid endarterectomy in patients with a carotid transient ischaemic attack?

- For patients with severe stenosis (70–99%) the risks of surgery are significantly outweighed by the later benefits.
- For patients with mild stenosis (0–50% of cases) there is little 3-year risk of ipsilateral ischaemic stroke, even in the absence of surgery; consequently, any 3-year benefits of surgery are small and outweighed by its early risks (N Engl J Med 2000;342:1743–5).
- For patients with moderate stenosis (50–69% of cases) the balance of surgical risk and eventual benefit is still being evaluated.

What is the role of carotid angioplasties in patients with recent carotid artery transient ischaemic attacks who have severe stenosis of the ipsilateral carotid artery?

Carotid angioplasty has not been adequately assessed in patients with recent carotid artery TIAs or non-disabling ischaemic stroke and severe stenosis of the ipsilateral carotid artery, and hence it is not recommended. However, registry data suggest that carotid artery stenting may be useful in carefully selected patients. The results of the CREST (Revascularization Endarterectomy Versus Stenting Trial) trial (randomized trial funded by the NIH examining the role of carotid stenting) showed similar net outcomes with carotid artery stenting and carotid endarterectomy for the treatment of carotid stenosis. Whereas the International Carotid Stenting Study (ICSS) interim safety results at 120 days appeared to favour carotid artery stenting over carotid endarterectomy for patients with symptomatic carotid stenosis only.

What to you understand by 'RIND'?

Reversible ischaemic neurological disease, in which symptoms and signs reverse within 1 week but not within 24 h.

What are lacunar infarcts?

Lacunar infarcts are seen in hypertensive patients and consist of small infarcts in the region of the internal capsule (causing partial hemiparesis or hemisensory impairment), pons (ataxia of cerebellar type, partial hemiparesis), basal ganglia or thalamus. They are often multiple. Lacunae are thought to be caused by occlusion of small branch arteries or by rupture of Charcot–Bouchard microaneurysms, producing a small haematoma that resolves leaving an area of infarction.

What are the deficits supplied by the anterior carotid artery?

The anterior carotid artery supplies the frontal lobes and the medial cerebral hemispheres with the exception of the visual cortex of the occipital lobes. Cortical areas supplied by this artery include the motor and sensory areas of the lower limbs, a 'micturition centre' and the supplementary motor cortex. Ischaemia in the territory of one anterior carotid artery produces weakness and mild sensory deficits in the opposite lower limb. Some patients with left anterior carotid artery ischaemia have a mild transient aphasia.

What do you understand by the term stroke?

Stroke is characterized by rapidly progressive clinical symptoms and signs of focal, and at times global, loss of cerebral function lasting >24 h or leading to death, with no apparent cause other than that of vascular origin (Bull Word Health Organ 1976;54:541–53).

How do you classify stroke?

The Bamford clinical classification of stroke has the following.
Total anterior circulation syndrome:

- Unilateral motor deficit of face, arm and leg
- Homonymous hemianopia
- Higher cerebral dysfunction (e.g. aphasia, neglect).

Parietal anterior circulation syndrome has any two of the following features:

- Unilateral motor and/or sensory deficit
- Ipsilateral hemianopia or higher cerebral dysfunction
- Higher cerebral dysfunction alone or isolated motor and/or sensory deficit restricted to one limb or the face.

Posterior circulation syndrome has one or more of the following features:

- Bilateral motor or sensory signs not secondary to brainstem compression by a large supratentorial lesion
- Cerebellar signs, unless accompanied by ipsilateral motor deficit (ataxic hemiparesis)

- Unequivocal diplopia with or without external ocular muscle palsy
- Crossed signs, for example left facial and right limb weakness
- Hemianopia alone or with any of the four items above.

Lacunar syndromes can be pure motor, pure sensory, ataxic hemiparesis or sensorimotor:

- Pure motor stroke:
  - Unilateral, pure motor deficit
  - Clearly involving two of three areas (face, arm and leg)
  - With the whole of any limb being involved.
- Pure sensory stroke:
  - Unilateral pure sensory symptoms (with or without signs)
  - Involving at least two of three areas (face, arm and leg)
  - With the whole of any limb being involved.
- Ataxic hemiparesis:
  - Ipsilateral cerebellar and corticospinal tract signs
  - With or without dysarthria
  - In the absence of higher cerebral dysfunction or a visual field defect.
- Sensorimotor stroke;
  - Pure motor and pure sensory stroke combined (i.e. unilateral motor or sensory signs and symptoms)
  - In the absence of higher cerebral dysfunction or a visual field defect.

What advice would you give a stroke patient regarding driving?
The patient should be informed about driving regulations and the legal requirement to inform the Driver and Vehicle Licensing Authority need to be explained.

M. Fischer wrote one of the earliest descriptions on the effect of 'occlusion of the internal carotid artery' including transient cerebral ischaemia and ischaemic stroke (Arch Neurol Psychiatry 1951;65:346–77).

---

38   PTOSIS AND HORNER SYNDROME

INSTRUCTION

Examine this patient's face.

SALIENT FEATURES

History

- Ask the patient whether or not there is absence of sweating on one side of the face
- History of lung cancer
- History of cervical sympathectomy
- Migraine.

Examination

In the examination if you notice **ptosis** then you must answer the following questions:

- Is ptosis complete or incomplete?
- Is it unilateral or bilateral?

- Is the pupil constricted (Horner syndrome) or dilated (third nerve palsy)?
- Are extraocular movements involved (third nerve palsy or myasthenia gravis)?
- Is the eyeball sunken or not (enophthalmos)?
- Is the light reflex intact (intact light reflex in Horner syndrome)?

If the patient has **Horner syndrome**, then quickly proceed as follows:

- Examine the supraclavicular area:
  - Percuss the supraclavicular area, looking for dullness of Pancoast's tumour
  - Look for scar of cervical sympathectomy (be prepared with indications for cervical sympathectomy)
  - Look for enlarged lymph nodes.
- Examine the neck:
  - for carotid and aortic aneurysms
  - for tracheal deviation (Pancoast's tumour).
- Examine the hands:
  - for small muscle wasting
  - for pain sensation with a pin
  - for clubbing.

These should help in making a diagnosis of syringomyelia or Pancoast's tumour.

If there is no clue so far about the cause, tell the examiner that you would like to examine for nystagmus, cerebellar signs, cranial nerves and pale optic discs, and pyramidal signs to ascertain brainstem vascular disease or demyelination.

DIAGNOSIS

This patient has Horner syndrome (lesion) associated with dullness in the supraclavicular area indicating a Pancoast's tumour (aetiology).

QUESTIONS

What causes Horner syndrome?

The syndrome is caused by the involvement of the sympathetic pathway. It starts in the sympathetic nucleus and travels through the brainstem and spinal cord to the level of C8/T1/T2 to the sympathetic chain, stellate ganglion and carotid sympathetic plexus (Am J Ophthalmol 1958;46:289–96)). Its significance requires an understanding of the oculosympathetic pathway 3-neuron chain. The first-order nerve (FON) fibres descend from the hypothalamus without decussation to the thoracic spinal cord before synapsing with the second-order neurons (SON). The SONs exit the spine at the C8, T1 and T2 levels to enter the sympathetic chain and travel over the pleural cap of the lung and loop around the subclavian artery before synapsing near the carotid bifurcation. The final third-order neurons (TON) travel along the internal carotid artery to innervate the eyelids and the eye and also along the external carotid artery to innervate facial sweat glands.

What are the features of Horner syndrome?

It is characterized by:

- miosis (resulting from paralysis of the dilator of the pupil) (Fig. 38.1)
- partial ptosis or pseudo-ptosis (caused by paralysis of the upper tarsal muscle)

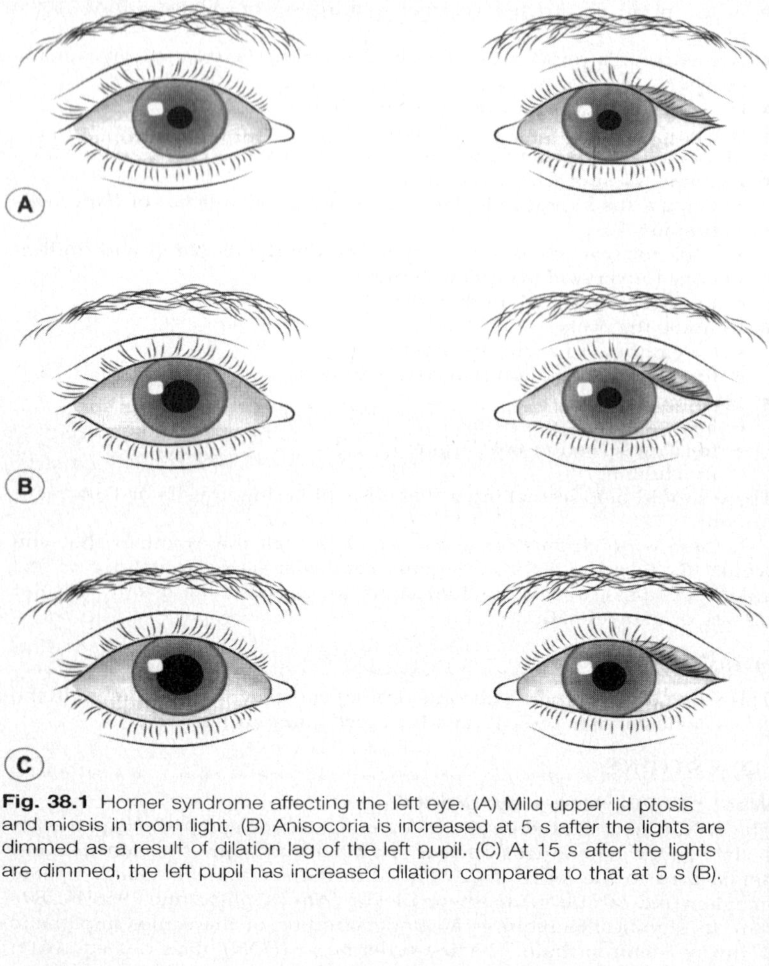

Fig. 38.1 Horner syndrome affecting the left eye. (A) Mild upper lid ptosis and miosis in room light. (B) Anisocoria is increased at 5 s after the lights are dimmed as a result of dilation lag of the left pupil. (C) At 15 s after the lights are dimmed, the left pupil has increased dilation compared to that at 5 s (B).

- enophthalmos (caused by paralysis of the muscle of Müller)
- often, slight elevation of the lower lid (because of paralysis of lower tarsal muscles).

What additional feature would you see in congenital Horner syndrome?

There would be heterochromia of the iris: the iris remains grey–blue.

How would you determine the level of lesion using only history?

The level of the lesion is determined by the distribution of the loss of sweating:

- Central lesion: sweating over the entire half of the head, arm and upper trunk is lost.
- Lesions of the neck:
  - Proximal to the superior cervical ganglion: diminished sweating on the face
  - Distal to the superior cervical ganglion: sweating is not affected.

ADVANCED-LEVEL QUESTIONS

How would you differentiate whether the lesion is above the superior ganglion (peripheral) or below the superior cervical ganglion (central)?

Test	Above	Below
Sweating	Such lesions may not affect sweating at all as the main outflow to the facial blood vessels is below the superior cervical ganglion	Such lesions affect sweating over the entire, head, neck and arm upper trunk Lesions in the lower neck affect sweating over the entire face
Cocaine 4% in both eyes	Dilates the normal pupil, no effect on the affected side	Dilates both pupils
Epinephrine (adrenaline, 1:1000) in both eyes	Dilates affected eye, no effect on normal side	No effect on both sides

Note: In peripheral lesions there is depletion of amine oxidase as a result of postganglionic denervation. As a result, this sensitizes the pupil to 1:1000 epinephrine (adrenaline), whereas it has no effect on the normal pupil or in central lesions (where the presence of the enzyme rapidly destroys the epinephrine).

Mention one cause of intermittent Horner syndrome
Migraine.

What are the causes of ptosis?
Unilateral:
- Third nerve palsy
- Horner syndrome
- Myasthenia gravis
- Congenital or idiopathic.

Bilateral:
- Myasthenia gravis
- Dystrophia myotonica
- Ocular myopathy or oculopharyngeal dystrophy
- Mitochondrial dystrophy
- Tabes dorsalis
- Congenital
- Bilateral Horner syndrome (as in syringomyelia).

If the patient has Pancoast's tumour, what is the most likely underlying pathology?

Squamous cell carcinoma.

JF Horner (1831–1886), Professor of Ophthalmology in Zurich, conceded that Claude Bernard had recognized the syndrome before him.

Henry K Pancoast (1875–1939) was the first Professor of Radiology in the USA at the University of Pennsylvania.

---

39 ARGYLL ROBERTSON PUPIL

INSTRUCTION

Examine this patient's eyes.

SALIENT FEATURES

History

- Ask the patient about lancinating pains
- History of multiple sclerosis, sarcoidosis or syphilis
- Difficulty in walking (remember the gait in tabes dorsalis).

EXAMINATION

- The pupils are small and irregular
- Light reflex is absent
- Accommodation reflex is intact (Fig. 39.1)
- There may be depigmentation of the iris
- Bilateral ptosis and marked overcompensation by frontalis muscle (in tabes doralis).

Proceed by telling the examiner that you would like to do the following:

- Examine for vibration and position sense
- Test for Romberg's sign and deep tendon reflexes (decreased)
- Check syphilitic serology
- Check urine sugar.

Remember that these pupils show little response to atropine, physostigmine or methacholine.

DIAGNOSIS

This patient has Argyll Robertson pupil (lesion) and you would like to investigate for underlying neurosyphilis or leutic infection (aetiology).

QUESTIONS

What are the causes of Argyll Robertson pupil?

- Neurosyphilis: tabes dorsalis
- Diabetes mellitus and other conditions with autonomic neuropathy

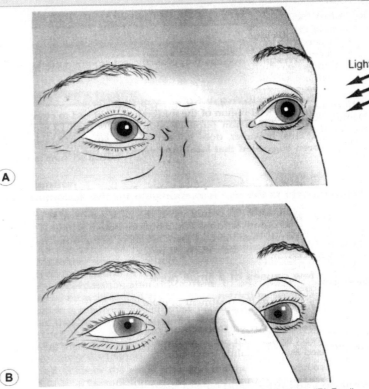

Fig. 39.1 Argyll Robertson pupil. (A) Pupil fails to constrict to light. (B) Pupil constricts to accommodation.

- Pinealoma
- Brainstem encephalitis
- Multiple sclerosis
- Lyme disease
- Sarcoidosis (BMJ 1984;289:356)
- Syringobulbia
- Tumours of the posterior portion of the third ventricle.

ADVANCED-LEVEL QUESTIONS

What do you know about the nerve pathways of the light reflex?

- The afferent is through the optic nerve and the efferent limb is through the third cranial nerve. Among the relevant optic nerve fibres responsible for the light reaction, those responsible for the perception of light terminate in the pretectal region of the midbrain, from whence a further relay passes to the Edinger–Westphal nucleus.

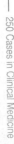

250 Cases in Clinical Medicine

- Disturbances of the pupillary right reflex occur when there is involvement of the following:
  - Superior colliculus
  - Decussation of Meynert
  - Edinger–Westphal nucleus (supplies the constrictor muscles of the iris).

Where is the lesion in Argyll Robertson pupil?

Damage to the pretectal region of the midbrain is believed to be responsible for the Argyll Robertson pupil of neurosyphilis (Am J Ophthalmol 1956;42:105). This, however, does not explain the small irregular pupils and it has been suggested that local involvement of the iris is a separate lesion.

Which muscle in the eye is responsible for the accommodation reflex?

Paralysis of accommodation occurs when the ciliary muscle is involved. Remember that accommodation is a much more potent stimulus for constriction of the pupils than light, as there are more nerve fibres mediating the accommodation reflex than the light reflex.

Mention a few causes of a small pupil

- Senile miosis
- Pilocarpine drops in the treatment of glaucoma.

What is 'reversed' Argyll Robertson pupil?

The pupils react to light but not to accommodation; this is seen in parkinsonism caused by encephalitis lethargica.

What do you understand by the term anisocoria?

Anisocoria is gross inequality of the pupils. Causes include:

- third nerve palsy
- iritis
- blind or amblyopia in one eye (pupil larger in the affected eye)
- cerebrovascular accidents
- severe head trauma
- hemianopia caused by optic tract involvement.

Notes

Anisocoria occurs also in about 20% of normal individuals.

Eccentric pupil occurs when the pupil is not in the centre of the iris. It may result from trauma or iritis and need not be pathognomonic of neurological disease.

Douglas MCL Argyll Robertson (1837–1909) of Edinburgh described these pupils in 1869 with neurosyphilis (Edinb Med J 1869;15:487). His studies on the effects of the extracts of the Calabar bean (*Physostigma venenosum*) on the pupil were widely acclaimed. He was the President of the Royal College of Surgeons of Edinburgh.

40 HOLMES-ADIE SYNDROME

INSTRUCTION

Examine this patient's eyes.

SALIENT FEATURES

History

- The patient is usually a young woman
- Impaired sweating
- Onset may be acute.

Examination

- The pupil is large, regular, irregular, oval, or circular
- The pupil will react sluggishly or fail to react to light (Fig. 40.1). However, if a strong and persistent stimulus is used it can be shown that the pupil contracts excessively to a very small size and when the stimulus is removed it returns to its former size gradually—this is known as the 'myotonic' pupil
- Delayed constriction in response to near vision
- Delayed re-dilatation after near vision
- Accomodation impaired (pupillary constriction secondary to accommodation is relatively less affected, because the ciliary muscle has innervation that is approximately 30 times as great as that of the iris sphincter)
- There is segmental palsy and segmental spontaneous movement of iris (Lancet 2000;356:1760–1)
- Proceed to check the ankle jerks and tell the examiner that you expect them to be absent. (The diminished reflexes result from dysfunction of the large sensory 1A afferent fibres involved in the spinal reflex arc, which is consistent with an underlying neuropathy.)

DIAGNOSIS

This woman has a sluggishly reacting pupil with absent ankle jerks (lesion) caused by Holmes–Adie syndrome (aetiology); this is a benign disorder (functional status).

QUESTIONS

What is the significance of this condition?
It is benign and must not be mistaken for Argyll Robertson pupil.

What are the causes of a dilated pupil?
- Mydriatic eye drops
- Third nerve lesion
- Holmes–Adie syndrome (degeneration of the nerve to the ciliary ganglion)
- Lens implant, iridectomy
- Blunt trauma to the iris (pupil may be irregular dilated and reacts sluggishly to light: post-traumatic iridoplegia)

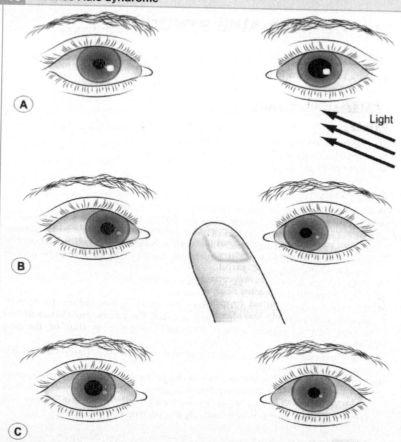

Fig. 40.1 Left tonic pupil. Little difference between the eyes is apparent in darkness as the normal right pupil is dilated. (A) Anisocoria is enhanced in bright light. (B) A near stimulus results in constriction of the tonic pupil, demonstrating light-near dissociation. (C) A few seconds after return of gaze to a distant target, the normal right pupil has redilated and the tonic pupil remains small.

- Drug overdose, e.g. cocaine, amphetamine
- Poisoning, e.g. belladonna
- Deep coma, death.

What are the causes of a small pupil?
- Old age
- Pilocarpine eye drops
- Horner syndrome
- Argyll Robertson pupil

- Pontine lesion
- Narcotics.

ADVANCED-LEVEL QUESTIONS

What do you know about the factors that control the size of the pupil?
The sphincter muscle of the pupil (causing miosis) is supplied by the cholinergic parasympathetic nerves, whereas the dilator of the pupil (causing mydriasis) is supplied by noradrenergic sympathetic fibres. The parasympathetic fibres arise from the Edinger–Westphal nucleus. They travel by the third cranial nerve to the ciliary ganglion. Postganglionic fibres arise from the ciliary ganglion and are distributed by the ciliary nerve.

Where is the lesion in Adie's tonic pupil?
It is caused by damage to the parasympathetic fibres from within the ciliary ganglion.

What is the difference between Adie's tonic pupil and Holmes–Adie syndrome?
Adie's tonic pupil with absent deep tendon jerks is called Holmes–Adie syndrome.

How does the Holmes–Adie pupil react to weak pilocarpine (0.125%) or 2.5% methacholine?
It usually constricts, indicating a supersensitivity to acetylcholine secondary to parasympathetic denervation resulting from degeneration of postganglionic neurons and neurons in the ciliary ganglion. There is no effect on a normal pupil.

Which conditions may accompany this syndrome?
Dysautonomias such as:
- Ross syndrome (segmental loss of sweating): the occurrence of Adie syndrome and segmental anhidrosis or hypohydrosis. It consists of cranial postganglionic parasympathetic and sympathetic dysfunction in association with more widespread autonomic failure that is rarely clinically relevant. The course is usually benign with a possible expansion of the dyshidrotic area.
- cardiac arrhythmias.

Further reading
Harriman DG, Garland H: The pathology of Adie's syndrome, *Brain* 91:401–418, 1968.
Miyasaki JM, Ashby P, Sharpe JA, Fletcher WA: On the cause of hyporeflexia in the Holmes–Adie syndrome, *Neurology* 38:262–265, 1988.

Sir Gordon M Holmes (1876–1965) and William J Adie (1886–1935) were London neurologists who described the condition independently in 1931 (Holmes: Trans Ophthalmol Soc 1931;41:209, Adie: Brain 1932;55:98, Br J Ophthalmol 1932;16:449).
The name Holmes–Adie syndrome was given by Bramwell in 1936.
Saenger and Strasburger independently described the syndrome in 1902; it was first recorded in English literature by Markus in 1905.

41 HOMONYMOUS HEMIANOPIA

INSTRUCTION

Examine this patient's eyes.
Examine this patient's visual fields.

SALIENT FEATURES

History

- Patient bumps into things on one side and may have a history of traffic accidents where one side of the car is damaged without the patient realizing.
- Patient may insist that they have one 'bad' eye (remember blindness in one eye causes impairment of perceiving distances but the normal eye will provide a full field of vision on both sides and hence patient will not bump into objects).
- Reading difficulty (suggests that the visual defect splits the midline: if the defect is on the right side, patient is unable to scan along the line to the next word and hence reading is almost impossible, whereas when the defect is on the left side the patient cannot find the beginning of the next line).
- Determine whether the patient is aware of his/her defect (if the patient is aware of the visual defect, it is likely the defect 'splits' the macula and bisects the central field; if the patient is unaware and bumps into things, then the defect is either macular sparing or an attention hemianopia).

Examination

- Homonymous hemianopia: examination includes:
  - testing for an attention field defect using both hands of the examiner and asking the patient to determine which finger is moving
  - testing the whole field in each eye using a white hat pin
  - re-evaluation of the field in each eye to determine whether there is macular sparing or macular splitting using a hat pin. If you are unable to determine, then tell the patient that you would like to do formal field testing with a tangent screen or using a perimeter.

Proceed as follows:

- Check the visual acuity; examine the fundus.
- Tell the examiner that you would like to do a full neurological examination to look for an underlying cause: stroke, intracranial tumour.

Remember: Homonymous hemianopic visual field defects with normal visual acuity are the hallmark of a unilateral retrochiasmal lesion.

DIAGNOSIS

This patient has a homonymous hemianopia (lesion) for which I would like to determine the aetiology, such as a stroke or tumour.

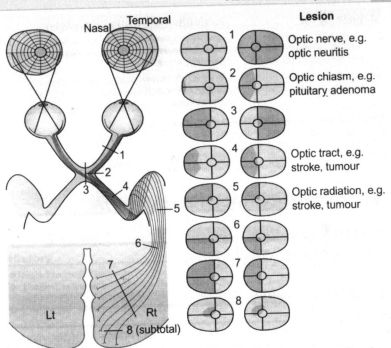

Fig. 41.1 Visual fields that accompany damage to the visual pathways. See the table for details.

ADVANCED-LEVEL QUESTIONS

Where is the lesion?

The lesion is in the optic tract and beyond (visual acuity is intact when the macula is spared). Figure 41.1 shows the sites of the lesions and the visual field effects.

	Site	Type of homonymous hemianopia
1	Optic nerve	Unilateral amaurosis
2	Lateral optic chiasm	Grossly incongruous, contralateral
3	Central optic chiasm	Bitemporal hemianopia
4	Optic tract	Incongruous, incomplete
5	Temporal lobe	Superior quadrantic defect, congruous partial or complete (contralateral
6	Posterior parietal lobe	Inferior quadrantic defect, congruous partial or complete

	Site	Type of homonymous hemianopia
7	Complete parieto-occipital interruption of the optic radiation	Complete congruous homonymous hemianopia with shift of foveal point, often sparing central vision
8	Incomplete damage to the visual cortex	Congruous homonymous scotomas, usually encroaching at least acutely on central vision

What further investigations would you do?

- Formal field testing: perimetry is particularly important if the patient holds a driver's licence
- MRI or CT.

42 BITEMPORAL HEMIANOPIA

INSTRUCTION

Examine this patient's eyes.
Examine this patient's visual fields.

SALIENT FEATURES

History

- Insidious onset of defects in visual field. Involvement of the macula is late and is associated with abrupt visual failure as the presenting feature
- Hypogonadism (may precede the visual failure many years): males have impotence and females have amenorrhoea.

Examination

- Bitemporal hemianopia, which is caused by a median lesion of the optic chiasma (see Fig. 41.1).
- Proceed by examining the hands and face for acromegaly.
- Tell the examiner that you would like to look for signs of hypopituitarism (p. 534). The probable causes are:
  - pituitary tumour (endocrine symptoms precede the visual symptoms; the upper temporal fields affected first and then defect spreads down)
  - craniopharyngioma (bitemporal hemianopia initially worse in the lower quadrants)
  - suprasellar meningioma
  - aneurysms
  - metastases
  - glioma.

DIAGNOSIS

This patient has bitemporal hemianopia (lesion) and I would like to investigate for a median mass lesion compressing the optic chiasma.

QUESTIONS

How would you investigate this patient?

- Formal field testing: perimetry
- Serum prolactin
- Skull radiography (calcification of craniopharyngioma and size of the pituitary fossa, which is best seen in the lateral skull radiograph)
- CT or MRI of head.

43   CENTRAL SCOTOMA

INSTRUCTION

Examine this patient's visual fields.

SALIENT FEATURES

History

- Sudden onset usually
- Patient notices a 'hole' in the vision while reading a poster or looking at a clock
- Difficulty performing in reading, driving, walking and recognizing faces.

Examination

- Central scotoma (allow the patient to find the defect by moving the white hat pin in his or her own visual field). Then determine:
  - the size and shape of the defect by moving the pin in and out of the blind area
  - whether the defect crosses the horizontal midline (vascular defects of retina do not do so)
  - whether the defect crosses the vertical midline (defects caused by pathway damage have a sharp vertical edge at the midline)
  - whether the defect extends to the blind spot: so-called caecocentral scotoma (seen in glaucoma, vitamin B_{12} deficiency) (Fig. 43.1)
  - whether there is a similar defect in the other eye (to exclude homonymous hemianopic scotomas).
- Examine the fundus; remember that the optic discs may be:
  - pale (optic atrophy)
  - normal (retrobulbar neuritis)
  - swollen and pink (papillitis).

DIAGNOSIS

This patient has a central scotoma (lesion) caused by optic atrophy (aetiology).

ADVANCED-LEVEL QUESTIONS

What do you understand by the term scotoma?

It is a small patch of visual loss within the visual field.

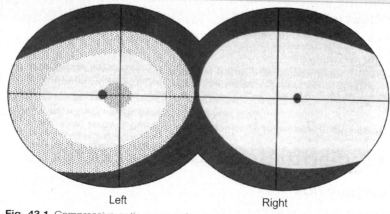

Left   Right

Fig. 43.1 Compressive optic neuropathy causing contraction of left visual field and cecocentral scotoma. Right visual field is normal.

Mention a few underlying causes for central scotoma

- Demyelinating disorders (multiple sclerosis)
- Optic nerve compression by tumour, aneurysm
- Glaucoma
- Toxins: methanol, tobacco, lead, arsenical poisoning
- Ischaemia, including central retinal artery occlusion caused by thromboembolism, temporal arteritis, syphilis, idiopathic acute ischaemic neuropathy
- Hereditary disorders: Friedreich's ataxia, Leber's optic atrophy
- Paget's disease
- Vitamin B deficiency
- Secondary to retinitis pigmentosa
- Late age-related macular degeneration: the patient usually has enough vision to be ambulatory because the peripheral visual field around a central scotoma is intact
- Valsalva retinopathy, which is characterized by a painless, sudden loss of vision in an otherwise healthy patient with no ocular history after activities such as vomiting, coughing and weight lifting. (The sudden rise in intrathoracic pressure increased the intraocular venous pressure, causing the rupture of perifoveal capillaries.) Visual loss can be marked but spontaneous recovery usually occurs (N Engl J Med 2005;352:e16)
- Bungee jumping.

44 TUNNEL VISION

INSTRUCTION

Examine this patient's eyes.
Examine this patient's visual fields.

SALIENT FEATURES

- Intact central vision with constriction of the peripheral fields
- Proceed by examine for the following:
  - optic atrophy (primary and secondary)
  - retinitis pigmentosa (p. 723)
  - choroidoretinitis (p. 726)
  - glaucoma.

DIAGNOSIS

This patient has tunnel vision (lesion) as a result of retinitis pigmentosa (aetiology).

ADVANCED-LEVEL QUESTIONS

What are the other causes of tunnel vision?
- Hysteria
- Slight contraction of field occurs when there is a significant refractive error.

Note: Before making a diagnosis of hysteria, contraction of the visual fields caused by extreme fatigue, poor attention, inadequate vision, diminished visual acuity or delayed reaction time must be excluded.

How would you differentiate hysteria from an organic cause of tubular vision?
In organic causes, the field of vision widens progressively as the test objects are held further away from the eye, but in the hysterical person this widening is not seen and the entire width of the field is as great at 1 foot (30 cm) from the eye as it is at 5, 10 or 15 feet (1.5, 3, or 4.5 m).

45 PARKINSON'S DISEASE

INSTRUCTION

Examine this patient.

SALIENT FEATURES

History

- Tremor: usually unilateral at onset; usually starts in upper limbs. Also seen in the legs and jaws
- Rigidity: ask about history of falls, poor balance, pain and muscle stiffness
- Poverty of movement: ask about drooling of saliva, difficulty in writing (micrographia), difficulty in turning in bed and change in voice (softness of voice)

- Family history of disease (susceptibility genes include α-synuclein, leucine rich repeat kinase 2 and glucocerebrosidase)
- History of encephalitis
- History of smoking (never smokers are twice as likely to develop disease) and caffeine intake (those who take no or very low quantities of daily caffeine, are at increased risk, ~25%) (Lancet 2009;373;2055–66)
- History of exposure to managanese dust, carbon disulfide or carbon monoxide
- Use of 1-Methyl-4-phenyl-1,2,3,6-tetrahydropyridine (MPTP) for recreational purposes
- Elicit a drug history, particularly regarding neuroleptics (reserpine, metoclopramide)
- History of herbal medications, particularly Pacific sedative kava kava and Indian snake root *Rauwolfia serpentina*
- History of severe head injury, encephalitis, hypertension or cerebrovascular disease.

Examination

- Usually florid cases are seen in the examination and the striking abnormalities (Fig. 45.1) are:
  - an expressionless or 'mask-like' face (fixed stare, infrequent blinking and ironed-out wrinkles)
  - drooling of saliva
  - resting or pill-rolling movement (most common in the distal extremities).

Proceed as follows:

- Comment on the expressionless face, pill-rolling movement and drooling of saliva so that the examiner knows that you have observed these abnormalities. Elicit bradykinesia by asking the patient to touch her thumb with each finger in turn.
- Examine the tone, in particular at the wrist for cog-wheel rigidity.
- Proceed to do the glabellar tap (tap the forehead just above the bridge of the nose repeatedly (about twice per second): in normal subjects, the blinking will stop whereas the patient with Parkinson's disease continues to blink: referred to as Myerson's sign. (It must be remembered that this sign is unreliable.)
- Ask the patient to walk and comment on the paucity of movement including the absence of arm swing and festinating gait (the patient walks with a stooped posture as if trying to catch up with her centre of gravity). The feet may scrape the floor in taking steps so the patient trips easily (be prepared to prevent the patient from falling when examining the gait).
- Tell the examiner that you would like to:
  - ask the patient a few questions with a view to assessing her speech
  - assess handwriting (tremulous and small, micrographia).
- Tell the examiner that you would like to look for:
  - postural hypotension (Shy–Drager syndrome, levodopa treatment)
  - impaired vertical gaze (Steele–Richardson–Olzewski syndrome)
  - check for anosmia (an early sign)
  - seborrhoea.

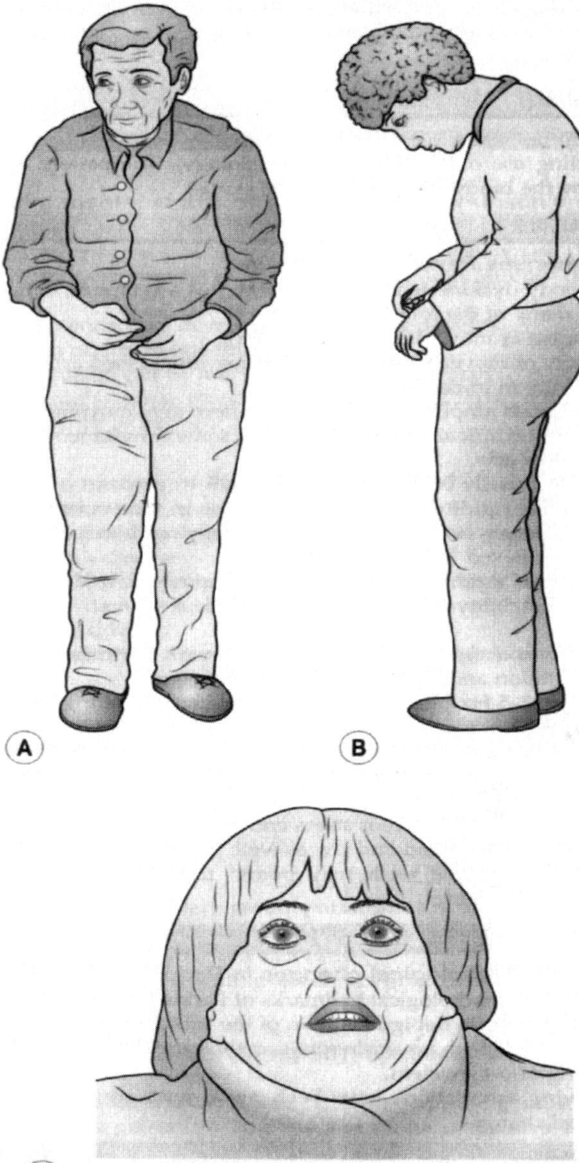

Fig. 45.1 Parkinson's disease. (A) The slightly anxious frozen face and characteristic flexed posture. (B) Development of anterocollis. (C) Typical facial expression of a patient with progressive supranuclear palsy, illustrating worried or surprised appearance, with furrowed brow and fixed expression of lower face.

Note: The diagnosis of Parkinson's disease is entirely clinical but the results of certain investigations may help in recognizing alternative causes for parkinsonism.

DIAGNOSIS

This patient has features of Parkinson's disease (lesion) that are caused by long-standing use of phenothiazines (aetiology). The patient is severely disabled by the bradykinesia (functional status).

QUESTIONS

What comprises Parkinson's disease?

- Upper body dyskinesia must be present; it is a symptom complex containing many of the following features:
  - Slowness of movement (bradykinesia)
  - Poverty of movement (mask-like facies, diminished arm swing)
  - Difficulty in initiating movement
  - Diminished amplitude of repetitive alternative movement
  - Inordinate difficulty in accomplishing some simultaneous or sequential motor acts.
- Rigidity is usually but not always present:
  - Lead-pipe rigidity is where the increase in tone is equal in flexors and extensors of all four limbs but slightly more in flexors, resulting in a part flexed 'simian' posture
  - Cog-wheel rigidity is caused by superimposed or underlying tremor.
- Postural instability is usually a late feature
- Tremor:
  - Absent in about one-third of patients with Parkinson's disease at presentation and throughout its course in some
  - Resting, 3–5 Hz pill, pronation and supination rolling tremor of the upper limb
  - Intermittent (can usually be brought about by getting the subject to count backwards with the eyes closed and hands dangling over the armrests of the seat)
  - Intensified by emotion or stress and disappearing during sleep
  - May affect legs, head and jaw as well; jaw tremor is rare but is most distressing as the teeth may pound together until they become unbearably painful.

ADVANCED-LEVEL QUESTIONS

What are the pathological changes in Parkinson's disease?

The most typical pathological hallmarks of Parkinson's disease are:

- neuronal loss with depigmentation of the substantia nigra
- Lewy bodies, which are eosinophilic cytoplasmic inclusions in neurons consisting of α-synuclein.

The following associations have been made with clinical features and pathological changes:

Clinical deficit	Pathology
Motor symptoms	Degeneration of dopaminergic nigrostnatal pathway
Cognitive defects	Degeneration of dopaminergic mesocortical and mesolimbic pathways

Clinical deficit	Pathology
Autonomic dysfunction	Dopamine depletion in the hypothalamus
'Freezing phenomenon'	Degeneration of the noradrenergic locus ceruleus
Dementia	Degeneration of the cholinergic nucleus

What is the mental status of patients with Parkinson's disease?

- In the initial stages, intellect and senses are usually preserved. Many patients have some intellectual deterioration — a slowness of thought and of memory retrieval (bradyphrenia), and subtle personality changes.
- Global dementia may develop in one-fifth of patients.
- Depression occurs in one-third of patients.
- Acute confusion can be precipitated by drug therapy.

Note: Parkinson's disease must be kept in mind in elderly patients presenting with a history of frequent falls.

What are the causes of Parkinson's disease?

- **True parkinsonism:**
- Idiopathic (caused by degeneration of the substantia nigra); also known as Parkinson's disease
- Drug induced (chlorpromazine, metaclopramide, prochlorperazine)
- Anoxic brain damage such as cardiac arrest, exposure to manganese and carbon monoxide
- Post-encephalitic, as a result of encephalitis lethargica or von Economo disease
- MPTP toxicity, seen in drug abusers
- Multiple system atrophy
- Progressive supranuclear atrophy
- Familial: mutation of the gene for α-synuclein or linkage to a region on chromosome 2.

- **Pseudoparkinsonism:**
- Essential tremor
- Atherosclerotic (vascular) pseudoparkinsonism (mention that in the past atherosclerosis was thought to be a cause of Parkinson's disease but this is no longer accepted as a cause)
- Hemiparkinsonism (presenting feature of a progressive space-occupying lesion)

What differences are seen in rigidity, spasticity and gegenhalten?

- Rigidity indicates increased tone affecting opposing muscle groups equally and is present throughout the range of passive movement. When smooth it is called lead-pipe rigidity and when intermittent is termed cog-wheel rigidity. It is common in extrapyramidal syndromes: Wilson's disease and Creutzfeldt–Jakob disease.
- Spasticity of the clasp-knife type is characterized by increased tone, which is maximal at the beginning of movement and suddenly decreases as passive movement is continued. It occurs chiefly in the

flexors of the upper limb and extensors of the lower limb (antigravity muscles).

- Gegenhalten, or paratonia, is where the increased muscle tone varies, and becomes worse the more the patient tries to relax.

What do you understand by the 'wheelchair sign' in Parkinson's disease?

Patients with advanced disease and 'on–off' motor fluctuations require a wheelchair when 'off' and when 'on' are seen to walk about (sometimes pushing the chair!). These patients are rarely permanently wheelchair bound; in contrast, those who never leave their wheelchair usually do not have Parkinson's disease.

What is the role of protein diets in patients who have episodes of sudden and substantial loss of mobility?

High-protein diets should be avoided in these patients because a large influx of dietary amino acids can interfere with the transport of levodopa into the brain (N Engl J Med 1967;276:374–9).

What do you understand by the term lower half parkinsonism?

It refers to vascular parkinsonism, which usually presents with severe failure to initiate gait, broad-based shuffling gait, mild bradykinesia, rigidity of the arms and subtle hypomimia. Risk factors include hypertension and history of ministrokes. There is no rest tremor; olfaction is normal and response to levodopa is usually poor (Lancet 2009;373;2055–66).

How is the severity of Parkinson's disease graded?

Hoehn–Yahr staging grades Parkinson's disease into five stages:
I: newly diagnosed disease
II and III: moderately severe disease
IV and V: advanced disease.

How would you manage a patient with Parkinson's disease?

Step I: replacing dopamine neurotransmitter that is lost as the dopamine neurons degenerate is the mainstay treatment. All drugs are started at low doses and doses are increased slowly to reduce adverse effects (start low, go slow). Withdrawal of therapy also should be done slowly to avoid worsening of parkinsonism or precipitating neuroleptic malignant syndrome:

- First-line dopaminergic agents: carbidopa plus levodopa (immediate release and controlled release), carbidopa plus levodopa plus entacoapone, dopamine agonists including non-ergot (pramipexole, ropinirole) and ergot (pergolide)
- Second-line alternatives: anticholinergic agents (trihexyphenidyl, benztropine), selective monoamine oxidase B inhibitors (selegiline) and N-methyl-D-aspartate (NMDA) antagonist (amantidine); anticholinergic drugs are more effective in alleviating tremor and rigidity rather than bradykinesia.

Step II: transplanting fetal nerve tissue to replace dopamine neurons that have been lost.

Step III: halting neuronal loss altogether with trophic factors; this is in the early stages of clinical testing. At present, there are no neuroprotective therapies, although clinical trials with monoamine oxidase B inhibitors, dopamine agoists and coenzyme Q_0 may slow progression. Glial cell line-derived neurotrophic factor (GDNF) is under investigation. Data are still needed to clarify neuroprotective therapies.

In which condition is levodopa absolutely contraindicated?
Melanoma.

What do you know about 'drug holidays' in levodopa therapy?
Drug holidays (i.e. discontinuation of therapy) was previously claimed to enhance the efficacy of treatment when it was resumed; it is now known to be dangerous (deaths have occurred) and of doubtful value.

What do you know about dopamine receptors?
At least four types of receptor have been reported: D_1 and D_2 are the two major families of dopamine receptors. For neurotransmission to occur, a complex consisting of a dopamine receptor and a G protein (guanine nucleotide-binding protein) must be formed. This complex then usually couples with the enzyme adenylate cyclase, which controls the formation of the second messenger cyclic AMP. Alteration of the second messenger leads to a cascade of events that ultimately determines the transfer of information between nerve cells. The D_{2A} receptor is involved in the therapeutic response elicited by dopaminergic agonists in parkinsonism, although the mechanism is not clear at a physiological level. The role of the D_1 family is unclear—whether the activation of these receptors leads to useful effects (i.e. reduction of parkinsonian deficits), undesireable effects (e.g. dyskinesia), or both. Bromocriptine, pergolide and lisuride all stimulate D_2 receptors, whereas bromocriptine and lisuride are D_1 receptor antagonists and pergolide is a D_1 receptor agonist.

What is the role of fetal tissue in potential treatment of Parkinson's disease?
Parkinson's disease is characterized by loss of the midbrain dopamine neurons that innervate the caudate and putamen. Patients tend to have a reduced response to levodopa after 5–20 years of therapy, with 'on–off' fluctuations consisting of dyskinesia alternating with immobility. Animal experiments have suggested that fetal dopaminergic neurons can survive transplantation and restore neurological function. Trials are underway to determine whether fetal grafts can improve motor function in patients with Parkinson's disease. Fetal ventral mesencephalic tissue is implanted in the patient's postcommissural putamen (N Engl J Med 1995;332:1118–24).

What is the role of thalamotomy in treatment of Parkinson's disease?
Thalamotomy used to be the main treatment until 1950, but with the introduction of levodopa it became less popular. However, there has been a revival of stereotactic surgery prompted by the failure of levodopa in four main aspects: in severe tremor, levodopa-induced dyskinesia, advanced Parkinson's disease and akinetic–rigid syndromes (BMJ 1998; 316:1259–60). Four types of stereotactic surgery are practised:
- Thalamotomy is used for intractable tremor and radiofrequency ablation of an area of the venterointermediate nucleus of the thalamus. It is

unsuitable for bilateral tremor as bilateral thalamotomy tends to cause impairment of speech.

- Thalamic stimulation is achieved with placement of a fine electrode in the venterointermediate nucleus and insertion of a pacemaker under the skin on the chest. This relieves tremor and can be performed bilaterally. Neither procedure improves akinesia, the most disabling aspect of Parkinson's disease.
- Deep-brain stimulation of the globus pallidus and subthalamic nucleus may result in striking improvements in parkinsonism and dyskinesia, resulting in large reductions of levodopa dose and thus improvements in levodopa-induced dyskinesias (Lancet 1995;345:91–5).
- Unilateral posteroventral medial pallidotomy ameliorates contralateral parkinsonian symptoms and medication-related dyskinesia and the effect is sustained for up to 5.5 years. Improvements in ipsilateral and axial symptoms are not sustained and many patients undergo, a second contralateral procedure (N Engl J Med 2000;342:1708–14).

Note: Patients with dementia and hallucinations tolerate all surgical procedures poorly and any benefit in patients with rapidly progressive parkinsonism is likely to be short lived.

What are Parkinson plus syndromes?

Some patients have other neurological deficits in addition to Parkinson's disease. Examples of these so-called Parkinson plus syndromes are:

- Steele–Richardson–Olszewski disease (akinesia, axial rigidity of the neck, bradyphrenia, supranuclear palsy)
- multiple system atrophy
- olivopontocerebellar degeneration
- strionigral degeneration.
- progressive autonomic failure (Shy–Drager syndrome)
- Basal ganglia calcification.

What is tardive dyskinesia?

Tardive dyskinesia is seen in patients taking neuroleptics. Its manifestations are orofacial dyskinesia such as smacking, chewing lip movements, discrete dystonia or choreiform movements and — rarely — rocking movements. Withdrawal of the offending drug will improve these symptoms over a period of 3–4 years, except in a small minority of patients. Drug-induced parkinsonism is usually bilateral with evident bradykinesia, rigidity and tremor. Tremor in drug-induced parkinsonism is often postural.

Mention some heredo-degenerative parkinsonian disorders

- Hallervorden–Spatz disease: autosomal recessive; patients also have dementia, dystonia, choreoathetosis, retinitis pigmentosa. There is increased iron deposition and increased cysteine in the globus pallidus.
- Fahr's disease or familial basal ganglia calcification: patients also have chorea, dementia and palilalia.
- Olivopontocerebellar and spinocerebellar degenerations: autosomal dominant; associated cerebellar ataxia and retinitis pigmentosa.

How would you manage autonomic and psychological symptoms?

- Insomnia: adjust Parkinson's disease drugs; use sleep hygiene techniques or clonazepam
- Depression: serotonin and noradrenergic reuptake inhibitors or amitryptiline
- Rapid eye movement behaviour disorders: adjust Parkinson's disease drugs or give clonazepam
- Fatigue: amantidine or selegiline
- Day time sleepiness: modafinil
- Psychosis and hallucinations: adjust Parkinson's disease drugs or use an antipsychotic (clozapine, quetiapine or aripiprazole). Quetapine typically does not worsen motor function and is often used as first-line therapy
- Constipation: osmotic laxatives (macrogol)
- Urinary urgency: check drugs; use anticholinergic bladder stabilizers, and desmopressin for nocturia
- Impotence: sildenafil, tadalafil and vardenafil
- Pain: adjust Parkinson's disease drugs and give muscle relaxants
- Restless legs: dopamine agonists
- Orthostatic hypotension: adjust Parkinson's disease drugs; increase water and salt intake; give fludrocortisone, ephedrine or midodrine
- Drooling: 0.5% atropine eye drops sublingually, scopoderm patch or botulinum toxin injections into salivary glands
- Excessive sweating: adjust Parkinson's disease drugs; give propantheline, propranolol or topical aluminium creams.

James Parkinson (1755–1824) first reported six cases of this syndrome in 1817 (at the age of 62 years).

Jean Martin Charcot (the father of neurology) proposed that this syndrome be called 'maladie de Parkinson'.

JC Steele, JC Richardson and J Olszewski were all US neurologists.

K von Economo (1876–1931), an Australian neurologist, also wrote on Wilson's disease.

Muhammed Ali (or Cassius Clay) the world heavy-weight boxing champion is reported to have premature of Parkinsons disease, the 'punch drunk' syndrome.

Professor K Ray Chaudhuri MD FRCP DSc is Consultant Neurologist and Professor in Neurology/Movement Disorders at Kings College Hospital NHS foundation Trust, University Hospital Lewisham, Kings College London and the Institute of Psychiatry. He is a recognized teacher and active researcher within the Guy's, King's and St Thomas' School of Medicine, London, UK and is the medical director of the National Parkinson Foundation International Centre of Excellence at Kings College, London.

Professor Christopher Mathias is Professor of Neurovascular Medicine in the University of London, with an appointment held jointly between Imperial College London and the Institute of Neurology, University College London. He has been a Consultant Physician at St Mary's Hospital since 1982 and at the National Hospital for Neurology and Neurosurgery, Queen Square, since 1985. His main interest is autonomic failure.

46 CEREBELLAR SYNDROME

INSTRUCTION

Examine this patient, who presented with a history of falling to one side. Demonstrate the cerebellar signs.

SALIENT FEATURES

History

- History of falls, wide-based gait, clumsiness and difficulty with fine coordinated movements
- Tremor
- Waxing and waning of symptoms (multiple sclerosis)
- Stroke (brainstem vascular lesion)
- Drug toxicity: phenytoin, alcohol abuse, lead poisoning and solvent abuse
- History of intracranial tumours (posterior fossa including cerebellopontine angle tumour)
- History of hypothyroidism (a reversible cause)
- Lung cancer (paraneoplastic manifestation)
- Family history (Friedreich's ataxia and other hereditary ataxias)
- Birth defects (congenital malformations at the level of the foramen magnum).

Examination

- Ask the patient a few questions to assess speech
- Ask the patient to keep his arms outstretched; then give them a small push downward and look for rebound phenomenon
- Examine for rapid alternating movements with the hand
- Do the finger–nose test: look for past-pointing and intention tremor
- Do the heel–shin test
- Examine the gait, in particular tandem walking. If ataxia is not marked, the patient's gait may be tested with eyes closed; patients will often progresses to the side of the lesion.
- Tell the examiner that you would like to examine the fundus for optic atrophy as demyelination is the commonest cause of cerebellar signs.

DIAGNOSIS

This patient has a cerebellar syndrome with optic atrophy (lesion) caused by multiple sclerosis (aetiology) and he is markedly ataxic (functional status).

QUESTIONS

How may cerebellar signs manifest?

- Disorders of movement:
  - Nystagmus: coarse horizontal nystagmus with lateral cerebellar lesions and its direction is towards the side of the lesion
  - Scanning dysarthria: a halting, jerking dysarthria, which is usually a feature of bilateral lesions
  - Lack of finger–nose coordination (past-pointing): movement is imprecise, in force, direction and distance (dysmetria)

- Rebound phenomenon: inability to arrest strong contraction on sudden removal of resistance (known as Holmes' rebound phenomenon)
- Intention tremor
- Dysdiadochokinesia: impairment of rapid alternating movements (clumsy)
- Dyssynergia: movements involving more than one joint are broken into parts.

● Hypotonia
● Absent reflexes or pendular reflexes
● Lack of coordination of gait: patient tends to fall towards the side of the lesion.

Notes

● The classical clinical triad of cerebellar disease is ataxia, atonia, asthenia.
● The cerebellum is not primarily a motor organ. It is developed phylogenetically from a primary vestibular area and is involved in modulation of motor activity. It receives afferents from the vestibular nuclei, spinal cord and cerebral cortex via the pontine nuclei.

What are the causes of cerebellar syndrome?

● Demyelination (multiple sclerosis)
● Brainstem vascular lesion
● Phenytoin toxicity
● Alcoholic cerebellar degeneration (there is atrophy of the anterior vermis of the cerebellum)
● Space-occupying lesion in the posterior fossa including cerebellopontine angle tumour
● Hypothyroidism (a reversible cause)
● Paraneoplastic manifestation of bronochogenic carcinoma
● Friedreich's ataxia (p. 267) and other hereditary ataxias
● Congenital malformations at the level of the foramen magnum.

ADVANCED-LEVEL QUESTIONS

How are cerebellar signs localized?

● Gait ataxia (inability to do tandem walking): anterior lobe (palaeocerebellum)
● Truncal ataxia (drunken gait, titubation): flocculonodular or posterior lobe (archicerebellum)
● Limb ataxia, especially upper limbs and hypotonia: lateral lobes (neocerebellum).

What is the difference between sensory ataxia and cerebellar ataxia?

	Cerebellar ataxia	**Sensory ataxia**
Site of lesion	Cerebellum	Posterior column or peripheral nerves
Deep tendon	Unchanged or pendular	Lost or diminished reflexes
Deep sensation	Normal	Decreased or lost
Sphincter disturbances	None	Decreased when posterior column involved, causing overflow incontinence

If you were allowed to do one investigation, which one would you choose in a patient with a suspected cerebellar lesion?
MRI.

Sir Gordon M Holmes (1876–1965) was consultant neurologist at the National Hospital for Nervous Diseases, London; his observations on wartime gunshot wounds allowed him to study cerebellar disease (Lancet 1922;ii:59,111, Brain 1939;62:1–30). He was the editor of the journal *Brain*.

47 JERKY NYSTAGMUS

INSTRUCTION

Examine this patient's eyes.
Test the patient's eye movements.

SALIENT FEATURES

History

- Obtain a history regarding cerebellar syndrome: multiple sclerosis, alcohol, etc. (case 46)
- Ear infections (vestibular involvement)
- Horizontal nystagmus with fast components to right or left side (when eliciting nystagmus take care to keep your finger at least 2 ft (60 cm) away from the patient and avoid going laterally beyond the extent of binocular vision)
- Proceed to look for other cerebellar signs (p. 201)
- Tell the examiner that you would like to do the following:
  - Examine the fundus for optic atrophy (Case 203) (multiple sclerosis)
  - Take a history of vertigo (vestibular nystagmus).

Note: If the patient has vertical nystagmus in addition to horizontal nystagmus, it is more likely to be vestibular nystagmus or brainstem disease.

DIAGNOSIS

This patient has a jerky nystagmus with optic atrophy (lesion) caused by multiple sclerosis (aetiology). I would like to examine her neurological system to evaluate the disability (functional status).

QUESTIONS

What do you understand by the term nystagmus?

Nystagmus is a series of involuntary, rhythmic oscillations of one or both eyes. It may be horizontal, vertical or rotator.

What are the types of nystagmus?

- Congenital
- Dissociated
- Gaze evoked
- Vestibular.

ADVANCED-LEVEL QUESTIONS

What is pendular nystagmus?

In pendular nystagmus, the oscillations are equal in speed and amplitude in both directions of movement. It may be seen on central gaze when the vision is poor, as in severe refractive error or macular disease.

What do you understand by the term jerky nystagmus?

Jerky or phasic nystagmus is a condition in which eye movement in one direction is faster than that in the other. This is usually seen in the horizontal plane and is brought out by lateral gaze to one or both sides. It is seen with lesions of the cerebellum, vestibular apparatus or their connections in the brainstem.

What is dissociated nystagmus?

Dissociated or ataxic nystagmus is irregular nystagmus in the abducting eye. It is bilateral in multiple sclerosis, brainstem tumour or Wernicke's encephalopathy. It is unilateral in vascular disease of the brainstem. It is caused by a lesion in the medial longitudinal fasciculus (which links the sixth nerve nucleus on one side to the medial rectus portion of the third nerve on the other).

Where is the lesion in vestibular nystagmus?

It may be in one of two locations:
- Peripheral (labyrinth or vestibular nerve), as in labyrinthitis, Ménière syndrome, acoustic neuroma, otitis media, head injury
- Central (affecting vestibular nuclei), as in stroke, multiple sclerosis, tumours, alcoholism.

What do you know about 'downbeat' and 'upbeat' nystagmus?

Downbeat nystagmus is associated with brainstem lesions, meningoencephalitis and hypomagnesaemia. Upbeat nystagmus is caused by lesions of the anterior vermis of the cerebellum.

Note: you may be asked about upward and downward gaze pathways

K Wernicke (1848–1904) graduated from Poland; although aware that a toxic factor was important in the aetiology, he did not realize that this syndrome was caused by a nutritional deficiency.

P Ménière (1799–1862), French ear, nose and throat specialist.

48 SPEECH

INSTRUCTION

Ask this patient some questions.

SALIENT FEATURES

Examination

- Proceed by asking the patient simple questions regarding personal details such as name, age, occupation, address and handedness (remember that over 90% of left-handed people have a dominant left hemisphere).

Test the following:

- *Comprehension*:
  - Put your tongue out
  - Shut your eyes
  - Touch your nose
  - Smile
  - Two-step commands, such as touch your left ear with your right hand.
- *Orientation*:
  - Time–date
  - Place.
- *Name familiar objects*:
  - Pen
  - Coin
  - Watch.
- *Articulation*, ask the patient to repeat the following:
  - British constitution
  - West Register Street
  - Baby hippopotamus
  - Biblical criticism
  - Artillery.
- *Abbreviated mental test*:
  - Address to recall: 42 West Street.
  - Age
  - Date of birth
  - Time
  - Year
  - Recognition of two persons such as doctor and nurse
  - Name of this place
  - Name of the monarch or prime minister
  - Year of World War I or World War II
  - Count backwards from 20 to 1
  - Serially subtract 7 from 200.
- Tell the examiner that you would like to check the 'primitive' reflexes:
  - *Snout reflex*: brought about by tapping the upper lip slightly; there is puckering or protrusion of the lips with percussion and the muscles around the mouth and the base of the nose contract.
  - *Palmomental reflex*: occurs when a disagreeable stimulus is drawn from the thenar eminence at the wrist to the base of the thumb (Arch

Neurol 1988;45:425–7); there is ipsilateral contraction of the orbicularis oris and mentalis muscles, the corner of the mouth elevates slightly and the skin over the chin wrinkles.

- *Sucking reflex*: elicited by tapping or lightly touching the lips with a tongue blade or the examiner's finger; sucking movements of the lips occur when they are stroked or touched.

Note: The above three reflexes are normal in infants, may be present in normal individuals and are said to be present in a larger number of patients with neurological disease. They are most often seen in those with diffuse cerebral conditions that affect the frontal lobes and pyramidal tracts. The occurrence of more than one reflex is more suggestive of disease than normality.

- *Grasp reflex*: obtained when the examiner's hand is gently inserted into the palm of the patient's hand (when the patient is distracted, usually by engaging him in conversation). With a positive response, the patient grasps the examiner's hand and continues to grasp it as it is moved. The presence of the grasp reflex indicates disease of the supplementary motor area of the frontal cortex.
- *Jaw jerk* (p. 156).

DIAGNOSIS

This patient has expressive dysphasia (lesion) caused by a stroke (aetiology) and is unable to express himself (functional status).

QUESTIONS

What do you understand by the term dysphasia?

Dysphasia is a disorder of the content of speech, which usually follows a lesion of the dominant cortex. The type of dysphasia indicates the site of the lesion in the cortex:

- Expressive, nominal or motor dysphasia: site is the posterior inferior part of the dominant frontal lobe of the cortex (i.e. Broca's area)
- Sensory or receptive dysphasia: site is the superior temporal lobe or *Wernicke's area*.

Note: Sites associated with speech function are variably located along the cortex and can go well beyond the classic anatomical boundaries of Broca's area. These sites typically involve an area contiguous with the face–motor cortex; however, they can be located several centimeters from the sylvian fissure (N Engl J Med 2008;358:18).

What do you understand by the term dysarthria?

Dysarthria is an inability to articulate properly caused by local lesions in the mouth or disorders of speech muscles or their connections. There is no disorder of the content of speech. The causes of dysarthria are:

- stutter
- paralysis of cranial nerves: Bell's palsy, ninth, tenth and eleventh nerves
- cerebellar disease: staccato, scanning speech
- Parkinson's speech: slow, quiet, slurred, monotonous
- pseudobulbar palsy: monotonous, high-pitched 'hot potato' speech
- progressive bulbar palsy: nasal.

ADVANCED-LEVEL QUESTIONS

What are the components of speech?
- Phonation: abnormality is called dysphonia
- Articulation: abnormality is called dysarthria
- Language: abnormality is called dysphasia.

What are the other dominant hemisphere functions?
- Right–left orientation
- Finger identification
- Calculation.

What are the non-dominant hemisphere functions?
- Drawing ability
- Topographic ability
- Construction
- Dressing
- Facial recognition
- Awareness of body and space
- Motor persistence.

What are the parietal lobe signs?
- Loss of accurate localization of touch, position, joint sense and temperature appreciation
- Loss of two-point discrimination
- Astereognosis
- Dysgraphaesthesia
- Sensory inattention
- Attention hemianopia, homonymous hemianopia, or lower quadrantic hemianopia.

What do you understand by the term agnosia?
Agnosia is a failure to recognize objects despite the fact that the sensory pathways for sight, sound or touch are intact. This is tested by asking the patient to feel, name and describe the use of certain objects.

What are the different types of agnosia?
- Tactile agnosia and astereognosis: the patient is unable to recognize objects placed in his or her hands despite the fact that the sensory system of the hands and fingers is intact and there is adequate motor function to allow examination of the object. The lesion is in the parietal lobe.
- Prosopagnosia: the inability to recognize a familiar face. The lesion is in the parieto-occipital lobe.
- Visual agnosia: the inability to recognize objects despite the fact that the main visual pathways to the occipital cortex are preserved. The lesion is in the parieto-occipital lobe.
- Anosognosia: the lack of awareness or realization that the limbs are paralysed, weak or have impaired sensation. The lesion is usually in the non-dominant parietal lobe.

What do you understand by the term apraxia?
Apraxia is the inability to perform purposeful volitional movements in the absence of motor weakness, sensory deficits or severe incoordination.

Usually the defect is in the dominant parietal lobe, with disruption of connections to the motor cortex and to the opposite hemisphere.

What are the different types of apraxia?

● Dressing apraxias: patient is unable to put on his clothes correctly.
● Gait apraxia: difficulty in walking, although patients may show intact leg movements when examined in bed.
● Ideomotor apraxia: patients are unable to perform movements on command, although they may do this automatically, e.g. lick their lips.
● Ideational apraxias: difficulty in carrying out a complex series of movements, e.g. to take a match from a box to light a cigarette.
● Constructional apraxia: patient has difficulty in arranging patterns on blocks or copying designs.

What do you know about dyslexia?

Reading difficulties, including dyslexia, occur as a part of a continuum that also includes normal reading ability. It is not an all-or-none phenomenon but, like hypertension, occurs in degrees. It has been defined as a disorder that is manifested by difficulty in learning to read despite conventional instruction, adequate intelligence and sociocultural opportunity.

Sir Charles Sherrington (1857–1952), Oxford University, and Lord Edgar Douglas Adrian (1889–1977), Cambridge University, were awarded the Nobel Prize in 1932 for their discoveries regarding the functions of neurons.

---

49 EXPRESSIVE DYSPHASIA

INSTRUCTION

Ask this patient a few questions.

SALIENT FEATURES

● Patient has difficulty in finding the appropriate words.

Examination

● Assess the patient's ability to find appropriate words, whether comprehension is intact (e.g. asking the patient to name geometric shapes, parts of the body, or components of common objects such as a pen).
● Repetition may or may not be intact.
● Proceed by telling the examiner that you would like to carry out a neurological examination of the patient for a right-sided stroke.

Remember: The neurologic basis of language is controlled by a network of neocortical areas centered in the perisylvian regions of the left hemisphere of the brain. This language network is almost always located in the left hemisphere of the brain and includes the perisylvian portions of the inferior frontal and temporoparietal regions, known as Broca's and Wernicke's (p. 205) areas, respectively, as well as surrounding regions of the frontal, parietal and temporal cortex. The term dysphasia denotes a disorder in language processing caused by damage to this network.

DIAGNOSIS

This patient has expressive dysphasia (lesion) caused by a right-sided stroke (aetiology).

QUESTIONS

Where is the lesion?
In Broca's area, which is located in the posterior portion of the third left frontal gyrus. It is the motor association cortex for face, tongue, lips and palate. It contains the motor patterns necessary to produce speech.

How would you manage this patient?
- CT or MRI head scan to localize the affected area (Fig. 49.1)
- Aspirin
- Referral to the speech therapist
- General rehabilitation of a patient with stroke.

ADVANCED-LEVEL QUESTIONS

What do you understand by stuttering?
- Stuttering is a disorder of fluency of speech fluency characterized by the involuntary repetition or prolongation of sounds, syllables, words or phrases, as well as frequent pauses, impeding the rhythmic flow of speech.
- Onset is typically between 3 and 6 years of age, and ~ 5% of preschool children may stutter. The majority of young children who stutter go on

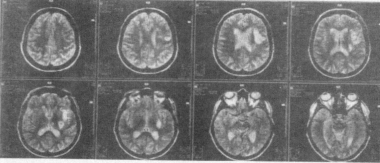

Fig. 49.1 MRI of the brain in Broca's aphasia. The infarct affects the cortical Broca's area, subcortical white matter, and the insula. (With permission from Bradley et al. 2008.)

to make a full recovery. The disorder may continue unabated in some, resulting in a prevalence of about 1% among adults.

What is the commonest sign of primary progressive aphasia?

The commonest clinical feature of primary progressive aphasia is anomia (the inability to retrieve the right word in conversation or to name objects as requested by an examiner). The early stages of anomia can be detected by asking the patient to name geometric shapes, parts of the body, or components of common objects (the cap of a pen or the wristband of a watch). Many patients remain in an anomic stage through most of the course of the disease, with a gradual intensification of word-finding deficits almost to the point of mutism. Occasionally, distinct forms of agrammatism or deficits in word comprehension develop.

What do you understand by the term agrammatism?

Agrammatism refers to inappropriate word order and the misuse of word endings, prepositions, pronouns, conjunctions and verb tenses.

What do you know about genetics of speech?

- Linkage studies of prevalent types of speech and language disorders have implicated several regions of the genome, most notably on chromosomes 3, 13, 16 and 19. The putative risk genes underlying these linkages have yet to be identified.
- Mutation in *FOXP2*, which is located in chromosomal band 7q31 and encodes a transcription factor, has been described in a British family with autosomal dominant transmission of oral motor and speech dyspraxia. These patients have problems sequencing the precise movements of tongue, lips, jaw and palate that contribute to intelligible speech (known as verbal dyspraxia or childhood apraxia of speech). They also have difficulties with learning and production of non-speech sequences involving the orofacial musculature (orofacial dyspraxia) and have a broad profile of linguistic deficits in expressive and receptive domains—problems that affect both oral and written language. The protein product, FOXP2, downregulates the expression of *CNTNAP2*, a gene that encodes a neurexin protein. The general relevance of *CNTNAP2* to speech dyspraxia remains to be determined. *CNTNAP2* is probably associated with disorders associated with nonsense-word repetition (e.g. autism).
- Genes at 7q11.23 are exquisitely sensitive to dosage alterations, which can influence human language and visuospatial capabilities.
- Genetic factors have been implicated in stuttering, with linkage to markers on chromosome 12 and variations in genes governing lysosomal metabolism (N Engl J Med 2010;362:677–85).

> Pierre Paul Broca (1824–1880) was Professor of Surgery in Paris. His notable achievements were in anthropology and his suggestion of cerebral localization of speech was first made at a French Anthropological Society meeting in 1861. He is reported to have described muscular dystrophy (before Duchenne), venous spread of cancer (before Rokitansky) and rickets as a nutritional disorder (before Virchow).

50 CEREBELLAR DYSARTHRIA

INSTRUCTION

Ask this patient a few questions.

SALIENT FEATURES

Examination

- The speech may be scanning (enunciation is difficult, words are produced slowly and in a measured fashion) or staccato (in bursts). Scanning speech is more common in multiple sclerosis, whereas staccato speech is more common in Friedreich's ataxia.
- Articulation is uneven, words are slurred and variations in pitch and loudness occur.
- Proceed by telling the examiner that you would like to carry out a neurological examination of the patient for cerebellar signs.

See Case 46 (Cerebellar syndrome) for discussion.

DIAGNOSIS

This patient has scanning speech (lesion) caused by cerebellar involvement secondary to chronic alcohol abuse (aetiology).

QUESTIONS

What do you understand by the term dysarthria?

Dysarthria is impaired articulation of speech. It may result from lesions of muscles, myoneural junctions or motor neurons of lips, tongue, palate and pharynx. Common causes include mechanical defects such as ill-fitting dentures or cleft palate. Dysarthria may also result from impaired hearing which begins in early childhood.

ADVANCED-LEVEL QUESTIONS

How would you test the different structures responsible for articulation?

- Lips: ask the patient to say, 'me, me, me'
- Tongue: ask the patient to say, 'la, la, la'
- Pharynx: ask the patient to say, 'kuh, gut'
- Palate, larynx and expiratory muscles: ask the patient to say, 'ah'. In palatal paralysis the patient's speech is worse when the head is bent forwards.

Articulation can also be tested by asking the patient to repeat the following:

- British constitution
- Hippopotamus
- Methodist episcopal
- Constantinople is the capital of Turkey.

What do you understand by 'top of the basiliar' syndrome?

Emboli to the rostral portion of the basilar artery usually produce this syndrome, with a myraid of possible symptoms characterized by visual, oculomotor and behavioural abnormalities, often without significant motor dysfunction. A top of the basilar syndrome is characterized by somnolence and sometimes, stupor; inability to make new memories; small, poorly reactive pupils; and defective vertical gaze. Patients with cerebellar infarcts often have dizziness, sometimes in conjunction with frank vertigo, blurred vision, difficulty walking and vomiting. These patients often veer to one side and cannot sit upright or maintain an erect posture without support. They may have hypotonia of the arm on the side of the infarct, a sign best elicited by having them hold their arms straight ahead and then rapidly lower them, quickly braking the movement. The hypotonic arm overshoots on both descent and rapid ascent. Nystagmus is common. Patients with pure cerebellar infarcts *do not* have hemiparesis or hemisensory loss.

What parts of the brain does the vertebrobasilar artery supply?

The vertebrobasilar arterial supplies the brainstem (medulla, pons and midbrain), cerebellum, occipital lobes, posterior temporal lobes and thalamus.

Remember: The vertebra-basilar arterial system consists of the extracranial and intracranial vertebral arteries; these unite to form the basilar artery, which runs midline along the ventral surface of the brainstem, feeding it with small, deep perforators until it merges with the circle of Willis to give off the posterior cerebral arteries.

What is the significance of anti-Yo antibodies in a patient with cerebellar syndrome?

The presence of anti-Yo antibodies in the serum of a woman with cerebellar symptoms is virtually conclusive evidence that she has paraneoplastic cerebellar degeneration and gynaecologic, usually ovarian, cancer.

What is the role of chaperones in cerebellar tumours?

A chaperone complex (which typically maintains cellular protein assembly and function) mediates the assembly of the von Hippel–Lindau tumour suppressor protein; when this protein is not assembled correctly, its tumour-suppressing activity is lost, permitting the development and growth of tumours. A mutation in or deletion of part of this tumoursuppressor protein is associated with von Hippel–Lindau disease (characterized by phaeochromocytoma, renal carcinoma and densely vascularized retinal and cerebellar tumours).

What is the role of Sonic hedgehog *Shh* pathway in pathogenesis of medulloblastoma?

Medulloblastoma arises through abnormalities of developmental pathways in a population of progenitor cells. These tumours aberrantly express multiple regulatory genes known to mediate the proliferation of neural stem cells. Activity in the *Shh* pathway is important for the self-renewal of progenitor cells and the proliferation of their progeny, and also in the initiation of brain tumours. Medulloblastoma cells die rapidly when cultured with cyclopamine, an antagonist of the hedgehog family of regulatory pathways.

51 THIRD CRANIAL NERVE PALSY

INSTRUCTION

Examine this patient's eyes.

SALIENT FEATURES
History

- Diplopia in all directions except on lateral gaze to the side of the third nerve lesion (because the lateral rectus muscle supplied by the sixth cranial nerve is intact)
- Painful onset (berry aneurysm or aneurysmal dilatation of the intracavernous part of the carotid artery causing third nerve palsy)
- Headaches (migraine, cranial arteritis)
- Obtain a history of diabetes or hypertension.

Examination

- Unilateral ptosis (from paralysis of the levator palpebrae superioris)
- Dilated pupil reacting slowly or incompletely to light (paralysis of the constrictor of the pupil)
- Paralysis of accommodation (from involvement of ciliary muscle)
- Squint and diplopia resulting from weakness of muscles supplied by the third cranial nerve (superior, inferior, medial recti and inferior oblique). The eye will be in the position of abduction (i.e. down and out) if the fourth and sixth nerves are intact
- Diplopia may not be obvious until the affected eyelid is elevated manually.

Proceed as follows:

- Exclude associated fourth cranial nerve lesion (supplies the superior oblique) by tilting the head of the patient to the same side – the affected eye will intort if the fourth cranial nerve is intact. Remember superior oblique intorts the eye (SIN). Inferior oblique externally rotates the eye.
- Tell the examiner that you would like to check:
  - urine for sugar (diabetes mellitus)
  - BP (hypertension).

Notes

- Vascular lesions (such as those associated with diabetes and arteritis) that infarct the third nerve may produce a complete oculomotor palsy with pupillary sparing. The pupillomotor fibres are around the periphery of the third nerve. Compression of the mass or aneurysm often involves the pupil.
- Be prepared to discuss the third cranial nerve anatomy.

DIAGNOSIS

This patient has a R/L third nerve palsy (lesion) caused by diabetes mellitus (aetiology).

QUESTIONS

What are the common causes of a third nerve palsy?

- Hypertension and diabetes are the most common causes of pupil-sparing third nerve palsy. (The presence of pain is not a good discriminating feature between diabetes and aneurysm, as pain is present in both.) Diabetic third nerve palsy usually recovers within 3 months
- Multiple sclerosis
- Aneurysms of posterior communicating artery (painful ophthalmoplegia)
- Trauma
- Tumours, collagen, vascular disorder, syphilis
- Ophthalmoplegic migraine
- Encephalitis
- Parasellar neoplasms
- Meningioma at the wing of sphenoid
- Basal meningitis
- Carcinoma at the base of the skull
- Rhinocerebral mucormycosis (in diabetic ketoacidosis, but about half the patients with diabetes who have this infection do not have ketoacidosis).

How would you investigate such a patient?

- Test BP and urine for sugar
- ESR to exclude temporal arteritis (in the elderly)
- Edrophonium test to exclude myasthenia if the pupil is not involved
- Thyroid function tests and orbital ultrasonography to exclude thyroid disease
- CT or MRI of the head
- Arteriography, especially when the pupil is involved and there is severe pain.

ADVANCED-LEVEL QUESTIONS

When would you suspect a lesion of the third nerve nucleus?

- Unilateral third nerve palsy with contralateral superior rectus palsy and bilateral partial ptosis
- Bilateral third nerve palsy (with or without internal opthalmoplegia associated with spared levator function).

What do you know about the muscles of extraocular movement?

Each eye is moved by three pairs of muscles and the precise action of these muscles depends on the position of the eye; the actions are as follows:

- Medial and lateral recti (first pair of muscles): adduct and abduct the eye, respectively
- Superior and inferior recti: elevate and depress the abducted eye
- Superior and inferior obliques: depress and elevate the adducted eye.

Note: Superior and inferior recti act in the abducted position (mnemonic RAB).

What do you know about the anatomy of the oculomotor nerve?

Midbrain. The third cranial nerve originates in the midbrain and courses through the cavernous sinus and superior orbital fissure into the orbit to innervate four muscles and provide parasympathetic fibres for pupillary constriction.

Cavernous sinus. In the cavernous sinus or at the superior orbital fissure, the third cranial nerve may lie very close to the optic nerve. The third cranial nerve divides into superior and inferior rami within either the anterior portion of the cavernous sinus or the posterior optic canal. The superior rami supply fibres to the levator palpebrae and superior rectus muscles, and the inferior rami supply the extraocular muscles innervated by this nerve and also carry the pupillomotor fibres, which are in the superomedial portion of the nerve.

Note: Ischaemic disease of the oculomotor nerve (e.g. in patients with diabetes mellitus or hypertension) typically spares the pupil, whereas compressive disease results in pupillary enlargement.

Do you know of any eponymous syndromes in which the third cranial nerve is involved?

- Weber syndrome: ipsilateral third nerve palsy with contralateral hemiplegia. The lesion is in the midbrain.
- Benedikt syndrome: ipsilateral third nerve palsy with contralateral involuntary movements such as tremor, chorea and athetosis. It is caused by a lesion of the red nucleus in the midbrain.
- Claude syndrome: ipsilateral oculomotor paresis with contralateral ataxia and tremor. It is caused by a lesion of the third nerve and red nucleus.
- Nothnagel syndrome: unilateral oculomotor paralysis combined with ipsilateral cerebellar ataxia.

M Benedikt (1835–1920), an Austrian physician, described this syndrome in 1889.

Sir HD Weber (1823–1918) qualified in Bonn and worked at Guy's Hospital, London.

Henri Claude (1869–1945), a French psychiatrist.

Carl Wilhelm Nothnagel (1841–1905), an Austrian physician.

---

52 SIXTH CRANIAL NERVE PALSY

INSTRUCTION

Examine this patient's eyes.

SALIENT FEATURES

History

- Diplopia in all directions of gaze except away from the affected side
- Patient may rotate the head towards the weak side to produce a single image
- Patient may intentionally close the affected eye to prevent diplopia (pseudo ptosis)

- Hearing loss (acoustic neuroma)
- Diabetes or hypertension.

Examination

- The eye is deviated medially and there is failure of lateral movement.
- The diplopia is maximal when looking towards the affected side. The two images are parallel and separated in the horizontal plane. The outer image comes from the affected eye and disappears when the eye is covered.
- Proceed by telling the examiner that you would like to check the following:
  - Blood pressure and urine sugar
  - Hearing and corneal sensation (early signs of acoustic neuroma).

DIAGNOSIS

This patient has a sixth nerve palsy (lesion) caused by diabetes mellitus (aetiology) and is having severe diplopia (functional status).

QUESTIONS

What are the causes of sixth nerve palsy?
- Hypertension
- Diabetes
- Raised intracranial pressure (false localizing signs)
- Multiple sclerosis
- Basal meningitis
- Encephalitis
- Acoustic neuroma, nasopharyngeal carcinoma
- Lyme disease (N Engl J Med 2007;356:1561).

ADVANCED-LEVEL QUESTIONS

Where is the nucleus of the sixth nerve located?
In the pons. (The nuclei of the first four cranial nerves are situated above the pons and those of the last four cranial nerves are situated below the pons.)

What are the structures in close proximity to the sixth nerve nucleus and fascicles?
These include:
- facial and trigeminal nerves
- corticospinal tract
- median longitudinal fasciculus
- parapontine reticular formation.

A combination of clinical findings pointing to the involvement of these structures indicates the presence of an intrapontine lesion.

What you know about the peripheral course of the abducens nerve?
It is lengthy: from the brainstem and base of the skull through the petrous tip and cavernous sinus to the superior orbital fissure and orbit. Lesions at any of these sites may affect the nerve.

Have you heard of Gradenigo syndrome?
Inflammation of the tip of the temporal bone may involve the fifth and sixth cranial nerves as well as the greater superficial petrosal nerve, resulting in unilateral paralysis of the lateral rectus nerve, pain in the

distribution of the trigeminal nerve (particularly its first division) and excessive lacrimation.

Do you know any eponymous syndromes where the pons is infarcted and consequently the sixth cranial nerve is involved?

- Raymond syndrome: ipsilateral sixth nerve paralysis and contralateral paresis of the extremities
- Millard–Gubler syndrome, in which there is ipsilateral sixth and seventh nerve palsy with contralateral hemiplegia
- Foville syndrome has all the features of Millard–Gubler paralysis with lateral conjugate gaze palsy.

Mention other syndromes with sixth nerve involvement

- Duane syndrome: widening of the palpebral fissure on abduction and narrowing on adduction
- Gerhardt syndrome: bilateral abducens palsy
- Möbius syndrome: paralysis of extraocular muscles, especially abducens, with paresis of facial muscles.

What do you know about Tolosa–Hunt syndrome?

It is a syndrome characterized by unilateral recurrent pain in the retro-orbital region with palsy of the extraocular muscles resulting from involvement of the third, fourth, fifth and sixth cranial nerves. It has been attributed to inflammation of the cavernous sinus.

C Gradenigo (1859–1926), an Italian otolaryngologist, described this syndrome in 1904.

    E Tolosa, a Spanish neurosurgeon.

    WE Hunt, an American neurosurgeon.

    ALJ Millard (1830–1915), a French physician.

    AM Gubler (1821–1915), Professor of Therapeutics in France.

    ALF Foville (1799–1878), Professor of Physiology at Rouen, described his syndrome in 1848.

---

53   SEVENTH CRANIAL NERVE PALSY: LOWER MOTOR NEURON TYPE

INSTRUCTION

Look at this patient's face.
Examine the cranial nerves.

SALIENT FEATURES

History

- Onset: whether abrupt followed by worsening over the following day (Bell's palsy)
- Pain over the preceding or accompanying the weakness (Bell's palsy)
- The face itself feels stiff and pulled to one side
- Ipsilateral restriction of eye closure

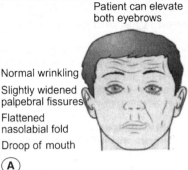
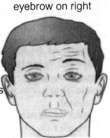

Patient can elevate both eyebrows

Unable to elevate eyebrow on right

Normal wrinkling

Forehead does not wrinkle

Slightly widened palpebral fissures

Markedly wider palpebral fissures

Flattened nasolabial fold

Flattened nasolabial fold

Droop of mouth

Droop of mouth

(A) (B)

Fig. 53.1 Facial weakness: central (A) and peripheral (B).

- Difficulty with eating
- Disturbance of taste (caused by chorda tympani fibres)
- Hyperacusis (involvement of stapedius muscle in the inner ear).

Examination

- Weakness of muscles of one half of the face; the patient is unable to screw his or her eyes tightly shut or move the angle of the mouth on the affected side (Fig. 53.1)
- Loss of facial expression
- Widened palpebral fissure.

Proceed as follows:

- Look for the following when the patient is unaware of being observed:
  - Flatter nasolabial folds on the affected side
  - Mouth on the affected side droops and participates manifestly less while talking
  - The eyelid on the affected side closes just after the opposite eyelid.
- Look at the external auditory meatus for herpes zoster (Ramsay Hunt syndrome)
- Look for parotid gland enlargement
- Examine for taste (loss of taste with the involvement of chorda tympani)
- Check for hearing (for hyperacusis resulting from involvement of the nerve to stapedius muscle)
- Examine tympanic membrane for otitis media
- Tell the examiner that you would like to test the urine for sugar (diabetes).

DIAGNOSIS

The patient has lower motor neuron seventh cranial nerve palsy (lesion), which is idiopathic (aetiology). She is distressed because the condition causes severe disfigurement while talking and has House Brackman grade VI facial palsy (functional status).

QUESTIONS

How would you differentiate between upper and lower motor neuron palsy?

In lower motor neuron palsy the whole half of the face on the affected side is involved. In upper motor neuron palsy the upper half of the face (the forehead) is spared (Fig. 53.1).

How is facial palsy graded?

House Brackman grades:

I: normal

II: mild dysfunction, slight weakness, slight synkinesis

III: moderate dysfunction, obvious weakness, incomplete eye closure, normal symmetry only at rest

IV: moderately severe dysfunction

V: severe dysfunction, barely perceptible movement, asymmetry at rest

VI: total paralysis.

ADVANCED-LEVEL QUESTIONS

What are the causes of bilateral facial nerve palsy?

- Guillain–Barré syndrome (p. 338)
- Sarcoidosis in the form of uveoparotid fever (Heerfordt's disease)
- Melkersson–Rosenthal syndrome, which is a triad of facial palsy, recurrent facial oedema and plication of the tongue (Hygiea 1928;90:737–41, Z Neurol Psychiatr 1931;131:475–501).

Note: Myasthenia may mimic bilateral facial nerve palsy.

What are causes of unilateral facial nerve palsy?

Causes can be idiopathic (Bell's palsy; 65%), infective (associated with Bell's palsy), trauma (25%), neoplasms (5%), metabolic and toxic, plus other rate causes.

- **Lower motor neuron** All the muscles of one half of the face are affected:
- Bell's palsy. Recent studies using a polymerase chain reaction (PCR) have implicated herpes simplex viral infection in Bell's palsy. The incidence of Bell's palsy is 23 per 100 000 individuals per year, or about 1 in 60–70 individuals per year. Men or women are affected equally and the peak incidence between the ages of 10 and 40. Both the right and left sides are affected with equal frequency
- Herpes zoster
- Cerebellopontine angle tumours
- Parotid tumours
- Old polio
- Otitis media
- Skull fracture.

- **Upper motor neuron** The forehead is spared:
- Stroke (hemiplegia).

Is the facial nerve a motor nerve or a sensory nerve?

The facial nerve is predominantly a motor nerve and supplies all muscles concerned with facial expression and the stapedius muscle. Uncommonly, it may have a sensory component, which is small (the nervus intermedius of Wrisberg). It conveys taste sensation from the anterior two-thirds of the tongue and, probably, cutaneous impulses from the anterior wall of the external auditory canal.

What do you know of nervus intermedius?

Nervus intermedius or pars intermedia of Wrisberg is the sensory or the parasympathetic root of the facial nerve and is lateral and inferior to the motor root. Inside the internal auditory meatus it lies between the motor root and the eighth cranial nerve. The sensory cells are located in the geniculate ganglion (at the bend of the facial nerve in the facial canal) and their nerve fibres enter the pons with the motor root. The geniculate ganglion is continued distally as the chorda tympani, which carries taste and preganglionic parasympathetic fibres. This nerve consists of contributions from three areas:

- Superior salivary nucleus (in the pons) supplies secretory fibres to the glands
- Gustatory or solitary nucleus (in the medulla) receives taste fibres via the chorda tympani
- Dorsal part of the trigeminal nerve receives cutaneous sensation from the external auditory meatus and the skin behind the ear (distributed with the facial nerve proper).

How would you manage Bell's palsy?

About 50–60% of patients recover spontaneously without deficits; others have considerable improvement, and about 10% have permanent residual deficits. Therefore, many physicians tend to initiate steroids only in those with clinically complete deficit or when there is severe pain. Treatment includes:

- physiotherapy: massage, electrical stimulation, splint to prevent drooping of the lower part of the face
- protection of the eye with lubricating eye drops and a patch during sleep
- early treatment (within 72 h) with prednisolone significantly improves the chances of complete recovery at 3 and 9 months (N Engl J Med 2007;357:1598)
- aciclovir–prednisone is more effective in improving volitional muscle activity and in preventing partial nerve degeneration than placebo–prednisone treatment (Ann Otol Rhinol Laryngol 1996;105:371).

What are the branches of the facial nerve?

- Greater superficial petrosal nerve (supplies lacrimal, nasal and palatine glands)
- Nerve to stapedius muscle
- Chorda tympani (supplies taste to anterior two-thirds of tongue, submaxillary and sublingual glands)
- Motor branches (exit from the stylomastoid foramen).

How would you localize facial nerve palsy?

- Involvement of the nuclei in the pons: associated ipsilateral sixth nerve palsy
- Cerebellopontine angle lesion: associated fifth and eighth nerve involvement
- Lesion in the bony canal: loss of taste (carried by the lingual nerve) and hyperacusis (caused by involvement of the nerve to stapedius).

Mention reflexes involving the facial nerve

- Corneal reflex (p. 156)
- Palmomental reflex (p. 204)
- Suck reflex

- Snout reflex (p. 204)
- Orbicularis oculi reflex or glabellar reflex (p. 194)
- Palpebral–oculogyric reflex
- Orbicularis oris reflex.

Mention a few examples of facial synkinesis

Facial synkinesis means that attempts to move one group of facial muscles result in contraction of associated muscles. It may be seen during anomalous regeneration of facial nerve. For example:

- if fibres originally connected with muscles of the face later innervate the lacrimal gland, anomalous secretion of tears (crocodile tears) may occur while eating
- if fibres originally connected with the orbicularis oculi innervate the orbicularis oris, closure of the eyelids causes retraction of the mouth
- opening of the jaw may cause closure of the eyelids on the corresponding side (jaw-winking).

Have you heard of Möbius syndrome?

It consists of congenital bilateral facial palsy associated with third and sixth nerve palsies and comprises congenital facial diplegia, congenital oculofacial paralysis and infantile nuclear aplasia.

What is the relationship between diabetes and Bell's palsy?

Diabetes is said to be an important cause in about 10% of cases of Bell's palsy. In one study, Bell's palsy was associated with abnormal glucose tolerance in two-thirds of patients (Lancet 1971;i:108, Arch Otolaryngol 1974;99:114).

What parts of the facial nerve must be imaged when facial nerve palsy is suspected?

Both MRI and CT of the temporal bone are used when the facial nerve must be examined.

The following anatomic areas must be imaged when the facial nerve is studied:

- The brain and pons (precentral, postcentral and central gyrus; posterior limb of the internal capsule)
- The cerebellopontine angle
- The internal auditory canal
- The labyrinthine part of the facial nerve canal (VII-1) and geniculate ganglion
- The tympanic part of the facial nerve canal (VII-2)
- The mastoid part of the facial nerve canal (VII-3)
- The stylomastoid foramen and the parotid gland.

Does the facial nerve communicate with other cranial nerves or cervical spinal nerves?

Yes, the facial nerve demonstrates clinically relevant communications with other cranial and cervical spinal nerves.

Site	Communication
Internal acoustic meatus	Vestibulocochlear nerve
Geniculate ganglion	Splenopalatine nucleus, otic ganglion, sympathetic nerves around the middle meningeal artery

Site	Communication
Facial canal	Auricular branche of the vagus nerve
Splenomastoid foramen	Glossopharnyngeal, vagus, great auricular, and auricular temporal nerves
Behind the ear	Lesser occipital nerve
On the face	Trigeminal
In the neck	Cutaneous cervical nerve

Sir Charles Bell (1774–1842) was Professor of Surgery in Edinburgh and a founder member of the Middlesex Hospital in London. He discovered that the anterior and posterior spinal nerve roots were motor and sensory respectively.

James Ramsay Hunt (1874–1937), Professor of Neurology in New York.

PJ Möbius (1853–1907), a German neurologist.

54 TREMORS

PATIENT 1

INSTRUCTION

Look at this patient's hands and demonstrate tremors.

SALIENT FEATURES

Examination

- Coarse resting tremor that is slow (4–6 per second)
- Adduction–abduction of the thumb with flexion–extension of fingers (pill-rolling movement)
- The tremor is halted by purposive movements of the hands. The upper limb tremor often increases as the patient walks
- Tell the examiner that you would like to do the following:
  - Look for cog-wheel rigidity
  - Comment on mask-like facies
  - Check gait for festinant gait
  - Ask the patient's relatives whether sleep relieves the tremor and whether emotion makes it worse
  - Examine the handwriting (Fig. 54.1).

DIAGNOSIS

This patient with resting tremor and mask-like facies (lesion) has Parkinson's disease (aetiology) and is severely disabled by the tremor (functional status).

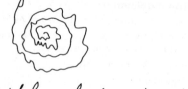 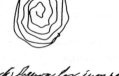

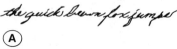

(A)   (A)

Fig. 54.1 Handwriting and spiral drawing reflects tremor type. (A) Large scrawl in essential tremor. (B) Cramped, parkinsonian writing and spiral shows little tremor; writing is an action.

PATIENT 2

INSTRUCTION

Look at this patient's hands and demonstrate tremors.

SALIENT FEATURES

Examination

- There is a 10-s physiological tremor that is brought on when the arms are outstretched. It can be amplified by laying a sheet of paper on the hands.
- Tell the examiner that you would like to do the following:
  - Check for thyrotoxicosis
  - Take a history for alcoholism
  - Take a drug history (salbutamol, terbutaline, lithium)
  - Take an occupational history to mercury (hatters' shakes)
  - Find out whether tremor runs in the family and is relieved by alcohol (benign essential tremor).

DIAGNOSIS

This patient has fine tremor with an enlarged thyroid gland (lesion), which could be from hyperthyroidism (aetiology).

PATIENT 3

INSTRUCTION

Look at this patient's hands and demonstrate tremors.

SALIENT FEATURES

Examination

- The patient does not have a resting tremor or a tremor with outstretched hands.

Proceed as follows:
● Check the past-pointing: the intention tremor of cerebellar disease
● Tell the examiner that you would like to check for other cerebellar signs (p. 201).

DIAGNOSIS

This patient has an intention tremor (lesion) caused by cerebellar syndrome (aetiology).

INSTRUCTION

Look at this patient's hands and demonstrate tremors.

SALIENT FEATURES

Examination
● Unsteadiness when standing still; by contrast, the patient has little or no difficulty while walking, which relieves the symptoms.
● Fine rippling of the muscles of the legs may be seen or felt when the patient attempts to stand still; after a short interval, the patient becomes increasingly unsteady and is forced to take a step to regain balance.

Diagnosis
This patient has primary orthostatic tremor (lesion).

QUESTIONS

What are the tremors?
Involuntary movements that result from alternating contraction and relaxation of groups of muscles, producing rhythmic oscillations about a joint or a group of joints.

How would you classify tremors?
● Resting tremor, as in Parkinson's disease
● Postural tremor (also referred to as action tremor or kinetic tremor). It is brought on when the arms are outstretched and is caused by the following:
  • Exaggerated physiological tremor, caused by anxiety, thyrotoxicosis, alcohol, drugs
  • Brain damage, seen in Wilson's disease, syphilis.
● Intention tremor (aggravated by voluntary movements) in cerebellar disease
● Tremor from neuropathy (postural tremor; arms more than legs).

Mention a few involuntary movements
● Chorea
● Athetosis
● Hemiballismus
● Fasciculation

- Torticollis
- Clonus.

What are the causes of drug-associated tremors?

- Drug-induced tremors: beta-2 agonists (e.g. salbutamol), caffeine, theophylline, lithium, tricyclic antidepressants, serotonin reuptake inhibitors, neuroleptics, sodium valproate, corticosteroids.
- Tremors associated with drug withdrawal: alcohol (delirium tremens), benzodiazepines, barbiturates, opiates.

ADVANCED-LEVEL QUESTIONS

What do you know about the investigation and management of primary orthostatic tremor?

- In primary orthostatic tremor:
  - Electromyography (EMG) shows rhythmic activation of lower limb muscles at a frequency of 4–18 Hz
  - PET shows increased activity in the cerebellum.
- Treatment is supportive and patient is often relieved to know the diagnosis, especially when a psychiatric cause has been suspected previously.

What is the pathophysiology of tremor?

- Physiological tremor has both mechanical and central components.
- Symptomatic palatal tremor is most likely caused by rhythmic activity of the inferior olive.
- Essential tremor is also generated from within the olivocerebellar circuits. The most common action tremor is essential tremor, a tremor of the hands at 4–12 Hz.
- Rest tremor of Parkinson's disease arises from the basal ganglia loop, and dystonic tremor originates from within the basal ganglia.
- Orthostatic tremor originates from unidentified brainstem nuclei.
- Cerebellar tremor is in part caused by a cerebellar circuit that involves feedforward control of voluntary movements.
- Neuropathic tremor is believed to be caused by abnormally functioning reflex pathways.
- Toxic and drug-induced tremors have many underlying causes.
- Psychogenic tremor is thought to be mediated by reflex mechanisms.

What is the treatment for tremor?

- Tremor caused by Parkinson's disease: levodopa, anticholinergic agents, dopamine agonists or budipine. When all other types of medication are not effective, clozapine is often beneficial. More than 50% of patients respond to this treatment (N Engl J Med 2000;342:505).
- Essential tremor: beta-blockers, primidone or both; 40–70% of these patients have some improvement with this treatment (N Engl J Med 2001;345:887).
- Cerebellar tremor: no standard treatment; clonazepam is sometimes effective, as is treatment with levodopa, anticholinergic agents or clozapine.
- Drug resistant tremor: thalamic stimulation (continuous deep-brain stimulation) and thalamotomy are equally effective, but thalamic stimulation has fewer adverse effects and results in a greater improvement of function (N Engl J Med 2000;342:461–8).

Further reading

Fahn S: Differential diagnosis of tremors. *Med Clin North Am* 56:1363–1375, 1972. (good review on tremors).

Mercury poisoning was known as 'hatter's shakes' because workers involved in the manufacture of felt hats were exposed to mercury.

---

55 PERIPHERAL NEUROPATHY

INSTRUCTION

Examine this patient's legs.
Carry out a neurological examination of this patient's legs.

SALIENT FEATURES

History

- Progressive and symmetrical numbness in the hands and feet that spreads proximally in a glove and stocking distribution
- Distal weakness, which also ascends
- History of diabetes, alcohol, connective tissue disorder, malignancy.

Examination

- Bilateral symmetrical sensory loss for all modalities with or without motor weakness
- Proceed by looking for evidence of the following (mnemonic: DAD,RUM):
  - **D**iabetes mellitus (diabetic chart, insulin injection sites, insulin pump)
  - **A**lcoholic liver diease (palmar erythema, spider naevi, tender liver)
  - **D**rug history
  - **R**heumatoid arthritis
  - **U**raemia
  - **M**alignancy.
- Palpate for thickened nerves and look for Charcot's joints
- Tell the examiner that you would like to do the following:
  - Look for anaemia and jaundice (vitamin B_{12} deficiency)
  - Check urine for sugar
  - Take a history of alcohol consumption and a drug history.

DIAGNOSIS

This patient has symmetrical, bilateral sensory loss for touch and pain (lesion) caused by diabetes mellitus (aetiology).

QUESTIONS

How are polyneuropathies classified?

- Polyneuropathies can be classified as demyelinating or axonal
  - Demyelinated: acute inflammatory demyelinating polyradiculoneuropathy (subtype of Guillain-Barré syndrome), diphtheria, chronic

inflammatory polyradiculoneuropathy, Charcot-Marie-Tooth disease type 1
- Axonal: acute motor axonal neuropathy, acute motor and sensory axonal neuropathy, multifocal motor neuropathy, associated with HIV, diabetic, medications, toxins.

● They can also be classified according to the diameter of the affected nerve fibre. Larger fibres are heavily myelinated and, therefore, most subject to processes that damage myelin.

● Most polyneuropathies, including the diabetic type, are axonal.

Mention a few causes of thickened nerves
● Amyloidosis
● Charcot–Marie–Tooth disease
● Leprosy
● Refsum disease (retinitis pigmentosa, deafness and cerebellar damage)
● Déjérine–Sottas disease (hypertrophic peripheral neuropathy).

What are the causes of motor neuropathy?
● Guillain–Barré syndrome
● Peroneal muscular atrophy
● Lead toxicity
● Porphyria
● Dapsone toxicity
● Organophosphorous poisoning.

What are the causes of mononeuritis multiplex?
Mononeuritis multiplex is a neuropathy affecting several nerves and causes include (mnemonic: WARDS, PLC):
● **W**egener's granulomatosis
● **A**myloidosis
● **R**heumatoid arthritis
● **D**iabetes mellitus
● **S**LE
● **P**olyarteritis nodosa
● **L**eprosy
● **C**arcinomatosis, Churg–Strauss syndrome.

Mention a few causes of predominantly sensory neuropathy
● Diabetes mellitus
● Alcoholism
● Deficiency of vitamins B_{12} and B_1
● Chronic renal failure
● Leprosy.

What are the types of neuropathy described in diabetes mellitus?
● Symmetrical, mainly sensory, polyneuropathy
● Asymmetrical, mainly motor, polyneuropathy (diabetic amyotrophy)
● Mononeuropathy
● Autonomic neuropathy.
Be aware there are different classifications (Fig. 55.1).

What drugs are used for painful peripheral neuropathy of diabetes?
Tricyclic antidepressants, phenytoin, carbamazepine and topical capsaicin.

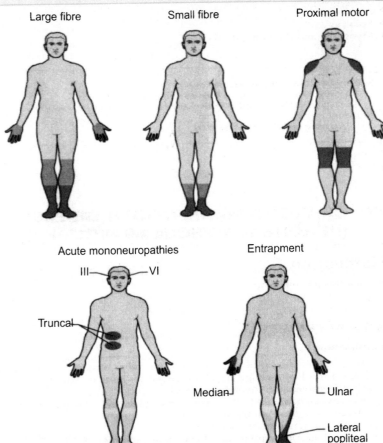

Fig. 55.1 Different clinical presentations of diabetic neuropathies.

ADVANCED-LEVEL QUESTIONS

What are the other effects of alcohol on the central nervous system?
- Wernicke's encephalopathy (ophthalmoplegia, nystagmus, confusion and neuropathy)
- Korsakoff's psychosis (recent memory loss and confabulation)
- Cerebellar degeneration
- Marchiafava–Bignami disease (symmetrical demyelination of corpus callosum)
- Central pontine myelinolysis

- Amblyopia
- Epilepsy
- Myopathy and rhabdomyolysis.

K Wernicke (1848–1904) worked in Poland.

SS Korasakoff (1853–1900), a Russian neuropsychiatrist.

J Churg (b. 1910) qualified in Poland and was Professor of Pathology in New York.

L Strauss, a pathologist in New York.

---

56 CHARCOT–MARIE–TOOTH DISEASE (PERONEAL MUSCULAR ATROPHY)

INSTRUCTION

Examine this patient's legs.

SALIENT FEATURES

Examination

- Wasting of muscles of calves and thighs that stops abruptly, usually in the lower third of the thigh, and is described as 'stork' or 'spindle' legs, 'fat bottle' calves and 'inverted champagne bottles' (Fig. 56.1)
- Pes cavus (high arched foot) or pes planus (flat foot), clawing of toes, contractures of the Achilles tendon
- Weakness of dorsiflexion, foot drop
- Absent ankle jerks, plantars are downgoing or equivocal
- Mild sensory impairment or no sensory loss. Some patients have decreased responses to pain in the stocking distribution.

Proceed as follows:

- Feel for lateral popliteal nerve thickening (seen in some cases only)
- Look at the hands for small muscle wasting and clawing
- Tell the examiner that you would like to:
  - Know whether there is a family history of disease
  - Look for enlarged greater auricular nerves
  - Examine the spine for scoliosis
  - Examine the gait (high-steppage gait of foot-drop).

Note: There are two distinctive clinical features of this disease:

1. The muscular atrophy begins in the distal portions of the affected muscles in the lower and upper limbs, unlike the global atrophy of motor neuron disease or muscular dystrophy. The atrophy then creeps upwards, involving all muscles.
2. Second, the degree of disability is minimal in spite of marked deformity.

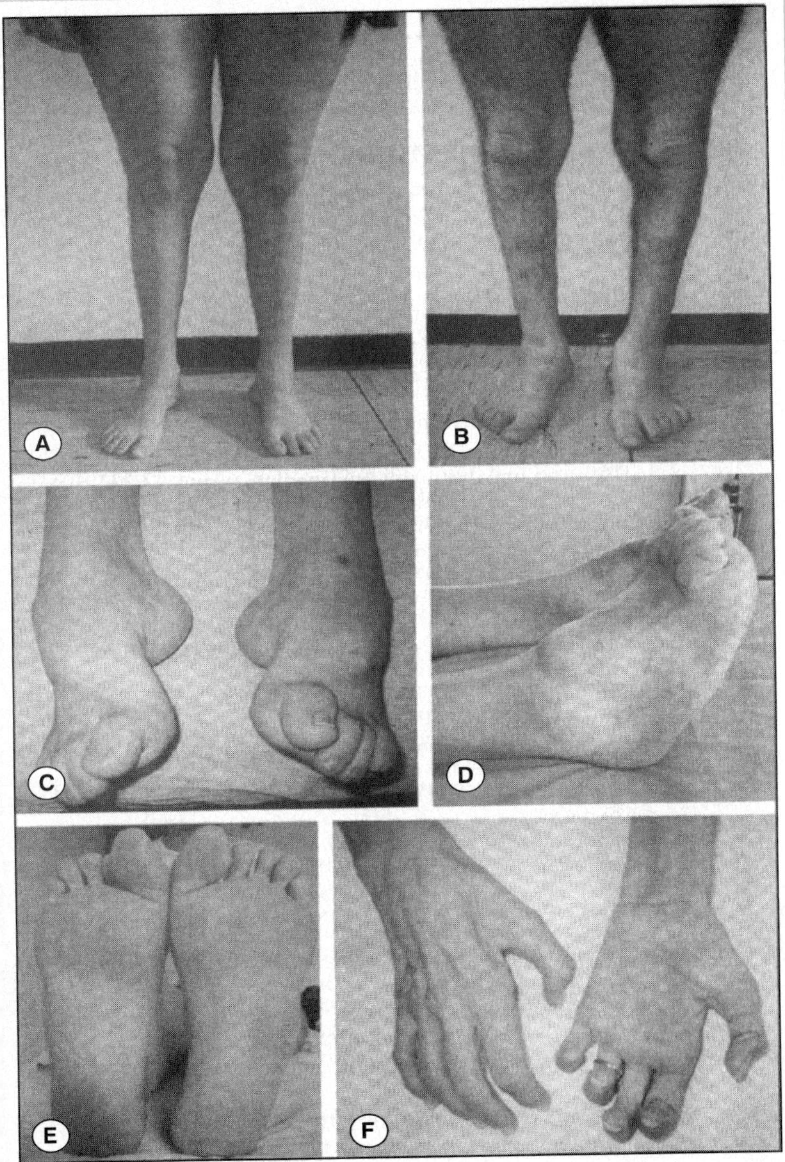

Fig. 56.1 Charcot–Marie–Tooth disease. (A,B) Muscle wasting of the legs and the lower third of the thigh. (C–E) Foot deformities of different severities, with high arches, hammer toes and callosities. (F) Severe atrophy of intrinsic hand muscles (main en griffe, claw hand). (With permission from Pareyson D, Marchesi C 2009.)

DIAGNOSIS

This patient has 'inverted champagne bottle' legs with sensory neuropathy (lesion), which is caused by hereditary Charcot–Marie–Tooth disease (aetiology). She has severe foot-drop and requires calipers (functional status).

ADVANCED-LEVEL QUESTIONS

What are the phenotypic types of Charcot–Marie–Tooth disease?

Charcot–Marie–Tooth disease (CMT) is divided in two major phenotypic types according to electrophysiological, clinical and nerve evaluations:

- Glial myelinopathy (type 1): a demyelinating neuropathy (marked slowing of conduction in motor nerves; absent deep tendon reflexes)
- Neuronal axonopathy (type 2): an axonal neuropathy (little or no slowing of nerve conduction; normal deep tendon reflexes)
- Distal spinal muscular atrophy.

What is the mode of inheritance?

- Each type can be inherited in a dominant, recessive or X-linked fashion. There are also autosomal dominant intermediate forms of CMT that can have features of both axonal and demyelinating neuropathies. Mutations in 31 known genes and additional unidentified loci can produce CMT:
  - Some common genes include *PMP22, MPZ, PRX, GDAP1,* and *EGR2*
  - *MPZ* (encoding myelin protein zero is a member of the immunoglobulin superfamily; it may be important not only in forming myelin but also in cell signalling), *GDAP1* and *GJB1* are known to be associated with CMT type 1, but select mutations in these genes can also cause CMT type 2
  - *NEFL* is known to be associated with CMT type 2, but select mutations convey a CMT type 1 phenotype
  - Dominant intermediate forms of CMT have been reported to be associated with *MPZ* mutations
  - Specific recessive alleles related to CMT have also been reported for *EGR2* and *PMP22*
  - Two mutations in *SH3TC2* (encoding the SH3 domain and tetratricopeptide repeats 2) cause autosomal recessive CMT (N Engl J Med 2010;362:1181–91)
  - Of the 31 genes in 39 known CMT loci, only 15 are currently available for clinical testing.
- Current evidence-based clinical guidelines for distal symmetric polyneuropathy recommend genetic testing consisting of screening for common mutations, including the *CMT1A* duplication copy-number variant and point mutations of the X-linked *GJB1*.
- Whole genome sequencing is emerging to be the diagnostic tool in this condition.

What other uncommon features may these patients have?

Optic atrophy, retinitis pigmentosa, spastic paraparesis.

In which other conditions is pes cavus seen?

Friedreich's ataxia.

What is the natural history of the disease?

The disease usually arrests in middle life.

How does the forme fruste of the disease manifest?

The forme fruste may be seen in family members of patients with CMT and manifests as pes cavus and absent ankle jerks.

Mention other hereditary neuropathies

- Roussy–Lévy syndrome (where features of progressive muscular atrophy may be combined with tremor and ataxia)
- Hereditary amyloidosis
- Refsum's disease (phytanic acid accumulates in the central and peripheral nervous systems)
- Fabry's disease (where there is a deficiency of α-galactosidase)
- Tangier disease
- Bassen–Kornzweig disease (abetalipoproteinaemia, absence of LDL, and vitamin E deficiency)
- Metachromatic leukodystrophy (where galactosyl sulfatide accumulates in the central and peripheral nervous systems).

Mention a few conditions that Charcot is credited to have described for the first time

- Ankle clonus
- Tabes dorsalis and Charcot's joints
- Multiple sclerosis
- Peroneal muscular atrophy
- Multiple cerebral aneurysms, called Charcot–Bouchard aneurysms
- Hysteria.

The syndrome was originally described by JM Charcot (1825–1923) and P Marie (1853–1940) in 1886 at the Saltpêtrière in Paris, and independently by HH Tooth at St Bartholomew's Hospital and the National Hospital for Nervous Diseases, Queen Square, London.

P Marie was a world-famed neurologist. He published extensively on aphasia. He succeeded Charcot's lineage of Raymond, Brissaud and Dejerine at the Saltpêtrière in 1918.

---

57 DYSTROPHIA MYOTONICA

INSTRUCTION

Look at this patient's face.
Examine this patient's cranial nerves.

SALIENT FEATURES

History

- Onset usually in the third and fourth decade. However, if the mother is the carrier then the disease may manifest in infancy and undergo rapid deterioration at the usual age of onset
- Onset dominated by weakness or myotonia or both
- Difficulty in releasing grip

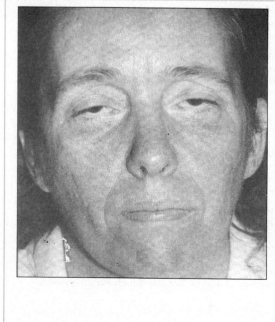

Fig. 57.1 Muscle wasting in myotonic dystrophy gives the characteristic drawn appearance of 'hatchet facies.' (With permission from Yanoff, Duker 2008.)

- Leg weakness (difficulty in kicking a ball)
- 'Pseudo-drop attacks' (caused by weakness of quadriceps muscle)
- Ask the patient if they have dysphagia (oesophageal involvement)
- Impotence (caused by gonadal atrophy)
- Recurrent respiratory infections (caused by weakness of muscles of bronchioles)
- Excessive urge to sleep (daytime somnolence is common).

Examination

- While shaking hands with the patient, note the myotonia
- Frontal baldness (the patient may be wearing a wig and it is important to mention if this is so)
- Ptosis (bilateral or unilateral) with a *smooth* forehead
- Cataracts (posterior capsular cataracts) or evidence of surgery for cataracts
- Difficulty in opening the eyes after firm closure
- Expressionless face ('hatchet face'; Fig. 57.1) with wasting of temporalis, masseters and sternomastoids and 'swan neck' caused by thinning of the neck.

Proceed as follows:
- Test:
  - Sternomastoids
  - Distal muscles of the upper limbs, wasting, percussion myotonia over thenar muscles and weakness
  - Deep tendon jerks (depressed).

- Tell the examiner that you would like to do the following:
  - Check the urine for sugar (diabetes mellitus)
  - Test higher intellectual function (low IQ)
  - Examine for gynaecomastia and testicular atrophy.

Remember: Respiratory failure is the commonest cause of death.

DIAGNOSIS

This patient has frontal balding, myotonia, cataracts and wasting of the sternomastoids (lesion) caused by dystrophia myotonica (aetiology). He has dysphagia and severe muscular weakness (functional status).

ADVANCED-LEVEL QUESTIONS

What is the inheritance of this condition?

Autosomal dominant inheritance. Myotonic dystrophy type 1 (the more common and typically the more severe of the two major types) is caused by an expanded cytosine–thymine–guanine (CTG) repeat on chromosome 19q13.3 in the 3'-untranslated region of *DMPK*, a gene for a dystrophia myotonica protein kinase (a serine–threonine protein kinase). The condition usually presents in the third and fourth decades. The disease tends to be worse in successive generations (known as anticipation). As a result, the grandparent may merely have cataracts while the grandchild develops a severe progressive form of the disease. Positional cloning has helped to identify the gene for myotonic dystrophy and localized a dynamic mutation with an increase in the number of trinucleotide repeats. The repeat size typically increases from generation to generation, providing a molecular basis for the clinical phenomenon of anticipation.

The less common form of the disease, myotonic dystrophy 2, is caused by an expanded CCTG repeat (with expansions ranging from 80 to 11 000 repeats) in the first intron of *ZNF9*, the gene for zinc finger protein 9.

Transcribed RNA repeats fold into a hairpin, and the RNA is retained in the nucleus, where it alters the ratio of CUG RNA-binding proteins, such as CUG-binding protein 1 (CUG-BP1) and muscleblind-like 1 (MBNL1). Splicing misregulation in myotonic dystrophy results from altered functions of these two RNA-binding proteins, which were identified because they bind CUG repeats in RNA. CUG-BP1 and MBNL1 are direct and antagonistic regulators of alternative splicing events that are normally regulated during development and misregulated in myotonic dystrophy. Increased activity of CUG-BP1 and decreased activity of MBNL1 induce 'embryonic pattern' splicing (i.e. isoforms typically expressed in the developing embryo and fetus predominate). The fact that MBNL1 colocalizes with nuclear RNA foci in the cells of patients with myotonic dystrophy suggests that MBNL1 is sequestered by mutant RNAs. Increasing the expression of MBNL1 in a mouse model of myotonic dystrophy restores the adult splicing pattern of the muscle-specific chloride channel (ClC-1) protein and reverses the myotonia associated with ClC-1 misregulated splicing (Proc Natl Acad Sci USA 2006;103:11748–53). These data support for a primary role of MBNL1 depletion in the pathogenesis of the disease.

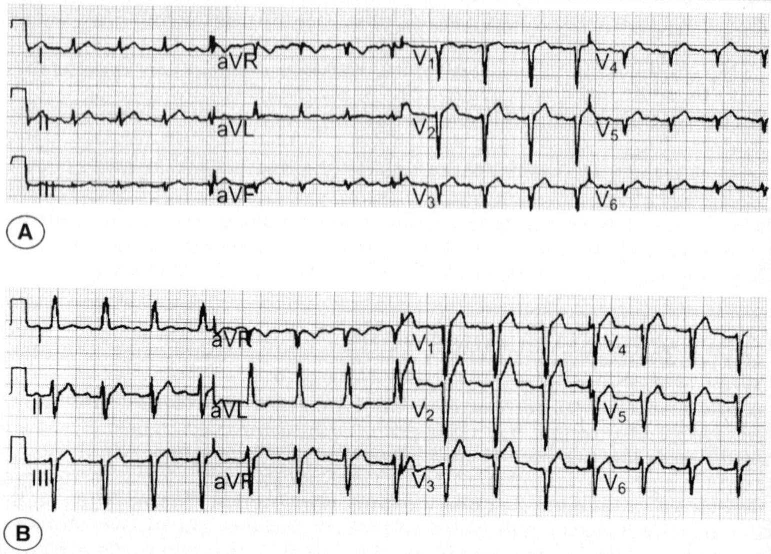

Fig. 57.2 ECG in myotonic dystrophy (A taken around a year before B). There are abnormal Q waves in the precordial leads. The increasing severity of conduction disease is indicated by increasing PR interval and QRS duration in (B).

What are the other features of this condition?
- Cardiomyopathy and cardiac conduction defects (Fig. 57.2). A severe abnormality on the ECG and a diagnosis of an atrial tachyarrhythmia predict sudden death (N Engl J Med 2008;358:2688–97). An implantable cardioverter defibrillator should be considered in all patients
- Respiratory infection (low serum immunoglobulin G levels)
- Somnolence
- External ophthalmoplegia (occasionally).

What do you understand by myotonia?
It is continued contraction of the muscle after voluntary contraction ceases, followed by impaired relaxation.

What therapeutic modalities are available?
Mexilitene, acetazolamide or phenytoin have been used in *disabling* myotonia. No treatment has altered the course of progressive weakness.

What other forms of myotonia do you know?
Myotonia congenita, or Oppenheim's disease, is an autosomal dominant condition that presents at birth with feeding difficulties. The myotonia improves with age and there is no dystrophy. Although this is considered to be a myopathy, changes have been reported in the motor nuclei of the spinal cord and motor cortex.

In which myopathies is distal weakness prominent?
- Myotonic dystrophy
- Welander's distal myopathy (more common in Scandinavians).

If this patient requires major surgery, what fact would you keep in mind?
Patients with dystrophia myotonica tend to do poorly after the administration of general anaesthetic (caused by impaired cardiorespiratory malfunction) and will require intensive postoperative observation.

Mention some causes of bilateral ptosis
- Myasthenia gravis
- Congenital muscular dystrophies
- Ocular myopathy
- Syphilis.

What is the pathognomonic pattern of cataract in dystrophia myotonica?
Stellate or 'christmas tree' cataract.

The patient's sister is worried about risks to her offspring. What tests would you do?
- Clinical examination
- Electromyography
- Slit-lamp examination for cataracts.

Is prenatal diagnosis available?
Yes – in some families. The myotonic dystrophy gene is linked to the *ABH* secretor gene. However, not all families are informative.

Remember: Babies born to mothers with myotonic dystrophy are prone to hypotonicity; in most instances there is a family history of this disease, which is dominantly inherited. The mother may have undiagnosed myotonic dystrophy.

What is the characteristic electromyography finding?
Waxing and waning of the potentials, known as the dive-bomber effect. Electromyography changes are found in almost any muscle.

How would you manage such patients?
- Foot drop is controlled by calipers or molded-foot orthoses.
- Myotonia when disabling may respond to phenytoin (avoid quinidine and procainamide as they can worsen cardiac conduction).
- Advanced heart block with or without syncope should be considered for pacemaker insertion.

Délége in 1890 first described the association of myotonia with muscular atrophy.

Batten and Gibb (Brain 1909;32:187) and Steinert (Dtsch Z Nervenheilk 1909;37:58.), in 1909, independently described the clinical features of the symptom complex.

Curschmann in 1912 emphasized the dystrophic symptoms and applied the term dystrophia myotonica.

58 PROXIMAL MYOPATHY

INSTRUCTION

Perform a neurological examination of this patient's arms or legs.

SALIENT FEATURES

History

- Weakness of proximal muscles
- Patient has difficulty in standing from the sitting position (getting up from chairs, getting off the commode) or difficulty in combing hair – elicit this history.

Examination

- Check the gait, looking for waddling gait (p. 251)
- Look for an underlying cause:
  - Diabetic amyotrophy (asymmetrical, usually in the lower limbs in non-insulin-dependent diabetes mellitus)
  - Cushing syndrome (characteristic facies, history of steroid ingestion; see p. 538)
  - Thyrotoxicosis (look for eye signs, goitre, rapid pulse, tremor)
  - Polymyositis (heliotropic rash, tender muscles)
  - Drug history (alcohol, steroids, chloroquine)
  - Carcinomatous neuropathy
  - Osteomalacia (bone pain)
  - Hereditary muscular dystrophy.

DIAGNOSIS

This patient has weakness of the proximal muscles of the lower limbs (lesion) caused by Cushing syndrome (aetiology) and is severely limited by the weakness (functional status).

QUESTIONS

What is Gowers' sign?

In severe proximal myopathy of the lower limbs, a patient on rising from the floor uses their hands against the body to climb up to vertical. It has been classically described in Duchenne muscular dystrophy.

What do you know about diabetic amyotrophy?

It is an asymmetrical motor polyneuropathy that presents with asymmetrical weakness and wasting of the proximal muscles of the lower limbs and sometimes upper limbs, diminished or absent knee jerk and sensory loss in the thigh. It is usually accompanied by severe pain in the thigh, often awakening the patient at night. The prognosis is good and most patients recover over months or years with diabetic control.

ADVANCED-LEVEL QUESTIONS

What is the difference between type 1 and type 2 muscle fibres?

- Type 1 muscle fibres are high in myoglobin and oxidative enzymes and have many mitochondria. They perform tonic contraction and are involved in weight bearing and movements requiring sustained force. Chloroquine causes vacuolation of myocytes, predominantly type 1 fibres.

- Type 2 muscle fibres are rich in glycolytic enzymes; they perform rapid phasic contractions and are involved in sudden movements and in purposeful motion. In steroid myopathy the muscle fibre atrophy predominantly affects these fibres.

Sir WR Gowers (1845–1915), Professor of Medicine at University College Hospital, London, invented a haemoglobinometer, personally illustrated an atlas of ophthalmology and wrote a book on spinal cord diseases and a manual on the nervous system. He also founded a society of medical stenographers.

Guillaume-Bejmanin-Amand Duchenne (1806–75) was first to describe Duchenne muscular dystrophy in 1868 in a paper where he described 13 cases of the disease; by 1870 he had seen about 40 cases.

---

59 DEFORMITY OF A LOWER LIMB

INSTRUCTION

Examine the lower limbs of this patient who has had this abnormality since childhood.

SALIENT FEATURES

History

- History of trauma to the spine and/or leg
- History of poliomyelitis
- History of weakness and fasciculations
- Bladder and bowel symptoms.

Examination

- Wasting and deformity of one lower limb (or both with one side being more affected than the other)
- Fasciculations
- Normal tone in both lower limbs
- Check the sensory system (L5 and/or S1 sensory loss in spina bifida)
- Examine the spine:
  - Kyphoscoliosis (seen in poliomyelitis, indicating involvement of trunk muscles)
  - Tuft of hair in the lower lumbosacral spine (closed spina bifida).
- Comment on bony deformity in the affected leg.

Note: Always check the gait and test for Romberg's sign.

DIAGNOSIS

This patient has unilateral wasting and deformity of the R/L leg (lesion) caused by poliomyelitis in childhood (aetiology) and wears calipers on that leg (functional status).

QUESTIONS

What is the differential diagnosis?
- Old poliomyelitis (Fig. 59.1)
- Spina bifida (Fig. 59.2).

What are the causes of lower motor neuron signs in the legs?
- Peripheral neuropathy
- Prolapsed intervertebral disc
- Diabetic amyotrophy
- Poliomyelitis
- Cauda equina lesions
- Motor neuron disease.

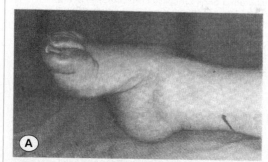

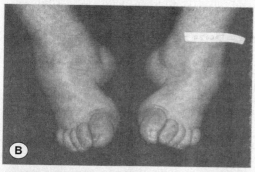

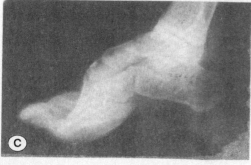

Fig. 59.1 Medial (A) and frontal (B) views and radiograph (C) of severe calcaneocavovarus deformities as sequelae of poliomyelitis. (With permission from Canale, Beaty 2007.)

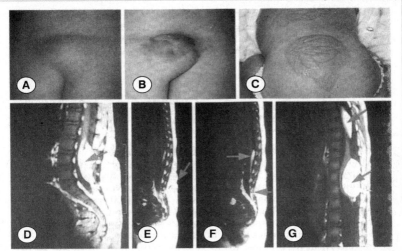

Fig. 59.2 Clinical features and corresponding occult spinal dysraphism detected by sagittal, T_1-weighted MRI studies of the spinal cord. (A) Sacral lipoma and deviated gluteal furrow. (B) Lumbar port-wine stain, lipoma, dermal sinus, and deviated gluteal furrow. (C) Dorsal and lumbar unclassified hamartomas. (D) Lipoma of the conus (arrow). (E) Dermal sinus (arrow). (F) Top of the lipoma of the filum terminale (upper arrow) and fistula (lower arrow). (G) Multiple lipomas of the thoracic cord (upper arrow) and posterior-conus (lower arrow). (With permission from Guggisberg et al: 2004.)

ADVANCED-LEVEL QUESTIONS

What is the cause of polio?

Polio is caused by a picornavirus of the genus *Enterovirus*; there are three antigenic types: I (Brunhilde), II (Lansing) and III (Leon).

Is the muscular involvement of polio in childhood progressive?

Usually paralytic polio remains stable after the initial attack. However, in some patients new muscle weakness and atrophy involving previously affected muscles or even unaffected muscles occurs and this deterioration can occur as long as 30 years after the first attack; this is known as post-poliomyelitis muscular atrophy (PPMA). The progression of this involvement is slow and is said to be distinct from motor neuron disease. It is not entirely clear why only some patients are affected but it has been reported that it is more likely to occur in those with widespread paralysis and poor immune status (N Engl J Med 1986;314:959).

Is poliomyelitis preventable?

Yes, three types of poliovaccine are available (each containing all three strains of the virus):

- Oral polio vaccine of Sabin consists of live attenuated virus
- Killed or inactivated vaccine of Salk
- Enhanced potency vaccine of van Wezel.

With which vaccine is paralytic poliomyelitis associated?

Vaccine-associated paralytic poliomyelitis (VAPP) is associated with oral polio vaccine, particularly in immunodeficient individuals (N Engl J Med 1995;332:500–6). Such individuals and their household contacts should be given inactivated vaccine.

What do you know about 'provocation poliomyelitis'?

Provocation poliomyelitis is caused by the administration of intramuscular injections during the incubation period of wild-type poliovirus or shortly after exposure to oral poliovaccine (either as a vaccine recipient or through contact with a recent recipient).

What do you understand by the term spina bifida?

Spina bifida means an incomplete closure of the bony vertebral canal and is commonly associated with a similar anomaly of the spinal cord. The commonest site is the lumbosacral region, but the cervical spine can be involved and may be associated with hydrocephalus. It results from failure of fusion of the caudal neural tube and is one of the most common malformations of human structure. The causes include single gene disorders, chromosome abnormalities and teratogenic exposures. Although the cause is not known in most cases, up to 70% of spina bifida cases can be prevented by maternal periconceptional folic acid supplementation. The mechanism underlying this protective effect is unclear, but it is probably related to genes that regulate folate transport and metabolism. Individuals with spina bifida often require both surgical and medical management. Surgical closure is usually done in the neonatal period. Medical management is a lifelong (Lancet, 2004;364:1885–95).

What are the features of closed spina bifida?

- Cutaneous: lumbosacral lipoma, hypertrichosis, sinus or dimple above the sacrum, naevus or scarring
- Unilateral shortening of one leg and foot with a deficiency of the muscles below the knee. There may be calcaneovalgus or equinovarus deformity. Sensory loss in the fifth lumbar and first sacral dermatome is common
- Neuropathic bladder, enuresis
- Bony changes on radiograph: sacral dysgenesis, scoliosis, laminar fusion of vertebral body, pedicle erosion and bony spurs.

Is the neurological deficit in closed spina bifida progressive?

This issue is contentious as much of the deficit is fixed antenatally and any progression is a result of growth and posture. However, in some patients the late appearance of bladder dysfunction indicates that the neurological deficit is progressive in these individuals.

Mention some teratogenic factors responsible for neural canal defects

- Maternal diabetes and sacral dysgenesis
- Sodium valproate in pregnancy and neural tube defects (Lancet 1982;ii:1282).

Mention some prenatal screening tests for spina bifida

- Amniotic α-fetoprotein levels
- Amniotic acetylcholinesterase estimation
- High-resolution diagnostic ultrasonography.

What is the basic mechanism of muscle atrophy?

Muscle atrophy (associated with disuse, nerve injury, fasting and many diseases including cancer, AIDS and TB) has a single basic mechanism: excessive activation of the ubiquitin–proteasome pathway in the muscle. The proteasome is a large protein complex that acts like a cell's garbage disposal by grabbing onto excess and damaged proteins and degrading them; ubiquitin is an enzyme (now called ATP-dependent protease) responsible for protein breakdown.

MH Romberg (1795–1873), German neurologist and Professor of Medicine in Berlin.

The 1952 Nobel Prize was jointly awarded to John F Enders (1897–1985), Thomas H Weller (b. 1915) both of Children's Medical Center and Harvard Medical School, Boston, and Frederick C Robbins (b. 1916) of Western Reserve University, Cleveland, Ohio, for their discovery of the ability of poliomyelitis viruses to grow in cultures of various types of tissue.

US President Franklin Delano Roosevelt is known for his defiant struggle with his permanent lower-limb paresis (caused by polio). In 1937, Roosevelt announced the formation of a National Foundation for Infantile Paralysis that would 'lead, direct, and unify the fight of every phase of this sickness'. Soon, millions of US citizens were responding to the pleas of the radio personality Eddie Cantor to 'send their dimes directly to the President at the White House' and now this movement is called 'the March of Dimes'.

---

60 MULTIPLE SCLEROSIS

PATIENT 1

INSTRUCTION

Examine this patient's eyes.

SALIENT FEATURES

History

- Remissions and relapses: visual loss, diplopia.

Examination

- Optic atrophy
- Nystagmus.
- Internuclearophthalmoplegia (see Fig. 81.1)
- Look for features of cerebellar syndrome (p. 200)
- Proceed by telling the examiner that you would like to do a full neurological examination.

DIAGNOSIS

This patient has optic atrophy (lesion) caused by multiple sclerosis.

INSTRUCTION

Examine this patient's legs.

SALIENT FEATURES

History

- Remissions and relapses: weakness, incoordination, pain, paraesthesias, urinary urgency, impotence. Steinberg's triad is history of incontinence of bladder, impotence or constipation.

Examination

- Spastic paraparesis (increased tone, upgoing plantars, weakness, brisk reflexes and ankle or patellar clonus). Spasticity is quantified using the Ashworth scale, which scores muscle tone on a scale of 0–4 with 0 representing normal tone and 4 severe spasticity
- Impaired coordination on heel–shin test (if there is marked weakness, this test may be unreliable).

Proceed as follows:

- Check abdominal reflexes (absent or diminished in over 80% of cases)
- Tell the examiner that you would like to look for optic atrophy and cerebellar signs.

Remember:

- in such patients, spinal cord compression should be excluded before making a diagnosis of multiple sclerosis
- some examiners may consider it insensitive to use the term multiple sclerosis in front of the patient and may prefer that the candidate uses the term 'demyelinating disorder' instead
- to be prepared to discuss the course and pathogenesis.

DIAGNOSIS

This patient has spastic paraparesis (lesion) caused by multiple sclerosis, and is wheelchair bound (functional status).

QUESTIONS

What investigations would you consider?

- Spinal radiography, including both cervical and thoracic regions
- Lumbar puncture: total protein concentration may be raised (in 60% of cases), with an increase in the level of immunoglobulin G (in 40%) and oligoclonal bands (in 80%) on electrophoresis
- Visual evoked potentials: despite normal visual function, there may be prolonged latency in cortical response to a pattern stimulus. This indicates a delay in conduction in the visual pathways
- MRI of brain: about 50% of patients with early multiple sclerosis in the spinal cord show abnormal areas in the periventricular white matter
- Serum vitamin B_{12} to exclude subacute degeneration of the spinal cord.

Mention a few causes of bilateral pyramidal lesions affecting the lower limbs

- Cord compression
- Multiple sclerosis

- Cervical spondylosis
- Transverse myelitis
- Motor neuron disease
- Vitamin B$_{12}$ deficiency
- Cerebrovascular disease.

ADVANCED-LEVEL QUESTIONS

How common is multiple sclerosis?
The prevalence in the UK is about 1 in 800 people, with an annual incidence of 2–10 per 100 000. The age of onset varies but peaks between 20 and 40 years of age (Brain 1980;112:133–6). Prevalence varies geographically.

What are the main ways in which multiple sclerosis can present?
- Optic neuritis (in 40%), resulting in partial loss of vision
- Weakness of one or more limbs
- Tingling in the extremities caused by posterior column involvement
- Diplopia
- Nystagmus, cerebellar ataxia
- Vertigo.

What is the natural history of multiple sclerosis?
The course of the disease is extremely variable and patients with multiple sclerosis face enormous prognostic uncertainty. The onset may be acute, subacute or insidious. The course may be rapidly downhill, or may spontaneously remit for periods lasting from days to years before a second exacerbation (N Engl J Med 2000;343:938–52).

What are the clinical categories of multiple sclerosis?
- Relapsing-remitting: episodes of acute worsening with recovery and a stable course between relapses
- Secondary progressive: gradual neurologic deterioration with or without superimposed acute relapses in a patient who previously had relapsing–remitting multiple sclerosis
- Primary progressive: gradual, nearly continuous neurologic deterioration from the onset of symptoms
- Progressive relapsing: gradual neurologic deterioration from the onset of symptoms but with subsquent superimposed relapses.

What is Lhermitte's sign?
A tingling or electric shock-like sensation that radiates to the arms, down the back or into the legs on flexion of the patient's neck. It has also been called the 'barber's chair' sign. It indicates disease near the dorsal column nuclei of the higher cervical cord. Causes include multiple sclerosis, cervical stenosis and subacute combined degeneration of the cord.

What is Uhthoff's symptom?
The exacerbation of symptoms of multiple sclerosis during a hot bath.

Do you know of any criteria for diagnosis of multiple sclerosis?
The revised **McDonald's criteria** are based on the clinical attacks and lesions initially, attempting to establish dissemination in time (have occurred at least 30 days apart) and place (affecting separate sites within the CNS) for lesions (Ann Neurol 2005;58:840–6, Lancet 2008; 372:1502–17). If the clinical features do not fit the criteria exactly, MRI can substitute for

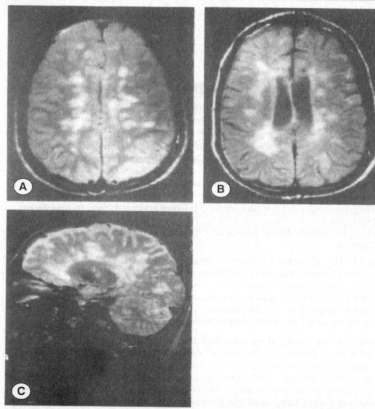

Fig. 60.1 MRI in in multiple sclerosis. (A) Multifocal lesions in the centrum semiovale (proton density image). (B) Multiple, at times confluent, white matter lesions abutting the lateral ventricles (proton density image). (C) Lesions distributed in a radiating fashion from the corpus callosum (Dawson's fingers) plus significant cerebral atrophy with ventriculomegaly and cortical atrophy (T_2-weighted image). (With permission from Bradley et al. 2008.)

one of these clinical episodes (Fig. 60.1): MR lesions are defined as occurring with:

- *dissemination in time*: one gadolinium-enhancing lesion at least 3 months after the onset of the clinical event *or* a new lesion identified by T_2-weighted imaging compared with a reference scan done at least 30 days after onset of the clinical event
- *dissemination in space*: three features from:
  - one gadolinium-enhancing lesion or T2 MRI lesions
  - one or more infratentorial lesions
  - one or more juxtacortical lesions
  - three or more periventricular lesions (a spinal cord lesion can replace some of these brain lesions).

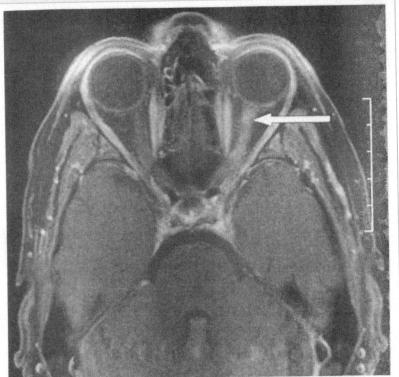

Fig. 60.2 Acute optic neuritis is associated with enhancement of the optic nerve in approximately two-thirds of the patients. Homogeneous enhancement of the left optic nerve can be seen in orbital view using axial T_1-weighted, postgadolinium infusion with fat suppression. (With permission from Courtney et al. 2009.)

Primary progressive multiple sclerosis can be diagnosed after 1 year of a progressive deficit and two of:
- a positive MRI of the brain
- a positive MRI of the spinal cord
- positive oligoclonal bands on examination of cerebrospinal fluid (CSF).

Possible multiple sclerosis: patients having an appropriate clinical presentation but who do not meet all of the diagnostic criteria can be classified as having possible multiple sclerosis.

Which conditions may be considered forme fruste of multiple sclerosis?
- Optic neuritis (Fig. 60.2)
- Single episode of transverse myelitis with optic neuritis.

What is the role of steroids in acute optic neuritis and the development of multiple sclerosis?

In acute optic neuritis, treatment with a 3-day course of high-dose intravenous methylprednisolone (followed by a short course of prednisone) reduces the rate of development of multiple sclerosis over a 2-year period (N Engl J Med 1990;326:581–8, N Engl J Med 1993;329:1764–9).

Does pregnancy affect the clinical features of multiple sclerosis?

Pregnancy itself may have a mildly protective effect but there is an increased risk of relapse during the puerperium; overall, the effect on the course of the disease is probably negligible.

What is the role of exercise in the treatment of such patients?

Patients should be encouraged to keep active during remission and to avoid excessive physical exercise during relapses.

What is the role of MRI in multiple sclerosis?

MRI can identify up to 80% of patients with multiple sclerosis. T_2-weighted images show hyperintense focal periventricular lesions. Although periventricular white matter lesions are typical of multiple sclerosis, they are not pathognomonic. Small infarcts, disseminated metastases, moya-moya disease and inflammatory diseases can produce a similar picture. High-resolution MRI may provide useful prognostic information in patients who present with an acute clinically isolated syndrome suggestive of multiple sclerosis. On 5-year follow-up, over half the patients who had asymptomatic white matter lesions at presentation had developed clinically definite multiple sclerosis, compared with 3% of patients with normal results at presentation. The disease progressed rapidly if the scan showed four or more lesions at presentation, and a greater number of lesions also correlated with development of moderate or severe disability (N Engl J Med 1993;116:135–6, Brain 1998;121:495–503).

Mention some other demyelinating disorders

- Devic's disease: optic neuritis with acute myelitis with MRI changes that extend over at least three segments of the spinal cord. It is associated with a specific antibody marker (NMO-IgG) targeting the water channel aquaphorin-4 (Curr Neurol Neurosci Rep 2008;8:427–33)
- Leukodystrophies
- Tuberous sclerosis (patchy demyelination; see p. 690)
- Schilder's disease (diffuse cerebral sclerosis; may present with cortical blindness when the occipital cortex is involved).

What are the prognostic markers that predict more severe multiple sclerosis?

- Progressive disease from the onset of symptoms
- Frequent relapses in the first 2 years
- Motor and cerebellar signs at presentation to neurologist
- Short interval between the first two relapses
- Male gender
- Poor recovery from relapse
- Multiple cranial lesions on T_2-weighted MRI at presentation.

Note: Women and patients with predominantly sensory symptoms and optic neuritis have a more favourable prognosis

What is the differential diagnosis of multiple sclerosis?

Systemic diseases complicated by CNS involvement that follow a relapsing–remitting course (e.g. systemic vasculitis) (Lancet 2008; 372:1502–17):

- Disorders affecting one anatomical site and with either a relapsing–remitting or progressive course (especially, tumours and other structural lesions)
- Monophasic disorders affecting several neuroantaomical locations (e.g. acute disseminated encephalomyelitis)
- Diseases of the spinal cord and brain confined to selected physiological systems and usually following a progressive course (e.g. the hereditary cerebellar ataxias)
- Non-organic symptoms that, intentionally or otherwise, mimic the clinical features of multiple sclerosis (so-called functional or somatization disorders).

Is there any treatment for multiple sclerosis?

- Immunomodulatory agents/approaches:
- Two forms of interferon-β (i.e. interferon beta-1b (Betaferon) and interferon beta-1a (Avonex, Rebif)) have been shown to reduce the relapse rate in relapsing–remitting (non-progressive) neurological deficit by one-third (Neurology 1993;43:655–67, Lancet 1998;352;1491–7). Whether reduction in relapse rate reduces or prevents later disability is not known; some evidence has been presented in favour. The Association of British Neurologists recommends interferon-β be prescribed for ambulant patients with at least two definite relapses in the previous 2 years followed by recovery (may or may not be complete).
- Interferon beta-1b has been reported to delay progression (for 9–12 months in a study period of 2–3 years) in secondary progressive multiple sclerosis of moderate severity (minimum walking distance of 20 m with assistance) and has been licensed for this indication. However, the SPECTRIMS study, which was a large trial, showed no significant benefit of interferon-1b therapy in delaying disability in secondary progressive multiple sclerosis.
- Intravenous methylprednisolone may hasten recovery from acute relapses but has no effect in the long term. A recent trial suggested intravenous methylprednisolone is no better than equivalent oral doses of methylprednisolone for acute relapses (Lancet 1997;349:902–6).
- Copolymer-1 (Neurology 1995;45:1268–76), glatiramer acetate (Copaxone) and pulsed intravenous immunoglobulin (Lancet 1997;349:589–93) like interferon-β, reduce the relapse rate. However, the role of immunomodulatory agents needs to be defined.
- Plasma exchange enhances recovery of relapse-related neurologic deficits in patients with no response to high-dose corticosteroids.
- Newer therapies: two oral agents, cladribine and fingolimod, have been used in the treatment of relapsing–remitting multiple sclerosis. Both reduce the number of potentially autoaggressive lymphocytes that are available to enter the central nervous system (CNS). Cladribine (in the CLARITY trial) and fingolimod (in the FREEDOMS trial) were highly effective against placebo over a 2-year period, and fingolimod was more effective than intramuscular interferon beta-1a over a 12-month period (in the TRANSFORMS trial).

- Alemtuzumab was more effective than interferon beta-1a in early, relapsing–remitting multiple sclerosis but was associated with autoimmunity, most seriously manifesting as immune thrombocytopenic purpura (N Engl J Med 2008;359:1786–1801).
- A single course of rituximab (by depleting B cells) reduces inflammatory brain lesions and clinical relapses for 48 weeks (N Engl J Med 2008;358:676–88).

- **Immunosuppression** Mitoxantrone hydrochorlide has been shown to reduce rate of clinical relapse and delay progression of disability in secondary progressive multiple sclerosis.

- **Selective adhesion molecule inhibitor** Natalizumab, an α_4-integrin antagonist (which targets the VLA-4 adhesion molecule) reduces development of brain lesions and reduces relapses rates. There is a small risk of developing progressive multifocal leukoencephalopathy and, therefore, requires participation in a safety surveillance programme (Lancet Neurol 2007;6:431–41).

- **Miscellaneous:**
- Fatigue is modestly reduced by amantadine (Neurology 1995;45: 1956–61).
- Bladder dysfunction usually consists of combined detrusor hyperreflexia and incomplete emptying volumes, with <100 ml urine remaining in the bladder after micturition, is managed with oxybutinin or detrusitol; retention of volumes >100 ml require clean, intermittent self-catheterization (J Neurol Neurosurg Psychiatry 1996;60:6–13).
- Sexual dysfunction (erectile failure) may be helped with the phosphodiesterase inhibitor sildenafil citrate (Viagra), yohimbine or other alpha-adrenergic blockers.
- Limb spasticity requires a multidisciplinary approach ensuring correct posture, prevention of skin ulceration from pressure, management of bladder and bowel dysfunction as well medications such as tizanidine (an α_2-adrenoreceptor antagonist) an antispastic agent (Neurology 1994;44(suppl 9):70S–8). Tizandine reduces spasticity but there is no beneficial effect on mobility.

Remember: There is no evidence to suggest that any treatment alters the long-term outcome in multiple sclerosis.

What do you know about the two-hit model in the pathogenesis of multiple sclerosis?

Grey matter atrophy proceeds three times faster in multiple sclerosis than in unaffected persons, and with progressive neurologic disability, this rate of atrophy increases to 14 times faster in affected patients than in unaffected persons. Grey matter atrophy correlates with physical disability and cognitive disability more strongly than white matter atrophy. The two-hit model for cortical demyelination posits that two separate pathogenic 'hits' — an activation hit and a demyelination hit — triggers the pathologic process in the cortex. An immune-mediated inflammation targets contactin 2 (expressed in specialized regions of myelinated fibres by oligodendrocytes, Schwann cells, and the axons of a subpopulation of neurons, including those in the hippocampus and spinal cord) on or near grey matter endothelial cells to open the blood–brain barrier or alter endothelial cells in the grey matter, permitting effectors of demyelination (such as antibodies to myelin proteins) to gain access to grey matter.

Note: Three patterns of demyelinating lesion have been described in the brain cortex in patients with multiple sclerosis:

I: lesions involve both white and grey matter
II: lesions are small perivascular areas of cortical demyelination
III: lesions are bands of cortical demyelination below the pial surface that often cover several gyri and stop at cortical layer three or four.

What do you understand by Pulfrich effect?

The Pulfrich effect is a stereo-illusion resulting from latency disparities in the visual pathways. It is a feature of optic neuritis but is also to be found with other conditions. The symptoms are often difficult for the patient to explain and for the physician to understand. Symptoms may be sufficiently disturbing to significantly interfere with activities of daily living (e.g. prevention of driving, crossing the road or playing ball games). Treatment with the use of monocular tints is simple and effective.

JL Lhermitte (1877–1959), a French neurologist and neuropsychiatrist, wrote exclusively on spinal injuries, myoclonus, internuclear ophthalmoplegia and chorea.

William Ian McDonald (1933–2006), native of New Zealand, was Head of the Department of Neurology at Queen Square, London. He delineated the pathophysiology of demyelination of peripheral nerve in 1963 (Brain 1963;86:481–500). His article on diagnostic criteria in multiple sclerosis in 1983 continues to this day to rank among the most cited and downloaded articles ever published in *Annals of Neurology*.

---

61 ABNORMAL GAIT

INSTRUCTION

Look at this patient walking.
Test this patient's gait.

SALIENT FEATURES

Examination

There are several types of abnormal gait. Keep in mind the phases and pathogenesis of gait (Fig. 61.1):

1. *Heel strike*: the lateral calcaneus makes contact with the ground and the muscles, tendons and ligaments relax, providing for optimal energy absorption.
2. *Midstance*: the foot is flat and is able to adapt to uneven terrain, maintain equilibrium and absorb the shock of touchdown; the calcaneus is just below the ankle, keeping the front and back of the foot aligned for optimal weight bearing.
3. *Heel rise*: the calcaneus lifts off the ground, the foot pronates, the muscles, tendons and ligaments tighten, and the foot regains its arch.
4. *Toe push-off*: the foot leaves the surface.

Stance phase

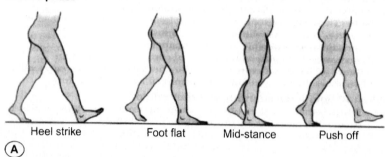

Heel strike   Foot flat   Mid-stance   Push off

(A)

Swing phase

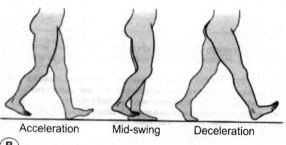

Acceleration   Mid-swing   Deceleration

(B)

Fig. 61.1 The phases of the normal gait cycle.

Cerebellar gait

The patient has a broad-based gait, reeling and lurching to one side:
- Proceed by telling the examiner that you would like to examine the patient for other cerebellar signs (p. 201).

Parkinsonian gait

Steps are small and shuffling, and the patient walks in a haste (festinates). The entire body stoops forwards, knees bent, head hunched forward and the feet must hurry to keep up with it as if trying to catch up with the centre of gravity. There is associated loss of arm swing and mask-like facies:
- Proceed by telling the examiner that you would like to look for other signs of Parkinson's disease (p. 191).

Hemiplegic gait

Gait is slow, spastic and shuffling. With each step the pelvis is tilted upward on the involved side to aid in lifting the foot off the ground, and the entire affected limb is circumducted, rotated in a semicircle at the pelvis. The upper limb is flexed, adducted and does not swing, and the lower limb is extended.

Sensory ataxia

The feet stamp, the movement of the legs bearing no relation to the position of the legs in space since proprioception is impaired or absent. The patient has to look down at the ground to compensate for the loss of proprioception. The patient walks on a wide base; the feet are lifted too high off the ground and are brought down too vigorously.

Proceed as follows:
- Check for Romberg's sign vibration and position sense
- Sensory ataxic gait may be caused by tabes dorsalis, subacute combined degeneration of the cord
- Tell the examiner that you would like to look for Argyll Robertson pupils and anaemia.

High steppage gait
Usually unilateral and results from foot drop. The patient has to lift the foot high in order to avoid dragging the forefoot. It is seen in:
- Lateral popliteal nerve palsy
- Poliomyelitis
- Charcot–Marie–Tooth disease
- Lead or arsenic poisoning.

Scissor gait
Seen in spastic paraplegia. The adductor spasm may be so severe as to lead to the legs crossing in front of one another. Short steps with the front of the feet clinging to the ground result in a wearing out of the toes of shoes:
- Proceed to tell the examiner that the underlying aetiology would probably be cord compression, multiple sclerosis or cerebral palsy.

Waddling gait
The legs are held wide apart and the patient shifts weight from one side to the other when walking:
- Comment on the lumbar lordosis
- Waddling gait is seen in advanced pregnancy and proximal weakness (Cushing syndrome, osteomalacia, thyrotoxicosis, polymyositis, diabetes, hereditary muscular dystrophies).

ADVANCED-LEVEL QUESTIONS

What do you understand by the term astasia abasia?
This is seen in psychogenic disturbances in which the patient is unable to walk or cannot stand. The patient falls far to the side on walking but usually regains balance before hitting the ground. The legs may be thrown out wildly or the patient may kneel with each step.

What do you understand by the term marche à petits pas?
This is to describe a gait in which the movement is slow and the patient walks with very short, shuffling and irregular steps with loss of associated movements. It is seen in normal-pressure hydrocephalus. This gait bears some resemblance to that seen in Parkinson's disease.

62 WASTING OF THE SMALL MUSCLES OF THE HAND

INSTRUCTION

Examine this patient's hands.
Ask the patient whether her hands are painful.

SALIENT FEATURES

History

- Rheumatoid arthritis
- Painful neck movements (cervical spondylosis)
- Fasciculations, weakness (motor neuron disease)
- Associated sensory loss (syringomyelia)
- Family history (Charcot–Marie–Tooth disease)
- Ascending muscle weakness (Guillain–Barré syndrome)
- Trauma to upper limbs (bilateral median and ulnar nerve lesions).

Examination

- Wasting of thenar and hypothenar eminences and dorsal interossei.

Proceed as follows:

- Look for deformity and swelling
- Look for fasciculations
- Check sensation over the hand, especially index and little fingers
- Test grip and pincer movements
- Test for median and ulnar nerve compression
- Ask the patient to unbutton clothes or to write
- Palpate for cervical ribs and compare radial pulses
- Look for Horner syndrome
- Examine the neck and test neck movements.

DIAGNOSIS

This patient has bilateral wasted hands (lesions) caused by cervical myelopathy (aetiology) and is unable to button her clothes (functional status).

Cause of wasted hands

Bilateral wasted hands:

- Rheumatoid arthritis
- Old age
- Cervical spondylosis
- Bilateral cervical ribs
- Motor neuron disease (Fig. 62.1)
- Syringomyelia
- Charcot–Marie–Tooth disease
- Guillain–Barré syndrome
- Bilateral median and ulnar nerve lesions.

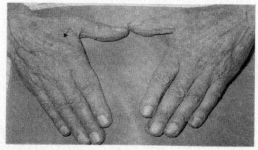

Fig. 62.1 Motor neuron disease. There is fasciculation and wasting of the muscles between the thumb and index finger on the dorsal (arrow) and palmar surfaces. (With permission from Goldman L, Ausiello DA 2007.)

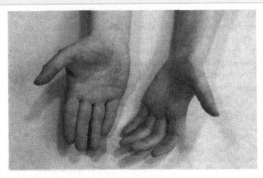

Fig. 62.2 True neurologic thoracic outlet syndrome with wasting of muscles clearly shown in the left hand. (With permission from Frontera et al. 2008.)

Unilateral wasting: causes additional to the above:
- Brachial plexus trauma
- Pancoast's tumour
- Cervical cord lesions
- Malignant infiltration of the brachial plexus
- Thoracic outlet syndrome (Fig. 62.2).

QUESTIONS

In unilateral wasting what is the level of the lesion?
C8, T1. These muscles are predominantly supplied by the ulnar nerve (the median nerve supplies the thenar eminence), the inner cord of the brachial plexus, the T1 spinal root and the anterior horn cells. Thus lesions of these structures may all produce wasting of the small muscles of the hand:
- Lesions of the radial, median and ulnar nerves (trauma)
- Brachial plexus (trauma, cervical lymph nodes, cervical ribs, tumour of superior sulcus of lung)
- Anterior root (cervical spondylosis)
- Anterior horn cell (motor neuron disease, tumours of spinal cord, syringomyelia, poliomyelitis).

63 DERMATOMYOSITIS

INSTRUCTION

Examine this patient.

SALIENT FEATURES

History

- The adult form usually occurs after the age of 40 years
- Weakness of proximal muscles evolving over weeks or months: difficulty in getting from a low chair or squatting position, climbing stairs, lifting and running
- Inability to raise head
- Dysphagia (caused by weakness of the muscles of the pharynx)
- Dysphonia
- Muscle pain and tenderness

- Raynaud's phenomenon
- Ask the patient whether the red rash is made worse by exposure to sunlight
- Skin features (Fig. 63.1):
  - Heliotrope rash or purplish-blue rash around the eyes, back of the hands, dilated capillary loops at the base of fingernails, erythema of knuckles accompanied by a raised violaceous scaly eruption (Gottron's sign); the erythema spares the phalanges (unlike that of SLE in which the phalanges are involved and the knuckles are spared)
  - Erythematous rash may be present on the neck and upper chest (often in the shape of a V), shoulders (shawl sign), elbows, knees and malleoli
  - Cuticles may be irregular, thickened and distorted; the lateral and palmar areas of the fingers become rough and cracked with irregular 'dirty' horizontal lines, resembling those in a mechanic's hands.

Note: In dermatomyositis, the myopathy is accompanied by a rash, which includes three classic types:
  - Gottron's sign: a papulosquamous eruption on the dorsum of the fingers
  - Heliotropic rash: a violaceous discoloration over the eyelids and face
  - 'Shawl' rash: an erythematous eruption over the anterior chest and upper torso.

- Muscle features:
  - Proximal muscle weakness and tenderness of muscles (muscle wasting absent or minimal)
  - Weakness of neck flexors in two-thirds of cases
  - Intact or absent deep tendon reflexes.

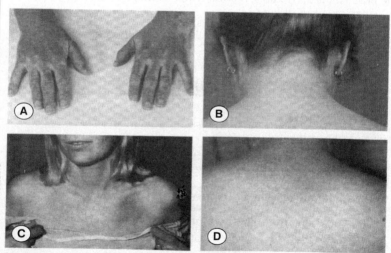

Fig. 63.1 Characteristic dermatomyositis skin changes. (A) Linear erythema (Gottron's sign). (B) Scalp rash. (C) V sign. (D) Shawl sign. (With permission from Firestein et al. 2008.)

Proceed as follows:
- If the patient is >40 years, tell the examiner that you would like to look for an underlying neoplasm.
- Look for interstitial lung disease (occurs in 5–10% of patients with polymyositis or dermatomyositis, especially in those with anti-Jo-1 antibody).

DIAGNOSIS

This patient has Gottron's papules and proximal muscle weakness (lesion) caused by dermatomyositis (aetiology).

QUESTIONS

What investigations would you like to do?
- Estimation of serum creatine kinase (also known as creatine phospho-kinase) levels (mirrors disease activity)
- Electromyography shows myopathic changes (spontaneous fibrillation, salvos of repetitive potentials, and short duration of polyphasic potentials of low amplitude)
- Muscle biopsy (will show necrosis and phagocytosis of muscle fibres, and interstitial and perivascular infiltration of inflammatory cells)
- MRI and MR spectroscopy of affected tissue may show abnormal signals in striated muscle and abnormalities of muscle metabolism.

In which other conditions is there proximal muscle weakness with high serum creatine kinase levels?
It may be caused by drugs such as lovastatin, chloroquine and colchicine, especially in patients on chronic haemodialysis. (Remember that steroids cause proximal muscle weakness with normal serum creatine kinase levels.)

How would you treat such patients?
- Most patients respond to steroids; prednisolone is the first-line drug for the empirical treatment of polymyositis and dermatomyositis.
- Resistant dermatomyositis may benefit from methotrexate, azathioprine and high-dose intravenous immunoglobulin.
- Those with an underlying neoplasm may see the dermatomyositis remit after treatment of the tumour.

ADVANCED-LEVEL QUESTIONS

How would you classify polymyositis–dermatomyositis?
The classification of Bohan et al. (Medicine 1977;56:255) is into five groups:
I: primary idiopathic polymyositis
II: primary idiopathic dermatomyositis
III: dermatomyositis (or polymyositis) associated with neoplasia (Mayo Clin Proc 1986;61:645)
IV: childhood dermatomyositis (or polymyositis) associated with vasculitis
V: polymyositis (or dermatomyositis) with associated collagen vascular disease.

Mention a few disorders associated with myositis
Sarcoid myositis, focal nodular myositis, infectious polymyositis (Lyme disease, toxoplasma), inclusion body myositis, eosinophilic myositis.

What do you know about inclusion body polymyositis?

Inclusion-body myositis usually occurs in men >50 years of age. It is characterized by indolent, progressive proximal muscle weakness, which may be asymmetric, that eventually also involves distal muscles. Both myopathic and neuropathic changes can be seen on electromyography studies. Muscle biopsy reveals mononuclear infiltrates and vacuoles in the muscle cells that contain inclusion bodies. Inclusion body myositis often responds poorly to conventional therapy with steroids.

What do you understand by the term overlap syndrome?

Overlap syndrome indicates that characteristics of two different disorders are common to both. Dermatomyositis overlaps with systemic sclerosis and mixed connective tissue disease. Specific signs of systemic sclerosis and mixed connective tissue disease, such as sclerotic thickening of the dermis, contractures, oesophageal hypomotility, microangiopathy and calcium deposits, are present in dermatomyositis. Patients with the overlap syndrome of dermatomyositis and systemic sclerosis may have a specific anti-nuclear autoantibody, anti-PM/Scl, directed against a nucleolar protein complex.

Further reading

Dalakas MC: Polymyositis, dermatomyositis, and inclusion-body myositis, *N Engl J Med* 325:1487, 1993 (review).

Heinrich Adolf Gottron (1890–1974), a German dermatologist.

---

64 FACIOSCAPULOHUMERAL DYSTROPHY (LANDOUZY–DÉJÉRINE SYNDROME)

INSTRUCTION

Perform a neurological examination of this patient's cranial nerves and upper limbs.

SALIENT FEATURES

History

- Age of onset (usually between 10 and 40 years of age)
- Family history (parents or siblings may only have facial weakness)
- Weakness begins in the face and affects the shoulder girdle subsequently (particularly the lower trapezii, pectoralis, triceps and biceps).

Examination

- In the face:
  - Prominent ptosis
  - Difficulty in closing the eyes
  - Marked facial weakness, resulting in a dull expressionless face with lips open and slack, and inability to whistle or puff the cheeks

- Speech is impaired owing to difficulty in articulation of labial consonants.
- In the neck:
  - Wasted sternomastoids and marked weakness of neck muscles.
- In the shoulder girdle (Figs 64.1 and 64.2):
  - Winging of the scapula
  - Lower pectorals and lower trapezii severely affected
  - Weakness of triceps and biceps
  - True hypertrophy of deltoids to compensate for other muscles
  - Absent biceps and triceps jerk.
- In the trunk:
  - Weakness (lower abdominal muscles are weaker than upper abdominal muscles, resulting in the *Beevor sign*; a physical finding very specific for this condition), which is a marked upward movement of the umbilicus following neck flexion of the patient in a lying position.

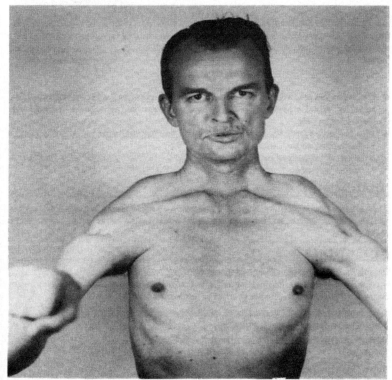

Fig. 64.1 Facioscapulohumeral dystrophy: the downward-sloping clavicles and bulge in the region of the trapezius muscle is caused by the scapula being displaced upward on attempted elevation of the arms. The patient also is attempting to purse his lips. (With permission from Bradley et al. 2008.)

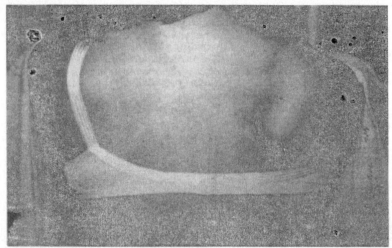

Fig. 64.2 Asymmetrical scapular winging in facioscapulohumeral muscular dystrophy. (With permission from Bradley et al. 2008.)

- Uncommon features: congenital absence of pectoralis, biceps or brachioradialis; tibialis anterior may be the only muscle involved outside the shoulder girdle
- Tell the examiner that you would like to evaluate for:
  - high-frequency hearing loss (in ~75%)
  - retinal telangiectasias (in ~60%)
  - sleep apnoea.

DIAGNOSIS

This patient has weakness of the muscles of the face, neck and shoulder girdle (lesion) caused by inherited facioscapulohumeral dystrophy (aetiology).

QUESTIONS

What is the mode of inheritance?

Autosomal dominant; both sexes are equally affected. The gene has been recently localized to the long arm of chromosome 4.

Are higher mental functions affected in this condition?

The IQ is normal in such patients.

What is the lifespan in such a patient?

Normal.

What is the age of onset of this disorder?

Between 10 and 40 years.

Are levels of muscle enzymes raised in this condition?

The enzyme levels remain normal usually. About half of those affected show a very slight increase.

What do you know about the genetics of this condition?

It results from a partial deletion of an integral number of 3.3 kb polymorphic D4Z4 repeats, within the subtelomeric region of chromosome 4q. Whereas healthy individuals normally have *Eco*RI digestion fragments of D4Z4 consisting of 11 to 150 U, patients with facioscapulohumeral dystrophy have fragments of 1 to 10 U. However, it has been noted that, although molecular diagnosis of the disease is often cited to be 98% accurate, the search for the gene during testing is sometimes hampered by sequence homologies between the suspected 4q35 region and other chromosomal regions. Although the genetic lesion is well described, the causal gene and the protein products are not known.

> Louis Théophile Joseph Landouzy (1845–1917), Professor of Therapeutics in Paris; although remembered for the description of the syndrome which bears his name, his major research interest was TB.
>
> Joseph Jules Déjérine (1849–1917), a French neurologist, was a pioneer in the localization of function in the brain. This syndrome was described in 1885.
>
> Charles Edward Beevor (1854–1908) first documented the finding of an upward deflection of the umbilicus on flexion of the neck in spinal cord injury at or below the level of Th10. Apart from positive Beevor's sign as a result of spinal cord lesions positive Beevor's sign has also been described in patients with facioscapulohumeral muscular dystrophy.

65 LIMB GIRDLE DYSTROPHY

INSTRUCTION

Perform a neurological examination of this patient's upper and lower limbs.

SALIENT FEATURES

History

- Age of onset (between 10 and 30 years of age)
- Onset may either be in the pelvic or shoulder girdle
- It may remain confined to the pelvic or shoulder girdle and may be static for years before peripheral weakness and wasting occur.

Examination

Upper limbs (Fig. 65.1):
- Biceps and brachioradialis are involved late; wrist extensors are first involved when it extends to the wrist.
- Deltoids may show pseudohypertrophy and are spared until late.

Lower limbs (Fig. 65.1):
- In the early stages of the disease, hip flexors and glutei are weak.
- There is early wasting of medial quadriceps and tibialis anterior.
- Lateral quadriceps and calves may show hypertrophy.

Note: The face is never affected.

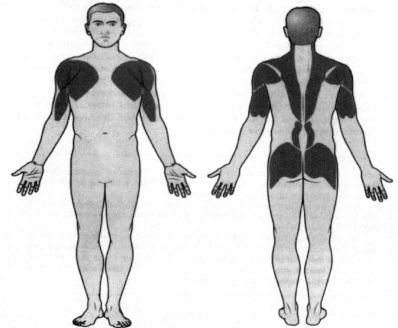

Fig. 65.1 Pattern of weakness in limb-girdle dystrophy.

DIAGNOSIS

This patient has weakness of the proximal muscles of the arms and legs (lesion) caused by limb girdle dystrophy (aetiology).

ADVANCED-LEVEL QUESTIONS

What is the mode of inheritance?

Traditionally, it was believed to be autosomal recessive, with males and females equally affected. More recently, the limb girdle muscular dystrophies (LGMDs) have been identified to be inherited either in an autosomal dominant (type 1) or autosomal recessive (type 2) pattern. Six subtypes of the dominant LGMDs (1A to 1F) and 11 subtypes of the recessive LGMDs (2A to 2K) have been reported. In four of the limb girdle dystrophies (2C, 2D, 2E and 2F), mutations affecting the *sarcoglycan complex of proteins* have been identified. These membrane proteins interact with dystrophin through another transmembrane protein, β-dystroglycan. Dysferlin is a sarcolemmal protein, and its deficiency causes proximal and distal forms of recessively inherited muscular dystrophies, designated as LGMD type 2B.

LGMD2A, the most prevalent form, accounts for at least 30% of all cases and is caused by mutations in *CAPN3* (also called *p94*), which encodes CAPN3, the largely skeletal-muscle-specific member of the calpain superfamily. These patients have symmetrical and selective involvement of proximal limb girdle muscles. They have normal intelligence and no cardiac or facial disturbances. The disease shows wide intrafamilial and interfamilial clinical variability. A dystrophic or myopathic process is seen on muscle biopsy. During the active phase, the serum level of creatine kinase is moderately or markedly increased; however, patients with a normal serum level of creatine kinase or a neurogenic pattern on electromyography have also been reported, suggesting that there is a spectrum of variability in this calpainopathy. Intramuscular administration of the synthetic calpain inhibitor leupeptin to dystrophic *Mdx* mice can prevent decreases in muscle fibre diameter (Muscle Nerve 2000;23:106–11). Calpain inhibitors, therefore, have the potential of being beneficial in this condition.

What is the age of onset?
Between 10 and 30 years, causing disability 10–20 years after onset.

How is the intelligence affected?
It is unaffected and IQ is normal.

Is the lifespan affected?
No.

What happens to the serum enzymes?
Levels of serum enzymes are slightly affected or normal.

John Walton, Professor of Neurology at Oxford and Newcastle, was made a peer following his retirement and carries the title of Lord Walton of Detchant. His chief interest was muscular diseases.

Sir Roger Bannister, Master of Pembroke College at Oxford, worked at the National Hospital for Nervous Diseases, Queen Square, and St Mary's Hospital, London, and his main interest was chronic autonomic failure. He was the first person to run the 4-minute mile.

---

66   MYASTHENIA GRAVIS

INSTRUCTION

This patient complains of drooping of the eyelids in the evenings; examine this patient.

SALIENT FEATURES

History

- Weakness in muscles is more marked in the evening
- Muscle weakness which increases with exercise (remember that *fatigability* is the hallmark of myasthenia gravis) and is painless
- Muscle weakness affects smiling (Fig. 66.1), chewing, speaking, muscles of the neck, walking, breathing, movements at the elbow and hand movements
- Obtain history of thyrotoxicosis, diabetes mellitus, rheumatoid arthritis, SLE and thymoma
- Ask about D-pencillamine treatment for rheumatoid arthritis (myasthenia gravis is sometimes caused by D-pencillamine).

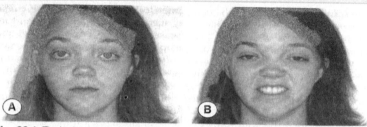

Fig. 66.1 Typical myasthenic facies. (A) At rest, there is slight bilateral lid ptosis, which is partially compensated by raising the right eyebrow. (B) During attempted smile, there is contraction of the medial portion of the upper lip and horizontal contraction of the corners of the mouth without the natural upward curling, producing a 'sneer'. (With permission from Bradley et al. 2008.)

Examination

- The patient may have obvious ptosis
- Check for worsening of ptosis after sustained upward gaze for at least 45 s
- Check extraocular movements for diplopia and variable squint
- Comment on snarling face when the patient attempts to smile
- Weakness without loss of reflexes or alteration of sensation or coordination. The weakness may be generalized; it may affect the limb muscles, often proximal in distribution, as well as the diaphragm and neck extensors
- Speech is nasal
- Muscle wasting is rare and when present inidicates it is late in the disease
- Ask the patient to count to 50 (voice may deteriorate).

Proceed as follows:

- Tell the examiner that myasthenia is associated with thyrotoxicosis, diabetes mellitus, rheumatoid arthritis, SLE and thymoma.

DIAGNOSIS

This patient has diplopia at the end of each day with ptosis; the weakness is marked on repeated exertion of the muscle (lesion) and is caused by myasthenia gravis (aetiology).

QUESTIONS

At what age is myasthenia common?

The incidence has two age peaks, with one peak in the second and third decades affecting mostly women and another peak in the sixth and seventh decades affecting mostly men.

What groups of muscles are commonly involved?

Muscles affected are as follows, in order of likelihood: extraocular, bulbar, neck, limb girdle, distal limbs and trunk.

What investigations would you like to do in this patient?

- Edrophonium (Tensilon) test. Edrophonium is a short-acting acetylcholinesterase inhibitor that gives an immediate increase in muscle strength (Fig. 66.2)

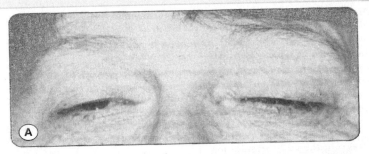

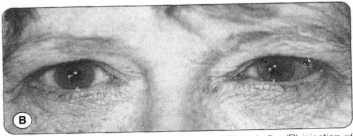

Fig. 66.2 The edrophonium (Tensilon) test before (A) and after (B) injection of edrophonium. (With permission from Currie, Douglas 2011.)

- Vital capacity
- Imaging of the mediastinum: chest radiography, CT or MRI of the chest
- Serum acetylcholine receptor antibodies (present in >80% of cases) (J Neurol Neurosurg Psychiatry 1985;48:1246–52). Remember that the basic deficit is a deficiency of acetylcholine receptors at the neuromuscular junction (Science 1973; 182:293–5); 50% have antibodies directed against muscle-specific kinase receptors
- Plasma thyroxine (to rule out an associated thyroid disorder)
- Anti-striated muscle antibody (seen in association with thymoma)
- Anti-nuclear antibody, rheumatoid factor and anti-thyroid antibodies may be positive
- Tuberculin test if immunosuppressive therapy is contemplated
- Electromyography (EMG): abnormalities include a decremental response to tetanic train stimulation at 5–10 Hz, and evidence of neuromuscular blockade in the form of jitter and blocking of motor action potentials in single-fibre EMG (Muscle Nerve 1992;15:720–4).

What is the differential diagnosis?
- Botulism
- Eaton–Lambert syndrome.

What are the treatment modalities available?
- Symptomatic treatment entails administration of an anticholinesterase drug (e.g. pyridostigmine) given up to five times per day.
- Definitive treatment entails immunosuppression, e.g. steroids, azathioprine, cylosporin, mycophenolate mofetil, rituximab, plasmapheresis, intravenous immunoglobulin, thymectomy.

Mention a drug that can cause myasthenia

D-Pencillamine therapy given for rheumatoid arthritis.

Why may a 'gin and tonic' exacerbate myasthenia?

The quinine in tonic water causes muscle weakness.

If this patient develops an infection, which group of antibiotics would you avoid?

Aminoglycosides.

Mention a few exacerbating features

Fatigue, exercise, infection, emotion, change of climate, pregnancy, magnesium enemas, drugs (aminoglycosides, propranolol, morphine, barbiturates, procainamide, quinidine).

ADVANCED-LEVEL QUESTIONS

How is the myasthenia graded?

The **Osserman grading** has four stages:

I: involves focal disease (e.g. restricted to ocular muscles, ocular myasthenia)

IIa: mild generalized myasthenia with slow progression, no crises and drug responsive

IIb: moderate generalized myasthenia with severe skeletal and bulbar involvement but no crises; drug response is less satisfactory

III: acute fulminating myasthenia with rapid progression of severe symptoms of respiratory crises and poor drug response; high incidence of thymoma and high mortality rate

IV: late severe myasthenia; same as grade III but takes 2 years to progress from class I to II; crises; high mortality rate with life-threatening respiratory impairment.

The Newsom-Davies clinical grading has three subgroups:

1. Patients with thymoma, equal sex incidence, peak age of onset 30–50 years, no HLA association and poor response to thymectomy.
2. Young onset (<40 years), typically female, thymic medullary germinal centres present, strong association with *HLA-B8* and *HLA-DR3* and usually a good response to thymectomy.
3. Older onset (>40 years), more common in males, thymic involution, an association with *HLA-B7* and *HLA-DR9* and doubtful response to thymectomy.

What do you know about Eaton–Lambert syndrome?

Eaton–Lambert syndrome (JAMA 1957;163:1117) is a myasthenic disorder associated with malignancy (Brain 1988;111:577; a review of 50 cases). It is associated with small cell carcinoma of the bronchus. Weakness of the truncal and proximal limb muscles is common. The pelvic girdle and thighs are almost invariably involved. Deep tendon reflexes are absent. Transient improvement in muscle strength and deep-tendon reflexes may follow brief exercise. Unlike myasthenia, bulbar symptoms are rare. Antibodies to calcium channels may be detected. Electromyography is diagnostic. In rested muscle, there is marked depression of neuromuscular transmission after a single submaximal stimulus and marked facilitation of response during repetitive stimulation at rates greater than 10 per second. Assays for P/Q-type calcium channel antibodies are positive.

What is myasthenic crisis?

Exacerbation of myasthenia. The need for artificial ventilation occurs in about 10% of patients with myasthenia. Those with bulbar and respiratory involvement are prone to respiratory infection. The crisis can be precipitated by respiratory infection and surgery. Such patients should be closely monitored for pulmonary function. Those with artificial ventilation are not given cholinergics as this avoids stimulation of pulmonary secretions and uncertainties about overdosage.

How does a cholinergic crisis manifest?

Excessive salivation, confusion, lacrimation, miosis, pallor and collapse. It is important to avoid edrophonium in such patients.

Mention a few associated disorders

Thyroid disorders (thyrotoxicosis, hypothyroidism), rheumatoid arthritis, diabetes mellitus, dermatomyositis, pernicious anaemia, SLE, Sjögren's disease, sarcoidosis, pemphigus.

What is the role of thymectomy in such patients?

In the case of thymoma, thymectomy is necessary to prevent tumour spread, although most thymomas are benign. In the absence of a tumour, thymectomy has been found to be beneficial in 85% of patients and 35% go into drug-free remission. The improvement is noticed for 1 to 10 years after surgery (Neurology 1990;40:1828–9). The role of thymectomy in ocular myasthenia, in adults over 55 years of age (Acta Neurol Scand 1994;12:343–68) and in children, is still under debate.

What is the role of immunomodulation in myasthenia gravis?

Intravenous immunoglobulin seems as efficacious as plasma exchange.

Myasthenia gravis was first described by Oxford physiologist Thomas Willis in 1672 and by Erb in 1878. It was also known as Hoppe–Goldflam disease after HH Hoppe (1867–1919), a US neurologist (Berl Klin Wochenschr 1892;29:332–6) and SV Goldflam (1852–1932), a Polish neurologist. In 1895, F. Jolly named the disease myasthenia gravis pseudoparalytica (Berl Klin Wochenschr 1895;32:1–7).

LM Eaton (1905–1958), Professor of Neurology at the Mayo Clinic, Rochester, Minnesota.

EH Lambert (b. 1915), Professor of Physiology, University of Minnesota.

Sir Samuel Wilks (1824–1911), physician, Guy's Hospital, London. Myasthenia gravis was known as Wilks syndrome.

John Newsom-Davies, FRS, contemporary Professor of Clinical Neurology, Oxford.

Alastair Composton, PhD, FRCP, contemporary Professor of Neurology, Cambridge.

---

67 THOMSEN'S DISEASE (MYOTONIA CONGENITA)

INSTRUCTION

Look at this patient.

SALIENT FEATURES

History

- Ask the patient whether or not there is any seasonal variation in symptoms: myotonia is worse in winter from the cold.
- Take a family history (inheritance is usually autosomal dominant; gene on long arm of chromosome 7).

Examination

- Diffuse muscle hypertrophy
- Myotonia, which may be apparent while shaking hands with the person. (The myotonia displays a *warm up phenomenon*, in which the myotonia decreases or vanishes completely when repeating the same movement several times.)

Note: Know the phenotypic patters of muscle disorders.

DIAGNOSIS

This patient has diffuse muscular hypertrophy with myotonia (lesion) caused by Thomsen's disease (aetiology).

ADVANCED-LEVEL QUESTIONS

How is the disease recognized in infancy?

Myotonia is present from birth and may be recognized by the child's peculiar cry. Also noticed in early infancy are difficulty in feeding and inability to reopen the eyes while having the face washed.

When does muscle hypertrophy manifest?

It is usually apparent in the second decade.

What is the cause of muscle hypertrophy?

It is caused by almost continual involuntary isometric exercise.

What is the life expectancy in such patients?

These patients have a normal life expectancy.

What drugs would you use to ameliorate the myotonia?

Procainamide, quinidine.

What do you know about genetics of this disease?

It can be inherited as either an autosomal dominant (Thomsen's disease) or recessive (Becker myotonia) trait. Myotonia congenita is a specific inherited disorder of muscle membrane hyperexcitability caused by reduced sarcolemmal chloride conductance as a result of mutations in *CLCN1*, the gene coding for the main skeletal muscle chloride channel ClC-1 (Neurology 2000;54:937–42). The disorder may be transmitted as either an autosomal dominant or recessive trait, with close to 130 currently known mutations.

In which other conditions is myotonia seen?

Myotonia can be a presenting sign of:
- myotonic dystrophy
- non-dystrophic myotonias, in which mytonia is caused by dysfunction of:
  - channels for chloride (in myotonia congenita) or
  - sodium channels (in paramyotonia congenita, potassium-aggravated myotonia and hyperkalaemic periodic paralysis with myotonia)

- myopathies (acid maltase deficiency, polymyositis, myotubular myopathy)
- following administration of drugs such as clofibrate, colchicine
- rarely, denervation of any cause.

AJT Thomsen (1815–1896) was a Danish physician who described this condition in his family and himself in 1876.

---

68 FRIEDREICH'S ATAXIA

INSTRUCTION

Perform a neurological examination of this patient's legs.

SALIENT FEATURES

History

- Age of onset (usually the same in each family and ranges from 8 to 16 years of age)
- High-arched foot in childhood in the family (Friedreich's foot) (Fig. 68.1)
- Scoliosis developing in childhood
- Cerebellar dysarthria (p. 210) and ataxia (p. 201).

Examination

- Pes cavus
- Pyramidal weakness in legs
- Cerebellar signs, ataxia being a constant sign
- Impaired vibration and joint sense
- Romberg's sign positive
- Absence of deep tendon reflexes (caused by degeneration of peripheral nerves)
- Distal muscle wasting (in 50% of cases), especially in the hands.

Proceed as follows:

- Check for nystagmus (present in 25% of the cases), scanning speech, intention tremor
- Examine the heart for hypertrophic cardiomyopathy (Fig. 68.2)

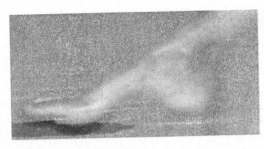

Fig. 68.1 Foot deformity in Friedreich's ataxia. (With permission from Bradley et al. 2008.)

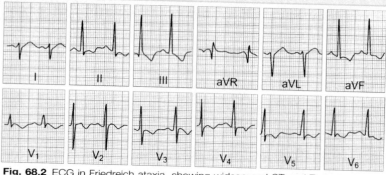

Fig. 68.2 ECG in Friedreich ataxia, showing widespread ST and T changes.

- Check the eyes for optic atrophy (present in 30% of cases)
- Check the spine for kyphoscoliosis
- Check the urine for sugar (10% of patients have diabetes)
- Check IQ, looking for intellectual deterioration
- Tell the examiner that you would like to do a 25 ft (7.5 m) walk test to determine ambulatory capacity.

Remember: Friedreich's ataxia is the most common genetic cause of ataxia, affecting approximately 1 : 30 000 people. Symptoms that affect mobility include ataxia, spasticity and peripheral neuropathy.

DIAGNOSIS

This patient has kyphoscoliosis, pes cavus and a combination of pyramidal, cerebellar and sensory deficits (lesions) in the lower limbs caused by Friedreich's ataxia (aetiology); he is severely disabled by his deformity.

ADVANCED-LEVEL QUESTIONS

What is the mode of inheritance?
Autosomal recessive or, rarely, sex linked.

Why are the deep tendon reflexes absent even though plantars are upgoing?
This is caused by a combination of pyramidal weakness with peripheral neuropathy.

In which other conditions is there a mixture of cerebellar, pyramidal and dorsal column signs?
Multiple sclerosis.

Mention a few conditions with absent knee jerks and upgoing plantars
- Peripheral neuropathy in a stroke patient
- Motor neuron disease
- Conus medullaris: cauda equina lesion
- Tabes dorsalis
- Subacute combined degeneration of the spinal cord.

What is the forme fruste of this condition?
Pes cavus or hammer toes, without any other signs, are seen in family members of such patients.

On which chromosome is the gene for this disorder localized?

The disease is caused by triplet repeat expansions on chromosome 9. The causative mutation is a GAA trinucleotide repeat expansion in the first intron of the gene *FRDA* (or *X25*), which encodes frataxin. The mitochondrial localization of frataxin and decreased oxidation activity suggest that this is a mitochondrial disease. Frataxin is involved in iron metabolism and may protect mitochondria from oxidative damage (Lancet Neurol 2002;1:370–74). Excessive free iron may damage proteins containing iron–sulfur groups, including complexes I, II and III and aconitase, a Krebs cycle enzyme.

What are the clinical criteria for diagnosis of Friedreich's ataxia?

Harding's criteria (Brain 1981;104:589):

- Essential criteria are onset before the age of 25 years, ataxia of limbs and gait, absent knee and ankle jerks, extensor plantars, autosomal recessive inheritance, motor conduction velocity greater than 40 m/s, small or absent sensory nerve action potentials, dysarthria within 5 years of onset.
- Additional criteria (present in two-thirds) are scoliosis, pyramidal weakness of lower limbs, absent upper limb reflexes, loss of vibration and joint position sense in the legs, abnormal ECG and pes cavus.
- Other features (present in <50%) are nystagmus, optic atrophy, deafness, distal muscle wasting and diabetes.

What is the prognosis of Friedreich's ataxia?

Friedreich's ataxia usually progresses slowly and few patients live longer than 20 years after the onset of symptoms. Occasionally, it may appear to be arrested, and abortive cases may be encountered in apparently healthy relatives of affected patients. Most patients will lose their ability to walk, stand or sit without support within 10 to 15 years of disease onset.

What are the pathological changes in Friedreich's ataxia?

- Marked loss of cells in the posterior root ganglia
- Degeneration of peripheral sensory fibres
- Involvement of the posterior and lateral columns of the cord.

What is the role of idebenone in Friedreich's ataxia?

Therapy with idebenone, an antioxidant, is associated with improvement in neurological function and activities of daily living in patients with Friedreich's ataxia. Idebenone also functions as an electron transport carrier (like coenzyme Q) and has various other effects, including stimulation of nerve growth factor production and blockade of voltage-sensitive calcium channels. In the murine conditional-knockout model of Friedreich's ataxia, oxidative stress is not observed, but idebenone exerts effects on cardiac measures and increases lifespan. Idebenone also enhances viability of Friedreich's ataxia fibroblasts in vitro (Lancet Neurol 2007; 6:878–86).

Name a few syndromes with spinocerebellar degeneration

- Roussy–Lévy disease: hereditary spinocerebellar degeneration with atrophy of lower limb muscles and loss of deep tendon reflexes
- Refsum's disease (p. 724)
- Bassen–Kornzweig syndrome (p. 724): caused by cellular deficiency of vitamin E (α-tocopherol) resulting from a defect in the α-tocopherol-transfer protein, and abetalipoproteinaemia associated with a defect of VLDL

- Olivopontocerebellar degeneration: first described in 1882. This has an autosomal dominant inheritance and has been mapped to the HLA loci on the short arm of chromosome 6 where a highly polymorphic CAG repeat sequence occurs. The CAG repeat sequence is longer than normal and unstable in affected patients
- Machado–Joseph disease: dominant inheritance, first described in families of Portuguese origin. Clinical features include progressive ataxia, ophthalmoparesis, spasticity, dystonia, amyotrophy and parkinsonism. This disorder has been linked to chromosome 14 and is caused by the expansion of unstable CAG repeat sequences
- Dentatorubral pallidoluysian atrophy is similar to Machado–Joseph disease but maps on the short arm of chromosome 12. The abnormally expanded CAG repeat sequences identified in the gene for olivopontocerebellar degeneration, Machado–Joseph disease and dentatorubral pallidoluysian atrophy each result in the expression of a specific ataxin.

Nikolaus Friedreich (1825–1882), Professor of Pathology and neurologist in Heidelberg, described this condition, in a series of papers from 1861 to 1876.
G Roussy (1874–1948), a French neuropathologist.
G Lévy (b. 1881), a French neurologist.
Sigvald Refsum (1907–1991), a Norwegian neurologist, was successively Professor of Neurology at Bergen University and at the National Hospital in Oslo (BMJ 1991;303:919).
Anita Harding (1953–1995) Professor of Neurology at the National Hospital, Queen Square, London, died at the age of 42 years from colonic cancer.

---

69 MOTOR NEURON DISEASE

INSTRUCTION

Examine this patient's cranial nerves.
Examine this patient's upper limbs.
Examine this patient's lower limbs.

SALIENT FEATURES

History

- Fasciculations and cramps: these may precede other symptoms by months
- Painless, asymmetrical weakness of muscles of the upper limb or lower limb
- Dysarthria and dysphagia
- Emotional lability if there is bulbar involvement.

Examination

- Fasciculations, absent reflexes and weakness in the upper limbs (see Fig. 62.1)

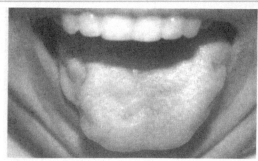

Fig. 69.1 Atrophy of the tongue in amyotrophic lateral sclerosis, a form of motor neuron disease. (With permission from Bradley et al. 2008.)

- Spasticity, exaggerated reflexes and upgoing plantars in lower limbs
- Sluggish palatal movements, absent gag reflex, brisk jaw jerk
- Check the tongue for fasciculations (Fig. 69.1)
- Check neck muscles; head droop is seen when there is weakness of the thoracic and cervical paraspinal muscles
- A combination of the above signs may be seen.

Remember: The therapy is generally palliative.

DIAGNOSIS

This patient has a combination of upper and lower motor neuron signs (lesions) caused by motor neuron disease (aetiology), although I would like to exclude cervical cord compression. The patient is wheelchair bound as a result of the disease (functional status).

QUESTIONS

What important cause should be ruled out before making a firm diagnosis of motor neuron disease?
Cord compression may produce a similar clinical picture and hence it is important to do an MRI scan of the spine and/or a myelogram to exclude it.

ADVANCED-LEVEL QUESTIONS

What are the symptoms attributable to motor neuron disease?
- Direct (owing to motor neuronal degeneration):
  - Weakness and atrophy
  - Fasciculations and muscle cramps
  - Spasticity
  - Dysarthria
  - Dysphagia
  - Dyspnoea
  - Emotional lability.
- Indirect (as a result of primary symptoms):
  - Psychological disturbances
  - Sleep disturbances
  - Constipation
  - Drooling

- Thick mucous secretions
- Symptoms of chronic hypoventilation
- Pain.

What are the characteristic features of this disease?
- It rarely begins before the age of 40 years
- Presence of upper and lower motor neuron involvement of a single spinal segment, and motor dysfunction involving at least two limbs or one limb and bulbar muscles
- Sensory symptoms or signs are not seen
- Ocular movements are not affected
- There are never cerebellar or extrapyramidal signs
- Sphincters are involved late, if at all
- Remission is unknown and the disease is fatal within 5 to 7 years (caused by bronchopneumonia).

What are the clinical patterns of motor neuron disease?
- Bulbar: bulbar or pseudobulbar palsy (in 25%)
- Amyotrophic lateral sclerosis (ALS; in 50%): flaccid arms and spastic legs
- Progressive muscular atrophy (in 25%): a lesion in the anterior horn cells affecting distal muscles. Characteristically there is retention of deep tendon reflexes in the presence of severe muscular atrophy
- Primary lateral sclerosis (rare): signs progress from an upper motor neuron to a lower motor neuron type
- Others conditions affect lower motor neurons:
  - Werdnig–Hoffman's disease: presents in the neonatal period as a 'floppy infant' and known as infantile progressive spinal muscular atrophy
  - X-linked spinal muscular atrophy: the patient has associated testicular atrophy resulting in oligospermia and gynaecomastia; it is associated with the amplification of a trinucleotide repeat in the coding sequence of the androgen receptor gene and disease severity is directly related to the number of repeats present
  - Spinal muscular atrophy: linked to locus on the large arm of chromosome 5.

What are the other types of motor neuron disease?
- Madras motor neuron disease, common in southern India, where the onset is early (before the age of 30), with asymmetrical limb weakness and wasting; bulbar and facial involvement occurs along with sensorineural deafness. The course is more benign than the disorder observed in Europe and America (Srinivas K, Jagannathan K, Valmikinathan K. The spectrum of motor neuron disease in Madras. In Rose FC (ed.) Research Progress in Motor Neuron Disease. London: Pitman, 1984, p. 142).
- ALS associated with a parkinsonism–dementia complex in Guam (Science 1987;237:517). It also tends to have an earlier onset and a more protracted course than the sporadic cases seen in Europe and America.

What are the criteria for diagnosis of amyotrophic lateral sclerosis?
Summary of revised **El Escorial criteria**:
- *Definite*: lower motor neuron and upper motor neuron signs in three regions

- *Probable*: lower motor neuron and upper motor neuron signs in two regions
- *Probable with laboratory support*: lower motor neuron and upper motor neuron signs in one region or upper motor neuron signs in one or more regions with electromyography evidence of acute denervation in two or more limbs
- *Possible*: lower motor neuron and upper motor neuron signs in one region
- *Suspected*: lower motor neuron signs only in one or more regions or upper motor neuron signs only in one or more regions.

All categories need evidence of disease progression and absence of sensory signs not explicable on the basis of comorbidity.

What is the pathology of motor neuron disease?

The clinical manifestations result from degeneration of Betz cells, pyramidal tracts, cranial nerve nuclei and anterior horn cells. Both upper and lower motor neurons may be involved, but sensory involvement is not seen.

What is the explanation for fasciculation?

It is the result of spontaneous firing of large motor units formed by branching fibres of surviving axons that are striving to innervate muscle fibres that have lost their nerve supply.

What are the cerebrospinal fluid changes in the disease?

Usually normal; protein may be slightly raised.

What do you know about the heredity of amyotrophic lateral sclerosis?

Most cases are sporadic but 5–10% are familial. Familial ALS is linked to a gene on the long arm of chromosome 21 (N Engl J Med 1991;324:1381), with various missense mutations identified in different families. This genetic locus appears to encode a copper–zinc-binding superoxide dismutase (SOD). Therapy that ameliorate symptoms in the *Sod1* mutant mouse have consistently failed in humans suggesting other mechanisms. It has been shown that a muscle-specific microRNA (miR-206) in the *Sod1* mouse delays disease progression and promotes regeneration of neuromuscular synapses by boosting the secretion of a growth factor-binding protein into the extracellular matrix indirectly; this, in turn, potentiates growth factors that promote presynaptic innervation at the neuromuscular junction (Science 2009;326:1549–54). [Micro-RNAs are endogenous, small RNAs (~22 nucleotides in length) that target and downregulate, in a sequence-specific manner, messenger RNA.]

Mutations in additional genes (encoding alsin, angiogenin, dynactin 1, senataxin and vesicle-associated protein B) have also been associated with a motor neuron disease (although often not a typical ALS phenotype) in a few families.

How are DNA chips (microarrays) used in genetic analysis?

The DNA chip or the microarray is able to genotype hundreds of thousands of single-nucleotide polymorphisms (SNPs) simultaneously in a single experiment. (SNPs are single-nucleotide variations in the DNA sequence that can be used as markers for neighboring genetic variation.) Comparing the prevalence of a specific SNP in patients and controls, the chromosomal region represented by the SNP associated with a disease can be determined. This approach is known as a high-density genomewide association study. Using one such study, a recent group of investigators reported that variants of *FLJ10986* may confer susceptibility to sporadic ALS. *FLJ10986* and 50 other candidate loci warrant further investigation for their potential role in conferring susceptibility to the disease (Lancet Neurol 2007;6:322–8, N Engl J Med 2007;357:775–88).

Is there any treatment for motor neuron disease?

No treatment has been shown to influence the course of the disease. Riluzole, a glutamate antagonist, is being used in limb or bulbar palsy (N Engl J Med 1994;330:585–91). Patients often require treatment for painful muscle cramps, constant drooling, severe fatiguability, sleep problems, incipient contractures, subluxation of the shoulder joint, dysphagia and neuralgia — all of which can be ameliorated. Patients often have extreme lability of emotion, particularly in the early stages of ALS. In order to alleviate distress before or during respiratory failure, which is usually the terminal event, narcotic drugs should not be withheld.

What is the rationale for using riluzole?

The suggestion that accumulation of toxic levels of glutamate at synapses may cause neuronal death through a calcium-dependent pathway. Riluzole has been shown to be useful in patients with disease of bulbar onset but not in those with disease of spinal onset. The risk of death or tracheostomy is lower with 100 mg riluzole than placebo in limb or bulbar onset disease (Lancet 1996;347:1425–31), but it is debatable whether this translates into an improved quality of life.

What is the role of beta-lactam antibiotics in amyotrophic lateral sclerosis?

More recently beta-lactam antibiotics have been shown to enhance astroglial transport of glutamate in vitro by enhancing the surface expression of the glutamate transporter GLT1 and they do so at levels that are routinely achieved during the treatment of CNS infections (Nature 2005;433:73–7). Long-term ceftriaxone treatment slows the course of disease in mouse models of ALS caused by transgenic expression of mutant SOD. When administered at high doses at the onset of the disease, ceftriaxone preserves grip strength, slows weight loss and increased the overall duration of survival from 122 to 132 days. The slowing of motor neuron death is accompanied by a marked increase in the expression of GLT1 protein in the mice. The US National Institutes of Health has approved funding for a multicentre trial of ceftriaxone in patients with ALS.

What is the role of microglia in motor neuron disease?

Recent data suggest that the expression of mutant SOD1 in microglia accelerates the death of motor neurons in murine models of SOD1-linked ALS (Science 2006;312:1389–92). The aetiology may be toxin production or the transfer of toxins to nearby motor neurons or astrocytes by mutant microglia, or the mutant protein may damage the microglia and prevent them from producing protective factors. Other possibilities exist, including the production of diffusible toxins (such as ions or cytokines) by damaged microglia.

What is the course of palliative care in motor neuron disease?

1. Counselling on diagnosis
2. Treatment of symptoms:

- Fasciculations:
  - Mild: magnesium, vitamin E
  - Severe: quinine, carbamazepine, phenytoin
- Spasticity:
  - Support: ankle–foot orthoses, wheelchair, home modification
  - Drug treatment: badofen, tizanidine, mementine, tetrazepam
- Drooling: amitriptyline, transdermal hyosine patches, glycopyrrolate, atropine, benzatropine
- Pathological laughing or crying: amitriptyline, fluvoxamine, lithium, levodopa
- Riluzole for disease of bulbar onset.

3. Support for vital functions:
   - Assisted ventilation
   - Nutritional support: percutaneous endoscopic or radiologically inserted gastrostomy.

4. End of life palliative care (any end-of-life directive?).

Is there any test to monitor the rate of disease progression?

Antibodies to L-type voltage-gated calcium channels are present in the serum of patients with sporadic AML, and antibody titres correlate with the rate of disease progression (N Engl J Med 1992;327:1721–8).

What is the role of magnetic cortical stimulation in amyotrophic lateral sclerosis?

Magnetic cortical stimlation uses time-varying magnetic fields to induce electrical currents within the brain painlessly. It is said to activate cortical motor neurons trans-synaptically through thalamocortical and corticocortical afferents, and allows detection of degeneration of cortical Betz cells. In patients with AML, the sensitivity of this technique to detect upper motor neuron involvement in those with clinical signs is high, but the sensitivity of the technique in those without clinical signs is unknown.

Is there any animal model for amyotrophic lateral sclerosis?

Transgenic mouse model possessing mutations in the gene encoding the cytosolic form of the enzyme copper–zinc SOD (Nature 1993;362:59).

Further reading

Radunović A, Mitsumoto H, Leigh PN: Clinical care of patients with amyotrophic lateral sclerosis, *Lancet Neurol* 6:913–925, 2007.

Lou Gehrig, the American baseball player, died from AML 50 years ago.
  Charcot gave a detailed clinical and pathological description of AML in 1865.
  Professor Stephen Hawking, the Cambridge theoretical physicist, is the most famous sufferer of motor neuron disease. It claimed the lives of the actor David Niven, the football manager Don Revie and the wartime pilot Sir Leonard Cheshire, VC.

70 NEUROFIBROMATOSIS

INSTRUCTION

Examine this patient.

SALIENT FEATURES

History

- Presents in childhood with cutaneous features including café-au-lait spots, axillary freckles and neurofibromas
- Obtain history of learning disabilities (about half the patients with neurofibroma 1 are affected; Nature 2000;403:846–7)
- Childhood leukaemia: the risk of malignant myeloid disorders, particularly juvenile myelomonocytic leukaemia and the monosomy 7 syndrome (a childhood variant of myeloid dysplasia) is 200 to 500 times the normal risk (N Engl J Med 1997;336:1713–20).

Examination

- Multiple neurofibroma and café-au-lait spots (brown macules, >2.5 cm diameter and >5 lesions)
- Examine the axilla for freckles
- Check visual acuity and fundus for optic glioma (Fig. 70.1)
- Hearing and corneal sensation for acoustic neuroma
- The iris for Lisch nodules (often apparent only by slit-lamp examination). The incidence of Lisch nodules in type 1 increases with age (at the age of 5 years only 22% have Lisch nodules, whereas at the age of 20 years 100% have them). Therefore, older individuals who do not have Lisch nodules are unlikely to have type 1 neurofibromatosis (Fig. 70.2)
- The spine for kyphoscoliosis
- Tell the examiner that you would like to check the BP for renal artery stenosis or phaeochromocytoma).

Remember the triad for neurofibromatosis — neurofibroma, café-au-lait spots and Lisch nodules — allows identification of virtually all patients with neurofibromatosis type 1.

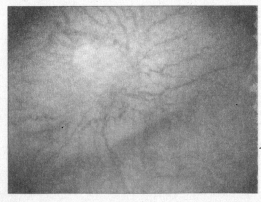

Fig. 70.1 Typical combined hamartoma of retina. Note typical juxtapapillary and epipapillary location of lesion. (With permission from Yanoff, Duker 2008.)

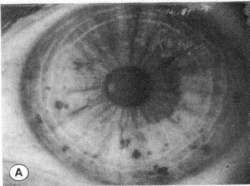

Fig. 70.2
Neurofibromatosis type 1.
Slit-lamp examination
(B) is essential for
differentiation of Lisch
nodules (iris hamartoma)
from iris freckles. Iris
freckles are flat and have
a lace-work structure;
Lisch nodules are raised,
round, fluffy, and light
brown. (Courtesy Lucian
Szmyd, with permission
from Habif 2009.)

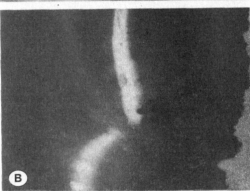

DIAGNOSIS

This patient has multiple café-au-lait spots and neurofibromas (lesion) caused by von Recklinghausen's disease (aetiology), which are cosmetically disfiguring (functional status).

ADVANCED-LEVEL QUESTIONS

What are the criteria for neurofibromatosis type 1 (von Recklinghausen's disease)?

Neurofibromatosis type 1 may be diagnosed when two or more of the following are present:

- Six or more café-au-lait spots, the greatest diameter of which is >5 mm in prepubertal patients and >15 mm in postpubertal patients
- Two or more neurofibromas or one plexiform neurofibroma. Plexiform neurofibroma is considered by some to be a defining lesion of neurofibroma type 1
- Freckling in the axilla or inguinal region (Crowe's sign)
- Optic glioma
- Two or more Lisch nodules (iris hamartoma)

- A distinctive osseous lesion such as sphenoid dysplasia or thinning of long bone cortex with or without pseudoarthroses
- A parent, sibling or child with neurofibromatosis according to the above criteria.

What are the criteria for neurofibromatosis type 2?
- Bilateral eighth nerve palsy confirmed by CT or MRI
- A parent, sibling or child with neurofibromatosis type 2 and either unilateral eighth nerve mass or any two of the following: neurofibroma, meningioma, glioma, schwannoma or juvenile posterior subcapsular lenticular opacity (N Engl J Med 1988;318:685).

Note: Blockade of vascular endothelial growth factor (VGEF) with bevacizumab improves hearing in some patients (not all) with neurofibromatosis type 2 and has been associated with a reduction in the volume of most growing vestibular schwannomas (N Engl J Med 2009;361:358–67).

What is the significance of the Lisch nodules?
Lisch nodules are melanocytic hamartomas that appear as well-defined, dome-shaped elevations projecting from the surface of the iris and are clear to yellow and brown. The incidence increases with age: at the age of 5 years only 22% have Lisch nodules, whereas at the age of 20 years, 100% have them. Therefore, older patients who do not have Lisch nodules are also unlikely to have neurofibromatosis 1. They are an important tool in establishing the diagnosis of neurofibromatosis type 1 and in providing accurate genetic screening (N Engl J Med 1991;324:1264).

What is the histology of the skin tumours?
The peripheral nerve tumours are of two types:
- Schwannomas: arise in cranial and spinal nerve roots and also in peripheral nerve trunks.
- Neurofibromas: composed of a proliferation of all elements of the peripheral nerve including neuritis, Schwann cells and fibroblasts. In sensory nerve twigs, they appear as subcutaneous nodules, while in peripheral nerve trunks they may appear as a fusiform enlargement or a plexiform neurofibroma.

Is a biopsy of the neurofibromas required to make a diagnosis?
No, as the diagnosis is usually evident on clinical grounds.

What are the associated abnormalities of neurofibroma?
- Lung cysts
- Retinal hamartomas
- Skeletal lesions: rib notching and other erosive bony defects, intraosseous cystic lesions, subperiosteal bony cysts, dysplasia of the skull, bowed legs and pseudoarthrosis of the tibia
- Intellectual disability
- Aqueductal stenosis
- Epilepsy
- Sarcomatous change

Is phaeochromocytoma common in this condition?
In neurofibromatosis type 1, phaeochromocytoma is relatively rare (<5%). Because of this, routine screening for the tumour is not generally recommended. Genetic testing in members of an affected family is possible.

Phaeochromocytomas in affected individuals usually produce both epine-phrine and norepinephrine.

What do you know about the inheritance of the two types?

Both are autosomal dominant syndromes, type 1 being carried on chromosome 17q11.2 and type 2 on chromosome 22 (Science1987;236:110, Nature 1993;363:515). The gene for neurofibromatosis type 1 encodes a protein called neurofibromin (GTPase-activating protein), which downregulates the function of the p21 Ras oncoprotein (Neuron 1993;10:335). Learning disabilities have been ascribed to abnormal brain development resulting from deficiency in neurofibromin signalling (Nature 2000;403:895–8). The gene for type 2 neurofibromatosis (locus is 22q11) also encodes a tumour suppressor protein (merlin or schwannomin), which links integral membrane proteins of the cytoskeleton. How this protein is involved in tumorigenesis is not clear. Family members at risk for type 2 neurofibromatosis should be screened regularly with hearing tests and brainstem auditory evoked responses.

How would you manage these patients?

- Most are asymptomatic and require no treatment
- Large plexiform neurofibromas should be usually left alone
- Small neurofibromas can be removed if painful
- Optic gliomas are treated with radiation.

What is the risk of a further child being affected in a family?

If one parent is affected then there is a 50% chance that another child will be affected, whereas when neither parent is affected then the risk of another child being affected is no more than the standard risk in the normal population.

The first case reports of probable neurofibromatosis appeared in the 16th century.

The first review of this condition was published in 1849 by Robert W Smith, Professor of Surgery in Dublin, who suggested that the tumours originated from connective tissue surrounding small nerves.

Friedreich Daniel von Recklinghausen (1833–1910) was Professor of Pathology successively at Könisberg, Wüurzburg and Strasbourg. He also described another disease, arthritis deformans neoplastica, to which his name is attached. Von Recklinghausen in 1882 was the first to recognize that the characteristic tumours arise from nervous tissue. He described in the report of his second case: 'His [a 47-year-old male] most striking abnormality consisted of innumerable tumours, running close to a thousand altogether, in the outer skin layer. ...The patient could only report that he had had them as long as he could remember ...and that they had increased markedly after his fifteenth year ...my interest turned understandably to the externally palpable peripheral nerve trunks. ...I was soon able clearly to recognise thickenings of these in their gross distribution' (Lancet 2003; 361:1552–4).

The elephant man, John Merrick, is commonly believed to have suffered from neurofibromatosis, but according to Wallace (Science 1994;264:188) a rare condition Proteus syndrome is the more likely diagnosis.

Professor Lisch first described the association of the Lisch nodule with neurofibromatosis in 1937 (Z Augenheilkd 1937;93:137–43). These nodules were first described by Waardenburg in 1918 but he did not appreciate the association with neurofibromatosis.

71 SYRINGOMYELIA

INSTRUCTION

Examine this patient's arms.

SALIENT FEATURES

History

- Classically patient has a history of painless trauma or burns with cigarettes, hot water
- Patient may have cuts that never seem to hurt
- Patient may have a long history of poorly localized unpleasant pain (although pain sensation is impaired these patients have severe pain)
- Patient may notice scoliosis during childhood.

Examination

- Wasting and weakness of the small muscles of the hands and forearm (if fasciculation is seen, then the other diagnosis that comes to mind at this stage is motor neuron disease (Case 69))
- Rarely patients may have hypertrophy in limbs, hand and feet (Lancet 1996;347:1593–5)
- Tone and deep tendon reflexes are diminished
- Loss of pain and temperature sensation with intact vibration, light touch and joint position sense: this deficit is the underlying cause for any burns present
- There may be Charcot's joints of the shoulder and elbow
- There may be signs of hemi-hypertrophy of the limbs.

Proceed as follows:

- Examine vibration sense over the fingers, lower end of radius, elbow and clavicles (note that vibration sense is impaired only at a later stage)
- Look for Horner syndrome
- Examine the neck posteriorly for scar of previous surgery
- Ask whether you may examine the following:
  - The lower limbs for pyramidal signs
  - The face for loss of temperature and pain sensation (starting from the outer part of the face and progressing forward, looking for the 'onion-skin pattern' of sensory loss caused by a lesion in the spinal nucleus of the fifth cranial nerve, which extends from the pons down to the upper cervical cord)
  - For lower cranial nerve palsy
  - For nystagmus and ataxia (caused by involvement of the medial longitudinal bundle from C5 upwards)
  - For kyphoscoliosis (caused by paravertebral muscle involvement).

DIAGNOSIS

This patient has dissociated sensory loss (lesion) caused by syringomyelia (aetiology) and has had severe painless trauma or burns (functional status).

QUESTIONS

How common is syringomyelia?

It is a rare disorder affecting both sexes equally; the usual age of onset is the fourth or fifth decade.

How do you explain the clinical features?

- At the level of the syrinx:
  - Anterior horn cell involvement causing a lower motor neuron lesion
  - Involvement of the central decussating fibres of the spinothalamic tract producing dissociated sensory loss and late development of neuropathic arthropathy and other trophic changes.
- Below the level of the syrinx:
  - Involvement of pyramidal corticospinal tracts resulting in spastic paraparesis (sphincter function is usually well preserved)
  - Involvement of cervical sympathetics:
    - Horner syndrome (miosis, enophthalmos, ptosis).

ADVANCED-LEVEL QUESTIONS

What is la main succulente?

In some patients with syringomyelia, the hands have an ugly appearance as a result of trophic and vasomotor disturbances; these commonly result in cold, cyanosed and swollen fingers and palms.

What are the other causes of dissociated sensory loss?

- Anterior spinal artery occlusion (affecting the dorsal horn and lateral spinothalamic tract)
- Diabetic small-fibre polyneuropathy
- Hereditary amyloidotic polyneuropathy
- Leprosy.

The last three affect small peripheral nerve axons.

What investigations would you do?

MRI scan (J Neurosurg 1988;68:726) (Fig. 71.1). In the past, myelography was performed to confirm the diagnosis but was associated with deterioration of the condition in a large number of patients.

What associated abnormalities may be present?

Arnold–Chiari malformation (Fig. 71.1), spina bifida, bony defects around the foramen magnum, hydrocephalus, spinal cord tumours.

What conditions may be present with a similar picture?

- Intramedullary tumours of the spinal cord
- Arachnoiditis around the foramen magnum obstructing the CSF pathway
- Haematomyelia
- Craniovertebral anomalies
- Late sequelae of spinal cord injuries (manifest as a painful ascending myelopathy).

What is the difference between hydromyelia and syringomyelia?

Hydromyelia is the expansion of the ependymal-lined central canal of the spinal cord, whereas syringomyelia is the formation of a cleft-like cavity in the inner portion of the cord. Both these lesions are associated with destruction of the white and grey matter and an accompanying reactive

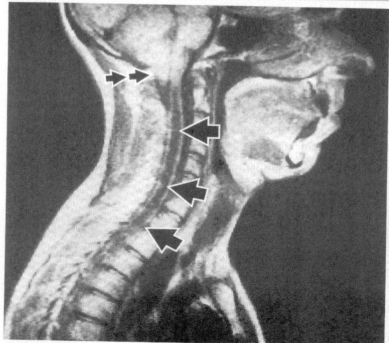

Fig. 71.1 Midsagittal MRI of Arnold-Chiari malformation (small black arrows) and syringomyelia (three large black arrows). Note the cerebellar tonsils extending below the posterior rim of the foramen magnum (dark structure immediately above the black arrow). The syrinx extends from the medulla well into the thoracic cord. (With permission from Andreoli 1997.)

gliosis. In syringomyelia the process generally begins in the cervical cord, and with expansion of the cavity the brainstem and distal cord also become affected.

What are the clinical features of syringobulbia?

- Dissociated sensory loss of the face in an 'onion-skin' pattern (extending from behind forwards, converging on the nose and upper lip)
- Vertigo (common symptom)
- Wasting of the small muscles of the tongue (important physical sign)
- The process may be limited to the medullary region
- The main cranial nerve nuclei involved are those of the fifth, seventh, ninth and tenth cranial nerves.

What does the cavity of the syrinx contain?

It contains a fluid similar to CSF but with a higher protein content.

What treatment is available?

- Syringoperitoneal shunting (particularly in patients with basal arachnoiditis and without tonsillar descent)
- Direct drainage of the syrinx into the subarachnoid space (in post-traumatic cavitation)
- When there is an association with Arnold–Chiari malformation, the pressure is relieved by removing the lower central portion of the occipital bone and cervical laminectomy to restore normal CSF dynamics.

(See J Neurol Neurosurg Psychiatry 1981;44:273–84.)

What other causes of Charcot's joints do you know?

- Diabetes mellitus, especially when toes and ankles are affected
- Tabes dorsalis, especially when knee and hip joints are affected.

What do you know about Morvan syndrome?

It was initially used to describe painless whitlows on the fingers but was subsequently applied to the progressive loss of pain sensation and its effects (such as ulceration, resorption of the phalanges and loss of soft tissue) in both hands and feet (Gaz Heb Med Chir 1883;35:580). These changes are now more commonly seen in leprosy.

Mention some theories of formation of syringomyelia

Gardner's hydrodynamic theory. This theory posits that syringomyelia is caused by a 'water hammer'-like transmission of pulsatile CSF pressure via a communication between the fourth ventricle and the central canal of the spinal cord through the obex. A blockage of the foramen of Magendie initiates this process (J Neurol Neurosurg Psychiatry 1965; 28:247–59.)

William's theory. William's theory posits that the development of the syrinx is caused by a differential between intracranial pressure and spinal pressure caused by a valve like action at the foramen magnum. The increase in subarachnoid fluid pressure from increased venous pressure during Valsalva maneuvers or coughing is localized to the intracranial compartment (Neurol Res 1986;8:130–45). This theory is particularly applicable to patients with Chiari malformation. The malformation of the hindbrain prevents the increased CSF pressure from dissipating caudally. During Valsalva maneuver or coughing, a progressive increase in cisterna magna pressure occurs simultaneously with a decrease in spinal subarachnoid pressure. This craniospinal pressure gradient draws CSF caudally into the syrinx.

Oldfield's theory. During dynamic MRI, downward movement of the cerebellar tonsils during systole can be visualized. A piston effect, created by oscillations, in the spinal subarachnoid space that acts on the surface of the spinal cord and forces CSF through the perivascular and interstitial spaces into the syrinx raising intramedullary pressure. The resulting compression of long tracts, neurons and microcirculation are responsible for the signs and symptoms of neurological dysfunction that appear with distension of the syrinx. Decompression of the syrinx, therefore, potentially reverses the symptoms referable to increased intramedullary pressure (J Neurosurg 1994;80:3–15).

The intramedullary pulse pressure theory. The intramedullary pulse pressure theory posits that syringomyelia is caused by increased pulse pressure in the spinal cord and that the syrinx consists of extracellular fluid. The distending force in the production of syringomyelia is a relative increase in pulse pressure in the spinal cord compared with that in the nearby subarachnoid space. The syrinix is formed by the accumulation of extracellular fluid in the distended cord.

What do you know about the management of syringomyelia?

- Arnold-Chiari malformation associated syringomyelia: suboccipital craniectomy and upper cervical laminectomy to decompress the malformation at the foramen magnum
- Intramedullary tumour: surgery with or without radiation therapy
- Post-traumatic syringomyelia: surgery when the neurologic deficits or pain is intolerable
- The term syringomyelia (from *syringx*, a pipe or tube) was first used by Ollivier in 1824, in his monograph on diseases of the spinal cord, to denote cavity formation. It denotes the presence of a large fluid-filled cavity in the grey matter of the spinal cord that is in communication with the central canal and contains CSF.

J Arnold (1835–1915), Professor of Pathology at Heidelberg.
 H Chiari (1851–1916), an Austrian pathologist.

---

72 SUBACUTE COMBINED DEGENERATION OF THE SPINAL CORD

INSTRUCTION

Carry out a neurological examination of the patient's legs.

SALIENT FEATURES

History

- Family history of pernicious anaemia
- History of alcohol consumption and previous gastrectomy
- History of chronic diarrhoea (Crohns' disease, etc.)
- Tingling distal paraesthesia (common presenting symptom)
- Whether the patient is a vegan.

Examination

- Absent ankle jerks (caused by peripheral neuropathy and motor involvement)
- Brisk knee jerks
- Upgoing plantars (usually first evidence of spinal cord lesion)
- Diminished light touch, vibration and posterior column signs
- Romberg's sign positive.

Proceed as follows:
- Examine:
  - mucous membranes for anaemia (pernicious anaemia)
  - abdomen for scars of previous gastrectomy (carcinoma of the stomach)
  - pupils (Argyll Robertson pupil (Case 39) because tabes is a differential diagnosis)
  - fundus for optic atrophy, seen in this condition.
- Tell the examiner that you would like to do the following investigations:
  - Mini-mental status examination for dementia
  - A 'red tongue and unsteady gait' is seen in the classic condition.

DIAGNOSIS

This patient has absent ankle jerks, brisk knee jerks and upgoing plantars with posterior column signs (lesion) caused by subacute combined degeneration of the spinal cord (aetiology) and paralysis (functional status).

QUESTIONS

Mention a few causes of vitamin B_{12} deficiency
- Vegan diet
- Impaired absorption:
  - from the stomach: pernicious anaemia, gastrectomy
  - from the small bowel: ileal disease, bacterial overgrowth, coeliac disease
  - from the pancreas: chronic pancreatic disease.
- As a result of fish tapeworm (rare).

ADVANCED-LEVEL QUESTIONS

What is the pathology of this condition?
There is degeneration of the axons in both the ascending tracts of the posterior columns (sensory) and the descending pyramidal tracts (motor), hence combined degeneration.

How would you investigate such a patient?
- FBC and reticulocyte count
- Vitamin B_{12} and folate concentrations
- Serum ferritin levels (since associated iron deficiency is common)
- Bone marrow examination
- Parietal cell and intrinsic factor antibodies
- Schilling test (no longer done because radioisotope is not available in UK)
- MRI findings are diverse (Fig. 72.1) but vitamin B_{12} deficiency should be considered in differential diagnosis of all spinal cord, peripheral nerve and neuropsychiatric disorders (J Neurol Neurosurg Psych 1998;65:822–7).

If this patient had a haemoglobin level of 6 g/l, how would you treat it?
Avoid giving packed cells before replacing vitamin B_{12} as this may irreversibly exacerbate the neurological manifestations. Furthermore, blood transfusion is reported to precipitate incipient heart failure and death.

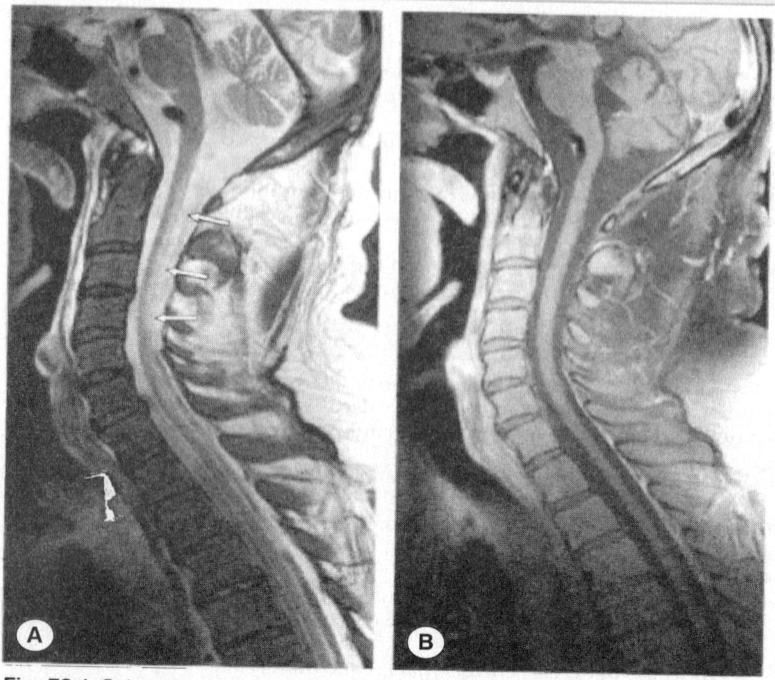

Fig. 72.1 Subacute combined degeneration of the spinal cord in vitamin B_{12} deficiency. (A) T_2-weighted MRI shows abnormal signal intensity of spinal cord extending from C1 toC6 (arrows). (B) There is no enhancement after application of gadolinium in the sagital T_1-weighted image. (With permission from Schöllhammer M et al. 2005.)

What type of anaemia may be seen in such patients?
Macrocytic anaemia.

Mention a few other causes of macrocytic anaemia
- With megaloblastic bone marrow: vitamin B_{12} deficiency, folate deficiency
- With normoblastic marrow: haemolytic anaemias, post-haemorrhagic anaemia, severe hypoxia, myxoedema, hypopituitarism, bone marrow infiltration, acute leukaemia and aplastic anaemia.

What do you know about intrinsic factor antibodies?
Intrinsic factor antibodies are seen in about 50% of patients with pernicious anaemia. About 45% of the patients have no antibody to intrinsic factor. There are two types of antibody:

Type 1: blocking antibody that prevents vitamin B_{12} from binding to intrinsic factor; occurs in 55% of patients

Type 2: binding or precipitating antibody, which reacts with intrinsic factor or with vitamin B_{12}–intrinsic factor complex and is seen in 35% of patients.

What is the relationship between pernicious anaemia and gastric carcinoma?

The incidence of gastric carcinoma in patients with pernicious anaemia is increased three-fold compared with that in the general population.

What gastrointestinal investigations would you do in an asymptomatic patient with pernicious anaemia?

In the absence of GI symptoms, gastroscopy or barium meal is not indicated, although many physicians tend to perform one of these investigations.

What do you understand by the term 'combined' degeneration of the cord?

This refers to the combined demyelination of both pyramids (or lateral columns) and posterior columns of the spinal cord.

What is the response of the neurological lesions to treatment with vitamin B$_{12}$?

The response to vitamin B$_{12}$ therapy is variable: it may improve, remain unchanged or even deteriorate. Sensory abnormalities improve more than motor abnormalities and peripheral neuropathy responds to treatment better than myelopathy.

Subacute combined degeneration is also known as Putnam–Dana syndrome or Lichtheim's disease. James Jackson Putnam (1846–1918) and Charles Loomis Dana (1852–1935) were both US neurologists. Ludwig Lichtheim (1845–1928), a German physician.

Pernicious anaemia was usually fatal, until 1926 when Whipple, Minot and Murphy described the beneficial effects of feeding liver. The 1934 Nobel Prize in Medicine was awarded jointly to George Whipple (1878–1976) of University of Rochester, New York, and to George Minot (1885–1950) and William P Murphy (1892–1987) of Harvard Medical School and Peter Brent Brigham Hospital, Boston, for their discoveries concerning liver therapy in anaemia. This condition is also known as Addison–Biermer's anaemia with reference to Thomas Addison and the German physician Anton Biermer.

William B Castle first found that oral administration of gastric juice (intrinsic factor) or beef (extrinsic factor, i.e. vitamin B$_{12}$) alone was not effective in the treatment of pernicious anaemia but that a mixture of both these factors rendered the patient erythropoietically active. Castle worked with Francis Peabody at the Harvard Medical School Unit at Boston City Hospital before he became Professor of Medicine at Harvard.

---

73 TABES DORSALIS

INSTRUCTION

Examine this patient with lightning pains (lightning denotes that the pains are fleeting and does not necessarily mean they are excruciating).

SALIENT FEATURES

History

● 'Lightening pains' are electrical shock like sensation in the limbs, throat, stomach or rectum

- High-stepping gait: patient may only hear their feet slapping the ground and feels as if they are walking on cotton-wool (caused by loss of joint position sense)
- Constipation (this is present as a rule).

Examination

- Examine the eyes:
  - Bilateral ptosis with frontalis overaction
  - Argyll Robertson pupil (irregular, small pupil which reacts sluggishly to light but reacts to accommodation; Case 39)
  - Optic atrophy (primary).
- Examine the sensory system:
  - Posterior column signs: look for loss of pain sensation but with normal touch and temperature sensation over the nose, cheeks, inner aspects of the arms and legs, a band across the nipple and in the anal area
  - Squeeze calf muscles and the Achilles tendon (evokes no pain as deep sensation is lost).
- Examine:
  - the ankle jerks (absent) and plantar response (normal)
  - the gait for ataxia (steppage gait) and Romberg's sign
  - the knees and hips for Charcot's joints
  - the feet for trophic ulcers.
- Tell the examiner that you would like to:
  - ask the patient about bladder sensation (lost), overflow incontinence and impotence (if male)
  - check testicular sensation (usually lost early).

Remember: As a rule, the lower limbs are affected before the upper limbs. Very rarely, the upper limbs may be affected first (cervical tabes).

DIAGNOSIS

This patient has posterior column signs and Argyll Robertson pupil (lesion) caused by tabes dorsalis (aetiology), and has severe ataxia (functional status).

ADVANCED-LEVEL QUESTIONS

What do you know about neurosyphilis?

Without treatment, early syphilis progresses (Fig. 73.1). Tertiary syphilis of the nervous system never develops in those who have received appropriate therapy in the early stages. There are five clinical patterns of neurosyphilis:

- Meningovascular disease, which occurs 3–4 years after primary infection
- Tabes dorsalis, which occurs 10–35 years after primary infection
- Generalized paralysis of the insane (GPI), which occurs 10–15 years after primary infection
- Taboparesis (a combination of tabes dorsalis and GPI)
- Localized gummata.

What is the underlying pathology?

It is caused by a combination of neuronal degeneration and/or arterial lesions.

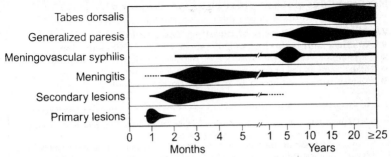

Fig. 73.1 Approximate time course of the clinical manifestations of early syphilis and neurosyphilis. Width of the areas indicates approximate proportion of patients with the syndrome.

How would you confirm the diagnosis?
The Wasserman reaction, Veneral Disease Reference Laboratory (VDRL), or *Treponema pallidum* haemagglutination assay (TPHA):
- Meningovascular syphilis: 70% positive, whereas CSF shows 90% positive
- Tabes dorsalis: 75% positive
- GPI: nearly 100% positive.

Note: Other tests include fluorescent treponemal antibody (FTA) and the treponemal immoblization test (TPI).

Mention a few conditions for which the Wasserman reaction may be falsely positive
Rheumatoid arthritis, SLE, chronic active hepatitis, infectious mononucleosis.

How would you treat the active syphilitic infection?
A course of parenteral penicillin.

How would you manage other symptoms of tabes?
- Lightning pains: simple analgesics, carbamazepine
- Sensory ataxia: re-educational exercises to improve limb coordination
- Bladder symptoms: avoid anticholinergics, employ urodynamic studies and intermittent self-catheterization
- Visceral crises: opiate analgesics; in recurrent cases, section of lower thoracic spinal dorsal roots
- Perforating ulcer: well-fitting shoes and regular foot care
- Charcot's arthropathy: symptomatic treatment, avoid insertion of prostheses as results are poor.

In which group of patients is syphilis now common?
In those with underlying HIV infection.

What is the Jarisch–Herxheimer reaction?
An acute hypersensitivity reaction seen when a patient with syphilis is treated with penicillin. Toxins from the killed spirochaetes cause this reaction, which can be fatal. Steroids are often given during the first few days of penicillin therapy.

How may this patient present to the surgeons?

With acute abdominal pain (lancinating pains).

What are the methods of eliciting deep pain?

- Abadie's sign is the loss of pain sense in the Achilles tendon
- Biernacki's sign is the absence of pain on pressure on the ulnar nerve
- Pitres' sign is loss of pain on pressure on the testes
- Haenel sign is analgesia to pressure on the eyeballs.

Tabes was first recognized by Romberg and Duchenne. Fournier was the first to suspect that it was caused by syphilis.

In the first half of the 19th century, three European physicians—namely Mortiz Romberg, Marshall Hall and Bernadus Brach described the loss of postural control in darkness of patients with severely impaired proprioceptive sensation (Neurology 2000;55:1201–6). Romberg and Brach showed the relationship between this sign and tabes dorsalis (Semin Neurol. 2002;22: 409–18).

Alphonse Daudet's (French novelist) experience of the agonies of tabes dorsalis has been well described.

AP Wassermann (1866–1925), a German physician.

A Jarisch (1850–1902), Professor of Dermatology in Austria.

K Herxheimer (1861–1944), a Jewish German dermatologist who died in a concentration camp.

---

74 ULNAR NERVE PALSY

INSTRUCTION

Carry out a neurological examination of this patient's upper limbs.

SALIENT FEATURES

History

- Repeated trivial trauma to the elbow; the patient feels the 'funny bone'
- Patient may be immobilized in the orthopaedic ward and use the elbows to shuffle in bed
- History of fracture of the upper arm in childhood (supracondylar fractures of humerus in childhood has an insidious course and can result in acute ulnar nerve palsy 20–30 years later: tardy-ulnar palsy).

Examination

- Generalized wasting of the small muscles of the hand.
- There may be features of ulnar claw hand: hyperextension at the metacarpophalangeal joints and flexion at the interphalangeal joints of the fourth and fifth fingers (Fig. 74.1).
- There is weakness of movement of the fingers, except that of the thenar eminence.
- There is sensory loss over the medial one and half fingers.

Proceed as follows:

- Examine the elbow for scars and signs of osteoarthrosis.

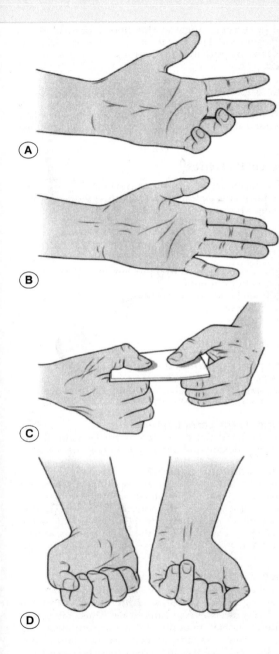

Fig. 74.1 (A) Benediction posture, with clawing of the fourth and fifth fingers while fingers and thumb are held slightly abducted. (B) Wartenberg' sign, abduction of the little finger with the hand at rest. (C) Froment's sign, seen when using the thumb and index finger to pinch an object. (D) Weakness of the ulnar flexor digitorum profundus, inability to completely flex the distal phalanx of the fourth and fifth digits.

● Comment on the large carrying angle at the elbow, particularly in women (repeated extension and flexion of the arm can result in damage of the olecranon and consequently the ulnar nerve).

DIAGNOSIS

This patient has wasting of the small muscles of the hand and claw hand with sensory loss over the medial one and half fingers (lesion) caused by ulnar nerve palsy following trauma (aetiology). She is unable to button her clothes (functional status).

ADVANCED-LEVEL QUESTIONS

What are the muscles supplied by the ulnar nerve?

The ulnar nerve is derived from the eighth cervical and first thoracic spinal nerves. It gives no branches above the elbow and supplies:
● in the forearm:
  • flexor carpi ulnaris
  • medial half of the flexor digitorum profundus
● in the hand:
  • movers of the little finger: abductor digiti minimi, flexor digiti minimi and opponens digiti minimi
  • adductor pollicis (oblique and transverse heads)
  • dorsal and palmar interossei
  • third and fourth lumbricals
  • palmaris brevis
  • inner head of flexor pollicis brevis.

How would you differentiate between a lesion above the cubital fossa and a lesion at the wrist?

● In lesions above the cubital fossa the flexor carpi ulnaris is involved.
● In lesions at the wrist, the adductor pollicis is involved.

How would you test the flexor carpi ulnaris?

Ask the patient to keep the hand flat on a table with the palm facing upwards and then to perform flexion and ulnar deviation at the wrist.

How would you test the adductor pollicis?

Ask the patient to grip a folded newspaper between the thumb and index finger of each hand so that the thumbs are uppermost — this causes the adductor to contract. When the muscle is paralysed, the thumb is incapable of adequate adduction and becomes flexed at the interphalangeal joint caused by contraction of the flexor pollicis longus (innervated by the median nerve). This is known as Froment's sign (Fig. 74.1C).

What is ulnar paradox?

The higher the lesion in the upper limb, the lesser is the deformity. A lesion at or above the elbow causes paralysis of the ulnar half of the flexor digitorum profundus, interossei and lumbricals. Thus, the action of the paralysed profundus is not unopposed by the interossei and lumbricals; as a result, the ring and little fingers are not flexed and hence there is no claw, whereas a lesion at the wrist causes an ulnar claw hand.

What causes the ulnar claw hand?

A lesion of the ulnar nerve at the wrist. The little and ring fingers are flexed at the interphalangeal joints and hyperextended at the metacarpophalangeal joints. The index and middle fingers are less affected as the first and second lumbricals are supplied by the median nerve.

What are the causes of claw hand?

True claw hand is seen in the following conditions:

● Advanced rheumatoid arthritis
● Lesion of both the median and ulnar nerves, as in leprosy
● Lesions of the medial cord of the brachial plexus
● Anterior poliomyelitis
● Syringomyelia
● Polyneuritis
● Amyotrophic lateral sclerosis
● Klumpke's paralysis (lower brachial plexus, C7–8 involvement)
● Severe Volkmann's ischaemic contracture.

How can the ulnar nerve be affected at the wrist?

The deep branch of the ulnar nerve is motor and may be compressed in Guyon's canal, which runs between the pisiform and hook of the hamate. This results in wasting and weakness of the interossei, particularly the first and the adductor pollicis, but sensation is spared. Also the hypothenar muscles are usually spared, although the third and fourth lumbricals may be affected. The nerve may be compressed in Guyon's canal by a ganglion, neuroma or repeated trauma. Surgical exposure of the nerve may be necessary when there is no history of trauma.

What is the most common cause of an ulnar nerve lesion at the elbow?

It is caused by compression of the nerve by the fibrous arch of the flexor carpi ulnaris (the cubital tunnel), which arises as two heads from the medial epicondyle and the olecranon.

What you understand by 'tardy ulnar nerve palsy'?

This occurs when injuries or arthritic changes at the elbow cause a delayed or slowly progressive involvement of the ulnar nerve.

How would you rapidly exclude an injury to a major nerve in the arm?

● Radial nerve: test for wrist drop
● Ulnar nerve: test for Froment's sign (see above)
● Median nerve: Ochsner's clasping test.

R von Volkmann (1830–1889), Professor of Surgery in Halle, Germany.

Augusta Déjérine-Klumpke (1859–1927), a French neurologist, was the first woman to receive the title 'Internes des Hôpitaux' in 1877.

Jules Froment (1876–1946), Professor of Clinical Medicine, Lyons, France.

AJ Ochsner (1896–1981), a US surgeon, also investigated the role of tobacco in lung cancer.

75 LATERAL POPLITEAL NERVE PALSY, L4, L5 (COMMON PERONEAL NERVE PALSY)

INSTRUCTION

Examine this patient's legs.
Test this patient's gait.

SALIENT FEATURES

History

- History of trauma to the nerve particularly when it winds around the neck of the fibula where it is protected by only skin and fascia
- Whether the symptoms occur after sitting crossed leg for prolonged periods
- Recent weight loss, particularly in those who have been confined to bed rest (nerve more vulnerable because the protective fat and muscle is lost)
- Plasters around the knee
- History of diabetes, polyarteritis nodosa, collagen vascular diseases (all causes of mononeuritis multiplex, p. 226).

Examination

- Wasting of the muscles on the lateral aspect of the leg, namely the peronei and tibialis anterior muscle
- Weakness of dorsiflexion and eversion of the foot
- Foot drop (Fig. 75.1A)
- High steppage gait (Fig. 75.1B)
- Loss of sensation on the lateral aspect of the leg and dorsum of the foot. If the deep peroneal branch is affected, the sensory loss may be limited to the dorsum of the web between the first and second toes.

Proceed as follows:
- Test the ankle jerk:
  - Absent ankle jerk: suspect an S1 lesion
  - Normal jerk: common peroneal nerve palsy
  - Brisk jerk: suspect an upper motor neuron lesion.
- Comment on calliper shoes by the bedside (if any).

DIAGNOSIS

This patient has wasting of the lateral aspect of the leg and sensory loss (lesion) caused by common nerve palsy after trauma to the head of the fibula (aetiology), and has to wear callipers (functional status).

QUESTIONS

Mention a few causes

- Compression resulting from application of a tourniquet or plaster of Paris casts. The nerve is vulnerable at the head of the fibula,

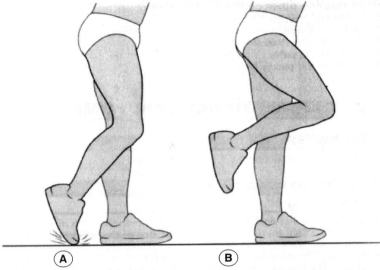

Fig. 75.1 Weakness of ankle dorsiflexors. (A) Foot drop. (B) Steppage gait.

where it lies on the surface of the hard bone with a covering of only skin
- Direct trauma to the nerve
- Leprosy (commonest cause worldwide)
- Ganglion arising from the superior tibiofibular joint may compress the nerve
- Compression of the nerve by the tendinous edge of the peroneus longus.

ADVANCED-LEVEL QUESTIONS

How would you manage such a patient?
- Nerve conduction studies: there may be a local conduction block or slowing in the region of the head of the fibula. There may denervation in the tibialis anterior and extensor digitorum profundus.
- If the intact nerve is severed: surgery.
- If the nerve is intact and concussed: 90 degree splint at night, calliper shoes with a 90 degree stop, and galvanic or faradic stimulation to maintain the bulk of the muscle until the nerve recovers.

What other types of nerve injury do you know?
- Neurapraxia: concussion of the nerve, after which a complete recovery occurs
- Axonotmesis: the axon is severed but the myelin sheath is intact; recovery may occur
- Neurotmesis: the nerve is completely served and the prognosis for recovery is poor.

What are the other causes of foot drop?

- Peripheral neuropathy (p. 225)
- L4, L5 root lesion
- Motor neuron disease
- Sciatic nerve palsy
- Lumbosacral plexus lesion.

76   CARPAL TUNNEL SYNDROME

INSTRUCTION

Examine this patient's hands.

SALIENT FEATURES

History

- Ask the patient about nocturnal pain (commonest cause of hand pain at night). Often the pain wakes up and shakes the hand to ameliorate symptoms: 'wake and shake'.
- Pain, tingling, burning, numbness or some combination of these symptoms on the palmar aspect of the thumb, index finger, middle finger and radial half of the ring finger (no such symptoms affect the fifth finger even on detailed questioning).
- History of oral contraceptives, rheumatoid arthritis, myxoedema, acromegaly, chronic renal failure or sarcoidosis.
- Take a family history (abnormally small size of carpal tunnel runs in families).

Examination

- Wasting of the thenar eminence (Fig. 76.1A)
- Weakness of flexion, abduction and opposition of thumb
- Diminished sensation over lateral three and half fingers
- Ask the patient, 'What do you actually do with your hand(s) when symptoms are at their worst?' If the patient makes flicking movement of the wrist and hand, similar to that employed in shaking down a clinical thermometer (the 'flick sign'), this had both a sensitivity and a specificity >90% in one study (J Neurol Neurosurg Psychiatry 1984;47: 870–2).

Proceed as follows:

- Look carefully for scar of previous surgery (hidden by the crease of the wrist).
- Percuss over the course of the median nerve in the forearm: patient may experience tingling (Tinel's sign (Fig. 76.1A). The sensitivity of Tinel's sign ranges from 25 to 60%, although its specificity is higher (67 to 87%).
- Ask the patient to hyperextend the wrist maximally for 1 min; this may bring on symptoms (dysaesthesia over the thumb and lateral two and half fingers): Phalen's test (Fig. 76.1B).
- Tell the examiner that you would like to:
  - examine for underlying causes such as myxoedema, acromegaly and rheumatoid arthritis

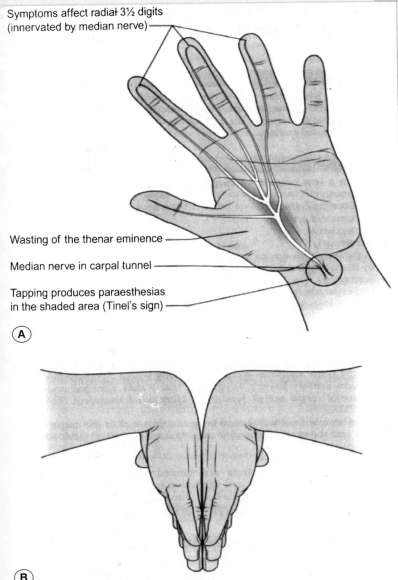

Symptoms affect radial 3½ digits
(innervated by median nerve)

Wasting of the thenar eminence

Median nerve in carpal tunnel

Tapping produces paraesthesias
in the shaded area (Tinel's sign)

(A)

(B)

Fig. 76.1 Carpal tunnel syndrome. (A) Distribution of pain and/or paraesthesias
(shaded area) when the median nerve is compressed by swelling in the wrist
(carpal tunnel). (B) Phalen's test.

- look for cervical spondylosis, frozen shoulder and tennis elbow (these may be associated)
- look for a Cimino–Brescia fistula for haemodialysis (J Neurol Neurosurg Psychiatry 1997;40:511).

DIAGNOSIS

This patient has median nerve involvement of the hand with Tinel's sign (lesion) caused by carpal tunnel syndrome as a complication of chronic haemodialysis (aetiology). The patient has disabling tingling and pain at night (functional status).

QUESTIONS

Mention a few causes of carpal tunnel syndrome

- Pregnancy
- Oral contraceptives
- Rheumatoid arthritis
- Myxoedema
- Acromegaly
- In patients with chronic renal failure on long-term dialysis, it is caused by β_2-microglobulin as amyloid deposition
- Sarcoidosis
- Hyperparathyroidism
- Amyloidosis (e.g. caused by multiple myeloma).

How would you treat this condition?

- Diuretics, NSAIDs, steroids have been studied in small trials but were not efficacious
- Wrist splint in neutral posture rather than in extension (80% report that a wrist splint alleviates symptoms, usually within days). Splinting also reduces sensory latency, suggesting that it may alter the underlying course of carpal tunnel syndrome. Ultrasound treatment (BMJ 1998; 316:731–5)
- Local steroid injection should be given proximal to the carpal tunnel (not into the tunnel because it may damage the nerve) (BMJ 1999;319: 884–6)
- Surgical decompression
- Alternative therapies. Data are limited: acupuncture, yoga-based stretching, strengthening and relaxation (greater improvement in grip strength and reduction of pain than with splinting), chiropractic therapy (was as effective for pain as splints and medication).

ADVANCED-LEVEL QUESTIONS

How would you confirm the diagnosis?

Nerve conduction studies: increased latency at the wrist on stimulation of the median nerve; the muscle action potential from abductor pollicis brevis is a valuable diagnostic sign. Rarely, the proximal latency may be normal with a prolonged distal latency caused by an anastomosis between the ulnar and median nerves in the forearm. Therefore, a negative test does not rule the syndrome out absolutely but calls it into question (J Neurol Neurosurg Psychiatry 1976;39:449).

Mention a few clinical diagnostic tests

- Wrist extension test: the patient is asked to extend the wrists for 1 min; this should produce numbness or tingling in the distribution of the median nerve.
- Phalen's test: the patient is asked to keep both hands with the wrist in complete palmar flexion for 1 min; this produces numbness or tingling in the distribution of the median nerve (Fig. 76.1B). Sensitivity and specificity ranges widely from 40 to 80%.
- Tourniquet test: the symptoms are produced when the BP cuff is inflated above the systolic pressure.
- Pressure test: pressure placed where the median nerve leaves the carpal tunnel causes pain.
- Luthy's sign: is regarded as positive if the skinfold between the thumb and index finger does not close tightly around a bottle or cup because of thumb abduction paresis.
- Durkan's test: direct pressure over the carpal tunnel (the carpal compression test); this is more sensitive and specific than Tinel's and Phalen's signs.

(See Lancet 1990;335:393.)

Mention other entrapment neuropathies

- Meralgia paraesthetica: lateral cutaneous nerve of the thigh trapped under the inguinal ligament
- Elbow tunnel syndrome: ulnar nerve trapped in the cubital tunnel (p. 290)
- Common peroneal nerve trapped at the head of the fibula (p. 295)
- Morton's metatarsalgia: trapped medial and lateral plantar nerves causing pain between third and fourth toes
- Tarsal tunnel syndrome: trapped posterior tibial nerve
- Suprascapular nerve trapped in the spinoglenoid notch
- Radial nerve trapped in the humeral groove
- Anterior interosseous nerve trapped between the heads of the pronator muscle.

Jules Tinel (1879–1952), a French neurologist, described it as the 'sign of formication' in his book on nerve wounds. He took an active part in the French resistance.
   TG Morton (1835–1903), a US surgeon, described this syndrome in 1876.

---

77   RADIAL NERVE PALSY

INSTRUCTION

Perform a neurological examination of this patient's arms.

SALIENT FEATURES

History

- An intoxicated person sleeping with the head resting in the upper arm, causing compression of the nerve over the middle third of the humerus; this is known as Saturday night palsy

- Trauma to the nerve while it courses through the axilla: crutch palsy, shoulder dislocation, fractures of humerus or radius
- History of exposure to lead (lead neuropathy).

Examination

- There is weakness of extension of the wrist and elbow (wrist flexion is normal).
- The patient is unable to straighten the fingers.
- However, if the wrist is passively extended, the patient is able to straighten the fingers at the interphalangeal joints (caused by the action of interossei and lumbricals) but is unable to extend the metacarpophalangeal joint.
- There appears to be a weakness in abduction and adduction of the fingers, but this is not present when the hand is kept flat on a table and the fingers are extended.

Proceed as follows:

- Test the brachoradialis, looking for weakened elbow flexion. When the patient attempts to flex the elbow against resistance, the brachioradialis no longer springs up.
- Test the triceps.
- Check sensation over the first dorsal interosseous (Fig. 77.1).

Note

1. The radial nerve gives off two branches at the elbow:
   - Superficial radial (entirely sensory)
   - Posterior interosseous (entirely muscular).
2. If the injury is situated above the junction of the upper and middle thirds of the humerus, the action of triceps is lost.
3. If the lesion is situated in the middle third of the humerus (frequent site of fracture of the humerus), the brachioradialis is spared.

Be prepared to differentiate from high and low radial nerve palsy (below).

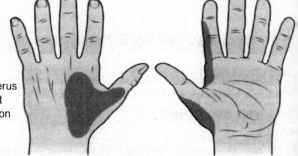

Compression at axilla or mid-humerus Weakness of wrist and finger extension

Fig. 77.1 Sensory impairment in radial nerve palsy.

DIAGNOSIS

This patient has features of radial nerve palsy with the brachioradialis remaining unaffected (lesion) resulting from a fracture located in the middle third of the humerus (aetiology); she is disabled by the deficits (functional status).

QUESTIONS

What are the features of high nerve palsy?
Anatomical:
- Motor deficits:
  - Accessory forearm flexion and supination
  - Wrist extension
  - Digital extension
  - Radial abduction of thumb
- Sensory deficits: radial 2/3 dorsal sensation.

Functional requirements:
- Wrist extension
- Digital extension
- Radial abduction of thumb.

What are the features of low nerve palsy?
Anatomical:
- Motor deficits:
  - Finger extension
  - Thumb extension/abduction
- Sensory deficits: dorsoradial forearm/hand.

Functional requirements:
- Digital extension
- Radial abduction of thumb.

ADVANCED-LEVEL QUESTIONS

What is the cutaneous supply of the radial nerve?
Because of overlap in the areas supplied by the median and ulnar nerves, only a small area of skin over the first dorsal interosseous is exclusively supplied by the radial nerve.

What do you know about the origin of the radial nerve?
The radial nerve is the termination of the posterior cord of the brachial plexus and is derived from the fifth, sixth, seventh and eighth cervical spinal nerves.

What are the branches of the radial nerve in the forearm?
The radial nerve enters the forearm and passes between the two heads of the supinator muscle to become the posterior interosseous nerve.

What muscles are supplied by the radial nerve?
The radial nerve supplies the triceps, anconeus, brachioradialis, extensor carpi radialis longus and, through the posterior interosseous nerve, extensor carpi radialis brevis, supinator, extensor digitorum, extensor digiti minimi, extensor ulnaris, the three extensors of the thumb and extensor indicis.

78 CHOREA

INSTRUCTION

Look at this patient.

SALIENT FEATURES

History

- Ask about sore throats if the patient is an adolescent, particularly if female; suspect Sydenham's chorea (St Vitus dance) in rheumatic fever.
- Take a family history (especially in the middle-aged adult) for Huntington disease.
- Take a history of oral contraceptive use in a young woman or recent pregnancy (chorea gravidorum).

Examination

- Irregular, jerking, ill-sustained, unpredictable, quasipurposive movements of the upper limbs
- The patient is clumsy and keeps dropping objects. Patients with mild disease may show increased fidgeting or restlessness.

Proceed as follows:

- Check the grip of the hands: ask the patient to squeeze your fingers. A squeezing and relaxing motion occurs, which has been described as a 'milkmaid's grip'.
- Look at the tongue for any involuntary movements: known as 'jack-in-the box' tongue or 'bag of worms'.
- Test deep tendon reflexes ('pendular' or 'hung-up' reflexes).
- Tell the examiner that you would like to make enquiries to assess mental status (to exclude premature dementia seen in Huntington disease).

DIAGNOSIS

This young patient has Sydenham's chorea (lesion) secondary to streptococcal sore throat (aetiology); this condition is usually self-limiting.

ADVANCED-LEVEL QUESTIONS

Mention a few more causes of chorea

- SLE
- Polycythaemia vera
- Chorea gravidorum, seen in pregnancy
- Idiopathic hypoparathyroidism
- Following a stroke
- Kernicterus.

What is the prognosis of patients with Sydenham's chorea?
Most patients recover within 1 month; a few may have relapses. A small proportion may develop valvular heart disease and hence should receive penicillin prophylaxis to prevent recurrence of rheumatic fever.

Is there any haematological disorder associated with chorea?
● Polycythaemia vera
● Neuroacanthocytosis or 'chorea–acanthocystosis', where >15% of the red blood cells are acanthocytes (Brain 1991;114:13).

PATIENT 2: HUNTINGTON DISEASE

INSTRUCTION

Look at this patient and ask him a few questions.

SALIENT FEATURES

History

● Tell the examiner that you would like to take a family history of dementia and chorea.

Examination

● Young adult (aged 30–50 years)
● Chorea
● Patient has dementia.

DIAGNOSIS

This patient has chorea (lesion) caused by Huntington disease, and is severely limited by the disease and chorea.

ADVANCED-LEVEL QUESTIONS

What do you know about Huntington disease?
It is an autosomal dominant disorder with a full penetrance characterized by progressive chorea and dementia in middle life. These characteristic findings are the result of severe neuronal loss, initially in the neostriatum and later in the cerebral cortex. The defect is on the small arm of chromosome 4. There is associated random repetition of a sequence of

There is a marked reduction in acetylcholine, substance P and γ-aminobutyric acid (GABA) activity in corpus striatum, whereas dopamine activity is normal and somatostatin is increased (Ann Neurol 1990;27:357).

Using neuropeptide immunochemistry, the chorea has been shown to be associated with damage to the lateral globus pallidus, whereas the parkinsonian signs are caused by additional damage in projections of the medial globus pallidus.

trinucleotides (CAG; normal chromosomes contain about 11–34 copies of this repeat). In Huntington disease, the greater the number of CAG repeats, the earlier the onset of disease (Cell 1993;72:971). The protein product for the gene has been termed huntingtin. It has been proposed that the huntingtin protein is cleaved to fragments that are conjugated with ubiquitin and carried to the proteasome complex. This huntingtin and proteasome component then translocates to the nucleus where it forms intranuclear inclusions; over time this process leads to cell death.

What is the advantage of assessing CAG expansion in persons at risk for Huntington disease?

It is a direct test allowing more accurate assessment of genetic risk, without the need to obtain DNA from family members. This also allows privacy and confidentiality to be maintained because of the reduced need for blood samples from relatives. However, since the misdiagnosis of other illnesses as Huntington disease may occur, the testing of DNA from at least one affected relative is recommended to confirm that CAG expansion is present in other affected persons in the family. This finding will allow the correct interpretation of a normal number of CAG repeats in a person at risk.

Notes

Transcriptional dysregulation and mitochondrial impairment are two important mechanisms in Huntingtons's disease and these are related (N Engl J Med 2007;356:518).

Transcriptional dysregulation. Mutant huntingtin may alter the complement of proteins that are synthesized in a cell, a change that may lead to the pattern of neurodegeneration that characterizes Huntington disease (it binds and sequesters the binding protein for cyclic AMP response-element-binding protein (CREB), which alters the expression of genes regulated by the transcription factor CREB. In a similar way, mutant huntingtin interferes with Sp1-mediated gene transcription.

Mitochondrial impairment. Activities of mitochondrial electron transport complexes II, III and IV are reduced in Huntington disease. Peroxisome proliferator-activated receptor-γ coactivator 1α (PGC-1α) is a transcriptional coactivator that controls many metabolic processes, including mitochondrial biogenesis, oxidative phosphorylation and adaptive thermogenesis (the body's response to cold temperatures). PGC-1α-regulated gene transcription is defective. As a result, there is reduced expression of mitochondrial and antioxidant genes regulated by PGC-1α.

Are any other diseases known to be associated with increased numbers of triplet repeats?

Yes, these include myotonic muscular dystrophy, spinocerebellar ataxia type 1, FRAXE mental retardation (a variant of fragile X syndrome) and hereditary dentatorubral pallidoluysian atrophy (DRPLA).

How would you manage this patient?

Management progresses from clinical suspicion and genetic testing. Once a diagnosis is confirmed, the treatment is symptomatic plus support for depression. A combination of valporate and olanzapine may help in relieving the psychosis and movements disorders associated with Huntington disease (N Engl J Med 2000;343:973).

Thomas Sydenham (1624–1689) was a Puritan from Dorset, and in 1666 published his first work on fevers, which he dedicated to Robert Boyle. Chorea in Greek means dance.

Gustav Mahler was diagnosed with a cardiac valve anomaly in 1907 and died of subacute bacterial endocarditis in 1911. It is possible that the composer suffered from rheumatic disease in childhood with carditis and Syndenham's chorea, which may have left him with cardiac valve disorder, obsessive–compulsive personality and persistent chorea.

George Summer Huntington (1851–1916) first documented (in 1909) the clinical and hereditary features of this condition in a family from Suffolk settled in Long Island in New York.

79 HEMIBALLISMUS

INSTRUCTION

Look at this patient.

SALIENT FEATURES

History
- Sudden onset
- Cardiovascular disease for source of emboli: atrial fibrillation, valvular heart disease or severe left ventricular dysfunction.

Examination
- Unilateral, involuntary, flinging movements of the proximal upper limbs.

DIAGNOSIS

This patient has hemiballismus (lesion) caused by a stroke (aetiology), and has severe exhaustion (functional status).

ADVANCED-LEVEL QUESTIONS

Where is the lesion?
It is often thought that hemiballismus is caused most commonly by a lesion in the contralateral subthalamic nucleus, but the localization is usually elsewhere. It may result from lesions affecting the afferent or efferent pathways of the subthalamic nucleus, corpus striatum, thalamus, parieto-temporal or frontal cerebral cortex.

What is the underlying cause?
- Vascular event, usually an infarct
- Rarely tumour, abscess, multiple sclerosis, arteriovenous malformation, cerebral trauma.

What investigations would you do?
- ECG for atrial fibrillation
- Echocardiogram to rule out source of emboli
- CT scan, but this is usually unhelpful because the lesion is small
- MRI of brain may be useful.

What is the prognosis?
The prognosis for recovery is usually good and most patients recover within 1 month. Hemiballismus may occasionally prevent the patient from eating and can be exhausting or even life threatening.

Which drug is usually used in ameliorating this condition?
Tetrabenazine haloperidol, or levetiracetam are useful. Prolonged and medically intractable hemiballism can be treated with contralateral thalamotomy or pallidectomy.

> JB Luys (1828–1897), a French neurologist who also studied insanity, hysteria and hypnotism.

80 OROFACIAL DYSKINESIA

INSTRUCTION

Look at this patient.

SALIENT FEATURES

History

- Ask the patient about removal of teeth and how long the patient has been edentulous
- History of date of onset and duration
- Drug history (phenothiazines, levodopa and related drugs).

Examination

- Smacking, chewing or chomping movement of the lips, seen particularly in elderly patients; it usually involves the masticatory, lower facial and tongue muscles.

Proceed as follows:

- Comment if the patient is edentulous (Ann Neurol 1983;13:97).

Remember: Orofacial dyskinesia is defined as involuntary, repetitive, stereotypical movement of the face, tongue and jaw that may be painful.

DIAGNOSIS

This patient has orofacial dyskinesia (lesion) caused by phenothiazines (aetiology) and is in considerable distress (functional status).

QUESTIONS

What is the workup for orofacial movement disorders?

After taking a history and examination, contrast MRI and CT can be used to exclude a CNS pathology.

Neurological workup assesses:

- sensory vs. motor conduction deficit
- central vs. peripheral disease
- electromyography to identify specific muscles
- consider central degenerative, demyelinating or sclerotic lesion
- consider infract or tumour of brain or spina cord.

ADVANCED-LEVEL QUESTIONS

What is Meige syndrome?

A combination of blepharospasm, oromandibular dystonia and cranial dystonia. There is spastic dysarthria when the throat and respiratory muscles are affected. The neck muscles are invariably involved.

What do you understand by tardive dyskinesia?

It represents rapid, repetitive, non-random, stereotypic movements involving the tongue, lips and jaw areas. It is a drug-induced dyskinesia that may appear long after drug therapy has been discontinued. It is troublesome and may resist all forms of treatment.

How would you manage such patients?

Anticholinergic drugs (baclofen, benzodiazepines and tetrabenazine) can be used but pharmacotherapy is usually ineffective. Injection of botulinum toxin into the masseter, temporalis and internal pterygoid muscles results in improvement in chewing and speech in approximately 80% of patients with jaw closure caused by oromandibular dystonia (Ophthalmology 1987;2:237–54).

Mention a few other dystonias

- Blepharospasm
- Spasmodic torticollis
- Laryngeal dystonias
- Writer's cramp.

> H Meige (1866–1940), a French physician, also wrote on ancient Egyptian diseases.

81 INTERNUCLEAR OPHTHALMOPLEGIA

INSTRUCTION

Examine this patient's eyes.

SALIENT FEATURES

History

- Diplopia
- History of multiple sclerosis

- Neurofibroma (causing pontine gliomas)
- Drugs (phenytoin, carbamezapine).

Examination

- Nystagmus is more prominent in the abducting eye (Harris' sign)
- Diverging squint
- Abduction in either eye is normal, whereas adduction is impaired (Fig. 81.1): there is dissociation of eye movements. On covering the abducting eye, the adduction in the other eye is normal.

Proceed as follows:

- Tell the examiner that you would like to look for other signs of demyelination: optic atrophy, pale discs, pyramidal signs.

Remember: Multiple sclerosis and microvascular brainstem ischaemia are the most common causes of internuclear ophthalmoplegia. The two causes may be distinguished by age at presentation, with younger patients likely to have demyelination and older patients ischaemia.

DIAGNOSIS

This patient has internuclear ophthalmoplegia (lesion), which is probably caused by multiple sclerosis (aetiology).

ADVANCED-LEVEL QUESTIONS

Where is the lesion?

In the medial longitudinal bundle, which connects the sixth nerve nucleus on one side to the third nerve nucleus on the opposite side of the brainstem. The eye will not adduct because the third nerve and, therefore, the

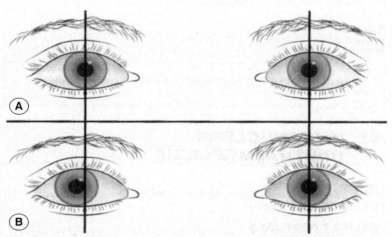

Fig. 81.1 Internuclear ophthalmoplegia. (A) Gaze straight ahead. (B) Attempted right gaze, the right abducting eye achieves the target earlier than the left adducting eye. The vertical line indicates the midpupillary point; the left pupil does not move off this when the gaze changes.

medial rectus have been disconnected from the lateral gaze centre and sixth nucleus of the opposite side.

What are the causes?
- Multiple sclerosis
- Vascular disease
- Tumour (pontine glioma)
- Inflammatory lesions of the brainstem
- Drugs (phenytoin, carbamezapine)

How would you investigate?
- MRI scan
- Edrophonium (Tensilon) test to exclude myasthenia (see Fig. 66.2).

What are the mechanisms to elicit conjugate gaze?
There are four mechanisms for eliciting conjugate gaze in any direction.

- *The saccadic system* involves voluntary gaze (even when the eyes are shut). Pathways mediating saccadic gaze arise in the frontal lobe and pass to the pontine gaze centre.
- *The pursuit system* allows the subject to follow a moving object. Pathways mediating pursuit movements arise in the parieto-occipital lobe and pass to the pontine gaze centre.
- *The optokinetic system* involves the restoration of gaze despite movements from the outside world (e.g. while a subject is sitting in a railway train and looking out of the window, the eyes move slowly as the train moves, to be followed by rapid corrective movement back to the initial position of gaze). This is tested with a hand-held drum bearing vertical black and white stripes. Optokinetic nystagmus is often disturbed even before damage to the pursuit system is apparent.
- *The vestibulo-ocular system* involves correction of gaze for movements of the head. This is achieved by inputs from the labyrinths and neck proprioreceptors to the brainstem. The patient is asked to fixate to the examiner's face and the head is briskly rotated by the examiner from side to side or up and down (doll's head manoeuvre). In supranuclear gaze palsy, these vestibulo-ocular reflex eye movements are preserved, despite the absence of both saccadic and pursuit movements. Caloric tests are used to demonstrate the vestibulo-ocular reflex.

Notes
1. Diplopia is not a feature of defects in conjugate gaze.
2. The centres for saccadic and pursuit movements in the cerebral hemispheres control deviation of the eyes towards the opposite side of the body. These pathways descend towards the brainstem and cross before they reach the pons.
3. The centres for conjugate vertical gaze lie in the midbrain.
4. The centres for conjugate downward vertical gaze are not well localized and lesions both in the midbrain and at the level of the foramen magnum can cause defects of voluntary downgaze.

What do you know about 'Fisher's one and a half syndrome'?
It is a syndrome in which horizontal eye movement is absent and the other eye is capable only of abduction — one and a half movements are paralysed. The vertical eye movements and the pupils are normal. The cause is a

lesion in the pontine region involving the medial longitudinal fasciculus and the parapontine reticular formation on the same side. This results in failure of conjugate gaze to the same side, impairment of adduction of the eye and nystagmus on abduction of the other eye. One and a half syndrome is most often caused by multiple sclerosis, brainstem stroke, brainstem tumours and arteriovenous malformations.

> Internuclear ophthalmoplegia was first reported by Bielschowsky (1902) and then subsequently by Lhermitte in 1922.
>   Spiller in 1924 described the necropsy findings, implicated the median longitudinal fasciculus and suggested the name 'ophthalmoplegia internuclearis anterior'.

82 CEREBELLOPONTINE ANGLE TUMOUR

INSTRUCTION

Examine this patient's cranial nerves.

SALIENT FEATURES

Examination

- Damage to the seventh and eighth cranial nerves is the hallmark of this lesion in this region.
- Obtain a history of hearing loss and tinnitus.

Proceed as follows:

- Check the corneal reflex and test the trigeminal nerve (p. 156).
- Tell the examiner that you would like to look for the following:
  - Cerebellar signs (p. 200)
  - Signs of neurofibroma type 2 (p. 278)
  - Papilloedema (seen uncommonly as a result of raised intracranial pressure).

DIAGNOSIS

This patient has features of cerebellopontine angle tumour (lesion) usually caused by an acoustic neuroma (aetiology), and has severe hearing loss (functional status).

ADVANCED-LEVEL QUESTIONS

Mention a few causes of cerebellopontine angle lesions

- Acoustic neuroma (now knowns as vestibular schwanommas) accounts for 70–80% of cerebellopontine angle tumours
- Meningioma, cholesteatoma, haemangioblastoma, aneurysm of the basilar artery
- Pontine glioma

- Medullablastoma and astrocytoma of the cerebellum
- Carcinoma of the nasopharynx
- Local meningeal involvement by syphilis and TB.

What do you understand by the term cerebellopontine angle?

It is the shallow triangular fossa lying between the cerebellum, lateral pons and the inner third of the petrous temporal bone. It extends from the trigeminal nerve (above) to the glossopharyngeal nerve (see below). The abducens nerve runs along the medial edge, whereas the facial and auditory cranial nerves transverse the angle to enter the internal auditory meatus.

> There is a wide range of pathologic processes within the cerebellopontine angle. These processes may present because of mass effect on local structures, such as the fifth to twelfth cranial nerves, or because of mass effect on the pons or cerebellum, which may result in fourth ventricular obstruction.

What is the histology of acoustic neurofibroma?

It consists of elongated cells similar to spindle fibroblasts with much collagen and reticulum. They are believed to arise from Schwann cells and are also known as schwannomas. These lesions most often arise from the inferior vestibular nerve within the internal auditory canal and present with hearing loss or tinnitus. Schwannomas can be entirely intracanalicular or have intracanalicular and cisternal components, resulting in the description of an 'ice-cream cone' tumour (Fig. 82.1).

How would you investigate such patients?

- Skull radiography, tomography of the internal auditory meatus and CT head scan
- Serology for syphilis
- Audiography
- Caloric test (which will reveal that the labyrinth is destroyed)
- Vertebral angiography
- CSF may be abnormal or have raised protein concentration
- MRI (Fig. 82.1).

What is the treatment in this condition?

- Microsurgical resection
- Stereotactic radiosurgery (N Engl J Med 1998;339:1426–33)
- Conservative approach.

Mention some tumours that occur in families with familial adenomatous polyposis

Papillary thyroid carcinoma, sarcomas, hepatoblastomas, pancreatic carcinomas, and medulloblastomas of the cerebellar–pontine angle of the brain.

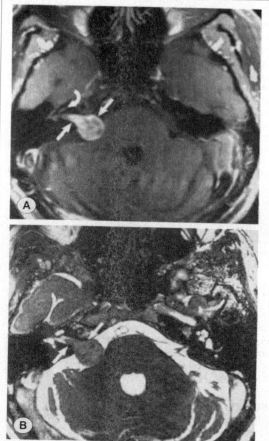

Fig. 82.1 (A) Axial T$_1$-weighted, postcontrast, fat-saturated imaging demonstrates a heterogeneously enhancing classic 'ice-cream cone' vestibular schwannoma of the right cerebellopontine angle and internal auditory canal (arrows). (B) Axial fast imaging using steady-state acquisition, thin-slice, T$_2$-weighted imaging of the same lesion (arrows) shows the contours of the schwannoma, clearly delineated from hyperintense CSF and with a 'cap' of CSF between the schwannoma and the cochlea. (With permission from Lakshmi, Glastonbury 2009.)

FT Schwann (1810–1882), a German anatomist, was Professor of Anatomy in the Louvain. He was one of the first to demonstrate that fermentation was associated with living organisms. Independently from Schleiden, he concluded that plants are formed of cells; this is known as the Schleiden–Schwann cellular theory. Schwann also discovered that the upper oesophagus contains striated muscle. He discovered pepsin and showed that bile was essential for digestion.

The first surgical removal of an acoustic neuroma was performed in 1894 (N Engl J Med 1998;339:1471).

L Leksell was the first to use radiosurgery, what he called the 'gamma knife' (Acta Chir Scand 1971;137:763–5).

83 JUGULAR FORAMEN SYNDROME

INSTRUCTION

Examine this patient's cranial nerves.

SALIENT FEATURES

History

- Clinical presentation reflects effects on a combination of the last four cranial nerves:
  - Hoarseness of voice
  - Nasal quality to the speech
  - Nasal regurgitation and dysphagia
  - Aspiration of food with choking attacks
  - Weakness of the sternomastoids and trapezii
  - Wasting of the tongue (often noticed by the dentist)
  - Pain in and around the ear (caused by damage of the ninth and tenth cranial nerves, which carries sensation to the external auditory meatus and behind the ear)
  - Headache
  - Ptosis (caused by Horner syndrome).

Examination

- Sluggish movement of the palate when the patient says 'aah' on the affected side
- Absent gag reflex on the same side
- Flattening of the shoulder on the same side
- Wasting of the sternomastoid (Fig. 83.1)
- Weakness when the patient moves her chin to the opposite side
- Difficulty in shrugging the shoulder on the same side (Fig. 83.2).

Proceed as follows:

- Look for wasting and deviation of the tongue (twelfth cranial nerve palsy)
- Tell the examiner that you would like to check for two signs:
  - Bovine cough
  - Husky voice.

DIAGNOSIS

This patient has features of jugular foramen syndrome (lesion) that could have several causes, including pharyngeal neoplasm (aetiology); she has difficulty in swallowing and requires a nasogastric tube (functional status).

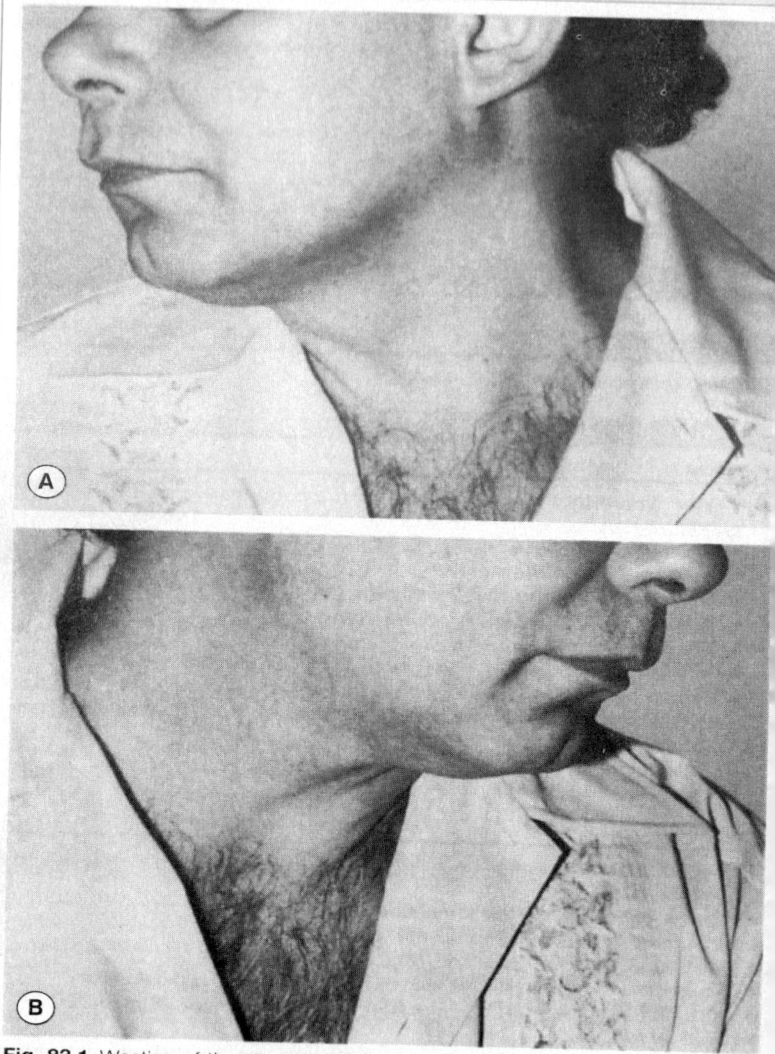

Fig. 83.1 Wasting of the sternomastoid. (A) Normal left muscle with forceful thrust of chin to the right. (B) Movement to the left shows loss of muscle bulk. (With permission from Bradley et al. 2008.)

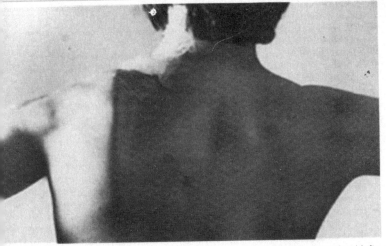

Fig. 83.2 Left spinal accessory palsy with scapular winging upon attempted left arm abduction. (With permission from Bradley et al. 2008.)

ADVANCED-LEVEL QUESTIONS

Where is the jugular foramen located?
Between the lateral part of the occipital bone and the petrous portion of the temporal bones.

Which cranial nerves leave the skull through the jugular foramen?
The ninth, tenth and eleventh cranial nerves.

Through which foramen does the twelfth cranial nerve leave the skull?
The anterior condylar foramen.

Mention a few causes of jugular foramen syndrome
- Carcinoma of the pharynx is the commonest cause
- Glomus jugulare paraganglioma (accounts for 80% of jugular foramen neoplasms)
- Fractured base of the skull
- Paget's disease
- Basal meningitis
- Neurofibroma or any tumour
- Thrombosis of jugular vein.

Do you know of any eponymous syndromes of the lower cranial nerves?
- Vernet syndrome: paresis of the ninth, tenth and eleventh cranial nerves caused by extension of tumour into the jugular foramen

- Collet–Sicard syndrome: fracture of the floor of the posterior crania fossa, causing palsy of the last four cranial nerves
- Villaret syndrome: ipsilateral paralysis of the last four cranial nerves and cervical sympathetics
- Syndrome of Schmidt: vagus and accessory nerve involvement
- Syndrome of Hughlings Jackson: accessory and hypoglossal nerve involvement.

What is the cause of the unilateral eleventh cranial nerve palsy?

- Trauma to the nerve in the neck
- In hemiplegia.

How would you test for eleventh cranial nerve palsy?

- Sternocleidomastoids are tested by having the patient turn the head forcibly against the examiner's hand in a direction away from the muscle being tested while the muscle is observed and palpated.
- Upper portion of the trapezii is tested by having the patient forcibly elevate (shrug) the shoulder while the examiner attempts to depress the shoulder.

FJ Collet (b. 1870), a French otolaryngologist, described his patient in 1915.

M Vernet (1887–1974), a French neurologist, described this syndrome in 1916.

JA Sicard (1872–1929), a French physician and radiologist, was the first to perform myelography, used alcohol in trigeminal neuralgia and injected a sclerosing substance in varicose veins. He described his patient in 1917.

M Villaret (1877–1946), Professor of Neurology in France, described this syndrome in 1918.

---

84 PSEUDOBULBAR PALSY

INSTRUCTION

Examine this patient's cranial nerves.

SALIENT FEATURES
History

- Ask the patient whether there is difficulty in swallowing or nasal regurgitation
- Any changes in speech
- Emotional lability
- History of stroke, multiple sclerosis or motor neuron disease.

Examination

- Spastic tongue
- Donald Duck speech

- Patient is emotionally labile (uncontrollable laughter, crying, irritability or anger)
- Sluggish movements of the palate when the patient is asked to say 'aah'

Proceed as follows:

- Check the jaw jerk
- Tell the examiner that you would like to do the following:
  - Check the gag reflex
  - Look for upper motor neuron signs in the limbs.

DIAGNOSIS

This patient has pseudobulbar palsy (lesion) caused by a stroke (aetiology); he has difficulty in swallowing and emotional lability (functional status).

QUESTIONS

What could be the underlying cause?

- Bilateral stroke
- Multiple sclerosis
- Motor neuron disease.

ADVANCED-LEVEL QUESTIONS

How would you differentiate bulbar palsy from pseudobulbar palsy?

	Pseudobulbar palsy	Bulbar palsy
Prevalence	Common	Rare
Type of lesion	Upper motor neuron	Lower motor neuron, muscular
Site of lesion	Bilateral, usually in the internal capsule	Medulla oblongata
Tongue	Small, stiff and spastic	Flaccid, fasciculations
Speech	Slow, thick and indistinct	Nasal twang
Nasal regurgitation	Not prominent	Prominent
Jaw jerk	Brisk	Normal or absent
Other findings	Upper motor neuron lesions of the limbs	Lower motor neuron lesions of the limbs
Effect	Emotionally labile	Normal effect
Causes	Stroke, multiple sclerosis, motor neuron disease, Creutzfeldt–Jakob disease	Motor neuron disease, poliomyelitis, Guillain-Barré syndrome, myasthenia gravis myopathy

How would you manage the swallowing and speech difficulties?

The patient would initially require assessment by a speech therapist for the difficulty in swallowing and speech deficits. Barium swallow with videofluoroscopy may be required to 'visualize' the swallowing.

Is there any therapy for emotional lability?

One study suggested that therapy with a combination of dextromethorphan and quinidine improves symptoms and quality of life in patients with emotional lability (Neurology 2004:63:1363–70).

What do you understand by the term CADASIL?

Cerebral autosomal dominant arteriopathy with subcortical infarcts and leukoencephalopathy (CADASIL) is the most common heritable cause of stroke and vascular dementia in adults. Clinical and neuroimaging features resemble those of sporadic small-artery disease, although patients with CADASIL have an earlier age at onset of stroke events, an increased frequency of migraine with aura and a slightly variable pattern of ischaemic white matter lesions on brain MRI. *NOTCH3* (Notch homolog 3), the gene involved in CADASIL, encodes a transmembrane receptor primarily expressed in systemic arterial smooth-muscle cells.

Charles Darwin described pseudobulbar affect in The Expression of Emotions in Man and Animals (1872): 'certain brain diseases, such as hemiplegia, brain wasting and senile decay, have a special tendency to induce weeping'.

---

85 BULBAR PALSY

INSTRUCTION

Examine this patient's cranial nerves.
Ask the patient a few questions.
Test this patient's speech.

SALIENT FEATURES

History

- Ask the patient about nasal regurgitation, dysphagia
- Slurring of speech (patient may sound as if they have been intoxicated)
- Difficulty in chewing and swallowing
- Choking on liquids.

Examination

- Nasal speech lacking in modulation and great difficulty with all consonants
- Wasting of the tongue with fasciculations (see Fig. 69.1)
- Weakness of the soft palate: ask the patient to say 'aah'
- There may be accumulation of the saliva
- Fasciculation elsewhere (particularly trunk muscles).

Proceed as follows:

- Check the jaw jerk (normal or absent)
- Tell the examiner that you would like to do the following:
  - Check gag reflex
  - Examine the hands for fasciculations, dissociated sensory loss.

DIAGNOSIS

This patient has bulbar palsy (lesion) caused by motor neuron disease (aetiology) and has difficulty in swallowing (functional status).

QUESTIONS

What may be the underlying cause?

- Motor neuron disease: after age 60 rapidly progressive bulbar palsy is the commonest presenting symptom (p. 270)
- Guillain–Barré syndrome
- Syringomyelia (p. 280)
- Poliomyelitis
- Nasopharyngeal tumour
- Neurosyphilis
- Neurosarcoid.

What are the stages of swallowing?

There are three phases to swallowing: oral, pharyngeal and oesophageal. Six events occur during the oropharyngeal phase of swallowing:

Elevation of the tongue: soft bolus preparation with saliva

Posterior movement of the tongue: movement of food bolus into the hypopharynx

Elevation of the soft palate: closes the passage into the nasopharynx as the food bolus reaches the hypopharynx

Elevation of the hyoid: helps to bring the epiglottis under the tongue

Elevation of the larynx: opens up the retrolaryngeal space, further facilitating the movement of the epiglottis under the tongue

Tilting back of the epiglottis: covers the opening of the larynx to prevent aspiration.

These rapid series of events last about 1.5 s and, once initiated, are completely reflexive.

Remember: 'Amyotrophic' refers to the muscle atrophy, weakness and fasciculation that signify disease of the lower motor neurons. 'Lateral sclerosis' refers to the hardness to palpation of the lateral columns of the spinal cord in postmortem specimens, where gliosis follows degeneration of the corticospinal tracts. The clinical results are upper motor neuron signs: overactive tendon reflexes, Hoffmann signs, clonus and Babinski signs.

86 WALLENBERG'S SYNDROME (LATERAL MEDULLARY SYNDROME)

INSTRUCTION

Examine this patient's cranial nerves.

SALIENT FEATURES

History

- Severe nausea, vomiting, nystagmus (involvement of the lower vestibular nuclei)
- Limb ataxia (involvement of the inferior cerebellar peduncle)

- Intractable hiccups, dysphagia (ninth and tenth cranial nerve involvement).

Examination

- Nystagmus
- Ipsilateral involvement of fifth, sixth, seventh and eighth cranial nerves
- Bulbar palsy: impaired gag, sluggish palatal movements
- Horner syndrome.

Proceed as follows:

- Tell the examiner that you would like to check for the following:
  - Cerebellar signs on the same side
  - Pain and temperature sensory loss on the opposite side (dissociated sensory loss).

Remember:

- The main features of this syndrome is *ipsilateral* Horner syndrome and *contralateral* loss of pain and temperature sensation.
- Wallenberg syndrome is an infarction of the lateral portion of the medullary tegmentum. The most common cause is occlusion of the intracranial vertebral artery.
- Neuroimaging: MRI is preferred because CT provides less complete visualization of the brainstem, owing to artefacts related to the skull. MRI with diffusion-weighted imaging is the most sensitive test available to detect acute infarcts.

DIAGNOSIS

This patient has lateral medullary syndrome (lesion) caused by a stroke (aetiology) and has dysphagia (functional status).

ADVANCED-LEVEL QUESTIONS

Which vessel is occluded?

Any of the following five vessels:

- Posterior inferior cerebellar artery
- Vertebral artery
- Superior, middle or inferior lateral medullary arteries.

How may these patients present?

With sudden onset of vertigo, vomiting and ipsilateral ataxia, with contralateral loss of pain and temperature sensations.

Where is the lesion in lateral medullary syndrome?

It results from infarction of a wedge-shaped area of the lateral aspect of the medulla and inferior surface of the cerebellum. The deficits are from involvement of one side of the nucleus ambiguus, trigeminal nucleus, vestibular nuclei, cerebellar peduncle, spinothalamic tract and autonomic fibres.

What is the medial medullary syndrome?

It is caused by occlusion of the lower basilar artery or vertebral artery. Ipsilateral lesions result in paralysis and wasting of the tongue. Contralateral lesions result in hemiplegia and loss of vibration and joint position sense.

Mention a few other eponymous syndromes with crossed hemiplegias

- Weber syndrome: contralateral hemiplegia with ipsilateral lower motor neuron lesion of the oculomotor nerve. The lesion is in the midbrain
- Millard–Gubler syndrome: contralateral hemiplegia with lower motor neuron lesion of the abducens nerve. The lesion is in the pons
- Foville syndrome: as Millard–Gubler syndrome with gaze palsy.

What is Benedikt syndrome?

It causes cerebellar signs on the side opposite the third nerve palsy (which is produced by damage to the nucleus itself or to the nerve fascicle). It is caused by a midbrain vascular lesion causing damage to the red nucleus, interrupting the dentatorubrothalamic tract from the opposite cerebellar signs.

Further reading

Savitz SI, Caplan LR: Vertebrobasilar disease, *N Engl J Med* 352:2618, 2005 (classic article).

Achille LF Foville (1799–1878), a Parisian neurologist.
   Auguste LJ Millard (1830–1915) and Adolphe Marie Gubler (1821–1879), Parisian physicians.
   Adolf Wallenburg (1862–1949), a German neurologist, described this syndrome in 1895.

---

87 WINGING OF THE SCAPULA

INSTRUCTION

Look at this patient's back.

SALIENT FEATURES

History

- Difficulty in raising the arms above the level of the shoulders
- Winging of the scapula.

Examination

- Winging of the scapula (see Fig. 83.2)
- Difficulty in raising the arms above the horizontal.

Proceed as follows:

- Check whether the winging is unilateral or bilateral
- Ask the patient to push the outstretched arm firmly against your hand and check whether or not the winging is more prominent
- Tell the examiner that you would like to examine the muscles in the arm to rule out muscular dystrophy.

DIAGNOSIS

This patient has winging of the scapula (lesion) caused by palsy of the long thoracic nerve of Bell (aetiology).

ADVANCED-LEVEL QUESTIONS

Which nerve lesion is responsible for these signs?

Long thoracic nerve of Bell arising from the anterior rami of C5, C6 and C7.

Which muscle is supplied by this nerve?

Serratus anterior.

What is the action of the serratus anterior?

It is responsible for the lateral and forward movement of the scapula, keeping it closely applied to the thorax.

Which other muscle palsy can cause winging of the scapula?

Paralysis of the trapezius.

How would you differentiate winging of the scapula caused by serratus anterior palsy from that of trapezius palsy?

In serratus anterior palsy, abduction of the arm laterally produces little winging of the scapula, whereas winging caused by weakness of the trapezius is intensified by abduction of the arm against resistance.

What do you know about brachial neuritis?

Brachial neuritis (neuralgic amyotrophy, Parsonage–Turner syndrome) often follows an infection or surgery. Diagnosis may be difficult initially when the patients have only pain. Later the patients have muscular weakness, affecting particularly the deltoid and serratus anterior (winging of the scapula). Atrophy often becomes prominent. In this syndrome there is often more than one lesion. The white cell count in the CSF is occasionally raised. Recovery occurs over the next year and may not be complete.

88　BECKER MUSCULAR DYSTROPHY

INSTRUCTION

Examine this patient's muscles.

SALIENT FEATURES

History

- Know whether there is a family history of the condition
- Age of onset
- Ask about shortness of breath (heart failure as a result of cardiomyopathy)
- History of mental retardation.

Examination

- Young adult male (>15 years)
- Proximal weakness of the lower extremities (in later stages more generalized muscle involvement)

- Pseudohypertrophy of calves
- Facial muscle weakness is characteristically absent or insignificant
- Kyphoscoliosis in late stages.

Proceed as follows:
- Tell the examiner that you would like to check the IQ (mental retardation may be seen).

DIAGNOSIS

This young patient has proximal muscle weakness and pseudohypertrophy (lesion) caused by Becker's dystrophy (aetiology). The patient has mild disability and the condition is usually progressive (functional status).

QUESTIONS

What is the difference between Duchenne and Becker muscular dystrophy?

By definition, patients with Becker muscular dystrophy can ambulate beyond the age of 15 years. The onset in Becker is usually between the ages of 5 and 15 years, but onset can occur in the third or fourth decades or even later. The majority survive into the fourth or fifth decades. Becker muscular dystrophy is less common (3 per 100000 live male births) and has a more variable presentation of skeletal muscle weakness (Fig. 88.1).

Is there any difference between the genetics of Duchenne and Becker muscular dystrophy?

No, both Duchenne and Becker muscular dystrophy are caused by mutations in the same gene, located at Xp21. Dystrophin, its protein product, is usually absent in patients with Duchenne muscular dystrophy but is reduced in amount or abnormal in size in people with Becker muscular dystrophy. Another protein, utrophin, closely related to dystrophin, is encoded by a second gene on chromosome 6. In normal muscle, utrophin is located predominantly in the neuromuscular junction, whereas dystrophin is found in the sarcolemmal surface.

How would you confirm the clinical diagnosis of Becker dystrophy?

It requires Western blot analysis of muscle biopsy samples, demonstrating abnormal or reduced dystrophin.

ADVANCED-LEVEL QUESTIONS

Mention other X-linked myopathies

- X-linked tubular myopathy linked to Xq28
- McLeod syndrome, where the responsible gene has been localized to Xp21 and the phenotype is characterized by mild, even subclinical, myopathy, acanthocytosis and haemolytic anaemia. The definitive diagnosis rests on determination of the Kell red cell antigen phenotype
- Emery–Dreifuss muscular dystrophy, first described in a large family in Virginia by Emery and Dreifuss in 1966. Known association with deutan colour blindness led to localization of the gene on Xq28. The weakness presents in early childhood and is slowly progressive. The

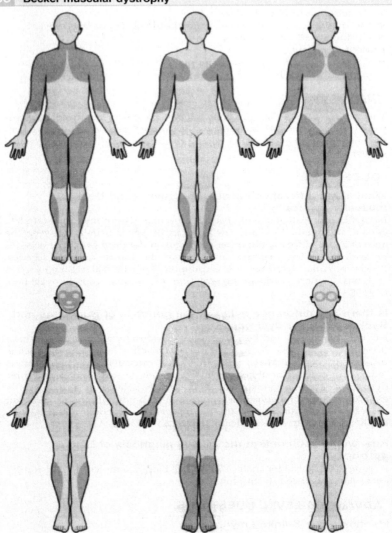

Fig. 88.1 Distribution of predominant muscle weakness (shaded) in different types of dystrophy. (A) Duchenne and Becker types; (B) Emery–Dreifuss; (C) limb-girdle; (D) facioscapulohumeral; (E) distal; (F) oculopharyngeal.

distribution of weakness is unique: an early humeral–peroneal pattern eventually evolves into a scapulo-humero-pelvo-peroneal distribution. Marked focal atrophy of the humeral and peroneal muscles is a consistent feature. Pseudohypertrophy is absent, except in extensor digitorum brevis.

What is the role of antisense-mediated exon skipping in Duchenne's muscular dystrophy?

Antisense-mediated exon skipping induces dystrophin synthesis in selected patients with Duchenne's muscular dystrophy (N Engl J Med 2007;357:2677–86). The skipping of the additional exon restores the reading frame of the mRNA, allowing new production of dystrophin. The dystrophin that is produced is not normal but probably retains considerable function (as seen in patients with clinically milder Becker's muscular dystrophy, who have similar or identically modified dystrophins).

What is the role of myogenic stem cell transplant in muscle degenerative disorders?

Prospectively isolatable muscle-forming stem cells are present in adult skeletal muscle and experimental studies have demonstrated the efficacy of myogenic stem cell transplant in therapy of muscle degenerative disease (Cell 2008;134:37–47). In particular, satellite cells reside beneath the basal lamina of skeletal muscle fibres and include cells that act as precursors for muscle growth and repair. Although they share a common anatomical localization and typically are considered a homogeneous population, satellite cells actually exhibit substantial heterogeneity. Cell-surface marker expression was utilized to purify from the satellite cell pool a distinct population of skeletal muscle precursors that function as muscle stem cells. When purified, these precursor cells were engrafted into muscle of dystrophin-deficient *Mdx* mice and were found to contribute up to 94% of myofibres, restoring dystrophin expression and significantly improving muscle histology and contractile function. Transplanted skeletal muscle precursors also entered the satellite cell compartment, renewed the endogenous stem cell pool and participated in subsequent rounds of injury repair.

Edward Meryon described Duchenne muscular dystrophy in 1852, 10 years before the French neurologist Guillaume Benjamin Amand Duchenne, with remarkably prescient pathological observations: '… the sarcolemma or tunic of the elementary fibre was broken and destroyed' (Emery AEH, Emery MLH. The History of a Genetic Disease: Duchenne Muscular Dystrophy or Meryon's Disease. London: Royal Society of Medicine Press, 1995).

PE Becker, Professor of Human Genetics at the University of Göttingen, Germany.

Duchenne is reported to have designed a version of the modern muscle biopsy needle, which he kept in alcohol to prevent rusting. He could not have known that this also prevented sepsis.

Newton Morton, a geneticist, was the first to introduce discriminant and segregation analysis into modern human genetics as a part of a large population study of Duchenne muscular dystrophy. Tony Murphy used the disease to develop bayesian risk-analysis procedures.

89 TETRAPLEGIA

INSTRUCTION

Carry out a neurological examination of this patient's lower limbs.

SALIENT FEATURES

History

- Ask about bladder symptoms and check sacral sensation
- Ask about radicular pain
- Ask whether the weakness was sudden or gradual
- History of trauma, multiple sclerosis.

Examination

- Increased or decreased tone in both lower limbs
- Hyperreflexia
- Ankle clonus
- Weakness in all four limbs
- Wasted hands (cervical spondylosis, motor neuron disease or syringomyelia).

Remember: The physical examination pertinent to spinal cord dysfunction involves testing in three areas: motor function, sensory function and reflexes.

Proceed as follows:

- Remember to check the sensory level and examine the spine.
- Tell the examiner that you would like to do the following:
  - Check for cerebellar signs (multiple sclerosis, Friedreich's ataxia)
  - Check BP (postural hypotension, autonomic dysreflexia).
- Try to localize the level of lesion using the following:
  - Spasticity of all four limbs: lesion above the C4 spinal cord segment
  - Spasticity of the lower limbs with flaccid weakness of some muscles of the upper limb: lesion of cervical cord enlargement (C5–T2)
  - Deep tendon reflexes: an absent biceps jerk with a brisk supinator jerk (inversion of the supinator jerk) or an absent biceps and supinator with a brisk triceps jerk localizes the lesion to C5–6
  - Radicular pain: useful early in the disease; with time becomes diffuse and ceases to have localizing value
  - Superficial sensation: not good for localizing as the level of sensory loss may vary greatly in different individuals and in different types of lesion.

Note: Be prepared to discuss the Frankel classification (below).

DIAGNOSIS

This patient has weakness in all four limbs (lesion) caused by spinal trauma (aetiology), and is wheelchair bound (functional status).

ADVANCED-LEVEL QUESTIONS

What is autonomic dysreflexia?

It is bradycardia, sweating, rhinorrhoea, pounding headaches and severe paroxysmal hypertension, which presents quickly and can rapidly precipitate seizures and death if not relieved. Precipitating factors include blockage of urinary catheter, visceral distension from full bowel, stimulation of the skin secondary to an irritative pressure sore and vesicoureteric reflux. Labour in a high-tetraplegic female may also be complicated by it.

What non-traumatic causes are there for spinal cord dysfunction?

● Processes affecting the spinal cord or blood supply directly:.
  ● Multiple sclerosis
  ● Transverse myelitis
  ● Spinal arteriovenous malformation/subarachnoid haemorrhage
  ● Syringomyelia
  ● HIV myelopathy
  ● Other myelopathies
  ● Spinal cord infarction.
● Compressive lesions affecting the spinal cord:
  ● Spinal epidural abscess
  ● Spinal epidural haematoma
  ● Discitis
  ● Neoplasm
  ● Metastatic
  ● Primary CNS.

Does ingestion of food affect blood pressure in tetraplegics?
The ingestion of food causes a small fall in BP and this exacerbates the postural hypotension in these patients.

How would you manage spasticity in these patients?
● Drugs: diazepam, baclofen
● Surgery: dorsal rhizotomy, neurectomy, myelotomy, orthopaedic procedures that divide and lengthen tendons of spastic muscles.

How do you localize the lesion to the fifth cervical root level?
● Muscular weakness: deltoid, supraspinatus, brachoradialis
● Deep tendon reflexes affected: biceps and supinator jerks
● Radicular pain/paraesthesia: neck, top of shoulder, outer aspect of the arm, forearm
● Superficial sensory deficit: outer aspect of the upper arm.

How do you localize the lesion to the sixth cervical root level?
● Muscular weakness: biceps, brachioradialis, extensor carpi radialis longus
● Deep tendon reflexes affected: biceps and supinator jerks
● Radicular pain/paraesthesia: neck, shoulder, outer arm, forearm, thumb and index finger
● Superficial sensory deficit: thumb and index finger.

How do you localize the lesion to the seventh cervical root level?
● Muscular weakness: triceps and most of the muscles on the dorsum of the forearm
● Deep tendon reflexes affected: triceps jerk
● Radicular pain/paraesthesia: neck, shoulder, arm, forearm to index and middle finger
● Superficial sensory deficit: mostly middle and index fingers.

How do you localize the lesion to the eighth cervical root level?

- Muscular weakness: flexors of the forearm
- Deep tendon reflexes affected: finger jerk
- Radicular pain/paraesthesia: neck, shoulder, arm, ring and little fingers
- Superficial sensory deficit: ring and little fingers.

How do you localize the lesion to the first thoracic root level?

- Muscular weakness: small muscles of the hand
- Deep tendon reflexes affected: finger jerk
- Radicular pain/paraesthesia: neck, axilla, medial aspect of the arm and forearm, little and ring finger
- Superficial sensory deficit: medial arm and little finger.

What precautions would you take when transporting patients with acute high-spinal injuries by air?

- Lung function should be stable before transfer
- Air humidifier and supplemental oxygen should be available
- Patient should be accompanied by someone trained in manoeuvres to clear airway secretions. Tracheal suction should be done regularly; this may be complicated by reflex bradycardia and cardiac arrest, and so atropine and orciprenaline should be readily available (BMJ 1990; 300:1498).

What is the mode of onset in patients with the classical syndrome of foramen magnum?

First, there is weakness of the shoulder and arm, followed by weakness of the ipsilateral leg, then contralateral leg and, finally, contralateral arm. Neoplasms in this region can cause suboccipital pain spreading to the neck and shoulders.

What is Raymond–Cestan syndrome?

Raymond–Cestan syndrome is the result of the obstruction of twigs of the basilar artery causing lesions of the pontine region; it is characterized by tetraplegia, nystagmus and anaesthesia.

Can you describe Frankel's classification of neurological deficit?

The classification is into five types:

A: absent motor and sensory function

B: sensation present, motor function absent

C: sensation present, motor function active but not useful (grades 2/5 to 3/5)

D: sensation present, motor function active and useful (grade 4/5)

E: normal motor and sensory function.

What is the role of robotics in such patients?

Animal experiments suggest that a robotic arm can be used through impulses generated by the motor cortex (Nature 2006;442:164–71, Nature 2008;453:1098–1101). Clinical trials for safety and feasibility are necessary to test the efficacy of these devices.

Sir Ludwig Guttman, FRS, fled from Nazi persecution and worked at the National Spinal Injuries Centre in Stoke Mandeville Hospital, Aylesbury. He was entrusted to look after the paraplegics and tetraplegics of the war. He was the first to show that pressure sores can be avoided by 2-hourly turning of patients.

Prof Hans Ludwig Frankel, OBE, contemporary Physician, National Hospital of Spinal Injuries, Stoke Mandeville Hospital, Aylesbury.

90 BROWN-SÉQUARD SYNDROME

INSTRUCTION

Examine this patient's neurological system.

SALIENT FEATURES

History

- Weak leg that feels normal whereas the other leg is moving perfectly but the patient cannot feel pain and temperature sensation (Fig. 90.1)
- Trauma to the spine, e.g. stab injury
- History of degenerative spine disease or multiple sclerosis
- Tell the examiner you would like also to take a history for bladder and bowel symptoms.

Examination

Deficits below the level of the lesion include:
- Ipsilateral monoplegia or hemiplegia
- Ipsilateral loss of joint position and vibration sense
- Contralateral loss of spinothalamic (pain and temperature) sensation; the latter is sometimes localized to one or two segments below the anatomical level of the lesion.

Deficits in the segment of the lesion:
- Ipsilateral lower motor neuron paralysis
- Ipsilateral zone of cutaneous anaesthesia and a zone hyperaesthesia just below the anaesthetic zone
- Segmental signs such as muscular atrophy, radicular pain or decreased tendon reflexes are usually unilateral.
- Tell the examiner you would like to:
  • examine the spine and exclude multiple sclerosis.

DIAGNOSIS

This patient has Brown–Séquard syndrome (or hemisection of the spinal cord) at the level of T8 (lesion) and is probably the result of a compressive or destructive lesion of the spinal cord (aetiology). The patient is limited by the weakness in one limb (functional status).

ADVANCED-LEVEL QUESTIONS

What are the causes of hemisection of the spinal cord?
- Syringomyelia (p. 280)
- Cord tumour

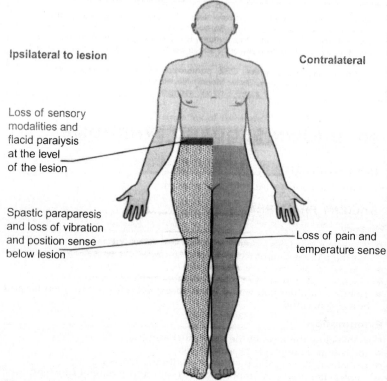

Ipsilateral to lesion

Contralateral

Loss of sensory
modalities and
flacid paralysis
at the level
of the lesion

Spastic paraparesis
and loss of vibration
and position sense
below lesion

Loss of pain and
temperature sense

Fig. 90.1 Sensory deficit in Brown–Séquard syndrome.

- Haematomyelia
- Bullet or stab wounds
- Degenerative disease of spine
- Multiple myeloma.

Charles-Edouard Brown-Séquard (1817–1894) was Professor of Physiology in
Virginia, USA, at the National Hospital, Queen Square, London, at Harvard,
and finally in Paris. He was the first physician-in-chief of the National Hospital
in Queen Square, which was founded in 1860. In 1889, he is said to have
drawn much attention and criticism for injecting himself with a testicular
extract (BMJ 1889;1:1416). Several nations lay claim to Brown–Séquard: he
was born in Mauritius, then a British colony, the son of a French woman and
an American sea captain (Lancet 2000;356:61–3). He is said to have crossed
the Atlantic more than 60 times and set up residence in the USA four times,
France six and England once.

91 CAUDA EQUINA SYNDROME

INSTRUCTION

This patient has bowel and bladder dysfunction; examine the lower limbs.

SALIENT FEATURES

History

- Ask the patient whether there is pain (usually projected to the perineum and thighs); these are root pain in the dermatomes L2 or L3 or S2 or S3 (whereas pain in L4, L5 or S1 distribution is commonly attributed to disc disease)
- Determine whether there is a history of trauma and 'neural claudication' (where the patient develops root pain and leg weakness, usually a foot drop while walking that rapidly recovers with resting)
- Pain in the anterior thigh, wasting of the quadriceps muscle, weakness of the foot invertors (caused by L4 root lesion) and an absent knee jerk
- Obtain history of leukaemia or prostatic carcinoma (primaries for bony metastases).

Examination

- Flaccid, asymmetrical paraparesis
- Knee and ankle jerks are diminished or absent
- Saddle distribution of sensory loss up to the L1 level
- Plantars downgoing.

DIAGNOSIS

This patient has flaccid paraparesis with saddle anaesthesia caused by cauda equina syndrome (lesion) caused by a compressive lesion (aetiology).

ADVANCED-LEVEL QUESTIONS

What is the relationship of the spinal cord to the vertebra?

The spinal cord extends from the foramen magnum to the interspace between the twelfth thoracic (dorsal) and first lumbar spines, although the thecal membranes may extend down the body of the second sacral vertebra. To determine the spinal segments in relation to the vertebral body:

- For cervical vertebrae add 1
- For thoracic 1–6 add 2
- For thoracic 7–9 add 3
- The lumbar segments lie opposite the tenth and eleventh thoracic spines and the next interspinal space
- The first lumbar arch overlies the sacral and coccygeal segments.

Remember: The sacral segments are compressed into the last inch of the cord known as the conus medullaris, which is located behind the T9 to the L1 vertebra.

At which vertebral level is the lesion in cauda equina syndrome?

A lesion in the spinal canal at any level below the T10 (dorsal) vertebra can cause cauda equina syndrome.

How would you differentiate between cauda equina and conus medullaris syndrome?

The cauda equina consists of lower spinal roots (T12 to S5) and hence a lesion causes lower motor neuron signs, whereas the conus medullaris is the lowest part of the spinal cord and lesions result in upper motor neuron signs. Both conus and cauda lesions result in a mixed picture. In its purest form, conus medullaris syndrome presents with sphincter disturbances, saddle anaesthesia (S3–S5), impotence and absence of lower extremity abnormalities.

What are the causes of cauda equina syndrome?

- Centrally placed lumbosacral disc or spondylolisthesis at the lumbosacral junction
- Tumours of the cauda equina (ependymoma, neurofibroma).

What are the types of cauda equina syndrome in adults?

- The lateral cauda equina syndrome: pain in the anterior thigh, wasting of the quadriceps muscle, weakness of the foot invertors (caused by L4 root lesion) and an absent knee jerk. Causes include neurofibroma, a high disc lesion.
- The midline cauda equina syndrome: bilateral lumbar and sacral root lesions. Causes include disc lesion, primary sacral bone tumours (chordomas), metastatic bone disease (from prostate) and leukaemia.

92 TORSION DYSTONIA (DYSTONIA MUSCULORUM DEFORMANS)

INSTRUCTION

Look at this patient.

SALIENT FEATURES

History

- Perinatal anoxia, birth trauma or kernicterus
- Family history
- Drug history (neuroleptics)
- The age of onset of clinical features (abnormal movements are usually present before the age of 5 years in birth anoxia).

Examination

- Dystonic movements of head and neck
- Torticollis
- Blepharospasm
- Facial grimacing
- Forced opening or closing of the mouth
- Limbs may adopt abnormal but characteristic postures.

DIAGNOSIS

This patient has torsion dystonia (lesion), which may be a result of birth anoxia (aetiology), and is confined to a wheelchair because of the disability (functional status).

QUESTIONS

What do you understand by the term dystonia?

It implies a movement caused by a prolonged muscular contraction when a part of the body is thrown into spasm. Dystonia is defined as a movement disorder that causes sustained muscle contractions, repetitive twisting movements, and abnormal postures of the trunk, neck, face, or arms and legs (Marsden CD, Fahn S (eds.) Movement Disorders 2. London: Butterworths, 1987, pp. 332–58).

ADVANCED-LEVEL QUESTIONS

What is the inheritance of dystonia?

Dystonia loci *DYT1* through *DYT13* include autosomal dominant, autosomal recessive, and X-linked causes of primary dystonia and dystonia-plus syndromes.

What are the other causes of dystonia?

- Birth anoxia (abnormal movements develop before the age of 5 years; often associated with a history of seizures and mental disability)
- Wilson's disease, Huntington disease or parkinsonism
- Drugs.

How would you treat such patients?

- Drugs: patients respond poorly to drugs. Occasionally helpful medications include diazepam, levodopa, amantidine, carbamezapine, tetrabenazine, phenothiazines and haloperidol.
- Stereotactic thalamotomy may be useful in predominantly unilateral dystonia.

What are the abnormal postures in dystonia?

- Cervical dystonia: combined head rotation and backward head deviation
- Blepharospasm: involuntary eye closure with reactive lower facial grimacing
- Oromandibular dystonia: involuntary jaw opening
- Lower-limb dystonia: involuntary ankle inversion and toe flexion
- Upper-limb dystonia (writers cramp): flexion dystonia of the wrist and digits while the patient is writing.

What is dopa-responsive dystonia?

Dopa-responsive dystonia is an inherited condition (now classified as *DYT5*) that results in dopamine deficiency in the basal ganglia, unaccompanied by neuronal degeneration. An important feature of this disorder is that the neurologic function is substantially improved in a sustained manner by means of orally administered dopaminergic therapy. Two biochemical pathway defects have been described in patients with dopa-responsive dystonia: autosomal dominant guanosine triphosphate cyclohydrolase 1 (GTPCH1) deficiency and autosomal recessive tyrosine hydroxylase deficiency. GTPCH1 is the rate-limiting enzyme in the synthesis of tetrahydrobiopterin, which has a central role as cofactor in the metabolic pathways, including the synthesis of the biogenic amine dopamine; in the hepatic metabolism of phenylalanine to tyrosine; and in the production of the serotonin precursor 5-hydroxytryptophan. The gene that encodes the 32 kDa GTPCH1 protein, *GCH1,* is located on chromosome 14q22.1. Because of incomplete penetrance and apparently high rate of sporadic mutation, many patients may have no family history of dystonia.

Further reading

Tarsy D, Simon DK: Dystonia, *N Engl J Med* 355:818–829, 2006 (classic article).

> Hermann Oppenheim (1858–1919), a German neurologist, coined the term dystonia in 1911 to describe a disorder causing variable muscle tone and recurrent muscle spasm.

93 EPILEPSY

INSTRUCTION

This patient is suspected to have seizures; ask her a few questions. The eye-witness (usually the spouse) of the suspected event is next to the patient and you may ask him or her any relevant questions.

SALIENT FEATURES

Examination

- Ask the patient about aura, whether she bit her tongue, whether she was incontinent during the attack, any hallucinations (déjà vu phenomenon). Ask the patient about triggering factors (including television, disco strobes, hypoglycaemia and alcohol ingestion) and whether they are recurrent. Take a family history (about 30% of patients with epilepsy have a history of seizures in relatives), and past history of head injury.
- Confirm this by asking the eye-witness about the description of seizures (note whether they were tonic–clonic), frothing at the mouth, whether the patient was unconscious or incontinent, how long the whole 'episode' lasted and how long she was unconscious after the attack, and whether there was any weakness after the attack (Todd's paralysis).
- Tell the examiner that you would like to evaluate for depression (~55% of patients with uncontrolled seizures are depressed. Patients with well-controlled seizures have rates of depression that are greater than rates the general population, and suicide rates are three-fold, with the highest rates in the 6 months after diagnosis). Since antiepileptic drugs cause mood changes, it is appropriate to evaluate mood before starting therapy.

Note: Epilepsy, which is defined as two or more seizures that are not provoked by other illnesses or circumstances, affects about 45 million people worldwide.

DIAGNOSIS

This patient has recent-onset grand mal epilepsy (lesion), which could be caused by an intracranial tumour (aetiology). The patient will have to give up her job as a truck-driver as a consequence of this (functional status).

QUESTIONS

How would you investigate the patient?
- FBC, urea and electrolytes, blood glucose, liver function tests
- Chest radiography
- Electroencephalography (EEG; Fig. 93.1)
- CT scan: appropriate for emergency situations
- MRI and telemetry: MRI of the brain is more sensitive than CT in identifying structural lesions causally related to epilepsy.

Mention some metabolic abnormalities found in these patients
Hypoglycaemia, hyponatraemia (e.g. syndrome of inappropriate antidiuretic hormone secretion (SIADH)), hypocalcaemia, hepatic failure, uraemia.

How would you classify seizures?
- Generalized seizures: grand mal (tonic–clonic) seizures, petit mal and atypical absences, myoclonus, akinetic seizures. Petit mal describes only 3 Hz seizures rather than clinically similar absence attacks, which are partial seizures.
- Partial or focal seizures (a partial seizure is epileptic activity confined to one area of cortex with a recognizable clinical pattern): simple partial seizures (no impairment of consciousness), complex partial seizures, partial seizures evolving to tonic–clonic.

ADVANCED-LEVEL QUESTIONS

What is Jacksonian epilepsy?
It is a simple partial seizure that usually originates in one portion of the prefrontal motor cortex so that fits begin in one part of the body (e.g. thumb) and then proceed to involve that side of the body and then the whole body. It suggests a space-occupying lesion.

What is Todd's paralysis?
Paresis of a limb or hemiplegia occurring after an epileptic attack, which may last up to 3 days.

How would you manage epilepsy?
- General advice: avoid ladders, heights, unsupervised swimming and cycling for 2 years from the last episode
- Antiepileptic drugs: the first-line drugs for epilepsy monotherapy remain carbamazepine and sodium valproate; phenytoin is now used less often. Although lamotrigine has a monotherapy licence, its place has still to be defined. Several new 'add on drugs' have been licensed in recent years including vigabatrin, gabapentin, lamotrigine and topiramate. An overview of trials in patients with refractory partial seizures suggests no major differences between these agents in either efficacy or tolerability (BMJ 1996;313:1169–74). Prolonged use of vigabatrin can result in severe visual field defects, prompting the development of guidelines for monitoring vision (BMJ 1998;317:1322). The SANAD trial

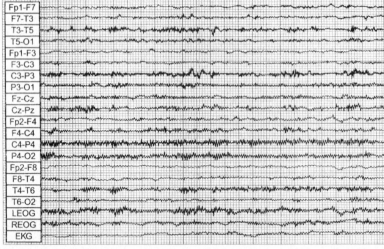

(A)

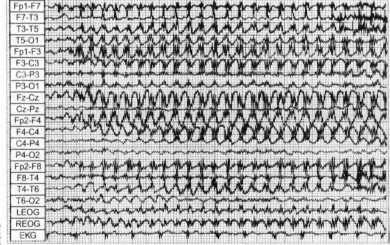

(B)

Fig. 93.1 Electroencephalography. (A) Normal awake adult. (B) Absence epilepsy showing a 3 Hz spike and wave activity.

suggested that lamotrigine is the drug of first choice in patients with partial seizures, and valproate for patients with generalized or unclassified seizures in the absence of factors that would lead to an alternative choice. Valproic acid was more effective than lamotrigine and topiramate in generalized seizures. Lamotrigine had almost twice the failure rate because of inadequate seizure control, whereas topiramate was similarly effective in controlling seizures but had a higher failure rate caused by discontinuation because of side effects (Lancet 2007;369:1016–26). Ethosuximide and valproic acid were more effective than lamotrigine in the treatment of childhood absence epilepsy. Valproate, compared with other commonly used antiepileptic drugs, was associated with an increased risk of impaired cognitive function at 3 years of age and risk of birth defects. Therefore, it should be avoided as a first-choice drug in women of childbearing potential; risks of valproate should be balanced with the risks of uncontrolled seizures.

- Vagal stimulation remains an experimental approach in seizure control (J Clin Neurophysiol 1997;14:358–68).
- Advice about driving: those who have had more than one seizure are unable to hold a driving licence in the UK unless they have been free from any form of epileptic attack while awake for a period of 1 year before the issue of a licence or, in the case of attacks while asleep, these attacks must have occurred only while asleep over a period of 3 years and no awake attacks before the issue of a licence. Drivers of heavy goods vehicles and public service vehicles must have been free of epileptic attacks for at least the last 10 years and must not have taken anticonvulsant medications during this 10-year period.
- Patients should be discouraged from participating in other activities for which a history of seizures increases the risk of injury or death, such as operating high-risk power equipment, working at heights and swimming or bathing alone.
- Women who intend to use oral contraceptive pills and are taking phenytoin, carbamazepine, phenobarbital, topiramate or oxcarbazepine (these drugs induce hepatic enzymes to increases clearance of oral contraceptives) should be advised to use preparations containing at least 50 µg ethinylestradiol in order to reduce the chance of pregnancy. Valproate should also be avoided because of the risk of teratogenicity.

What do you understand by the term status epilepticus?

It is a medical emergency where seizures follow each other without recovery of consciousness.

What is the prognosis in epilepsy?

Most individuals with newly diagnosed epilepsy enter prolonged seizure remission and have an excellent prognosis, but seizures remain refractory in 20–30%.

Up to 75% of patients with refractory partial epilepsy show evidence of abnormalities on MRI (J Neurol Neurosurg Psych 1995;59:384–7), some of which are amenable to surgery.

Population-based studies show that patients with epilepsy have an increased risk of sudden death compared with age- and sex-matched controls (J Neurol Neurosurg Psych 1995;58:462–4). Some of these deaths are related to epilepsy itself, for example as a consequence of accidents, but others are unexplained. This has been termed as SUDEP (sudden unexpected death in epilepsy) and is more common in refractory epilepsy (about 1 per 200 patients per year). Many of these deaths may be related to unwitnessed seizures, possibly associated with respiratory arrest, cardiac arrest or neurologically mediated pulmonary oedema. Therefore, a proportion of the patients with SUDEP can potentially be prevented by better control of seizures.

What is the mechanism of spike and wave electroencephalography pattern seen in absence seizures?

A burst firing of cortical neurons leads to recruitment of reticular thalamic neuronal network. Activation of low-threshold calcium currents results in burst firing of the network, releasing γ-aminobutyric acid (GABA) onto thalamocortical neurons, which are hyperpolarized through activation of GABA-B and GABA-A receptors. This hyperpolarization removes the inactivation of T type calcium channels. On repolarization, these channels open, resulting in a burst of action potentials from the thalamocortical neurons, which then drives the cortical neurons). In this way the cycle continues and generates the spike-wave discharges seen on scalp EEG (Lancet 2006;367:1087–100).

What do you know about the pathogenesis of epilepsy?

Generalized epilepsies originate from alterations in either neuronal networks or intrinsic neuronal function:

- Neuronal networks between thalamus and cerebral cortex, as in absence seizures
- Intrinsic neuronal function as in channelopathies: mutations in *SCN1B*, which encodes a voltage-gated sodium channel subunit, are associated with generalized epilepsy with febrile seizures; mutations in *KCNQ2* and *KCNQ3*, which both encode potassium channels, are associated with benign familial neonatal convulsions.

Partial epilepsy syndromes probably arise from a focal lesion. Hippocampal sclerosis is the most common pathological finding in adults with the most common partial epilepsy, but its aetiological role, if any, in epileptogenesis is still unclear.

Robert B Todd FRS (1809–1860), an Irish physician, graduated from Pembroke College, Oxford, and was Professor of Physiology at King's College, London (J Neurol Neurosurg Psychiatry 1994;57:359). He was founder of King's College Hospital.

J Hughlings Jackson (1835–1911), an English neurologist, worked at the National Hospital, Queen Square, London.

---

94 GUILLAIN–BARRÉ SYNDROME

INSTRUCTION

Examine this patient's lower limbs, whose weakness began distally.

SALIENT FEATURES

History

- Weakness: difficulty in rising up from standing position or climbing stairs, legs usually affected before upper limbs

- Dyspnoea: late in the course suggesting diaphragmatic and intercostals muscle weakness
- Cranial nerve involvement: diplopia, drooling of saliva, regurgitation of food
- Paraesthesias
- Urinary symptoms
- Systemic symptoms: fatigue
- Ascertain whether the onset was preceded by a trivial viral illness.

Examination

- Weakness of distal limb muscles
- Distal numbness
- Areflexia.

Proceed as follows:
- Tell the examiner that you would like to:
  - assess respiratory function (forced vital capacity)
  - check BP (for labile BP).

Remember: Polyneuropathies can be classified as demyelinating or axonal. They can also be classified according to the diameter of the affected nerve fibre. Larger fibres are heavily myelinated and, therefore, most subject to processes that damage myelin. Most polyneuropathies, including the diabetic type, are axonal.

DIAGNOSIS

This patient has Guillain–Barré syndrome (lesion) and is currently experiencing weakness of the distal limb muscles (functional status).

QUESTIONS

What features are required for diagnosis?
- Progressive weakness in both arms and legs (might start with weakness only in the legs)
- Areflexia (or decreased tendon reflexes).

What features strongly support diagnosis?
- Progression of symptoms over days to 4 weeks
- Relative symmetry of symptoms
- Mild sensory symptoms or signs
- Cranial nerve involvement, especially bilateral weakness of facial muscles
- Autonomic dysfunction
- Pain (often present)
- High concentration of protein in CSF
- Typical electrodiagnostic features.

What feature should raise doubt about the diagnosis?
- Severe pulmonary dysfunction with limited limb weakness at onset
- Severe sensory signs with limited weakness at onset
- Bladder or bowel dysfunction at onset

- Fever at onset
- Sharp sensory level
- Slow progression with limited weakness without respiratory involvement (consider subacute inflammatory demyelinating polyneuropathy or chronic inflammatory demyelinating polyradiculoneurtopathy (CIDP)
- Marked persistent asymmetry of weakness
- Persistent bladder or bowel dysfunction
- Increased number of mononuclear cells in CSF ($>50 \times 10^6/l$)
- Polymorphonuclear cells in CSF.

What is the pathology?

It is a demyelinating neuropathy. Infections (e.g. with *Campylobacter jejuni*) might induce an immune response that finally leads to Guillain–Barré syndrome. The immune response depends on certain bacterial factors, such as the specificity of lipooligosaccharide, and on patient-related (host) factors. Genetic polymorphisms in the patients might partially determine the severity of Guillain–Barré syndrome. Antibodies to lipooligosaccharides can cross-react with specific nerve gangliosides and can activate complement. The extent of nerve damage depends on several factors. Nerve dysfunction leads to weakness and might cause sensory disturbances (Lancet Neurol 2008; 7:939–50).

ADVANCED-LEVEL QUESTIONS

How is the diagnosis confirmed?

- Nerve conduction studies demonstrate slowing of conduction or conduction block
- CSF shows albumino-cytological dissociation: a normal cell count but protein concentration is frequently raised.

What is Miller–Fisher syndrome?

A rare proximal variant of Guillain–Barré syndrome that initially affects the ocular muscles and in which ataxia is prominent.

What is the differential diagnosis?

Poliomyelitis, botulism, primary muscle disease or other neuropathy (porphyric, diphtheric heavy metal or organophosphorous poisoning).

How would you treat such patients?

- High-dose intravenous gammaglobulin during the acute phase to reduce the severity and duration of symptoms (N Engl J Med 1992; 326:1123–9). This is equivalent to plasma exchange in effectiveness in reducing disability, but the combination of intravenous immunoglobulin and plasma exchange offers no significant additional advantage (Lancet 1997;349:225–30)
- Ventilatory support if respiratory muscles are affected
- Physiotherapy and occupational therapy for muscle weakness.

What is the prognosis?

Despite medical therapy, this syndrome often remains a severe disease: 3–10% of patients die and 20% are still unable to walk after 6 months.

In addition, many patients have pain and fatigue that can persist for months or years. Outcome in patients with Guillain–Barré syndrome can be determined with the Erasmus GBS Outcome Scale (EGOS). Using EGOS, the chance of walking unaided after 6 months can be calculated on the basis of the age of the patient, the presence of diarrhoea and the severity of weakness in the first weeks. Despite treatment with intravenous immunoglobulin, many patients only partially recover and have residual weakness, pain and fatigue (Lancet Neurol 2008; 7:939–50).

What do you know about chronic inflammatory demyelinating polyradiculoneuropathy CIDP?

- This is the most common demeylinating neuropathy (N Engl J Med 2010;362:929–40).
- It is an idiopathic multifocal inflammation of the nerves that can occur at any age in the form of a subacute sensorimotor polyneuropathy.
- It is diagnosed by the findings of electrical conduction block (segmental demyelination at areas of inflammation, as seen on nerve-conduction studies) and by a high level of protein in the CSF.
- CIDP is usually idiopathic but also can occur as a feature of some connective tissue diseases.
- Corticosteroids, intravenous immunoglobulin and plasma exchange are usually effective therapies; when these are not effective, immunosuppressive drugs are often added.
- CIDP is clinically similar to Guillain–Barré syndrome except for the differing time course, and was at one time called chronic Guillain–Barré syndrome.

What do you know about POEMS syndrome?

The acronym POEMS (polyneuropathy, organomegaly, endocrinopathy, M protein and skin changes) was introduced by Bardwick et al. Polyneuropathy and polyclonal plasma cell proliferation is present in all patients. In the POEMS syndrome, a clonal expansion of plasma cells occurs in association with sclerotic bone lesions (osteosclerotic myeloma). The syndrome may also involve lymph nodes in the form of angiofollicular hyperplasia, also known as Castleman disease. A moderately increased level of CSF protein in this patient is typical of the POEMS syndrome but does not distinguish it from CIDP. A low level of monoclonal IgG with lambda light chain is also characteristic of the POEMS syndrome, whereas kappa light chain predominates in monoclonal gammopathy of unknown significance (MGUS). However, in contrast to multiple myeloma, the levels of other immunoglobulin subclasses are not reduced in the POEMS syndrome.

C Guillain (1876–1961), Professor of Medicine in Paris.
JA Barré (1880–1967), Professor of Neurology in Strasbourg, trained in Paris.

95 MULTIPLE SYSTEM ATROPHY

INSTRUCTION

Perform a neurological examination on this patient.

SALIENT FEATURES

History

- Dizziness when standing up (caused by postural hypotension)
- Dysphagia
- Ataxia
- Symptoms of Parkinson's disease (p. 191)
- Impotence, bladder disturbances (p. 346)
- Anhidrosis.

Examination

- Mask-like facies and other features of bradykinesia
- Increased tone (rigidity)
- Cerebellar signs.

Proceed as follows:

- Tell the examiner that you would like to:
  - look for postural hypotension (a fall in systolic BP of at least 20 mmHg or in diastolic BP of at least 10 mmHg within 3 min after standing), the hallmark of this condition (caused by autonomic failure)
  - look for signs of autonomic dysfunction (pupillary asymmetry, Horner syndrome).

DIAGNOSIS

This patient has cerebellar and Parkinson's signs (lesion) caused by multiple system atrophy, a degenerative disorder (aetiology), and has marked disability including incontinence (functional status).

ADVANCED-LEVEL QUESTIONS

What are the types of multisystem atrophy?

Striatonigral degeneration. Clinical picture resembles Parkinson's disease but without tremor. These patients do not respond to antiparkinsonian medications and often develop adverse reactions to these agents.

Shy–Drager syndrome. Clinical picture consists of Parkinson's disease combined with severe autonomic neuropathy (particularly postural hypotension). Other important clinical features are impotence and bladder disturbances.

Olivopontocerebellar atrophy. Combination of extrapyramidal manifestations and cerebellar ataxia. Patients may also have autonomic neuropathy and anterior horn cell degeneration.

Parkinsonism and motor neuron disease. Rare.

What is the pathology in Shy–Drager syndrome?

In 1960, Shy and Drager described changes in the brainstem and ganglia; subsequently, loss of neurons has been shown in the autonomic nervous system and in the cells of the intermediolateral column of the spinal cord. PET shows decreased uptake of dopamine in the putamen and caudate lobe.

What factors can lower blood pressure in these patients?

Standing up: orthostatic hypotension, a hallmark of this condition.
Food and exercise can produce hypotension even in the supine position (J Neurol 1990;237(suppl 1):S24, J Am Coll Cardiol 1993;21:97A).

What is the morbidity of this condition?

It is tends to disable most patients severely by the end of 5–7 years.

How would you treat these patients?

Treatment is symptomatic and supportive for hypotension and neurological deficits. Symptoms of postural hypotension may be ameliorated by antigravity stockings and fluorohydrocortisone.

How does pure autonomic failure differ from multisystem atrophy?

Pure autonomic failure differs in its lack of any sensory, cerebellar, pyramidal or extrapyramidal dysfunction. Afferent pathways and somatic neurons are not affected. It is less progressive than multisystem atrophy, and patients usually have a prolonged and sometimes stable course. Pure autonomic failure affects postganglionic neurons and autonomic impairment is the principal clinical feature (orthostatic hypotension, bladder incontinence and impotence in men are the major signs).

What are the radiological signs of multisystem atrophy?

- The more common typical radiological findings in multisystem atrophy include atrophy of the cerebellum, most prominently in the vermis, middle cerebellar peduncles, pons and lower brainstem (Neuroimag Clin North Am 2010;20: Issue 1; on imaging of movement disorders).
- In addition to putaminal atrophy, a characteristic hypointense signal in T_2 with hyperintense rim, corresponding to reactive gliosis and astrogliosis, can be observed in the external putamen and is termed the 'slit-like void sign' (Fig. 95.1B). This combination of hypointense and hyperintense putaminal signal change is specific for multisystem atrophy and its finding can be used to differentiate multisystem atrophy from progressive supranuclear palsy and Parkinson's disease.
- The 'hot-cross bun' sign is characterized by cruciform signal hyperintensity on T_2-weighted images in mid pons (Fig. 95.1A). This finding is said to correspond to the loss of pontine neurons and myelinated transverse cerebellar fibres with preservation of the corticospinal tracts. However, this sign is not specific to multisystem atrophy and has been reported in other conditions such as spinocerebellar ataxia.
- Hypointensity alone without hyperintense rim is a sensitive radiological feature but non-specific for multisystem atrophy.

What are the diagnostic criteria for *probable* multisystem atrophy?

A sporadic, progressive, adult-onset (>30 years) disease characterized by:
- autonomic failure involving urinary incontinence (with erectile dysfunction in males) *or*
- orthostatic decrease of BP within 3 min of standing by at least 30 mmHg systolic or 15 mmHg diastolic *and either*

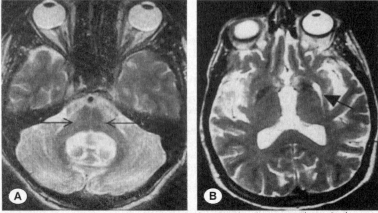

Fig. 95.1 Axial T$_2$-weighted MR images showing the 'hot-cross bun sign' (A) and the 'slit-like void sign' (B). (With permission from Ling, Lees 2010.)

- poorly levodopa-responsive parkinsonism (bradykinesia with rigidity, tremor, or postural instability) *or*
- a cerebellar syndrome (gait ataxia with cerebellar dysarthria, limb ataxia or cerebellar oculomotor dysfunction).

What are the diagnostic criteria for *possible* multisystem atrophy?

A sporadic, progressive, adult-onset (>30 years) disease characterized by:
- parkinsonism (bradykinesia with rigidity, tremor, or postural instability) *or*
- a cerebellar syndrome (gait ataxia with cerebellar dysarthria, limb ataxia or cerebellar oculomotor dysfunction) *and*
- at least one feature suggesting autonomic dysfunction (otherwise unexplained urinary urgency, frequency or incomplete bladder emptying, erectile dysfunction in males, or significant orthostatic BP decline that does not meet the level required in probable MSA) *and*
- at least one of the additional features:
  - Possible MSA-P or MSA-C (parkinsonian subtype or cerebellar dysfunction subtype, respectively, see below)
  - Babinski sign with hyper-reflexia
  - Stridor.

Possible MSA-P is indicated by:
- rapidly progressive parkinsonism
- poor response to levodopa
- postural instability within 3 years of motor onset
- gait ataxia, cerebellar dysarthria, limb ataxia or cerebellar oculomotor dysfunction
- dysphagia within 5 years of motor onset
- atrophy on MRI of putamen, middle cerebellar peduncle, pons or cerebellum

- hypometabolism on fludeoxyglucose PET (FDG-PET) in putamen, brainstem or cerebellum.

Possible MSA-C is indicated by:

- parkinsonism (bradykinesia and rigidity)
- atrophy on MRI of putamen, middle cerebellar peduncle or pons
- hypometabolism on FDG-PET in putamen
- presynaptic nigrostriatal dopaminergic denervation on single photon emission CT (SPECT) or PET.

What are features supporting a diagnosis of multisystem atrophy?

- Orofacial dystonia
- Disproportionate antecollis
- Camptocormia (severe anterior flexion of the spine) with or without Pisa syndrome (severe lateral flexion of the spine)
- Contractures of hands or feet
- Inspiratory sighs
- Severe dysphonia
- Severe dysarthria
- New or increased snoring
- Cold hands and feet
- Pathological laughter or crying
- Jerky, myoclonic postural or action tremor.

What are features that do not support a diagnosis of multisystem atrophy?

- Classic pill-rolling rest tremor
- Clinically significant neuropathy
- Onset after age 75 years
- Family history of ataxia or parkinsonism
- Dementia (on Diagnostic and Statistical Manual of Mental Disorders, 4th edition (DSM-IV))
- White matter lesions that suggest multiple sclerosis
- Hallucinations not induced by drugs.

What do you know about the pathogenesis of multisystem atrophy?

In transgenic mouse models of oligodendroglial α-synucleinopathy, sickle-shaped glial cytoplasmic inclusions composed of misfolded α-synuclein can be seen. The dying neuron contains condensed chromatin; the nuclear membrane is disrupted and there is cell shrinkage. These findings indicate three possible pathogenic pathways in multiple system atrophy:

- Inclusions could trigger microglial activation, which causes chronic oxidative stress and ultimately leads to neuronal cell death
- Inclusions could exacerbate susceptibility to exogenous oxidative stress and lead to neuronal cell death in striatonigral and olivopontocerebellar systems
- Inclusions could lead to secondary axonal α-synuclein aggregation or oligodendroglial mitochondrial dysfunction, which eventually lead to neuronal cell death.

Bradbury and Eggleston in 1925 first described the combination of postural hypotension, incontinence, impotence and abnormality of sweating (anhidrosis). Neurological manifestations were identified later.

GM Shy (1919–1967), a US neurologist who obtained his MRCP in London in 1947.

GA Drager (1917–1967), a US neurologist.

Christopher J Mathias, FRCP, DSc, contemporary Professor of Medicine, St Mary's Hospital Medical School and National Hospital, Queen Square, London, whose chief interest is the autonomic control of the cardiovascular system.

In 1969 Graham and Oppenheimer introduced the term multiple system atrophy to combine the entities of striatonigral degeneration, olivopontocerebellar ataxia, and Shy–Drager syndrome.

96   NEUROLOGICAL BLADDER

INSTRUCTION

This patient is suspected to have difficulty in micturition accompanying paraparesis. Would you like to ask him a few questions?

SALIENT FEATURES

Examination

Ask the patient the following questions:
- Do you get a sensation when the bladder is full?
- Do you feel the urine passing?
- Are you able to stop urine passing in midstream at your own will?
- Does the bladder leak continually?
- Do you suddenly pass large volumes?
- Is there any difficulty in defaecation?
- Is there any numbness in the perineal region?

Proceed as follows:
- The examination should concentrate on the legs, because the segments that innervate the bladder are caudal to those that innervate the lower limbs, and spinal cord involvement that affects the innervation of the bladder almost always results in lower limb signs. (Possible exceptions are lesions of the low sacral cord or conus, but only the most caudal lesions fail to produce some overactivity in the legs and extensor plantar responses.)
- Tell the examiner that in male patients you would like to take a history of impotence and examine the neurological system and spine.

Note: Cauda equina lesions at S1 and S2 may impair the ankle reflexes, and those at S3 may affect the intrinsic muscles of the foot, causing foot deformities and fasciculation of the muscles. Saddle anaesthesia is a feature of cauda equina (p. 331) or conus medullaris lesions (p. 332).

DIAGNOSIS

This patient has a spastic bladder (lesion) accompanying his paraparesis, which is the result of trauma (aetiology) and he requires an indwelling urinary catheter (functional status).

ADVANCED-LEVEL QUESTIONS

What are the types of neurogenic bladder?

Spinal or spastic bladder. The bladder is small and spastic and holds <250 ml. A hyper-reflexive bladder usually occurs when the spinal cord lesion is at the level of T5 or higher. It is seen in lesions of the spinal cord secondary to trauma, multiple sclerosis and tumour (upper motor neuron lesion). On a contrasted study, a spastic bladder has the shape of a Christmas tree, with little outpouchings along the lateral margins (Fig. 96.1). These areas of outpouching of contrast or urine are pseudo-diverticula caused by hypertrophy of the bladder musculature. Bladder fullness is not appreciated and the bladder tends to empty reflexly and suddenly — the automatic bladder. Evacuation may be incomplete unless it is massaged by pressure in the suprapubic region. These patients are prime candidates for urinary infection, calculi and bilateral collecting system dilatation.

Autonomous bladder. This results from damage to the cauda equina (i.e. lower motor neuron lesion; p. 237). These bladders are usually the result of a herniated disc, multiple sclerosis, diabetic neuropathy or lower spinal cord tumour. The patient is incontinent with continual urine dribbling and there is no sensation of bladder fullness. Despite the dribbling, there is considerable residual urine. There is loss of perineal sensation and sexual dysfunction. (In conus medullaris–cauda equina lesions, it is possible to have a flaccid lower motor neuron detrusor, with a spastic sphincter. The reverse may also occur.) Although these patients may demonstrate a large bladder, the upper urinary collecting systems are usually within normal limits, and vesicoureteral reflux is rare.

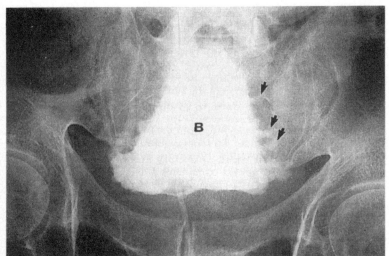

Fig. 96.1 Spastic bladder, showing the typical 'Christmas tree' deformity of the bladder with lateral diverticula (arrows). (With permission from Mettler 2004.)

Sensory bladder. Similar to autonomous bladder and seen in tabes dorsalis, subacute combined degeneration of the cord and multiple sclerosis. There is loss of awareness of bladder fullness with a loss of spinal reflex. This results in retention of large quantities of urine, incontinence with dribbling; the high volume of residual urine can be voided by considerable straining.

Uninhibited bladder. This occurs with lesions affecting the second gyrus of the frontal lobe (e.g. frontal lobe tumours, parasagittal meningiomas, aneurysms of the anterior communicating arteries and some dementia disorders). Patient has urgency despite low bladder volumes and has sudden uncontrolled evacuation. There is no residual urine. When there is deterioration of the intellect, the patient may pass urine at any time without concern.

What do you know about the neurological control of the bladder?

- As the bladder fills, distention stimulates low-level firing of vesical afferents (pelvic nerve), which, in turn, stimulate sympathetic outflow to the bladder outlet (hypogastric nerve to contract the internal sphincter and inhibit detrusor activity) and pudendal outflow to the external urethral sphincter. These responses occur by spinal reflex pathways that promote continence.

- As the bladder becomes fuller, afferents fire more intensely and activate spinobulbospinal reflex pathways passing through the pontine micturition centre. Micturition follows activation of the parasympathetic pathways to the detrusor muscle and inhibition of the somatic input to the external urethral sphincter. The parasympathetic reflex is based in the S3 roots and S3 segments of the cord.

- Ascending afferent input from the spinal cord may pass through the periaqueductal grey matter before reaching the cortex, thereby leading to the sensation of urgency.

- The sympathetic system promotes urinary storage by increasing urethral resistance and depressing detrusor contractions. The sympathetic supply descends into the pelvis from the hypogastric reflex.

- A cortical representation of the bladder is present in the paracentral lobule, stimulation of which may evoke bladder contractions. It may play a part in initiating voluntary contractions and in stopping micturition by initiating contraction of the external sphincter.

What investigations are done to evaluate bladder function?

Cystometry, sphincter electromyography, uroflowmetry with measurement and recording of urinary flow, urethral pressure profiles and electrophysiological tests of bladder wall innervation.

What are the different types of urinary incontinence?

Urinary continence requires a compliant reservoir (the bladder) and sphincter efficiency; the latter depends on its two components: the involuntary smooth muscle of the bladder neck and the voluntary skeletal muscle of the external sphincter. Urinary incontinence occurs when urine leaks involuntarily and is of five types:

- Total incontinence where the patient loses urine at all times and in all positions. It occurs when the sphincter is damaged (surgery, cancerous infiltration and nerve damage) or when there is a fistula between the urinary tract and the skin, or ectopic ureters

- Stress incontinence: occurs when there is an increase in intra-abdominal pressure (on coughing, sneezing, lifting, exercising); it is seen in patients with a lax pelvic floor (e.g. multiparous women, patients who have undergone pelvic surgery) and urine is not lost in the supine position
- Urge incontinence: loss of urine preceded by a strong, unexpected urge to void urine; it occurs with inflammation or neurogenic disorders
- Overflow incontinence: occurs in chronic urinary retention from a chronically distended bladder
- Enuresis: a form of involuntary nocturnal incontinence, usually seen in children.

Respiratory system
History and examination of the chest

INSTRUCTION

Introduce yourself to the patient.

SALIENT FEATURES

History

- Cough
- Sputum
- Haemoptysis (acute infection, including in chronic obstructive airways disease (COPD), pulmonary infarction, bronchogenic carcinoma, bronchiectasis, TB, Goodpasture's syndrome, pulmonary haemosiderosis, mitral stenosis)
- Degree of dyspnoea: what the patient can do without becoming breathless:
  - Normal
  - Walk normally on the level but not on stairs or hills
  - Walk on the level for 1.5 km (1 mile) but cannot keep up with people of a similar ages
  - Walk about 1.5 km (110 yards) on the level
  - Breathless at rest or on minimal effort.
- Onset of dyspnoea:
  - Intermittent: asthma, recurrent pulmonary oedema, exacerbations of COAD
  - Over days: pleural fluid, carcinoma of bronchus, heart failure
  - Over months to years: COAD, fibrosing alveolitis, anaemia, fibrotic lung disease
  - Over a few hours: pulmonary oedema, bronchial asthma, pneumonia
  - Acute or sudden: pneumothorax, pulmonary oedema, inhaled foreign body.
- Wheezing: airways limitation including asthma, COAD
- Chest pain: pleurisy, tracheitis
- Smoking
- Family history.

Examination

- Place the patient in a sitting position and ask whether he or she is comfortable.
- Examine the sputum cup and comment on the sputum.
- Examine the patient from the foot end of the bed and comment as follows:
  - Whether the patient is breathless at rest
  - On wasting, if any, in the infraclavicular region
  - On diminished movement on the right or left side
  - Count the respiratory rate
  - Comment on pattern of breathing (Fig. III.1).

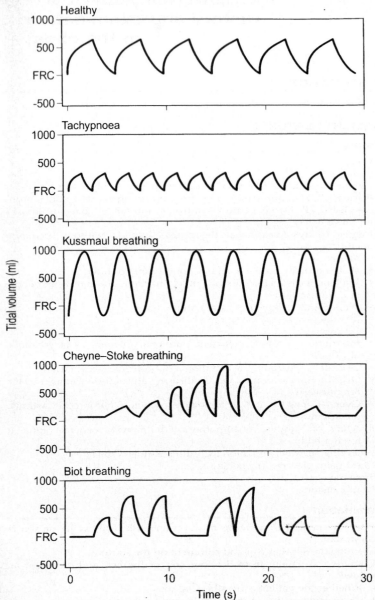

Fig. III.1 Different patterns of breathing. FRC, functional residual capacity.

- Examine the hands:
  - Clubbing
  - Cyanosis
  - Tar staining (the yellow 'nicotine' staining is actually tar).
- Examine the pulse for bounding pulse and asterixis: signs of carbon monoxide narcosis.
- Examine the face:
  - Comment on the tongue, looking for central cyanosis
  - Comment on the eyes, looking for pallor and evidence of Horner's syndrome (see p. 176).
- Examine the neck:
  - Comment on neck veins
  - Check for cervical lymphadenopathy
  - Comment on the trachea: any deviation, distance between the cricoid cartilage and suprasternal notch.
- Palpate:
  - Apex beat
  - Movements on both sides with the fingers symmetrically placed in the intercostal spaces on both sides
  - Vocal fremitus (tell the examiner that you would prefer to do vocal resonance because it gives the same information and is more reliable).
- Percussion: percuss over supraclavicular areas, clavicles, upper, middle and lower chest on both sides.
- Auscultation:
  - Over supraclavicular areas, upper, middle and lower chest on both sides: comment on breath sounds (whether vesicular or bronchial) and on adventitious sounds (wheeze, crackles or pleural rub)
  - If crackles are heard, ask the patient to cough and then repeat auscultation. It is important to time the crackles to ascertain whether they occur in early, mid or late inspiration
  - While auscultating the front of the chest, seize the opportunity to listen to the second pulmonary sound
  - Check for vocal resonance by asking the patient to repeat 'one, one, one'
  - Check for forced expiratory time (FET) if your diagnosis is COAD by asking the patient to exhale forcefully after full inspiration while you are listening over the trachea: if the patient takes more than 6 s, airway disease is indicated (be prepared to discuss spirometry findings; Fig. III.2).
- Ask the patient to sit forward:
  - Palpate: assess expansion posteriorly
  - Percuss: on both sides including axillae
  - Auscultate: posteriorly including the axillae.
- Remember to look for signs of middle lobe disease in the right axilla and correlate your findings with common clinical conditions.
- Tell the examiner you would like to do a chest X-ray or chest CT (and be prepared to comment on the findings:
  - Normal: airways disease, neuromuscular disease, pulmonary emboli, amaemia

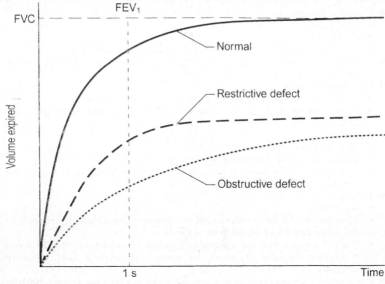

Fig. III.2 Typical spirometry. FVC, forced vital capacity; FEV1, forced expiratory volume in 1 s.

- Abnormal lung fields: pleural thickening, effusion, tumar, lobar collapse, diffuse infiltration
- Abnormal mediastinum: lymphadenopathy, large pulmonary vessels
- Cardiomegaly with upper lobe blood diversion: pericardial infusion, LV failure.

97 PLEURAL EFFUSION

INSTRUCTION

Examine this patient's chest.
Examine this patient's chest from the back.
Examine this patient's chest from the front.

SALIENT FEATURES

History

- Fever
- Pleuritic pain (made worse on coughing or deep breathing)
- Cough (pneumonia, TB)
- Haemoptysis (associated parenchymal involvment in bronchogenic carcinoma or TB)
- Shortness of breath (large effusions, cardiac failure)
- Exposure to asbestos (mesothelioma)
- Nephrotic syndrome.

Examination

- Decreased movement on the affected side
- Tracheal deviation to the opposite side
- Stony dull note on the affected side
- Decreased vocal resonance and diminished breath sounds on the affected side.

Proceed as follows:
- Comment on aspiration marks
- Percuss for the upper level of effusion in the axilla
- Listen for bronchial breath sounds
- Listen for aegophony at the upper level of the effusion
- It is important to elicit any evidence of an underlying cause, such as clubbing, tar staining, lymph nodes, radiation burns and mastectomy, raised JVP, rheumatoid hands or butterfly rash.

Remember:
For clinical detection, 500 ml of pleural fluid should be present.
There are five major types of pleural effusion: exudate, transudate, empyema, haemorrhagic pleural effusion or haemothorax and chylous effusion.
The most common causes of pleural effusion in the Western world are congestive heart failure, pneumonia and cancer.
The first step in developing a differential diagnosis of a pleural effusion is to establish whether the effusion is a transudate or an exudate by analysis of fluid obtained at thoracentesis.

DIAGNOSIS

This patient has a pleural effusion (lesion) probably caused by bronchogenic carcinoma and is short of breath at rest (functional status).

QUESTIONS

How would you investigate this patient?

- Chest radiography: standard posteroanterior and lateral films detect pleural fluid in excess of 175 ml. Obliteration of costophrenic angle to hemithorax suggest fluid. Subpulmonic effusion can simulate an elevated diaphragm (Fig. 97.1).
- Pleural tap:
  - Pleural fluid for determination of the levels of protein, albumin, lactate dehydrogenase (LDH), glucose, cholesterol and cytology; a simultaneous blood sample should be obtained for estimation of glucose, protein, albumin and LDH
  - When empyema is suspected or seen, pleural fluid pH should be obtained

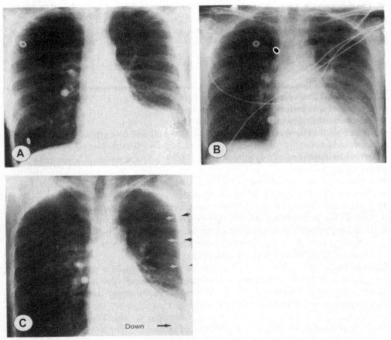

Fig. 97.1 The appearance of pleural effusions in chest radiography depend on patient position (also shown in diagramatic form). (A) Upright posteroanterior: a large left pleural effusion obscures the left hemidiaphragm, the left costophrenic angle and the left cardiac border. (B) Supine anteroposterior view: fluid runs posteriorly, causing a diffuse opacity over the lower two-thirds of the left lung, the left hemidiaphragm remaining obscured (this can easily mimic left lower lobe infiltrate or left lower lobe atelectasis). (C) Left lateral decubitus view: pleural effusion can be seen to be freely moving and layering (arrows) along the lateral chest wall. (With permission from Mettler 2004.)

- When TB is suspected, pleural fluid adenosine deaminase or lysozyme levels should be determined and Ziehl–Neelsen staining and pleural fluid mycobacterial cultures should be done
- Pleural fluid amylase levels should be estimated when malignancy, pancreatitis or oesophageal rupture is suspected
- In autoimmune disorders, pleural fluid rheumatoid factor or antinuclear antibodies should be tested.
- Pleural biopsy: the biopsy specimen is sent for histopathological examination and mycobacterial culture.

What are the causes of dullness at a lung base?
- Pleural effusion
- Pleural thickening
- Consolidation and collapse of the lung
- Raised hemidiaphragm.

How would you differentiate between the above?
- Pleural effusion: stony dull note; trachea may be deviated to the opposite side in large effusions
- Pleural thickening: trachea not deviated; breath sounds will be heard
- Consolidation: vocal resonance increased; bronchial breath sounds and associated crackles
- Collapse: trachea deviated to the affected side; absent breath sounds.

How would you differentiate between an exudate and a transudate?
- The protein content of an exudate is >3 g/l. However, if this criterion alone is applied, about 10% of the exudates and 15% of the transudates will be wrongly classified. A more accurate diagnosis is made when Light's criteria (Ann Intern Med 1972;77:507–13) for an exudate are applied: (1) the ratio of the pleural fluid to serum protein is greater than 0.5; (2) the ratio of pleural fluid to serum LDH is greater than 0.6; (3) pleural fluid LDH is greater than two-thirds the upper normal limit for blood LDH. Light's criteria have been shown to have a sensitivity of 100% but a low specificity of 72% (Chest 1990;98:546–9). This was because many patients with effusion caused by chronic cardiac failure have protein values in the exudate range, particularly when on chronic diuretic therapy. Serum–effusion albumin gradient (i.e. serum albumin minus pleural fluid albumin) was 95% sensitive but a more specific (100%) marker of exduative effusion. A gradient of <12 g/l indicates an exudative effusion whereas a gradient >12 g/l indicates a transudative effusion. Measuring the difference between the serum and the pleural-fluid albumin levels is useful in patients with heart failure who are taking diuretics since a difference >12 g/l is consistent with a transudative effusion, even though other Light's criteria for an exudative effusion have been met.
- The pleural fluid cholesterol level is <600 mg/l in transudates. All malignant effusions have a pleural cholesterol level greater than this value, and therefore this test is useful to separate these two categories of effusion (Chest 1987;92:296–302, Chest 1991;99:1097–102).

Mention a few causes for an exudate and a transudate
Exudate:
- Bronchogenic carcinoma (presence of effusion is an ominous sign)
- Secondaries in the pleura (lung, breast, ovary and pancreas)

- Pneumonia
- Pulmonary infarction
- TB
- Rheumatoid arthritis
- SLE
- Lymphoma (in young individuals)
- Mesothelioma.

Transudate:
- Nephrotic syndrome
- Cardiac failure
- Liver cell failure
- Hypothyroidism.

ADVANCED-LEVEL QUESTIONS

Mention a few conditions in which the pleural fluid pH and glucose levels are low but lactate dehydrogenase is raised

Empyema, malignancy, TB, rheumatoid arthritis, SLE and oesophageal rupture.

What is the value of measuring pleural fluid pH and glucose concentrations in malignant effusions?

It is of value in determining the prognosis (Ann Intern Med 1988;108:345–9). Patients with a low pleural fluid pH (<7.3) or low glucose concentration (<600 mg/l) have a shorter life expectancy than those with higher values: 2.1 months versus 9.8 months. The low pH group tends to have more extensive pleural involvement as determined by thoracoscopy and a higher failure rate for chemical pleurodesis.

What further investigation would you do to determine the underlying cause of the pleural effusion?

- Pleural biopsy
- CT chest scan
- MRI of the chest: although this technique has limited value owing to motion artefacts caused by cardiac and respiratory movements, radiologists were able to differentiate transudates, simple exudates and complex exudates.

What is the role of pleural fluid cytology in the diagnosis of pleural effusion?

- Pleural fluid usually contains about 1.5×10^9 cells/l (predominantly mononuclear cells). Counts above 50×10^9 cells/l are seen in parapneumonic effusions, whereas transudates usually have counts of $<1 \times 10^9$ cells/l.
- Pleural fluid eosinophilia (i.e. greater than 10%) suggests a benign disease, including pneumothorax, asbestos-related effusions and post-haemothorax, although malignancy cannot be excluded.
- Pleural fluid lymphocytosis is seen in about one-third of transudates, in malignancy, TB, lymphoma, collagen vascular diseases and sarcoidosis.
- Computed interactive morphometry (analyses the size and nuclei of cells in a stained centrifuged specimen) differentiates between malignant cells and reactive lymphocytosis. This method is particularly useful when differentiating between benign reactive mesothelial cells from malignancy.

What characteristics of the pleural fluid in a parapneumonic effusion indicate a need for closed-tube drainage?

A pleural fluid glucose concentration of <400 mg/l or a pH<7.0 indicates the need for closed-tube drainage.

What does a pleural fluid total neutral fat level greater than 4.0 g/l suggest?

It suggests chylothorax and is seen most often in patients with lymphomas, solid tumours, nephrotic syndrome and cirrhosis, and occasionally in rheumatoid arthritis.

What is the significance of pleural fluid amylase levels?

A pleural fluid amylase level greater than the serum amylase concentration is seen in patients with pancreatitis, carcinoma, bacterial pneumonia and oesophageal rupture. In malignant effusions, when cytology cannot differentiate adenocarcinoma from mesothelioma, a raised amylase level suggests the presence of the former. Amylase-rich pleural effusions occur frequently, and pleural fluid isoamylase determination can be useful; the finding of a pleural effusion rich in salivary isoamylase should prompt an evaluation for carcinoma (particularly a lung primary), but may also be seen in other pleural inflammatory conditions (Chest 1992;102:1455–9).

What are the causes of an exudate with negative cytology findings and pleural fluid lymphocytosis?

Possible causes include TB, collagen vascular diseases and tumours, including lymphoma.

In such patients what other tests could you perform on the pleural fluid to determine the underlying cause?

- *Pleural fluid adenosine deaminase concentration* (an enzyme involved in purine metabolism and found in T lymphocytes) is markedly raised in tuberculous and rheumatoid effusions compared with malignant effusions.
- *Increased pleural fluid lysozyme concentration (muramidase)* is used to differentiate TB, rheumatoid arthritis and empyema from malignant effusions.
- Combined use of these two tests yields a sensitivity and specificity of 100% for tuberculous effusions if empyema is excluded.
- *Gamma-interferon and soluble interleukin 2 receptor levels* are also raised in tuberculous effusions compared with malignant effusions.
- *Estimation of pleural fluid rheumatoid factor and anti-nuclear antibodies* is useful in confirming the diagnosis of rheumatoid and lupus erythematosus, respectively.

In which conditions is the pleural fluid bloody?

Haemorrhagic fluid is seen in malignancy, pulmonary embolus, TB and trauma to the chest.

What are the earliest radiological signs of pleural fluid?

The earliest radiological signs are blunting of the costophrenic angle on the anterior–posterior view or loss of clear definition of the diaphragm posteriorly on the lateral view (Fig. 97.1).

When in doubt of a small effusion, how would you confirm your suspicions?

Either by a lateral decubitus view (which shows a layering of the fluid along the dependent chest wall unless the fluid is loculated) or by ultrasonography.

What are the other uses of ultrasonography in the diagnosis of pleural effusion?

Ultrasonography is also useful for loculated effusions, for guided thoracocentesis, closed pleural biopsy or insertion of a chest drain, and to differentiate pleural fluid from pleural thickening.

What is a pseudotumour?

It is the accumulation of fluid between the major or minor fissure or along the lateral chest wall, which can be mistaken for a tumour on the radiograph. Such loculated effusions can be confirmed with ultrasonography.

What do you know about pleural disease in rheumatoid arthritis?

About 70% of patients with rheumatoid arthritis have pleural inflammation at postmortem and about 5% have radiological evidence of pleural inflammation at some time. Pleural involvement is associated with male sex, rheumatoid factor in serum, the presence of nodules and other systemic manifestations. The effusion is thought to develop as an inflammatory response to the presence of multiple subpleural nodules. For reasons that are entirely unclear, the left side is the more common site of unilateral rheumatoid pleural effusions. The pleural fluid glucose level is characteristically low and is said to be caused by an 'entrance block' in which glucose is unable to enter the pleural space, unlike in empyema and malignant effusions where the low pleural fluid glucose concentration is attributed to the increased use of glucose by cells. Cytological appearances of slender and elongated macrophages, round giant multinucleated macrophages, presence of very few mesothelial cells and necrotic background material are thought to be pathognomonic of rheumatoid pleuritis.

What are the complications of thoracocentesis?

Pneumothorax, haemothorax, intravascular collapse and unilateral pulmonary oedema (the last after withdrawal of large quantities of fluid).

What do you know about Meigs syndrome?

Meigs syndrome comprises pleural effusion (usually right sided and a transudate) and ovarian malignancy (usually benign ovarian fibroma).

Mention some causes of drug-induced pleural effusion

Procainamide (associated with a lupus-like reaction), nitrofurantoin, dantrolene, methysergide, procarbazine, methotrexate, bromocriptine, practolol, amiodarone, mitomycin, bleomycin and minoxidil

The patient used to be a shipbuilder: what diagnosis would you consider?

It is most likely that this patient has malignant mesothelioma because he was exposed to asbestos (amphibole asbestos confers a higher risk of mesothelioma (dose for dose) than the more commonly used chrysotile or white asbestos, although the latter is as potent at causing carcinoma lung). Serum osteopontin levels may be used to distinguish individuals with exposure to asbestos who do not have cancer from those with exposure to asbestos who have pleural mesothelioma (N Engl J Med 2005;353:1564–73). If the diagnosis is confirmed, he should be advised to apply for industrial injuries benefit.

What are the mechanisms for abnormal accumulation of pleural fluid?

There are three main mechanisms:

- An abnormality of the pleura itself, such as neoplasm or inflammatory process, usually associated with increased permeability (e.g. increased vascular permeability in pneumonia)
- Disruption of the integrity of a fluid-containing structure within the pleural cavity, such as the thoracic duct, oesophagus, major blood vessels or tracheobronchial tree, with leakage of the contents into the pleural space (e.g. decreased lymphatic drainage as in mediastinal carcinomatosis)
- Abnormal hydrostatic or osmotic forces operating on an otherwise normal pleural surface and producing a transudate (e.g. increased hydrostatic pressure in heart failure, decreased osmotic pressure in nephrotic syndrome, increased intrapleural pressure as in atelectasis).

Further reading

Light RW: Pleural effusion, *N Engl J Med* 346:1971–1977 (classic article), 2002.

98 PLEURAL RUB

INSTRUCTION

This patient presented with sudden onset of lateral chest pain aggravated by deep inspiration and coughing.
Listen to this patient's chest.
Examine her chest.

SALIENT FEATURES

History

- Sharp localized pain worse on coughing or deep respiration
- Nature of the sputum (purulent expectoration in a patient with chest infection, haemoptysis in pulmonary embolism)
- Drug history (oral contraceptives).

Examination

- Pleural rub (superficial, scratchy, grating sound heard on deep inspiration).

Proceed as follows:

- Differentiate between pleural rub and crackles by asking the patient to cough and check whether or not there is any change in the nature (no change with the pleural rub).
- Tell the examiner that you would like to proceed by listening for tachycardia and right ventricular gallop (pulmonary embolism).

DIAGNOSIS

This patient has a pleural rub (lesion), which is caused by either underlying infection or pulmonary embolism (aetiology). You would like to analyse blood gases to determine whether she is hypoxic (functional status).

Be prepared to discuss prophylaxis of pulmonary embolism.

QUESTIONS

How would you investigate this patient?

- FBC
- Sputum cultures
- D-dimer: Plasma D-dimers are cross-linked fibrin derivatives produced when fibrin is degraded by plasmin. D-dimers are not specific for pulmonary embolism and are seen myocardial infarction, pneumonia, sepsis, cancer, during the second and third trimesters of pregnancy and after surgery. Therefore, this test is most useful in the emergency department, because most patients already in hospital have elevated D-dimers
- Blood gases
- ECG–RV strain (McGinn-White pattern). A normal electrocardiogram is very unusual in patients with massive acute pulmonary embolism (Fig. 98.1)
- Chest radiography: small wedge-shaped density at the periphery of the lungs indicates pulmonary infarction ('Hampton's hump'; Fig. 98.2)

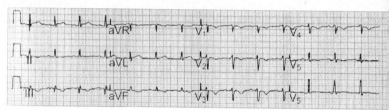

Fig. 98.1 ECG showing acute pulmonary embolism and moderately severe right ventricular dilatation and dysfunction on echocardiography (the McGinn-White pattern).

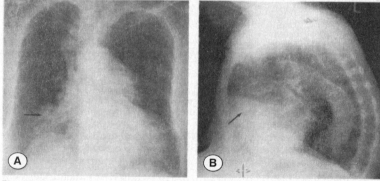

Fig. 98.2 Chest radiography showing a wedge-shaped pulmonary infarct (Hampton's hump) secondary to a pulmonary embolism (arrows). (With permission from Albert et al. 2008.)

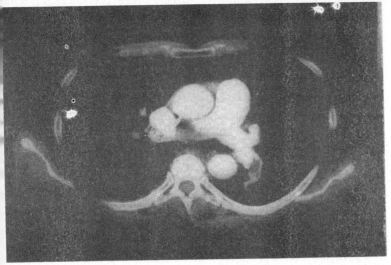

Fig. 98.3 CT shows bilateral central pulmonary embolism, with larger thrombus burden in the left than in the right pulmonary artery. (With permission from Goldhaber 2004.)

- Ventilation–perfusion scan: most scans are, however, of intermediate or indeterminate probability and, therefore, CT is increasingly becoming the test of choice
- CT chest has now emerged as the main imaging test in the work up of pulmonary embolism (Fig. 98.3). Chest CT has two advantages: thrombus can be directly visualized and alternative diagnoses can be established on lung parenchymal images that are not evident on chest radiography. It takes <30 s with a single breath-hold to minimize respiratory motion

ADVANCED-LEVEL QUESTIONS

What would you expect to see in the ventilation–perfusion scan in a patient with pulmonary embolism?

In acute pulmonary embolism the area of decreased perfusion usually has normal ventilation, whereas in pneumonia there are abnormalities in both the ventilation and perfusion scan.

How would you treat a patient with pulmonary embolism?
- Anticoagulation, thrombolysis, or IVC filter
- Pain relief for pleurisy.

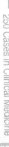

99 ASTHMA

INSTRUCTION

Examine this patient's chest.

SALIENT FEATURES

History

- Determine whether there is a reversible airway obstruction by history: whether the wheezing and breathlessness is reversible
- Tightness in the chest
- Recurrent cough
- Exacerbation of the cough or wheeze at night or after exercise
- Improvement of the cough or wheeze with bronchodilator therapy
- Fever, yellowish sputum
- History of atopy (eczema, hay fever)
- History of rhinitis, nasal polyps
- History of trigger factors such as cold air, emotion, vapors, dust, drugs (e.g. beta-blockers), pollution, viral infections, pets, pollen.

Examination

- Bilateral scattered wheeze
- Examine the sputum cup.

Comment on accessory muscles of respiration, tachycardia, pulsus paradoxus and whether the patient can speak sentences without stopping to take a breath.

DIAGNOSIS

This patient has a history of hay fever and bilateral scattered wheeze (lesion) caused by bronchial asthma (aetiology), and is breathless at rest (functional status).

QUESTIONS

Mention a few trigger factors known to aggravate asthma

- Infection
- Emotion
- Exercise
- Drugs, e.g. beta-blockers
- External allergens.

What do you understand by the term asthma?

Asthma is an inflammatory disorder characterized by hyper-responsiveness of the airway to various stimuli, resulting in widespread narrowing of the airway. The changes are reversible, either spontaneously or through therapy. The inflammatory response includes T lymphocytes, mast cells and eosinophils, and it is associated with exudation of plasma, oedema, smooth muscle hypertrophy, deposition of matrix, mucus plugging and epithelial damage.

ADVANCED-LEVEL QUESTIONS

What do you understand by intrinsic asthma?

Intrinsic asthma is of non-allergic aetiology and usually begins after the age of 30 years. It tends to be more continuous and more severe; status asthmaticus is common in this group.

What do you understand by extrinsic asthma?

Extrinsic asthma has a clearly defined history of allergy to a variety of inhaled factors and is characterized by a childhood onset and seasonal variation.

What are the indications for steroids in chronic asthma?

- Sleep is disturbed by wheeze
- Morning tightness persists until midday
- Symptoms and peak expiratory flows progressively deteriorate each day
- Maximum treatment with bronchodilators
- Emergency nebulizers are needed.

What is the effect of reducing or discontinuing inhaled budesonide in patients with mild asthma?

Early treatment with inhaled budesonide results in long-lasting control of mild asthma (i.e. the forced expiratory volume is >85% of predicted value). Maintenance therapy can usually be given at a reduced dose, but discontinuation of treatment is often accompanied by exacerbation of the disease.

How would you manage a patient with acute asthma?

- Nebulized beta-agonists, e.g. terbutaline or salbutamol
- Oxygen, using a high concentration
- High-dose steroids: intravenous hydrocortisone or oral prednisolone or both
- Blood gases
- Chest radiography to rule out pneumothorax (Fig. 99.1)
- *When life-threatening features* are present:
  - add ipratropium to nebulized beta-agonist
  - intravenous aminophylline or salbutamol or terbutaline.

What do you know about the British Thoracic Society step care regimen for the management of chronic asthma in adults?

Patients should be started on treatment at the step most appropriate to the initial severity (Thorax 1997;52:S1–24). A rescue course of prednisolone may be needed at any time and at any step. Stepwise reduction in treatment should be undertaken after the asthma has been stable over a period of 3–6 months.

Step 1, mild intermittent asthma: inhaled short-acting beta2-agonist used as required for symptom relief. If required more than once, go to step 2.

Step 2, regular preventer therapy: step 1 plus inhaled steroid therapy (200–400 µg/day).

Step 3, initial add on therapy: long-acting beta2-agonist (LABA) and assess control of asthma:

(a) If good response, continue LABA

(b) If some response, increase inhaled steroid to 400 µg/day (if not already on dose

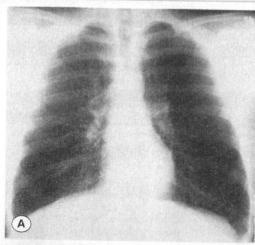

Fig. 99.1 Asthma. During a severe attack, hyperinflation (arrows) occurs, similar to that seen in COPD. Most patients with asthma have normal chest radiographs when not in an attack (compare with COPD in Fig. 100.1). (With permission from Mettler 2004.)

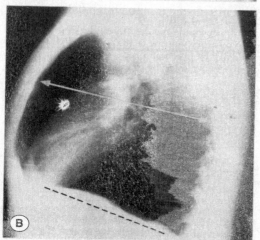

(c) If no response, stop LABA and increase steroids to 400 μg/day
(d) If control still inadequate consider sustained-release theophylline or leukotriene receptor antagonist.

Step 4, persistent poor control:
- Consider trial of inhaled steroid 2000 μg/day
- Consider adding a fourth drug such as leukotriene receptor antagonist (e.g. montelukast), sustained-release theophylline
- Consider adding tablet of beta2 agonist.

Step 5, continuous use of oral or frequent steroids:
- Consider low-dose oral steroids
- Maintain inhaled steroid at 2000 μg/day
- Consider other therapies to minimize steroid therapy
- Refer to respiratory physician.

What are the features of acute severe asthma?
- Inability to complete a sentence in one breath
- Respiration rate >25 breaths/min
- Pulse rate >110 beats/min
- Peak expiratory flow rate <50% of predicted or best.

What are the life-threatening indicators in acute asthma?
- Peak expiratory flow rate <33% of predicted or best
- Exhaustion, confusion, coma
- Silent chest, cyanosis or feeble respiratory effort
- Bradycardia or hypotension.

Note: Arterial blood gases should be measured if *any* of these features are present or if oxygen saturation is <92%.

What are the indicators of a very severe, life-threatening attack?
- Normal (5–6 kPa, 36–45 mmHg) or increased carbon dioxide tension (>6 kPa or 45 mmHg)
- Severe hypoxia of <8 kPa (60 mmHg)
- Low or falling arterial pH.

What is the value of assessing pulsus paradoxus in a patient with acute severe asthma?
It is a poor guide to the severity of acute asthma as it compares poorly with the measurement of peak flow.

In which other conditions is wheeze a prominent sign?
COPD, left ventricular failure (cardiac asthma), polyarteritis nodosa, eosinophilic lung disease, recurrent thromboembolism, tumour causing localized wheeze.

What are the indications for mechanical ventilation with intermittent positive pressure ventilation?
- Worsening hypoxia (arterial partial pressure of oxygen (PaO) <8 kPa) despite 60% inspired oxygen
- Hypercapnia ($PaCO_2$ >6 kPa)
- Drowsiness
- Unconsciousness
- Intermittent positive pressure ventilation.

What do you understand by the term severe brittle asthma?
This condition is characterized by life-threatening attacks, which can develop within hours or sometimes even within minutes and can lead to sudden death.

What do you know about Beta receptor polymorphisms in asthma?
Glycine homozygous patients do well on regular beta2-agonists whether short or long acting.

Long- and short-acting beta2-agonists produce disparate responses: for example a lack of increased bronchial hyper-responsiveness associated with long-acting beta2-agonists but is commonly seen with short-acting beta2-agonists.

All genotypes and beta2-agonists are associated with receptor desensitization but not associated with worsening asthma.

Specific label changes for long-acting beta-agonists

1. The use of LABAs for asthma in patients of all ages is contraindicated without concomitant use of an asthma-controller medication such as an inhaled corticosteroid.
2. Stop use of the LABA, if possible, once asthma control is achieved and maintain the use of an asthma-controller medication, such as an inhaled corticosteroid.
3. Recommend against LABA use in patients whose asthma is adequately controlled with a low- or medium-dose inhaled corticosteroid.
4. Recommend that a fixed-dose combination product containing a LABA and an inhaled corticosteroid be used to ensure compliance with concomitant therapy in pediatric and adolescent patients who require the addition of a LABA to an inhaled corticosteroid.

100   CHRONIC BRONCHITIS

INSTRUCTION

Examine this patient's chest.

SALIENT FEATURES

History

- Productive cough
- Increasing dyspnoea
- Weight loss
- History of smoking
- History of α_1-antitrypsin deficiency.

Examination

- Begin with examination of the *sputum pot*.

Observe the patient:

- From the end of the bed: for obvious breathlessness, pursed lip breathing and symmetrical chest movements—and count respiratory rate.
- Look for nail changes such as tar staining.
- Feel the palms for warmth and the pulse for rapid bounding pulse (signs of carbon dioxide retention).
- Look at the lips and tongue for central cyanosis.

Examine the neck:

- Comment on the active contractions of the accessory muscles of respiration such as sternocleidomastoids, scaleni and trapezii.
- Palpate for tracheal deviation and measure the distance between the cricoid cartilage and suprasternal notch (less than three fingers' breadth in emphysema).
- Comment on the raised JVP.

Examine the chest:

- Comment on barrel-shaped chest
- Inspiratory retraction of the lower ribs (Hoover's sign)

- Use of accessory muscles of respiration.
- Palpate for:
  - apex beat
  - chest expansion
  - vocal fremitus.
- Percuss looking for:
  - hyper-resonance and obliteration of cardiac and liver dullness.
- Auscultate for:
  - breath sounds (diminished breath sounds)
  - vocal resonance
  - forced expiratory time (FET): the end-point is detected by auscultating over the trachea in the suprasternal notch; normal individuals can empty their chest from full inspiration in ≤4 s and prolongation to >6 s indicates airflow obstruction.
  - loud pulmonary second heart sound.

Examine the abdomen:
- Palpable liver to look for hepatic displacement (comment on upper border of liver by percussion).

Finally:
  Tell the examiner that this patient is at increased risk for cardiovascular disease, osteoporosis, lung cancer and depression.

  Remember: Airflow obstruction as measured by spirometry is defined as a ratio of the postbronchodilator forced expiratory volume in 1 s (FEV_1) to forced vital capacity (FVC) of <0.70.

DIAGNOSIS

This patient has features of COPD (lesion) caused by cigarette smoking (aetiology) and is very cyanosed at rest (functional status).

QUESTIONS

What do you understand by the term chronic bronchitis?
Chronic bronchitis is cough with mucoid expectoration for at least 3 months in a year for 2 successive years.

What is the definition of emphysema?
Emphysema is the abnormal permanent enlargement of the airway distal to the terminal respiratory bronchioles with destruction of their walls. Clinical, radiological and lung function tests give an imprecise picture in an individual case but a combination of all these features gives a reasonable picture.

What do you understand by the term chronic obstructive pulmonary disease?
COPD is a condition characterized by airflow limitation that is not fully reversible and is usually progressive and associated with an abnormal inflammatory response. The term COPD encompasses chronic obstructive bronchitis (with obstruction of small airways) and emphysema (with destruction of lung parenchyma, loss of lung elasticity and closure of small airways). Most patients also have mucus plugging (N Engl J Med 2000;343:269).

ADVANCED-LEVEL QUESTIONS

What is the mechanism reduction in expiratory capacity in chronic obstructive pulmonary disease?

Dynamic hyperinflation is considered to be an important factor in the reduction of exercise capacity and the development of dyspnoea.

COPD is caused by a variable mixture of three processes including loss of alveolar attachments, inflammatory obstruction of the airway and luminal obstruction with mucus. Alveolar attachments ensure a radial tethering effect, which is important for keeping small airways patent in the normal lung. At smaller lung volumes, airways narrow because of decreased lung elasticity and weaker tethering effects. As a result, maximal expiratory airflow decreases as the lung empties and ceases at 25 to 35% of total lung capacity. The remaining air (or residual volume) may account for as much as 60 to 70% of predicted total lung capacity. Patients with COPD must breathe at larger lung volumes to optimize expiratory airflow, but this requires greater respiratory work because the lungs and chest wall become stiffer at larger volumes. These effects are worse with exercise. A normal lung meets the increased ventilatory demands of exercise by increasing both tidal volume and respiratory rate, with little change in the final end-expiratory lung volume. Whereas in COPD the respiratory rate does increase in response to exercise, but with insufficient expiratory time, breaths become increasingly shallow and end-expiratory lung volume progressively enlarges, a phenomenon called dynamic hyperinflation (N Engl J Med 2010;362:1407–16).

What is the role of inflammatory mechanisms in chronic obstructive pulmonary disease?

In COPD, reactive oxygen species (ROS), pathogen associated molecular patterns (PAMPs), and damage-associated molecular patterns (DAMPs) activate families of pattern recognition receptors (PRRs) that include the toll-like receptors (TLRs). This understanding has led to the hypothesis that COPD is also a disease of innate immunity. COPD is characterized by abnormal response to injury, with altered barrier function of the respiratory tract, an acute phase reaction and excessive activation of macrophages, neutrophils and fibroblasts in the lung. Macrophages and epithelial cells in airways are activated by cigarette smoke and other irritants (in developing countries, the inhalation of smoke from biomass fuels is an important cause of COPD, particularly among women who cook in poorly ventilated homes) and these release neutrophil chemotactic factors including interleukin-8 and leukotriene B_4. Neutrophils and macrophages then release proteases that break down connective tissue in the lung parenchyma, resulting in emphysema, and also stimulate hypersecretion of bronchial mucus. The chronic inflammatory process in COPD differs markedly from that seen in bronchial asthma, with different inflammatory cells, mediators, inflammatory effects and responses to treatment.

What is the role of proteolysis in chronic obstructive pulmonary disease?

In COPD, the protease-antiprotease balance is tipped in favour of proteolysis because of either an increase in proteases (including neutrophil elastase, proteinase 3, cathepsins, matrix metalloproteases 1, 2, 9 and 12) or a deficiency of antiproteases (including α_1-antitrypsin, elafin, secretory leukoprotease inhibitor and tissue inhibitors of matrix metalloproteases).

What is the main cause of death and disability in chronic obstructive pulmonary disease?

Mortality and disability from COPD is related to an accelerated decline in lung function over time, with a loss of >50–60 ml/year in the forced expiratory volume in 1 s (FEV_1), compared with a normal loss of 20–30 ml/year. The progressive reduction in FEV_1 and increasing severity of disease over time result in increasing dyspnoea on exertion, which slowly advances to respiratory failure.

What is explanation for the cardiac silhouette on chest radiography in patients with emphysema?

In patients with emphysema, the cardiac silhouette on chest radiography is typically long and narrow (Fig. 100.1). The common explanation for this

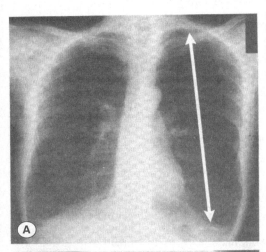

Fig. 100.1 COPD.
(A) The superior aspect of the hemidiaphragms is at the same level as the posterior aspect of the twelfth ribs.
(B) Hyperinflation. (With permission from Mettler 2004.)

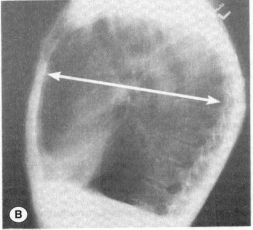

finding is the altered, more vertical position of the heart in the thoracic cavity. A recent study suggested an alternative explanation for this finding: a decreased left ventricular volume (N Engl J Med 2010;362:217). This study also reported a linear relation to impaired left ventricular filling, reduced stroke volume and lower cardiac output without changes in the ejection fraction.

What is the role of high-resolution CT in the diagnosis of emphysema?

It is the most sensitive technique for the diagnosis of emphysema. It is useful in evaluating symptomatic patients with almost normal pulmonary function except for a low carbon monoxide diffusing capacity — a combination of findings that occurs in emphysema, interstitial lung disease and pulmonary vascular disease (Radiology 1992;182:817–21).

How would you differentiate emphysema from chronic bronchitis?

	Predominant bronchitis	Perdominant emphysema
Age (years)	40–45	50–75
Appearance	Blue bloater	Pink puffer
Dyspnoea	Mild; late	Severe; early
Cough	Early; copious sputum	Late; scanty sputum
Infections	Common	Occasional
Respiratory insufficiency	Repeated	Terminal
Cor pulmonale	Common	Rare; terminal
Airway resistance	Increased	Normal or slightly increased
Elastic recoil	Normal	Low
Chest radiograph	Prominent vessels; large heart	Hyperinflation; small heart

From Kumar et al. Pathologic Basis of Disease, 8th edn. Saunders.

If the patient was between the ages of 30 and 45 years, what would you consider to be the underlying cause of the emphysema?

Smoking, α_1-antitrypsin deficiency.

What medications are commonly used in outpatient treatment of chronic obstructive pulmonary disease?

- Short-acting bronchodilators:
  - Beta2-adrenergic agonist: albuterol
  - Anti-cholinergic agent: ipratropium
  - Combination: albuterol–ipratropium.
- Long-acting bronchodilators:
  - Beta2-adrenergic agonists: salmeterol, formoterol, arformoterol
  - Anticholinergic agent: tiotropium.

- Inhaled corticosteroids: fluticasone, budesonide, beclomethasone, mometasone
- Combination beta2-adrenergic agonist bronchodilator with inhaled corticosteroid:
  - Fluticasone–salmeterol
  - Budesonide–formoterol.
- Methylxanthine: 24-hour sustained-release theophylline.

Note: Influenza and pneumococcal vaccinations and pulmonary rehabilitation (including education, exercise, behaviour modification and interventions to improve social and psychological functioning) are important therapeutic measures in COPD.

How would you treat an acute exacerbation?

- Nebulized bronchodilators: terbutaline, ipratropium bromide
- Intravenous antibiotics (BMJ 1994;308:871–872), initially with amoxicillin and, if no clinical response, then with a second-generation cephalosporin, quinoline or co-amoxiclav. Antibiotics decrease the relative risk of treatment failure by approximately 50% in exacerbations (Cochrane Database Syst Rev 2006;2:CD004403)
- Oxygen (24%)
- Intravenous hydrocortisone and oral steroids (steroids useful in only acute exacerbations and, unlike in asthma, do not influence the course of chronic bronchitis). Systemic steroids reduced the relative risk of treatment failure (as defined by intensification of therapy, rehospitalization or return to the emergency department) by about 30% in patients with acute exacerbations who were hospitalized or seen in the emergency department (N Engl J Med 1999;340:1941–7; N Engl J Med 2003;348:2618–25).

What is the role of inhaled steroids in chronic obstructive pulmonary disease?

Inhaled steroids reduce the frequency of exacerbations by 15–20%. The combination of an inhaled corticosteroid with a long-acting beta-agonist reduces exacerbations compared with either therapy alone.

What are the organisms commonly associated with exacerbations of chronic obstructive pulmonary disease?

Haemophilus influenzae and *Streptococcus pneumoniae* are the commonest organisms identified in the sputum during exacerbations of COPD, accounting for 43% and 25%, respectively, of positive cultures in one study. *Moraxella* (previously *Branhamella*) *catarrhalis* is also frequently isolated from sputum during exacerbations. Less commonly, *Chlamydia pneumoniae* or *Pseudomonas aeruginosa* has been associated with some exacerbations.

What clinical features would suggest that this patient is suitable for long-term domiciliary oxygen therapy?

- COPD: FEV_1 <1500 ml, FVC <2000 ml and stable chronic respiratory failure (PaO <7.3 kPa, that is, 55 mmHg or oxygen saturation <88% at normal blood pH) in patients who have (1) had peripheral oedema or (2) not necessarily had hypercapnia or oedema (New Engl J Med 1995;333:710–14); carboxyhaemoglobin of <3% (i.e. patients who have stopped smoking)
- Terminally ill patients of whatever cause with severe hypoxia (PaO <7.3 kPa).

Note: If the patient's oxygen saturation is ≤88% at rest in a clinical stable state, long-term oxygen therapy should be prescribed and used for at least 18 h each day.

How can the sensation of breathlessness be reduced?
By the use of either promethazine or dihydrocodeine.

How would you treat acute respiratory failure?
If PaO is <8 kPa, administer 24% oxygen. There is no need for oxygen when PaO is >8 kPa. Monitor blood gases after 30 min. If $PaCO_2$ is rising (by 1 kPa), monitor blood gases hourly. If $PaCO_2$ continues to rise, administer doxapram. If, in spite of this, the patient continues to deteriorate, artificial ventilation may be called for.

What do you know about non-invasive ventilation?
Non-invasive ventilation is an alternative approach to endotracheal intubation to treat hypercapnic ventilatory failure, which occurs in COPD. It reduces the complications of endotracheal intubation such as infection and injury to the trachea. Non-invasive ventilation is pressure-support ventilation delivered with a face mask and a piece of white foam placed in the face mask to reduce the amount of internal dead space. In a recent randomized trial, non-invasive ventilation was shown to reduce the need for endotracheal intubation, length of hospital stay and in-hospital mortality rate in selected patients with acute exacerbations of COPD (N Engl J Med 1995;333:817–22).

What do you know about the BODE index?
The BODE index combines information about several predictors in a score ranging from 0 to 10, including:
- **b**ody mass index (BMI)
- **a**irflow obstruction (FEV_1)
- **d**yspnoea (Medical Research Council dyspnoea scale)
- **e**xercise capacity (6 min walk distance) in a score ranging from 0 to 10.

This prognostic index predicts mortality significantly better than FEV (the traditional prognostic COPD indicator) alone.

What do you know about molecular genetics of chronic obstructive pulmonary disease?
- Deficiency of α_1-antitrypsin:
- It was first described in Sweden. The patient is deficient in α_1-antitrypsin, with activity approximately 15% of normal values; concentrations of 40% or more are required for health. The patient is homozygous for the gene (Z) encoding a protease inhibitor (Pi). Other genetic combinations and their percentage normal activity are MS (80%), MZ (60%), SS (60%), SZ (40%). Six per cent of the population is heterozygous for S(PiMS) and 4% for Z(PiMZ), making an overall frequency of 1 in 10 for the carriage of the defective gene. Liver transplantation results in conversion to the genotype of the donor.
- In the lung α_1-antitrypsin inhibits the excessive actions of neutrophil and macrophage elastase, which cigarette smoke promotes. When the lung is heavily exposed to cigarette smoke, the protective effect of α_1-antitrypsin may be overwhelmed by the amount of elastase released or by a direct oxidative action of cigarette smoke on the α_1-antitrypsin molecule. The emphysema is panacinar and is seen in the lower lobes

of the lungs. Smoking increases the severity of, and decreases the age of onset of, emphysema. Liver disease is a much less common complication. Human α_1-antitrypsin prepared from pooled plasma from normal donors is recommended for patients over 18 years with serum levels below 11 µmol/l and abnormal lung function.

- The siblings of an index case should be screened for this disorder. Their identification should be followed by counselling to avoid smoking and occupations with atmospheric pollution. Children of homozygotes will inherit at least one Z gene and hence will be heterozygotes. They should avoid pairing with another heterozygote if they wish to avoid the risk of producing an affected homozygote.

- **Tumour necrosis factor-alpha** COPD is 10 times more common in Taiwanese with a polymorphism in the promoter region of the gene for Tumour necrosis factor-alpha, resulting in its increased production (Am J Respir Crit Care Med 1997;156:136–9). However, the same polymorphism in the UK population is not associated with increased risk of COPD (Eur Respir J 2000;15:281–4).

- **Microsomal epoxide hydrolase** A polymorphism variant of microsomal epoxide hydrolase, an enzyme involved in the metabolism of the epoxides that may be generated in tobacco smoke, has been associated with a quintupling of the risk of COPD (Lancet 1997;350:663).

What is the role of surgery in chronic obstructive pulmonary disease?

- Bullectomy may improve gas exchange and airflow, and reduce dyspnoea in selected patients with bullae larger than one-third of the hemithorax and accompanying lung compression.
- Lung-volume reduction surgery (N Engl J Med 2000;343:239–45) results in functional improvements including increased FEV_1, reduced total lung capacity, improved function of respiratory muscles, improved exercise capacity and improved quality of life (J Thorac Cardiovasc Surg 1999;112:1319–29, Am J Respir Crit Care Med 1999;160:2018–27). The National Emphysema Treatment Trial Group found that lung-volume reduction surgery increased the chance of improved exercise capacity but did not confer a survival advantage over medical therapy. It did yield a survival advantage for patients with both predominantly upper-lobe emphysema and low baseline exercise capacity. Patients previously reported to be at high risk and those with non-upper-lobe emphysema and high baseline exercise capacity are poor candidates for lung-volume reduction surgery because of increased mortality and negligible functional gain (N Engl J Med 2003;348:2059–73).
- Single lung transplantation has been successful for at least 3–4 years in patients with COPD. The criteria for selecting patients for transplantation have not been established. It does not improve survival but improved quality of life (J Thorac Cardiovasc Surg 1991;101:623–32, J Heart Lung Transplantation 2006;25:75–84).

What is the best method for communicating spirometry findings to patients?

Results from studies suggest that providing feedback on lung age with graphic displays may be the best option so far for communicating the results of spirometry. More patients are likely to stop smoking when spirometry results, as communicated using Fletcher and Peto's diagram (a pictorial representation of how smoking ages the lungs), are shared with the patient (Thorax 2006;61:869–73, BMJ 2008;336:567–8).

What are the general indications for lung transplantation?

The general indication is end-stage lung disease without alternative forms of therapy. Patients should be <60 years of age and should have a life expectancy of <12–18 months; they should not have an underlying cancer or other serious systemic illness. The most common lung diseases are pulmonary fibrosis, emphysema (particularly α_1-antitrypsin deficiency), bronchiectasis, cystic fibrosis and primary pulmonary hypertension.

What is the role of nutrition in chronic obstructive pulmonary disease?

Undernutrition is associated with reduced respiratory muscle function and an increased mortality rate. A high dietary intake of n-3 fatty acids may protect cigarette smokers against COPD.

Mention some newer treatments for chronic obstructive pulmonary disease

- Antagonists of inflammatory mediators: 5-lipoxygenase inhibitors, leukotriene B_4 antagonists, interleukin-8 antagonists, tumour necrosis factor inhibitors and antioxidants
- Protease inhibitors: neutrophil elastase inhibitors, cathepsin inhibitors, non-selective matrix metalloprotease inhibitors, elafin, secretory leukoprotease inhibitor, α_1-antitrypsin
- New anti-inflammatory agents: phosphodieasterase-4 inhibitors, nuclear factor-κB inhibitors, adhesion molecule inhibitors and p38 mitogen-activated protein kinase inhibitors (N Engl J Med 2000; 343:1960–1).

Further reading

American Thoracic Society (ATS)/European Respiratory Society (ERS): Standards for the diagnosis and treatment of COPD. www.ersnet.org.

Cochrane Airways Group (up-to-date, accurate systematic reviews and meta-analyses). www.cochrane-airways.ac.uk.

United Kingdom National Institute for Clinical Excellence (NICE). COPD guidelines. www.nice.org.uk.

World Health Organization Global Initiative for Obstructive Lung Disease (GOLD) resources. www.goldcopd.com.

Peter Howard, contemporary chest physician, Sheffield; his chief interest is long-term domiciliary oxygen therapy.

Peter Barnes, contemporary physician and professor, National Heart and Lung Institute London.

Sir Michael Rawlins is the founding chairman of National Institute for Health and Clinical Excellence (NICE). From 1973 to 2006, Rawlins was the Ruth and Lionel Jacobson Professor of Clinical Pharmacology University of Newcastle. Rawlins obtained his medical degree at St Thomas' Hospital. His post-graduate training in clinical pharmacology and general medicine was completed at St Thomas' http://en.wikipedia.org/wiki/Hammersmith_ Hospital" \o "Hammersmith Hospital" Hammersmith hospitals, with a year at the Karolinska Institute in Stockholm.

101 BRONCHIECTASIS

INSTRUCTION

Examine this patient's chest.
Listen to this patient's chest.

SALIENT FEATURES

History

- Cough with copious purulent sputum, recurrent haemoptysis
- Intermittent fever and night sweats
- History of recurrent chest infections
- Weight loss.

Examination

- Copious purulent expectoration (remember to check the sputum cup in a chest case)
- Finger clubbing
- Bilateral coarse, late, inspiratory crackles.

Proceed as follows:

- Comment on kyphoscoliosis if any
- Tell the examiner that you would like to know whether the bronchiectasis is long standing; if so, you would like to examine the abdomen for splenomegaly (amyloidosis).

In addition there may be signs of collapse, fibrosis or pneumonia.

DIAGNOSIS

This patient has bilateral, coarse, late inspiratory crackles with purulent sputum (lesion) caused by bronchiectasis (aetiology), and is cyanosed.

QUESTIONS

What do you understand by bronchiectasis?

It is a chronic necrotizing infection of the bronchi and bronchioles leading to abnormal, permanent dilatation of the airways.

Mention the causes of bronchiectasis

- Postpneumonic, measles, pertussis, TB
- Mechanical bronchial obstruction, as in TB, carcinoma, nodal compression
- Allergic bronchopulmonary aspergillosis
- Gammaglobulin deficiency, congenital, acquired
- Immotile cilia syndrome (Kartagener syndrome)
- Cystic fibrosis
- Neuropathic disorders (namely Riley–Day syndrome, Chagas' disease)
- Inflammatory bowel disease, rheumatoid arthritis
- Idiopathic.

What investigations would you do in such a patient?

FBC
Sputum culture
Chest radiography

Bronchography
CT scan of the chest.

ADVANCED-LEVEL QUESTIONS

How can CT assess bronchiectasis?

High-resolution CT performed at the end of expiration suggests that small airways disease may be an early feature of bronchiectasis, which then leads to more progressive injury and bronchiolar distortion. Larger studies with long-term follow-up are required to confirm this. Conventional CT has a sensitivity of 60–80% for detecting bronchiectasis, whereas high-resolution CT has a sensitivity of >90%, using bronchography as the 'gold standard'.

Specific abnormalities found on high-resolution CT (Fig. 101.1) include:
- dilatation of an airway lumen (rendering it >1.5 times as wide as a nearby vessel)
- lack of tapering of an airway toward the periphery
- varicose constrictions along airways
- ballooned cysts at the end of a bronchus (the bullae found in patients with emphysema have thinner walls and are away from an airway).

Non-specific findings include:
- consolidation or infiltration of a lobe with dilatation of the airways
- thickening of the bronchial walls, mucous plugs
- enlarged lymph nodes

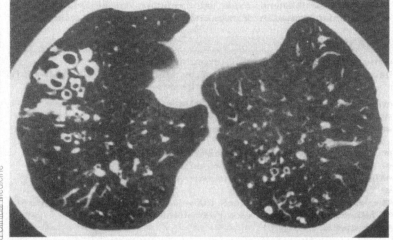

Fig. 101.1 Severe bronchiectasis in the right lower lobe with plugging of the dilated bronchi. Mild, cylindric bronchiectasis in the left lower lobe showing the signet ring sign. (With permission from Albert et al. 2008.)

● a reduction in vascular markings similar to that seen in emphysema (probably as a result of the inflammatory destruction of smaller airways and vessels).

Note: Cystic fibrosis and allergic bronchopulmonary aspergillosis involve an upper-lobe distribution, and *Mycobacterium avium* complex infection often involves the middle lobe or lingula. Bronchiectasis usually affects the lower lobe.

What is the difference between standard and high-resolution CT?

In standard CT, the resolution is 10 mm thick whereas with high-resolution CT the slices are 1–1.5 mm thick and high spatial resolution algorithms are used to reconstruct images (Radiology 1994;193:369–74).

What do you know about spiral CT?

This is a rapidly evolving technique to image the chest and has the advantage of creating truly contiguous sections; consequently totally seamless reconstructions are possible. This may allow virtual-reality bronchoscopy imaging. Spiral CT may elucidate additional subtle changes, because it reduces motion artefact, but it requires a larger dose of radiation.

What are the complications of bronchiectasis?

● Pneumonia, pleurisy, pleural effusion, pneumothorax
● Sinusitis
● Haemoptysis (life-threatening haemoptysis is >600 ml/day)
● Brain abscess
● Amyloidosis.

What are the major respiratory pathogens in bronchiectasis?

Staphylococcus aureus, Haemophilus influenzae, Pseudomonas aeruginosa.

How would you treat such patients?

● Identification of acute exacerbations and administration of antibiotics
● Suppression of the microbial load
● Treatment of underlying conditions
● Reduction of the excessive inflammatory response
● Promotion of bronchial hygiene:
  • Postural drainage
  • Bronchodilators.
● Control of bronchial haemorrhage
● Surgery in selected cases: surgical removal of extremely damaged segments or lobes that may be a nidus for infection or bleeding.

What abnormalities may be associated with bronchiectasis?

● Congenital absence of bronchial cartilage (Williams–Campbell syndrome)
● Tracheobronchomegaly (Mounier–Kuhn syndrome)
● Obstructive azoospermia and chronic sinopulmonary infection (Young syndrome), said to be caused by mercury intoxication. It was first described in the north of England by Young in 1970
● Congenital kyphoscoliosis
● Situs inversus and paranasal sinusitis (Kartagener syndrome) (p. 117)
● Unilateral absence of pulmonary artery.

What is the indication for surgery in bronchiectasis?

Bronchiectasis localized to a single lobe or a segment without clinical, bronchographic or CT evidence of bronchiectasis or bronchitis affecting other parts of the lung.

What are the common sites for localized disease?

Left lower lobe and lingula.

What do you understand by the term bronchiectasis sicca?

Bronchiectasis or 'dry' bronchiectasis is that which presents with recurrent dry cough associated with intermittent episodes (months or years apart) of haemoptysis. The haemoptysis can be life threatening as bleeding is from bronchial vessels with systemic pressures. There is usually a past history of granulomatous infection, particularly TB. The upper lobes are often primarily affected, allowing good drainage.

What do you know about bronchiectasis in allergic bronchopulmonary aspergillosis?

The bronchial dilatation occurs in more proximal bronchi as a result of type III immune complex reactions.

What do you know about Reid's classification of bronchiectasis?

In 1950, Reid correlated pathological changes with bronchography and described three different appearances:

- Cylindrical bronchiectasis: bronchi that are uniformly dilated (to >2 mm but can be so large as to admit a finger) and do not taper but rather end abruptly; caused by plugging of smaller bronchi by thick mucus and casts
- Varicose bronchiectasis: dilated bronchi with irregular bulging contours similar to a varicose vein and no tapering; terminations are bulbous and bronchial subdivisions are reduced
- Cystic or saccular bronchiectasis is the most severe form and is characterized by sharply reduced bronchial subdivisions and dilated bronchi ending in cystic pus-filled cavities.

All the three types can be present in the same patient.

What are the modes of presentation of the bronchiectasis?

Bronchiectasis may be diffuse or focal disease. There are three types of focal airway obstruction that may lead to bronchiectasis:

- Luminal blockage by a foreign body, broncholith or slowly growing beinign tumour
- Extrinsic narrowing caused by enlarged lymph nodes (e.g. in middle lobe syndrome, which involves a small angulated orifice surrounded by a collar of lymph nodes that may enlarge and encroach on the main airway after granulomatous disease caused by infection with mycobacteria or fungi
- Twisting or displacement of the airways after a lobar resection (e.g. the occasional cephalad displacement of a lower lobe after surgery for the resection of the upper lobe).

Note: Recurrent or persistent lobar pneumonia is a key distinguishing feature of the first two types of focal bronchiectasis and is important to recognize because interventional bronchoscopy or surgery may result in palliation and sometimes cure.

Laennec was the first to describe bronchiectasis in 1819.

M Kartagener (1897–1975), a Swiss physician.

CM Riley and RL Day, both US paediatricians. Riley–Day syndrome consists of dysautonomia and lack of coordination in swallowing.

CJR Chagas (1879–1934) a Brazilian physician.

102 COR PULMONALE

INSTRUCTION

Examine this patient's chest.

SALIENT FEATURES

History

- Symptoms of COPD (p. 369)
- Easy fatiguability, shortness of breath on exertion, weakness
- Leg oedema, and right upper quadrant pain.

Examination

- Patient is short of breath at rest and is centrally cyanosed
- Tar staining of the fingers
- JVP is raised: both 'a' and 'v' waves are seen, 'v' waves being prominent if there is associated tricuspid regurgitation
- On examination of the chest, there is bilateral wheeze and other signs of chronic bronchitis (p. 368).

Proceed as follows:

- Examine the cardiovascular system for signs of pulmonary hypertension:
  - Left parasternal heave (often absent when the chest is barrel shaped)
  - Right ventricular gallop rhythm
  - Loud P and a loud ejection click
  - Pansystolic murmur of tricuspid regurgitation
  - Early diastolic Graham Steell murmur in the pulmonary area.
- Look for signs of:
  - Hepatomegaly
  - Pedal oedema.

DIAGNOSIS

This patient has chronic cor pulmonale (lesion) caused by long-standing COAD (aetiology) and is in congestive cardiac failure (functional status).

QUESTIONS

What do you understand by the term cor pulmonale?

Cor pulmonale is right ventricular enlargement caused by the increase in afterload that occurs in diseases of the lung, chest wall or pulmonary circulation.

Mention a few causes of cor pulmonale

Respiratory disorders:
- Obstructive:
  - COAD
  - Chronic persistent asthma.
- Restrictive:
  - Intrinsic: interstitial fibrosis, lung resection
  - Extrinsic: obesity, muscle weakness, kyphoscoliosis, high altitude.

Pulmonary vascular disorders:
- Pulmonary emboli (Fig. 102.1)
- Vasculitis of the small pulmonary arteries
- Adult respiratory distress syndrome
- Primary pulmonary hypertension.

ADVANCED-LEVEL QUESTIONS

How would you manage a patient with cor pulmonale?

- Treat the underlying cause
- Treat respiratory failure. If PaO is <8 kPa, administer 24% oxygen. There is no need for oxygen if PaO is >8 kPa. Monitor blood gases after 30 min. If $PaCO_2$ is rising (by 1 kPa), monitor blood gases hourly. If $PaCO_2$ continues to rise, administer doxapram. If, in spite of this, the deterioration continues, the patient may merit artificial ventilation
- Treat cardiac failure with furosemide
- Consider venesection if the haematocrit is >55% (*Lancet* 1989;ii:20–1)
- Consider heart–lung transplantation in young patients.

What is the prognosis in cor pulmonale?
Approximately 50% of patients succumb within 5 years.

What is the relationship between chronic obstructive pulmonary disease and left ventricular function?

Even early-stage COPD influences stroke volume and left ventricular size. Left ventricular volume and stroke volume are decreased in COPD without changes in the LV ejection fraction. This decrease is related to the percent emphysema and to the degree of airway obstruction (N Engl J Med 2010;362:217–27). This impairment in left ventricular filling is probably caused by endothelial dysfunction (and not just loss) of the pulmonary microvasculature as a result of smoking.

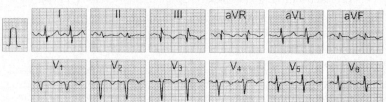

Fig. 102.1 Acute cor pulmonale secondary to pulmonary embolism simulating inferior and anterior infarction. An S1Q3T3, a QR in V₁ with poor R wave progression in the right precordial leads ('clockwise rotation'), and right precordial to midprecordial T wave inversion (V₁ to V₄). The S1Q3 pattern is usually associated with a QR or QS complex, but not an rS, in aVR. Furthermore, acute cor pulmonale per se does not cause prominent Q waves in II (only in III and aVF).

103 CONSOLIDATION

INSTRUCTION

Examine this patient's chest.

SALIENT FEATURES

History

- Abrupt onset of symptoms
- Cough with purulent sputum
- Fever with sweating or rigors
- Pleuritic chest pain (p. 355)
- Shortness of breath
- Haemoptysis
- Nausea, vomiting, diarrhoea (consider legionella infection)
- Mental status changes (especially in the elderly).

Examination

- Purulent sputum (if bacterial in aetiology)
- Tachypnoea
- Reduced movement of the affected side
- Trachea central
- Impaired percussion note
- Bronchial breath sounds
- Crackles.

DIAGNOSIS

This patient has left lower lobe consolidation with purulent sputum (lesion) indicating a bacterial pneumonia (aetiology) and her CURB65 score is zero (functional status).

QUESTIONS

What is the aetiology?

- Bacterial pneumonia
- Bronchogenic carcinoma
- Pulmonary infarct.

How would you investigate suspected bacterial pneumonia?

- FBC, serum urea, electrolytes and liver function tests
- Sputum and blood cultures
- Arterial blood gases
- Chest radiography (Fig. 103.1)
- Test for *Legionella* (culture, direct fluorescent-antibody test or urinary antigen assay), mycoplasma immunoglobulin M
- Consider serological testing for HIV (for patients 15–54 years, particularly when there is lymphopenia or a low CD4 cell count).

ADVANCED-LEVEL QUESTIONS

How do you determine the severity?

Using the CURB65 severity score, 1 point for each feature present:

- Confusion
- Urea> 7 mmol/l

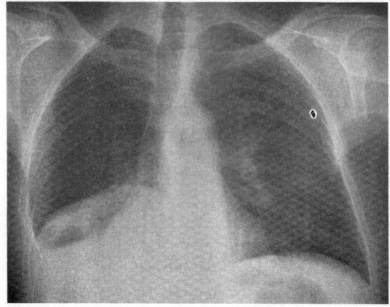

Fig. 103.1 Air bronchograms in a collapsed and consolidated right lower lobe. (With permission from Adam et al. 2008.)

- Respiratory rate ≥30/min
- BP (systolic <90 mmHg or diastolic ≤60 mmHg)
- Age ≥**65** years.

The prognosis based on CURB65 score:

4 or 5: assess with specific consideration to the need for transfer to a critical care unit

≥3: high risk of death

2: moderate risk of death; considered for short-stay inpatient treatment or hospital-supervised outpatient treatment

0 or 1: low risk of death; may be suitable for therapy at home.

The CURB65 severity score should be interpreted in context of the overall clinical picture.

What are the causes of a poorly resolving or recurrent pneumonia?

- Carcinoma of the lung
- Aspiration of a foreign body
- Inappropriate antibiotic
- Sequestration (rare; suspect if left lower lobe is involved).

What do you know about atypical pneumonias?

Typical pneumonia is caused by the pneumococcus (*Streptococcus pneumoniae*), whereas atypical pneumonia is that *not* resulting from pneumococcus infection; it may be caused by *Mycoplasma*, *Legionella*, *Chlamydia*,

Coxiella spp. The clinical picture in atypical pneumonia is dominated by constitutional symptoms, such as fever and headache, rather than respiratory symptoms.

What do you know about mycoplasma pneumonia?

Mycoplasma pneumoniae is an important cause of atypical pneumonia. It is important community-acquired pneumonia and epidemics are seen every 4 years or so. Its incubation is 2–3 weeks and it is usually seen in children and young adults. Reinfection can occur in older patients with detectable *M. pneumoniae* antibody. Like all other pneumonias, mycoplasma pneumonia is common in winter months.

What are the extrapulmonary manifestations of mycoplasma pneumonia?

- Arthralgia and arthritis
- Autoimmune haemolytic anaemia
- Neurological manifestations involving both central and peripheral systems
- Pericarditis, myocarditis
- Hepatitis, glomerulonephritis
- Non-specific rash, erythema multiforme and Stevens–Johnson syndrome
- Disseminated intravascular coagulation (DIC).

What are the complications of pneumonia?

- Septicaemia
- Lung abscess
- Empyema
- Adult respiratory distress syndrome
- Multiorgan failure, renal failure
- Haemolytic syndrome
- Death.

Which antibiotics would you use in a patient with community-acquired pneumonia where the pathogen is not known?

The British Thoracic Society recommends that empirical therapy 'should always cover' *S. pneumoniae*. The preferred regimen is amoxicillin or penicillin; when *Legionella* sp. or *M. pneumoniae* is specifically suspected, erythromycin should be given, and antibiotics directed against *Staphylococcus aureus* should be considered during epidemics of influenza.

What are the poor prognostic factors in patients with community-acquired pneumonia?

- Age >65 years
- Coexisting conditions such as cardiac failure, renal failure, COPD, malignancy
- Clinical features: respiratory rate >30 breaths/min, hypotension (systolic BP <90 mmHg or diastolic BP <60 mmHg), temperature >38.3°C, impaired mental status (stupor, lethargy, disorientation or coma), extrapulmonary infection (e.g. septic arthritis, meningitis)
- Investigations: haematocrit <30%, white cell count <4 or >30 × 10⁶ cells/l, azotaemia, arterial blood gas <60 mmHg while breathing room air, chest radiograph showing multiple lobe involvement, or rapid spread or pleural effusion
- Microbial pathogens: *S.*, *Legionella* sp., *S. pneumoniae*.

What do you know about Panton–Valentine leukocidin-producing *Staphylococcus aureus*?

Panton–Valentine leukocidin-producing *S. aureus* (PVL-SA) infection causes very severe pneumonia, resulting in rapid lung cavitation and multiorgan failure. Affected patients often require admission to the critical care unit. In patients with suspected necrotizing pneumonia, the antibiotic regimen should include include a combination of intravenous linezolid 600 mg twice daily, intravenous clindamycin 1.2 g four times a day and intravenous rifampicin 600 mg twice daily in addition to the initial empirical antibiotic regimen. As soon as PVL-SA infection is either confirmed or excluded, antibiotic therapy should be narrowed accordingly.

What do you know about pulmonary eosinophilic disorders?

Crofton et al. (1952) described five classes of pulmonary eosinophilic disorder (Thorax 1952;7:1–35).

Löffler syndrome. This is characterized by transient pulmonary infiltrates and peripheral eosinophilia. It is associated with parasitic infections, drug allergies and exposure to inorganic chemicals such as nickel carbonyl. The course is benign and respiratory failure almost unknown.

Eosinophilia in asthmatics. The most common cause is allergic bronchopulmonary aspergillosis. This condition is benign but chronic.

Tropical eosinophilia. This is secondary to filarial infection (*Wuchereria bancrofti* or *W. malayi brugi*).

Churg–Strauss syndrome. Diagnosis requires four of the following features: asthma; eosinophilia >10%, mononeuropathy or polyneuropathy; paranasal sinus abnormality; non-fixed pulmonary infiltrates visible on chest radiographs; and blood vessels with extravascular eosinophils found on biopsy.

Chronic eosinophilic pneumonia. This chronic debilitating illness is characterized by malaise, fever, weight loss and dyspnoea. The chest radiograph shows a peripheral alveolar filling infiltrate predominantly in the upper lobes (the 'photographic negative' of pulmonary oedema).

What do you know about bronchopulmonary sequestration?

It is an uncommon congenital lesion in which a portion of non-functioning lung tissue is detached from the normal lung and supplied by an anomalous systemic artery, usually arising from the aorta or one of its branches. The tissue has no communication with the bronchopulmonary tree. Two types of sequestration have been described: extralobar and intralobar. An extralobar sequestration has its own pleural lining, which separates it from the remaining lung tissue, and the intralobar type shares its pleura with the adjacent normal lung. Patients usually present in childhood with cough and recurrent pneumonia, and occasionally present with haemoptysis.

What is the pathogenesis of ventilator-acquired pneumonia?

Hospital-acquired pneumonia. *Micro-aspiration* is the primary route of bacterial entry into the lower respiratory tract. Risk factors include sedation, intubation for operative procedures, vomiting and impaired swallowing.

Ventilator-associated pneumonia. Leakage of bacteria and oral secretions around the endotracheal cuff, inhalation of contaminated aerosols, or reflux of contaminated ventilator tubing condensate are the primary routes of bacterial entry into the lower respiratory tract. Promising biomarkers include procalcitonin, C-reactive protein and soluble triggering receptor expressed on myeloid cells (sTREM-1).

Outcomes. The 'battlefield' between the pathogens entering the lower respiratory tract and the host defences determines possible outcomes: colonization, tracheobronchitis or hospital/ventilation-acquired pneumonia.

● **What do you understand by the term healthcare-associated pneumonia?** Pneumonia acquired in the community by patients who have had direct or indirect contact with a healthcare or long-term care facility and are subsequently hospitalized. These patients are more likely to have a coexisting illness and to receive ineffective empirical antibiotic therapy and are at greater risk for mortality than patients who have true community-acquired pneumonia. Therefore, a broader spectrum of antibiotics (especially against *Pseudomonas aeruginosa,* other multidrug-resistant Gram-negative bacilli, and drug-resistant *S. aureus*) may be needed.

Further reading

Bartlett JG, Mundy LM: Community-acquired pneumonia, *N Engl J Med* 333:1618–1624, 1995.

British Thoracic Society: Guidelines for the management of community-acquired pneumonia in adults admitted to hospital, *Br J Hosp Med* 49:346–350, 1993.

104 BRONCHOGENIC CARCINOMA

INSTRUCTION

Examine this patient's chest.

SALIENT FEATURES

History

● Symptoms related to primary tumour: cough, dyspnoea, haemoptysis, postobstructive pneumonia)
● Symptoms related to mediastinal spread:
  • Hoarseness with left-sided lesions (caused by recurrent laryngeal nerve palsy)
  • Obstructive of the superior vena cava with right-sided tumours or associated lymphadenopathy
  • Elevation of the hemidiaphragm from phrenic nerve paralysis
  • Dysphagia from oesophageal obstruction and pericardial tamponade.
● Symptoms related to metastases:
  • Sites include liver, brain, pleural cavity, bone, adrenal glands, contralateral lungs and skin
  • Initial presentation with symptoms from a metastatic focus is particularly common with adenocarcinoma.

- Paraneoplastic syndrome:
  - Pain or arm in legs caused by hypertrophic osteoarthropathy
  - Symptoms of hypercalcaemia caused by squamous cell carcinoma
  - Neurological syndromes.
- Systemic effects: anorexia, weight loss, weakness and profound fatigue.
- History of smoking

Examination

Patient 1
- Clubbing and tar staining the fingers
- Dull percussion note at the apex with absent breath sounds.

Look for Horner syndrome and wasting of the small muscles of the hand.

Patient 2
- Signs of pleural effusion on one side.

Patient 3
- Signs of unilateral collapse or consolidation of the upper lobe on one side.

Note: If you suspect bronchogenic carcinoma, always look for clubbing, tar staining, cervical lymph nodes and radiation marks, and comment on cachexia.

DIAGNOSIS

This patient with marked clubbing and large pleural effusion (lesion) probably has bronchogenic carcinoma (aetiology) and is very short of breath because of the large effusion (functional status).

QUESTIONS

How may patients with bronchogenic carcinoma present?

- Cough (in 80%), haemoptysis (70%) and dyspnoea (60%); loss of weight, anorexia
- Skeletal manifestations: clubbing (in 30%)
- Local pressure effects: recurrent laryngeal palsy, superior vena caval obstruction, Horner syndrome
- Endocrine manifestations (12% of the tumours)—in particular small cell tumours—present with syndrome of inappropriate antidiuretic hormone (SIADH), hypercalcaemia, adrenocorticotrophic hormone (ACTH) secretion or gynaecomastia. SIADH does not usually cause symptoms. When Cushing syndrome occurs, the manifestations are primarily metabolic (hypokalaemic alkalosis)
- Neurological manifestations: Eaton–Lambert syndrome, cerebellar degeneration, polyneuropathy, dementia, proximal myopathy, encephalomyelitis, subacute sensory neuropathy, limbic encephalitis, opsoclonus, myoclonus
- Cardiovascular: thrombophlebitis migrans, atrial fibrillation, pericarditis, non-bacterial thrombotic endocarditis
- Cutaneous manifestations: dermatomyositis, acanthosis nigricans, herpes zoster

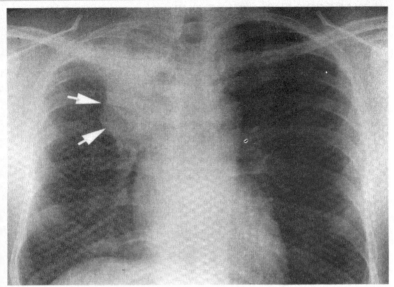

Fig. 104.1 Right upper lobe collapse with peripheral concavity and central convexity (arrows) caused by an underlying bronchogenic carcinoma resulting in a reverse S shape (Golden's 'S' sign). (With permission from Adam et al. 2008.)

- Anaemia, disseminated intravascular coagulation, thrombotic thrombocytopenic purpura. Hypercoagulatopathy in the form of venous thromboembolism is seen especially with adenocarcinoma
- Membranous glomerulonephritis.

How would you investigate this patient?

- Sputum cytology: high yield for endobronchial tumours such as squamous cell and small cell carcinoma) but the yield is poor for adenocarcinoma
- Chest radiography (Fig. 104.1)
- Pleural fluid cytology
- Bronchoscopy gives a high yield in excess of 90%, particularly when the tumour is viewed endobronchially. For tumours that are not visualized, the yield for washing and brushing is about 75% in central lesions and 55% in peripheral lesions. The yield in small cell and squamous cell carcinomas is higher than adenocarcinomas
- CT scan of the chest and upper abdomen (to image the liver and adrenals)
- Bone scan for metastases (helpful in staging)
- PET scanning is highly sensitive and specific for mediastinal staging
- Pulmonary function tests (most surgeons aim for a FEV_1 of about 1000 ml after planned resection), a DLCO (carbon monoxide diffusing capacity of the lung) <60% predicted is associated with a mortality rate as high as 25% as a result of respiratory complications.

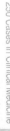

ADVANCED-LEVEL QUESTIONS

What is the aim of staging?

The main aim of staging is to identify candidates for surgical resection, since this approach offers the highest potential cure for lung cancer. The staging assessment covers three major issues: distant metastases, the state of chest and mediastinum and the condition of the patient.

What is the role of surgery in lung carcinoma?

Surgery is beneficial in peripheral non-small cell carcinoma. Its role is limited in small cell carcinoma as >90% would have metastasized by the time of diagnosis. Surgery should include resection (pneumonectomy or lobectomy) and mediastinal node mapping. Complete lymph node dissection should be performed if the tumour is resectable and mediastinal nodes are involved.

Which tumours respond well to chemotherapy?

Small cell carcinoma: cyclophosphamide, doxorubicin, cisplatin, etoposide and vincristine are some of the drugs used. The combination of etoposide and cisplatin appears to have the best therapeutic index of any regimen. A meta-analysis on the role of chemotherapy in non-small cell lung cancers suggested that the benefits are small.

What are the drugs used in non-small-cell lung cancer?

- Old agents: cisplatin, carboplatin, etopside, vinblastine, vindesine
- Newer agents: docetaxel, paclitaxel, irinotacen, vinorelbine, gemcitabine
- Vascular endothelial growth factor (VEGF) inhibitors: bevacizumab
- Epidermal growth factor receptor (EGFR) tyrosine kinase inhibitors (e.g. gefitinib, erlotinib. cetuximab): most effective in women, patients who have never smoked, patients with pulmonary adenocarcinomas and patients of Asian origin.

The EGFR family of surface-receptor tyrosine kinases contains four members, which can form homodimers or heterodimers after ligand binding. Dimerization results in the activation of tyrosine kinases, which is followed by stimulation of three major signalling pathways, eventually leading to the activation of five of the six hallmarks of cancer: angiogenesis, resistance to antigrowth signals, invasion and metastasis, self-sufficiency in growth signals, and evasion of apoptosis (the sixth hallmark being limitless replication). The vast majority of *EGFR* mutations are either a deletion of a conserved sequence in exon 19 or a single point mutation in exon 21 (L858R).

What are the indications for radiotherapy?

Radiotherapy is administered for palliation in the following circumstances:

- Pain: either local or metastatic
- Breathlessness caused by bronchial obstruction
- Dysphagia
- Haemoptysis
- Superior venal caval obstruction
- Pancoast's tumour
- Before and after operation in selected patients
- Cerebral metastases.

What are the contraindications for surgery?
- Metastatic carcinoma
- FEV$_1$ <1500 ml
- Transfer factor <50%
- Severe pulmonary hypertension
- Uncontrolled major cardiac arrhythmias
- Carbon dioxide retention
- Myocardial infarction in the past 3 months.

Is the progression of cancer associated with genetic change?
Yes: it is accompanied by a mutation in the p53 gene and loss of a portion of the short arm of chromosome 3 in small cell cancer; the functional significance of this is not clear.

What is the prognosis?
Survival after diagnosis for small cell carcinoma is 3 months if untreated and 18 months with treatment.

Survival after diagnosis for non-small cell carcinoma is 50% if there are no metastases and 10% with metastasis.

105 CYSTIC FIBROSIS

INSTRUCTION

Examine the chest of this male patient who has had a good appetite, poor weight gain and foul fatty stool.

SALIENT FEATURES

History

- Cough with purulent and viscous expectoration
- Diabetes mellitus
- GI symptoms (steatorrhoea, failure to thrive in childhood, rectal prolapse, meconium ileus or distal intestinal obstruction)
- Heat stroke, salt depletion
- Sterility in men and decreased fertility in women.

Examination

- Sputum is purulent
- Patient is short of breath
- Central cyanosis
- Finger clubbing
- Bilateral coarse crackles.

Proceed as follows:
- Tell the examiner that you would like to check the following:
  - Urine sugar
  - Faecal fat
  - Sweat sodium.

Remember: Cystic fibrosis is defined as the presence of a coherent clinical syndrome, plus either evidence of cystic fibrosis transmembrane conductor regulator (CFTR) dysfunction (an abnormal value for sweat chloride or nasal potential difference) or confirmation of cystic fibrosis-causing mutations on both alleles.

DIAGNOSIS

This patient has bilateral coarse crackles, asthenia and foul fatty stool (lesion) caused by cystic fibrosis (aetiology) and requires continuous oxygen, indicating respiratory failure (functional status).

QUESTIONS

What are the chances of this male patient having a child?
Males are sterile through the failure of development of the vas deferens and epididymis.

What are the clinical manifestations of this condition?
- Neonates: recurrent chest infections, failure to thrive, meconium ileus and rectal prolapse
- In childhood and young adults:
  - Respiratory: infection, bronchiectasis (Fig. 105.1), pneumothorax, haemoptysis, nasal polyps, allergic bronchopulmonary aspergillosis, deterioration during and after pregnancy
  - Cardiovascular: cor pulmonale. (see Fig. 102.1)

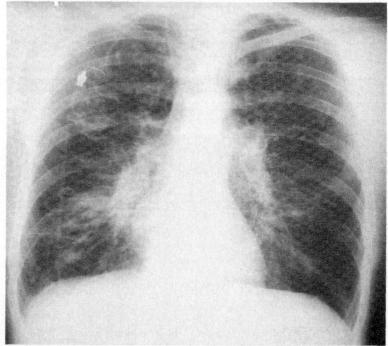

Fig. 105.1 Cystic fibrosis. There is slight overinflation and multiple thin-walled ring shadows in the right lung and the upper part of the left lung, reflecting cystic bronchiectasis. Some ring shadows contain air–fluid levels. (With permission from Adam et al. 2008.)

- GI: rectal prolapse, distal ileal obstruction (meconium ileus equivalent), cirrhosis, gallstones, intussusception
- Miscellaneous: male infertility, diabetes mellitus, hypertrophic pulmonary osteoarthropathy.

How would you treat steatorrhoea?
- Low-fat diet
- Pancreatic supplements
- H_2-receptor antagonist.

How would you treat chest complications?
- Postural drainage
- Antibiotics
- Bronchodilators
- Heart–lung transplantantion.

What is the role of physiotherapy?
Physiotherapy has shown to be useful, but there is considerable debate regarding the effectiveness of different techniques, including traditional postural drainage and percussion, forced expiratory technique, positive expiratory pressure masks, autodrainage and flutter valves.

ADVANCED-LEVEL QUESTIONS

What is the inheritance in cystic fibrosis?
Autosomal recessive. On the long arm of chromosome 7 resides the gene encoding CFTR, a protein of 1480 residues that acts as a cyclic AMP-regulated chloride channel. This gene is carried by 1 in 20 Caucasians and its incidence is about 1 in 2000 live births. There is a mutation on the long arm of chromosome 7 in 70% of patients. There is a deletion of the codon for phenylalanine at position 508 (Δ508). This defect leads to a failure of the chloride channel to open in response to cyclic AMP. More than 175 other lesions in the cystic fibrosis gene are responsible for the disease in the remaining 30% of patients.

How is this condition diagnosed in infancy?
Immunoreactive trypsin (IRT) assay in dried blood in neonates. A very high IRT concentration suggests pancreatic injury consistent with (but not specific for) cystic fibrosis. This assay is useful for screening rather than diagnosis. Infants who have a high IRT concentration on initial testing undergo further assessment via a repeat IRT 1–3 weeks later (IRT/IRT), or by analysis of the initial blood spot for a specified group of CFTR mutations (IRT/DNA).

What do you know about sweat testing?
A sweat sodium concentration >60 mmol/l is indicative of cystic fibrosis. It identifies over 75% by the age of 2 years and about 95% by the age of 12 years. It is more difficult to interpret in older children and adults.

What is the basic defect in the airways of these patients?
The opening of chloride channels at the luminal surface of the airway epithelial cells in normal individuals allows the passive transport of chloride along an electrochemical gradient from the cytoplasm to the lumen. In patients with cystic fibrosis, there is a defect in these channels that prevents this normal secretion. Simultaneously, there is a

three-fold increase in the reabsorption of sodium from the airway lumen into the cytoplasm of the epithelial cell. As the movement of water into airway secretions follows the movement of salt, it is believed that a decreased secretion of chloride into the airway lumen and the increased reabsorption of sodium from the airway lumen combine to reduce water content and increase the viscosity and tenacity of the airway secretions.

If the patient has persistent purulent cough, which organisms are usually responsible?

Staphylococcus aureus, Haemophilus influenzae, Burkholderia cepacia and *Pseudomonas aeruginosa*. The last is associated with poor prognosis as this organism is almost impossible to eradicate.

What is the risk of cancer in patients with cystic fibrosis?

The overall risk of cancer is similar to that of the general population, but there is an increased risk of digestive tract cancers. Persistent or unexplained GI symptoms in these patients should be investigated carefully.

What is the lifespan in such patients?

The median age of survival is currently in the late 30s. It is possible that a child born today will have a median survival into the 50s.

What is the cause of death in cystic fibrosis?

Death occurs from pulmonary complications, such as pneumonia, pneumothorax or haemoptysis, or from terminal chronic respiratory failure.

What parameters can predict death in cystic fibrosis?

Prediction of death within 2 years can be made for 50% of the patients whose FEV_1 is <30%. Thus the necessity for referral for transplantation can be anticipated about 1 year in advance of death.

How would you manage a patient who has been accepted for transplantation?

The aim is to sustain life by aggressive therapy with nocturnal oxygen, continuous intravenous antibiotics, enteral feeding, respiratory stimulants and nasal intermittent positive pressure ventilation.

If this patient requires lung transplantation, which type of transplantation is the treatment of choice?

Bilateral lung transplantation is necessary for patients with chronic bronchial infection such as cystic fibrosis (or bronchiectasis) to avoid contamination of the donor lung by spillover of infected material from the recipient's remaining lung.

What are the complications of lung transplantation?

Early post-transplantation lung oedema, infection and rejection (including obliterative bronchiolitis).

What are the indications for a combined heart–lung transplantation?

The combined heart–lung transplantation has relatively few indications, the primary one being congenital heart disease with Eisenmenger syndrome.

What are the new methods of treatment available for cystic fibrosis?

- High-dose ibuprofen in patients with mild disease (FEV_1 of at least 60% of the predicted value), taken consistently for 4 years, significantly slows the progression of lung disease without serious adverse effects.
- Aerosolized recombinant human DNAse (dornase-alpha), which is capable of degrading DNA in the bronchial secretion, has been shown to improve FEV_1 by 20% when given by aerosol.
- Gene therapy: the gene is transferred in a 'carrier' (either in a cationic lipid envelope known as a liposome, or in an adenovirus). On transferring the gene for cystic fibrosis to the nasal epithelium using a cationic liposome, the deficit has been partly removed without provoking a local inflammatory response.
- Inhalation of hypertonic saline produces a sustained acceleration of mucus clearance and improved lung function. This treatment may protect the lung from insults that reduce mucus clearance and produce lung disease.
- Improvement of the hydration of secretion by:
  - blocking the reabsorption of sodium from the airway lumen with amiloride
  - stimulating the secretion of chloride with triphosphate nucleotides (of adenosine or uridine) through nucleotide receptors by a pathway independent of cylic AMP metabolism.
- Immunization to various components of *Pseudomonas*.

What advice would you give a patient with cystic fibrosis who wishes to become pregnant?

- The couple will be offered genetic counselling and the man will be offered testing to determine his genetic status. If he is a carrier, chorionic villous sampling will be considered, as the risk of the couple conceiving an infant with cystic fibrosis is 1 in 2 and they may wish to consider selective termination in the first trimester. The hazards of general anaesthesia (as lung function is impaired) for termination of pregnancy will be brought to their attention. Termination of pregnancy either with spinal anaesthesia or medications is an alternative.
- Women with severe disease will be informed that they may be unable to complete pregnancy and that their premature demise may leave a motherless child.
- In women with an FEV_1 <60% of the predicted value there is an increased risk of premature delivery, an increased rate of caesarean section, some loss of lung function and risk of respiratory complications, and early death of the mother.
- Pregnancy after heart–lung transplantation offers better health and increased longevity in the mother, but the risk of organ rejection and exposure of the fetus to potentially teratogenic immunosuppressants means that pregnancy should not be attempted by women with transplants.

What is the *forme fruste* of cystic fibrosis?

Increasingly, with the availability of neonatal screening with immunoreactive trypsin and thorough diagnosis by genetic studies, milder forms of disease have been recognized without the increase in sweat sodium. It is predicted that a considerable number will present with a pattern of disease in adult life that has not been recognized in the past as being caused by cystic fibrosis.

Quinton established that sweat ducts are impermeable to chloride in 1986.

Sir Magdi H Yacoub, contemporary Egyptian-born cardiothoracic surgeon, popularized cardiac transplantation in the UK at Harefield Hospital, London.

The first successful pregnancy in a woman with cystic fibrosis was reported in 1960.

---

106   FIBROSING ALVEOLITIS

INSTRUCTION

Examine this patient's chest.
Examine the respiratory system from the back.

SALIENT FEATURES

History

- Progressive exertional dyspnoea (occurs in 90%)
- Chronic cough (occurs in 74%)
- Arthralgia/arthritis (occurs in 19%)
- Obtain a drug history (amiodarone, nitrofurantoin and busulfan).

Examination

- Clubbing (Fig. 106.1; see also Case 218)
- Central cyanosis
- Bilateral, basal, fine, end-inspiratory crackles that disappear or become quieter on leaning forwards. Furthermore, the crackles do not disappear on coughing (unlike those of pulmonary oedema). The crackles have been called 'velcro' or 'cellophane' crackles
- Tachypnoea (in advanced disease).

Proceed as follows:

- Examine the following:
  - Hands (for rheumatoid arthritis, systemic sclerosis)
  - Face (for typical rash of SLE, heliotropic rash of dermatomyositis, typical facies of systemic sclerosis, lupus pernio of sarcoid)
  - Mouth (for aphthous ulcers of Crohn's disease, dry mouth of Sjögren syndrome).
- Look for signs of pulmonary hypertension: 'a' wave in the JVP, left parasternal heave and P_2.

DIAGNOSIS

This patient has bilateral, basal, fine end-inspiratory crackles (lesion) caused by fibrosing alveolitis (aetiology) and is tachypnoeic at rest (functional status).

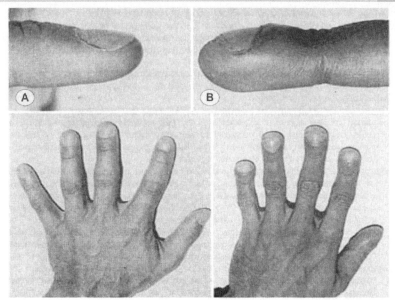

Fig. 106.1 Hands and index fingers of a normal person (A) and a person with clubbing of the digits (B) secondary to severe diffuse pulmonary interstitial fibrosis. (With permission from Mason RJ et al. 2005.)

QUESTIONS

In which other conditions is clubbing associated with crackles?
- Bronchogenic carcinoma (crackles are localized)
- Bronchiectasis (coarse crackles)
- Asbestosis (history of exposure to asbestos).

ADVANCED-LEVEL QUESTIONS

Mention possible aetiological factors
Metal dust (steel, brass, lead), wood dust (pine), wood smoke and smoking.

Mention other conditions which have similar pulmonary changes
- Rheumatoid arthritis, SLE, dermatomyositis, chronic active hepatitis, ulcerative colitis, systemic sclerosis
- Pneumoconiosis
- Granulomatous disease: sarcoid, TB
- Chronic pulmonary oedema
- Radiotherapy
- Lymphangitis carcinomatosa
- Extrinsic allergic alveolitis: farmer's lung, bird fancier's lung.

What is the pathology in fibrosing alveolitis?

Fibrosing alveolitis is characterized by the presence of connective tissue matrix proteins within the acinar regions of the lung in association with a variable cellular infiltrate within the alveoli and in the interstitium.

What are the types of interstitial pneumonitis?

Liebow and Carrington in 1969 described five subgroups depending on histology.

Classical (usual) interstitial pneumonia (UIP). This is characterized by thickening of the alveolar interstitium by fibrous tissue and mononuclear cells; characteristically varying in severity from one focus to another. The mean survival is 2.8–5.6 years; 12% respond to steroids and spontaneous improvement does not occur.

Desquamative interstitial pneumonia (DIP). There is a marked accumulation of macrophages in the alveolar airspaces associated with a relatively mild but uniform thickening of the interstitial space caused by mononuclear inflammatory cells. The mean survival is 12.4–14 years. The response to steroids is 62% and spontaneous improvement is 22%.

Non-specific interstitial pneumonia (NSIP). The survival is 14 years and therapeutic response is similar to DIP. This is a a diffuse lesion similar to UIP but with superimposed bronchiolitis obliterans.

Lymphoid interstitial pneumonia (LIP). There is marked infiltration of interstitium by lymphocytes that may be indistinguishable from lymphoma.

Giant-cell interstitial pneumonia. Consists of a mononuclear cell infiltrate in the interstitium associated with large numbers of multinucleated giant cells.

How would you investigate this patient?

- Chest radiography: typically shows small lung volumes and bilateral basal reticulonodular shadows, which progress upwards as the disease progresses. In advanced disease, there is marked destruction of the parenchyma, causing 'honeycombing' (caused by groups of closely set ring shadows), and nodular shadows are not conspicuous. The mediastinum may appear broad as a result of a decrease in lung volume.
- Blood gases: arterial desaturation worsens while upright and improves on recumbency. There is arterial hypoxaemia and hypocapnia.
- Pulmonary function tests: in the early stages lung volumes may be normal, but there is arterial desaturation following exercise. Typically there is a restrictive defect with reduction of both the gas transfer factor and gas transfer coefficient.
- Blood tests: high ESR, raised immunoglobulins, raised anti-nuclear factor and rheumatoid factor positive.
- Bronchial lavage: a large number of lymphocytes indicates a good response to steroids and a good prognosis. A large number of neutrophils and eosinophils indicates a poor prognosis (5-year survival rate of 60% for steroid responders versus 25% for non-responders). The patients are more likely to respond to cyclophosphamide if the number of neutrophils is increased (Am Rev Respir Dis 1987;135:26).
- Lung biopsy: in early stages there is mononuclear cell infiltration in the alveolar walls, progressing to interstitial fibrosis (UIP); in later stages, fibrotic contraction of the lung, honeycombing, bronchial dilatation and cysts are seen. The DIP form, with alveolar macrophages and little

mononuclear infiltration or fibrosis, has a better prognosis than UIP as it responds to steroids.

- MRI: useful in determining disease activity without ionizing radiation but it is an expensive method.
- High-resolution CT: useful to assess the pattern and extent of disease. A heterogeneous distribution of patchy, peripheral reticular densities, broad bands of fibrosis and honeycombing are typical features seen on high-resolution CT. Patients with a predominantly ground-glass appearance in the lungs are treated whereas those with a predominantly reticular appearance undergo technetium diethylenetriamine pentaacetate scanning (DPTA) to assess the probability of deterioration. It may avoid the need for biopsy especially if predominantly reticular shadowing. It acts as a guide for ideal biopsy site.
- DPTA scanning in non-smokers is of value in identifying which patients are more likely to deteriorate. Therapy can be postponed when there is slow clearance, whereas those with fast clearance should receive treatment (Eur Respir J 1993;6:797–802).

Mention prognostic factors

Good prognostic factors:
- Short duration of disease
- Young age of patient at onset
- Female
- Predominantly ground glass shadowing on radiographs
- Presence of little fibrosis on lung biopsies.

How would you manage this patient?

- Approximately 30% of patients treated with prednisone have had objective evidence of improvement. Therefore, all patients should be considered for a course of steroids (unless there are contraindications): prednisolone 40 mg/day for 6 weeks. Monitor symptoms and do a chest radiography and lung function tests. If response is good, continue; if no response then taper over 1 week.
- Steroid non-responders may benefit from a course of cyclophosphamide. Occasionally, patients who are unresponsive to prednisolone and cyclophosphamide will respond to prednisolone and azathioprine. Colchicine, penicillamine, interferon-gamma-1b and pirfenidone have also been used alone or as corticosteroid-sparing drugs. No well-controlled, randomized, and blinded studies have shown any of these medications to be efficacious
- High dose of acetylcysteine, administered over a period of 1 year, in addition to prednisone and azathioprine preserves vital capacity and diffusing capacity of the lung in patients with idiopathic pulmonary fibrosis better than standard therapy alone. The administration of acetylcysteine has no effect on survival.
- Identify the underlying cause and manage accordingly.

What is the prognosis?

The median survival of patients with the disease is about 3 years after diagnosis or 5 years after the onset of symptoms. The 5-year overall survival rate is 50%, 65% in steroid responders and 25% in steroid non-responders. The average life expectancy of patients with usual interstitial pneumonia is 2–5 years after diagnosis, regardless of treatment.

What are the causes of death in such patients?

- Respiratory failure or cor pulmonale precipitated by chest infection
- Bronchogenic carcinoma, 10-fold increase compared with normal controls.

What is the role for lung transplantation?

Single lung transplantation is now an established and effective form of treatment for certain individuals. Current survival rate at 1 year is approximately 60% (N Engl J Med 1986;314:1140–5).

What do you know about the Hamman–Rich syndrome?

The Hamman–Rich syndrome is a rapidly progressive and fatal variant of interstitial lung disease (Bull Johns Hopkins Hosps 1944;74:177).

Mention indications for transbronchial and open lung biopsy

- Transbronchial biopsy: sarcoidosis, TB, berylliosis, lymphangitis carcinomatosa, extrinsic allergic alveolitis
- Open lung biopsy: fibrosing alveolitis, rheumatological disease, pulmonary vasculitis, lymphangioleiomyomatosis, Langerhan cell histiocytosis.

Mention some genetic disorders with pulmonary fibrosis

- Dyskeratosis congenital: pulmonary fibrosis is present in 20% of patients. Dyskeratosis congenita is also typically associated with a triad of mucocutaneous manifestations: skin hyperpigmentation (p. 400), oral leukoplakia (p. 637) and nail dystrophy (p. 673)
- Hermansky–Pudlak syndrome: oculocutaneous albinism, a bleeding diathesis and pulmonary fibrosis.

What is the role of caveolin in pulmonary fibrosis?

Caveolin-1 (the most abundant protein found within caveolae, which are flask-shaped invaginations of the plasma membrane abundantly present in many terminally differentiated cells) is a protective regulator of pulmonary fibrosis and it limits transforming growth factor-β_1-induced production of extracellular matrix and restores alveolar epithelial repair processes. It attenuates the development of pulmonary fibrosis in a mouse model of the disease. Therapeutic approaches that augment caveolin-1 bioavailability may help to restore normal alveolar epithelial repair and regeneration and may help patients with idiopathic pulmonary fibrosis to breathe more easily and live longer.

LV Hamman (1877–1946), physician, and AR Rich (1893–1968), pathologist, worked at the Johns Hopkins Hospitals, Baltimore (Hamman L, Rich AR. Acute diffuse interstitial fibrosis of the lungs Bull Johns Hopkins Hosps 1944;74:177).

Dame Margaret Turner-Warwick, contemporary chest physician, was the first woman President of the Royal College of the Physicians of London; her chief interest is fibrotic lung disease.

107 PULMONARY FIBROSIS

INSTRUCTION

Examine this patient's chest.

SALIENT FEATURES

History

- History of TB, ankylosing spondylitis, radiation
- History of phrenic nerve crush, plombage, thoracotomy.

Examination

- The fibrosis is usually apical
- Flattening of the chest on the affected side
- Tracheal deviation to the affected side
- Reduced expansion on the affected side
- Dull percussion note
- Presence of localized crackles; bronchial breathing may be present.

Proceed as follows:

- Look for the following signs:
  - Scars of phrenic nerve crush, plombage, thoracotomy
  - Radiation scars.

DIAGNOSIS

This patient has flattening of the R/L side of the chest with diminished movements on that side, tracheal deviation and localized crackles (lesion) caused by pulmonary fibrosis secondary to TB (aetiology), and is comfortable at rest (functional status).

QUESTIONS

Mention a few causes of upper lobe fibrosis

- TB (Fig. 107.1)
- Ankylosing spondylitis
- Radiation-induced fibrosis.

ADVANCED-LEVEL QUESTIONS

Which is the best imaging procedure for the upper lobe lesions?

MRI is better for upper lobe lesions than CT of the chest.

What is the role of MRI of the thorax?

MRI of the thorax is less useful than CT scanning because of poorer imaging of the pulmonary parenchyma and inferior spatial resolution. However, MRI can provide images in multiple planes (e.g. sagittal, coronal as well as transverse), which CT cannot. MRI is excellent for evaluating processes near the lung apex, spine and thoracoabdominal junction.

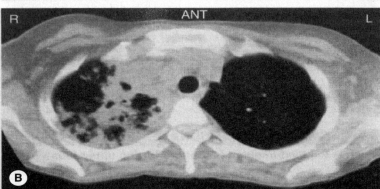

Fig. 107.1 Tuberculosis. (A) Fibrosis pulls the hilum up on the affected side. (B) CT shows the cavitation of the infitrate. (With permission from Mettler 2004.)

On 8 November 1895 Röntgen discovered what he called
X-rays. In the subsequent 7 weeks he meticulously performed experiments,
and a picture of his wife's hand convinced him about the potential role of the
new ray. In 1901 he was awarded the Nobel Prize for physics.

Hounsfield's work on CT in the EMI laboratories at Hounslow made it
possible to obtain detailed cross-sectional views of
the soft tissues, particularly brain. Sir Godfrey N Hounsfield (1919–2004) and
Alan M Cormack (1924–1998), the latter of Tufts University, Boston, were
jointly awarded the 1979 Nobel Prize for Medicine for the development of
computer-assisted tomography.

108 PNEUMOTHORAX

INSTRUCTION

Examine this patient's chest.

SALIENT FEATURES

History

- Sudden onset or rapidly progessive dyspnoea
- Ipsilateral acute pleuritic pain: either sharp or a steady ache
- A small pneumothorax may be asymptomatic
- Obtain history of:
  - recent pleural aspiration or insertion of subclavian line (J R Soc Med 1997;90:319–21)
  - recent surgeries in head and neck
  - abdominal procedures using bowel or peritoneal distension.
- History of asthma, COPD, acute respiratory distress syndrome, pneumonia, trauma to chest
- History of Marfan syndrome
- History of HIV
- History of positive pressure ventilation.

Examination

- Decreased movement of the affected side
- Increased percussion, note:
  - trachea may be central (small pneumothorax) or deviated to the affected side (underlying collapse of lung) or the opposite side (large pneumothorax)
  - increased vocal resonance with diminished breath sounds.

Proceed as follows:

- Look for clues regarding aetiology:
  - Pleural aspiration site
  - Infraclavicular region for a bruise of the central line
  - Comment if the patient is thin or has marfanoid features
  - Inhaler or peak flow meter by the bedside (asthma, COPD).
- Tell the examiner that you would suspect tension pneumothorax when there is tachycardia (>135 beats/min), hypotension and pulsus paradoxus.

DIAGNOSIS

This patient has diminished breath sounds and hyper-resonant note on R/L side of the chest (lesion) caused by pneumothorax secondary to Marfan syndrome (aetiology), and is not breathless at rest (functional status).

QUESTIONS

What do you understand by the term pneumothorax?
Air in the pleural cavity.

How would you investigate this patient?
- Chest radiography, both inspiratory and expiratory phases. In critically ill patients, pneumothorax is suspected when:
  - the costophrenic angle extends more inferiorly than usual because of air: the 'deep sulcus sign' (Fig. 108.1; Radiology 1980;136:25–7)
  - the liver appears more radiolucent as a result of air in the cerebellopontine angle, or on the left side, when the air will outline the medial aspect of the hemidiaphragm under the heart.
- Blood gases if the patient is breathless: hypoxaemia depending on the shunting, whereas hypercapnia does not develop.

ADVANCED-LEVEL QUESTIONS

How would you grade the degree of collapse?
British Thoracic Society of grading:
- *Small*: where there is a small rim of air around the lung
- *Moderate*: when the lung is collapsed towards the heart border
- *Complete*: airless lung, separate from the diaphragm (aspiration is necessary)
- *Tension*: any pneumothorax with cardiorespiratory distress (rare and requires immediate drainage).

How do you estimate the size of the pneumothorax?
The classic chest radiographic appearance is that of a thin, visceral pleural line lying parallel to the chest wall, separated by a radiolucent band devoid of lung markings. The average width of this band can be used to estimate the size of the pneumothorax with a fair degree of accuracy. However, it is usually clinically more convenient to characterize the pneumothorax as small, moderate, large or complete. The estimated size of the pneumothorax and the patient's clinical status can be useful in guiding management decisions.

How would you manage this patient?
- Small pneumothoraces (<20% in size) spontaneously resolve within weeks.
- Larger ones (irrespective of size) with normal lungs are managed by simple aspiration rather than an intercostal tube as the initial drainage procedure. Aspiration is less painful than intercostal drainage, leads to a shorter admission and reduces the need for pleurectomy, and has no increase in recurrence rate at 1 year.
- When there is rapid re-expansion following simple aspiration, an intercostal tube with underwater seal drainage is used. The tube should be left in for at least 24 h. When the lung re-expands, clamp the tube for 24 h. If repeat radiography shows that the lung remains expanded, the

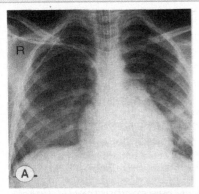

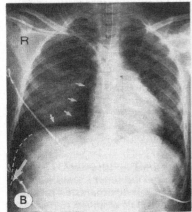

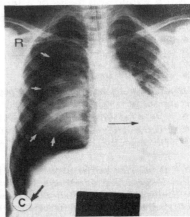

Fig. 108.1 Deep sulcus sign of pneumothorax. (A) On posteroanterior chest radiograph, the costophrenic angle is normally acute (arrow). In a supine patient, a pneumothorax will often be anterior, medial, and basilar. (B) On supine film, the dark area along the right cardiac border and lung base appeared larger (small arrows), and the costophrenic angle much deeper and more acute than normal (large arrow). (C) Tension pneumothorax, with an extremely deep costophrenic angle (large black arrow), an almost completely collapsed right lung (small white arrows) and shift of the mediastinum to the left. (With permission from Mettler 2004.)

tube can be removed. If not, suction should be applied to the tube. If it fails to resolve within 1 week, surgical pleurodesis should be considered. Video-assisted thoracoscopic surgery with several chest ports allows clear visualization of the pleural cavity for resection of bullae and pleurodesis.

What are the causes of pneumothorax?
- Spontanenous (usually in thin males)
- Trauma
- Bronchial asthma
- COPD: emphysematous bulla (JAMA 1975;234:389–93)

- Carcinoma of the lung
- Cystic fibrosis
- TB (the original descriptions of pneumothorax is commonly associated with TB, JAMA 1931;96:653–7)
- Mechanical ventilation
- Marfan syndrome, Ehlers–Danlos syndrome
- Catamenial pneumothorax: pneumothorax that occurs in association with menstruation.

How would you do a pleurodesis?
By injecting talc into the pleural cavity via the intercostal tube.

In which patients would you avoid doing a pleurodesis?
In patients with underlying cystic fibrosis. These patients may require lung transplantation in the future and pleurodesis may make this procedure technically not feasible.

When would you suspect a tension pneumothorax?
Tension pneumothorax should be suspected in the presence of any of the following:
- Severe progressive dyspnoea
- Severe tachycardia
- Hypotension
- Marked mediastinal shift.

When should open thoracotomy be considered?
It should be considered if there is one of the following present:
- A third episode of spontanenous pneumothorax
- Any occurrence of bilateral pneumothorax
- Failure of the lung to expand after tube thoracostomy for the first episode.

What do you know about *Birt–Hogg–Dubé* syndrome?
Birt–Hogg–Dubé syndrome is an autosomal dominant condition that includes skin fibrofolliculomas, pulmonary cysts, spontaneous pneumothorax and renal cancer. The condition is a result of germline mutations in the gene *FLCN*, which encodes folliculin; the function of this protein is largely unknown, although FLCN has been linked to the mTOR pathway. The availability of DNA-based diagnosis has allowed insight into the great variation in expression of *FLCN*, both within and between families.

Further reading

Sahn SA, Heffner J: Spontaneous pneumothorax, *N Engl J Med* 342:868–874 (review), 2000.

OK Williamson (1866–1941), an English physician, described the Williamson sign: BP in the leg is lower than that in the upper limb on the affected side in pneumothorax.

The use of simple aspiration to manage pneumothorax was first reported by OG Raja in 1981 when he was a medical registrar (Br J Dis Chest 1981;75:207–8).

. In 1995, a surgeon on a flight from Hong Kong undertook a life-saving, emergency operation on a woman with a spontaneous pneumothorax. The hero, Angus Wallace, was described by emeritus professor of surgery Miles Irving as 'a typical professor of surgery: ebullient, extrovert, and confident. It was a brilliant piece of improvisation' (Lancet, 2009;374:1055–6).

109 OLD TUBERCULOSIS

INSTRUCTION

Examine this patient's chest.

SALIENT FEATURES

History

- Fever and night sweats
- Malaise, fatigue, anorexia
- Weight loss
- Cough with sputum.

Examination

These patients tend to have signs of common chest diseases but signs are not cut and dried. There are several reasons for this, such as pleural thickening (Fig. 109.1), thoracotomy and pneumonectomy, associated COPD, associated chest infection, plombage or phrenic nerve crush.

DIAGNOSIS

Following are two examples of findings and diagnosis.

- **Patient 1** The candidate was asked to examine the chest from the front, as a result of which the old thoracotomy scar was not seen. The patient was wheezy. The trachea was deviated to the right. Percussion note was stony dull from the right second intercostal space downwards. Wheeze was present on the left side. This patient had a right pneumonectomy with COPD in the left lung. The candidate's diagnosis of right-sided pleural effusion with underlying collapse and left-sided COPD was accepted.

- **Patient 2** The trachea was central. A phrenic nerve crush scar was seen. Percussion note was dull in the left infra-axillary region and there were associated crackles. The diagnosis of pleural thickening with associated chest infection was accepted; that of pleural effusion was not.

QUESTIONS

How would you manage a patient with old tuberculosis?
Old TB requires no antituberculosis treatment. However, the patient may require symptomatic treatment for wheeze and shortness of breath.

In which groups of patients is the risk of tuberculosis high?
- Asian and Irish immigrants
- The elderly
- Immunocompromised individuals, particularly those with AIDS
- Alcoholics
- Occupations at risk: doctors, nurses, chest physiotherapists.

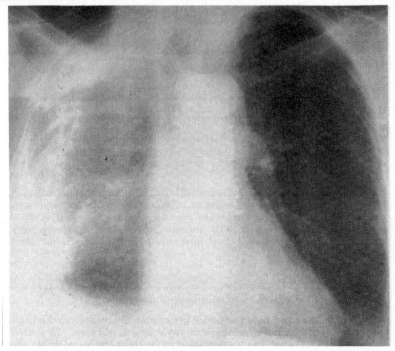

Fig. 109.1 Right-sided pleural thickening and calcification, with reduction in volume of the right hemithorax, in previous tuberculosis. (With permission from Albert et al. 2008.)

ADVANCED-LEVEL QUESTIONS

Would you isolate a patient with newly diagnosed, sputum-positive, pulmonary tuberculosis?

Yes. Segregation in a single room for 2 weeks is recommended for patients with smear-positive TB. Barrier nursing, however, is unnecessary. Adults with smear-negative or non-pulmonary disease may be in a general ward. A child with TB should be segregated until the source case is identified, as this person may be visiting the child.

How are contacts investigated?

● Inquiry into bacille Calmette–Guérin (BCG) vaccination site
● Tuberculin test or Mantoux. The test consists of 0.1 ml (5 tuberculin units) of PPD (purified protein derivative) administered intracutaneously, usually in the volar surface of the forearm. The reaction is read 48 to 72 h after injection (although a reading obtained up to 1 week later is accurate). The size of the reaction is determined by measurement of the induration (not erythema) across the forearm at the site of the injection. This test is not 100% sensitive for infection with *Mycobacerium tuberculosis*, and even among patients with confirmed TB and no

apparent immunosuppression, 10–20% will have negative results on tuberculin skin tests.

- Whole-blood interferon-γ assay (based on the release of interferon-γ from T lymphocytes in response to stimulation with *M. tuberculosis* PPD).
- Chest radiography examination. A chest radiography is considered abnormal if it reveals parenchymal abnormalities; chest radiographys showing pleural thickening or isolated calcified granulomas are not considered to be suggestive of previous TB. Patients with abnormal chest radiography , especially those with opacities occupying >2 cm^2 of the upper lobe, should be evaluated for active TB by sputum examination before therapy for latent TB is initiated.

How is latent tuberculosis diagnosed?

High risk patients. Induration of ≥5 mm in diameter on a tuberculin skin test is used to diagnose latent TB. This group includes persons with HIV infection, close contacts of persons with active TB, persons with an abnormal chest radiography showing upper-lobe fibrosis consistent with previous TB, and immunosuppressed patients who have been receiving the equivalent of at least 15 mg/day prednisone for at least 1 month.

Intermediate risk patients. Induration of ≥10 mm should be used to define latent infection.

To whom would you offer BCG vaccination?

BCG vaccination is offered to previously unvaccinated, persistently Heaf test-negative or grade 1 contacts aged <35 years unless there is a special occupational, travel or ethnic risk. Patients with known or suspected HIV infection should not be offered the vaccination.

What are the indications for chemoprophylaxis?

- Chemoprophylaxis may be given to those with strongly positive Heaf test reactions but no clinical or radiological evidence of TB (Thorax 1994;49:1193–1200).
- Chemoprophylaxis should be given to children <5 years who are close contacts of a smear-positive adult irrespective of their tuberculin test result.
- If chemoprophylaxis is not undertaken, follow-up with periodic chest radiography examinations for 2 years is recommended in all these groups.

Which rapid test allows early diagnosis of tuberculosis?

Polymerase chain reaction.

What questions would you ask an HIV-positive patient to exclude tuberculosis?

If they have cough (of any duration), fever (of any duration) or night sweats lasting 3 weeks or more during the previous 4 weeks. This accurately rules out TB in majority of HIV-positive patients. Adding chest radiography to symptom screening further improves sensitivity (N Engl J Med 2010;362:707)

When should antiretroviral therapy be started in a patient with tuberculosis and HIV infection?

Initiation of antiretroviral treatment during TB therapy in patients with confirmed TB and HIV coinfection reduces mortality by ~56%. The death rate rose from 5.4/100 person-years to 12.1/100 person-years when initiation of antiretroviral therapy was delayed until the completion of TB therapy. The interval between the completion of TB therapy and the initiation of antiretroviral therapy is important; a considerable number of deaths in a sequential therapy group occurs during this period.

What do you know about genes encoding interleukin and susceptibility to tuberculosis?

Human genetic studies have implicated both *IL12B* (the gene encoding interleukin-12β) and *NOD2* in increased susceptibility to mycobacterial disease, and mouse mutants lacking *Nod2, Ripk2* or *Infg* (encoding interferon-γ) are highly susceptible to TB. (**Note**: *Mycobacterium tuberculosis* induces mainly Th17 responses. To rid the body of fungi and certain extracellular bacteria requires inflammation of the type engendered by Th17 cells).

Robert Koch (1843–1910), Institute for Infectious Diseases, Berlin, was awarded the 1905 Nobel Prize for Medicine for his investigations and discoveries in relation to TB.

Kary Mullis of the USA was awarded the Nobel Prize for developing the technique of PCR.

---

110   PICKWICKIAN SYNDROME

INSTRUCTION

Look at this patient.

SALIENT FEATURES

History

- Daytime somnolence
- Unrefreshing sleep
- Daytime fatigue
- Snoring
- Shortness of breath
- Headache particularly in the morning
- Decreased libido
- Swelling of feet
- Poor concentration
- Systemic hypertension
- Family history of obesity
- Gastroesophageal reflux
- Poor quality of life
- History of stroke: obstructive sleep apnoea significantly increases the risk of stroke or mortality from any cause, and the increase is independent of other risk factors, including hypertension.

Examination

- Obese patient who is plethoric and cyanosed
- Maxillary or mandibular hypoplasia:
  - Short of breath at rest
  - May be nodding off to sleep.
- Systemic hypertenion
- Nocturnal angina
- Look for signs of pulmonary hypertension and right heart failure
- Tell the examiner that you would like to measure the neck circumference

Remember: Nearly 50% of patients with sleep apnoea syndrome are *not* obese.

DIAGNOSIS

This patient has marked obesity and hypersomnolence with signs of pulmonary hypertension (lesion), which indicate she has Pickwickian syndrome. The patient is in cardiac failure (functional status).

ADVANCED-LEVEL QUESTIONS

What is the cause of cyanosis in such a patient?

A mixture of obstructive apnoea and sleep-induced hypoventilation (Fig. 110.1). The blood gas picture is hypoxia and carbon dioxide retention.

Where is the obstruction?

It is caused by the apposition of the tongue and the palate of the posterior pharyngeal wall.

What is the significance of neck circumference?

A prediction rule based on neck circumference is used to estimate a patient's probability of having a sleep test result that is diagnostic of sleep apnoea. Neck circumference (measured in centimeters) is adjusted if the patient has hypertension (4 cm is added), is a habitual snorer (3 cm is added) or is reported to choke or gasp most nights (3 cm is added). Adjusted neck circumference of:

 <43 cm: low clinical probability
 43–48 cm: intermediate probability (4–8 times as probable as a low probability)
 >48 cm: high probability (20 times as probable).

How would you treat such a patient?

- Weight reduction
- Avoidance of smoking and alcohol
- Continuous nasal positive airway pressure (CPAP) delivered by a nasal mask (Lancet 1999;353:2100–5). CPAP is recommended even if the

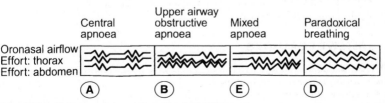

Fig. 110.1 Patterns of sleep-disordered breathing.

apnoea–hypopnoea index is in the mild range (5 to 15), although evidence for the efficacy of CPAP is strong for patients with an apnoea–hypopnoea index >15. CPAP acts like a pneumatic splint (resulting in patency of the upper airway during inspiration and expiration). The resultant reductions in gas-exchange perturbations, respiratory effort, abrupt arousals and BP surges all probably ameliorate symptoms

- Home oxygen
- Surgery. Tracheostomy, uvulopalatopharyngoplasty, linguoplasty, mandibular advancement, plastic remodelling of the uvula (laser-assisted or radiofrequency ablation), tonsillectomy, reconstruction of maxillae
- Drugs: serotonin, receptor blockade, acetazolamide, methylxanthines, weight loss medications
- Atrial overdrive pacing may benefit selected patients (the vagal tone that accompanies bradycardia also causes the sleep apnoea, so prevention of the enhanced vagal tone prevents the apnoea) (N Engl J Med 2002;346:404–12).

William Howard Taft, US President from 1909 to 1913, had a minimum body mass index of 42 kg/m2, wore size 54 pajamas, had a neck size of 19 inches (47.5 cm), snored and had hypersomnolence. He appears to have become symptomatic at approximately 300 lb (140 kg). Within 12 months of leaving office, Taft permanently lost over 60 lb (27 kg). His somnolence resolved. As Chief Justice of the United States from 1921 to 1930, he was not somnolent.

Mr Pickwick is a character in the novel 'Pickwick papers', written by Charles Dickens, and this term was applied by Sir William Osler. In Charles Dickens' The Posthumous Papers of the Pickwick Club', Dickens describes the first meeting of Mr Wardle with his servant:

'Damn that boy,' said the old gentleman, 'he's gone to sleep again.'

'Very extraordinary boy, that,' said Mr. Pickwick, 'does he always sleep in this way?'

'Sleep!' said the old gentleman, 'he's always asleep. Goes on errands fast asleep, and snores as he waits at the table.'

'How very odd!' said Mr. Pickwick

'Ah! Odd indeed,' returned the old gentleman; 'I'm proud of that boy—wouldn't part with him on any account—damme, he's a natural curiosity!'

---

111 COLLAPSED LUNG

INSTRUCTION

Examine this patient's chest.

SALIENT FEATURES

History

- Sudden onset of breathlessness
- History of cough
- History of asthma, TB, lung cancer.

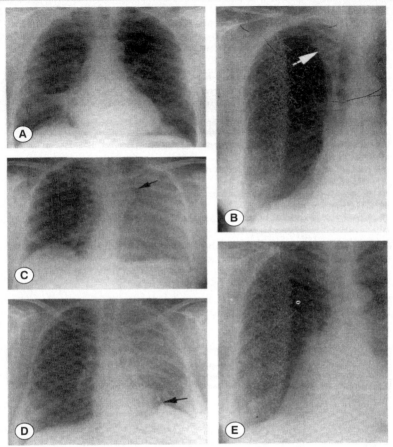

Fig. 111.1 Collapsed lung. (A) Triangular-shaped density adjacent to the right heart border in right middle lobe collapse. (B) Superior triangle sign in right lower lobe collapse (arrow). (C) Paramediastinal lucency (Luftsichel sign; arrow) in left upper lobe collapse. (D) A small triangular density (juxtaphrenic peak sign; arrow) in left upper lobe collapse (indicates reorientation of an inferior accessory fissure). (E) Shifting granuloma sign in right lower lobe collapse. (With permission from Adam et al. 2008.)

Examination

- Trachea deviated to the affected side
- Movements decreased on the affected side
- Percussion note dull on the affected side
- Breath sounds diminished on the affected side.

Proceed as follows:

- Tell the examiner that you would like to look for tar staining (tobacco smoking), clubbing and cachexia (bronchogenic carcinoma; see p. 387).
- Be prepared to discuss the patients chest radiography (Fig. 111.1).

DIAGNOSIS

This patient has a collapsed lung (lesion); he is breathless at rest (functional status). You would like to exclude malignancy (aetiology).

QUESTIONS

What are the causes of lung collapse?

- Bronchogenic carcinoma
- Mucus plugs (asthma, allergic bronchopulmonary aspergillosis) (BMJ 1982;285:552)
- Extrinsic compression from hilar adenopathy (e.g. primary TB)
- TB (Brock syndrome)
- Other intrabronchial tumours including bronchial adenoma
- Ventilation-induced lung injury.

What are the chest radiograph findings of collapse of the right middle lobe?

The loss of definition of the right heart border (Fig. 111.1A) reflects collapse (or consolidation) affecting the right middle lobe.

What is Brock syndrome?

It is collapse caused by compression of the right middle lobe bronchus by an enlarged lymph node.

Sir Russel C Brock (1903–1980) graduated from Guy's Hospital and was surgeon at Guy's and Brompton Hospitals. His interests included both thoracic and cardiac surgery. He was the President of the Royal College of Surgeons, 1963–1966.

History and examination
of the abdomen

SALIENT FEATURES

History

- Fever, loss of weight, fatigue, lassitude
- GI symptoms: dysphagia, nausea, vomiting, altered bowel movement, jaundice
- Renal symptoms: oliguria, history of renal failure
- History of diabetes, hypertension
- History of ascites, swelling of feet, mass abdomen.

Examination

1. Ensure the patient is lying flat (remove any extra pillows, if present, with the permission of the patient); the hands should by the patient's side with the abdomen exposed from the inframammary region to just above the genitalia. Do not expose the genitalia.
2. Begin with the hands, looking for the following signs:
   - Clubbing, leukonychia (white chalky nails)
   - Palmar erythema
   - Duputryen's contracture (feel for thickening of the fascia)
   - Hepatic flap.
3. Examine the arms:
   - Look for arteriovenous fistula, haemodialysis catheters, spider naevi.
4. Comment on the skin:
   - Pigmentation
   - Scratch marks.
5. Examine the following:
   - Supraclavicular and cervical lymph nodes
   - Tongue for pallor
   - Eyes for anaemia, jaundice, xanthelasma
   - Upper chest and face for spider naevi
   - Axilla for hair loss, acanthosis nigricans
   - Breast for gynaecomastia.
6. Inspect the abdomen, looking for the following signs:
   - Skin, e.g. ecchymosis (Fig. IV.1)
   - Movements
   - Any obvious mass
   - Visible veins (check direction of flow, which is usually away from the umbilicus)
   - Visible peristalsis
   - Hernial orifices (ask the patient to cough at this stage)
   - Expansile pulsations of aortic aneurysm.
7. Ask the patient whether the abdomen is sore at any part.
8. Palpation: kneel on the floor or sit on a chair before you begin palpation. At all times look at the patient's eyes to check whether he or she winces in pain. Begin with superficial pain and begin in the least tender

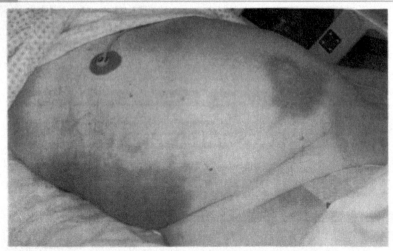

Fig. IV.1 Skin features. (A) Cullen's sign (periumbilical ecchymosis). (B) Grey–Turner's sign (ecchymosis on the abdominal flank). (With permission from Bosmann M et al. 2009.)

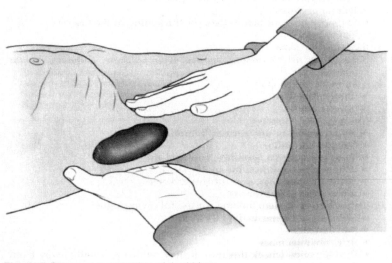

Fig. IV.2 Bimanual examination of the kidney.

area. Palpate in all the quadrants (remember that there are four quadrants). Palpate:

- for mass, determine its characteristics
- liver (percuss for upper border using heavy percussion, for lower border using light percussion)
- kidneys (bimanual palpation, demonstrate ballottement) (Fig. IV.2)

- groin for lymph nodes
- check hernial orifices
- test for expansile pulsation of an aortic aneurysm.

9. Percuss, looking for shifting dullness (at this stage, when the patient is lying on his or her right side, seize the opportunity to examine for a small spleen and for pitting oedema over the sacral region). Remember that abdominal percussion should follow adequate inspection and percussion.

10. Auscultate:
    - Over an enlarged liver for bruit
    - Over a suspected aortic aneurysm
    - For bowel sounds.

11. Tell the examiner that you would like to perform a rectal examination and examine the external genitalia.

12. Examine the legs for oedema.

112 HEPATOMEGALY

INSTRUCTION

Examine this patient's abdomen.

SALIENT FEATURES

History

- Shortness of breath, leg oedema (heart failure)
- History of alcohol ingestion, cirrhosis
- History of malignancies (secondaries in the liver)
- History of leukaemia or lymphoma.

Examination

- Enlarged liver: comment on its size, tenderness, surface (smooth or irregular)
- Percuss the upper border (normally in the fifth intercostal space in the right midclavicular line) and auscultate for bruit (N Engl J Med 1962;266:554–5, JAMA 1968;206:2518–20, Postgrad Med 1977;62:131–4).

Remember

- How far the liver extends below the costal margin is of less importance than 'liver span' particularly in patients with emphysema or flattened diaphragms.
- By percussion, the mean liver size is 7 cm for women and 10.5 cm for men. A liver span 2–3 cm larger or smaller than these values is considered abnormal. The liver size depends on several factors including age, sex, body size, shape and the examination technique utilized (e.g. palpation versus percussion versus radiographic) (Ann Intern Med 1969;70:1183–9).

Proceed as follows:

- Look for the following signs:
  - Spleen for ascites
  - Signs of cirrhosis
  - Lymph nodes
  - Raised JVP
  - Hepatic flap.
- Tell the examiner you would order an ultrasound of the abdomen.
- At this stage you may be asked to look for nervous system signs of alcoholism (peripheral neuropathy, proximal myopathy, cerebellar syndrome, bilateral sixth cranial nerve palsy as in Wernicke's encephalopathy, recent memory loss and confabulation in Korsakoff's psychosis).

DIAGNOSIS

This patient has a nodular, hard hepatomegaly (lesion), which indicates secondaries in the liver. I would like to look for a primary, particularly in the GI tract (aetiology).

QUESTIONS

How would you investigate hepatomegaly?

Once physical examination or radiography has suggested this diagnosis, the next step is percutaneous abdominal ultrasound; this should distinguish a dilated biliary system, nodular liver, heterogeneity, fatty liver or space-occupying lesion. Conditions to be excluded include viral hepatitis, alcohol- and drug-induced liver disease, steatohepatitis, autoimmune liver diseases and metabolic disorders, including haemochromatosis, Wilson's disease, and α_1-antitrypsin deficiency. Systemic and infiltrative diseases include amyloidosis, lymphoma, sarcoidosis and infectious processes such as disseminated tuberculosis and fungaemia.

What does a tender liver indicate?
A stretch of its capsule caused by a *recent* enlargement, as in cardiac failure or acute hepatitis.

What are the common causes of a palpable liver in the UK?
- Cardiac failure (firm, smooth, tender, mild to massive enlargement)
- Cirrhosis (non-tender, firm; in later stages the liver decreases in size)
- Secondaries in the liver (enlarged with rock-hard or nodular consistency).

ADVANCED-LEVEL QUESTIONS

Mention some less common causes of hepatomegaly
- Leukaemia and other reticuloendothelial disorders
- Infections: glandular fever, infectious hepatitis
- Primary biliary cirrhosis
- Haemochromatosis
- Sarcoid, amyloid
- Tumours: hepatoma, hydatid cysts.

Note: The liver may be felt without being enlarged in the following circumstances: increased diaphragmatic descent, presence of emphysema with an associated depressed diaphragm, thin body habitus with a narrow thoracic cage, presence of a palpable Riedel's lobe and right-sided pleural effusion.

In which condition does a pulsatile liver occur?
Tricuspid regurgitation.

What does a hepatic arterial bruit over the liver indicate?
The hepatic arterial bruit has been described in alcoholic hepatitis, primary or metastatic carcinoma. Although reported to occur in cirrhosis, it is rare without associated alcoholic hepatitis (Lancet 1966;ii:516–19).

What does the presence of an abdominal venous hum indicate?
It is virtually diagnostic of portal venous hypertension (usually caused by cirrhosis) (Br Heart J 1950;12:343–50). When present together with the hepatic arterial bruit in the same patient, it suggests cirrhosis with either alcoholic hepatitis or cancer.

What do you know about Cruveilhier–Baumgarten syndrome?
It is the presence of the abdominal venous hum in portal hypertension secondary to cirrhosis (Am J Med 1954;17:143–50).

What does a hepatic friction rub indicate?
In a young woman, it could be caused by gonococcal perihepatitis (Fitz–Hugh–Curtis syndrome); in others it could indicate hepatic neoplasm with inflammatory changes or infection in or adjacent to the liver. The presence

of a hepatic rub with a bruit usually indicates cancer of the liver (JAMA 1979;241:1495), whereas the presence of the hepatic rub, bruit and abdominal venous hum indicates that a patient with cirrhosis has developed a hepatoma.

Dame Sheila Sherlock, Emeritus Professor of Medicine, Royal Free Hospital, London, is a doyen of liver diseases.

Hans Popper (1903–1988), Professor of Pathology at Chicago and the founding dean of Mount Sinai School of Medicine in New York; he is regarded as the founding father of hepatology.

Professor Humphrey Humphrey, Vice President Royal College of Physicians of London graduated from the University of Oxford and he has been the Sheila Sherlock professor of medicine at the Royal Free and University College, School of Medicine and director of the Royal Free's Centre for Hepatology since 1999. He was also vice-dean and campus director at the Royal Free from 2000 until his recent retirement.

Humphrey has published numerous research papers relating to many aspects of liver disease, and is chairman of the Medical Advisory Committee of the British Liver Trust.

---

113 CIRRHOSIS OF THE LIVER

INSTRUCTION

Examine this patient's abdomen.

SALIENT FEATURES

History

- History of fatigue, weight loss, jaundice
- History of alcohol abuse
- History of hepatitis B, intravenous blood products
- History of intravenous drug abuse
- Mental status changes (hepatic encephalopathy)
- History of drugs: methyldopa, amiodarone, methotrexate
- History of Wilson's disease, α_1-antitrypsin deficiency
- History of hepatitis C.

Examination

- Hands:
  - Clubbing, leukonychia
  - Dupuytren's contracture (see Fig. 219.1), palmar erythema
  - Spider naevi, tattoos, hepatic flap, pallor
  - Scratch marks, generalized pigmentation.
- Eyes and face:
  - Icterus, cyanosis, parotid enlargement.
- Chest:
  - Spider naevi, loss of axillary hair, gynaecomastia.

- Abdomen:
  - Splenomegaly (seldom >5 cm below the costal margin)
  - Ascites
  - Hepatomegaly (particularly in alcoholic liver disease).
- Legs:
  - Loss of hair on the shins
  - Oedema.
- Tell the examiner that you would like to look for testicular atrophy.

DIAGNOSIS

This patient has spider naevi, gynaecomastia, splenomegaly and parotid enlargement (lesions) from cirrhosis caused by alcohol abuse (aetiology). The patient has hepatic flap, indicating liver cell failure (functional status).

QUESTIONS

What is cirrhosis?
Cirrhosis is defined pathologically as a diffuse liver abnormality character-ized by fibrosis and abnormal regenerating nodules.

Mention a few causes of cirrhosis
- Alcohol dependence
- Hepatitis B virus infection (look for tattoos)
- Lupoid hepatitis
- Primary biliary cirrhosis
- Haemochromatosis
- Drugs: methyldopa, amiodarone, methotrexate
- Metabolic: Wilson's disease, α_1-antitrypsin deficiency
- Cryptogenic.

How would you investigate this patient?
- FBC including haemoglobin and platelet count
- Liver function tests including γ-glutamyltransferase (GGT)
- Prothrombin time
- Hepatitis B markers
- Serum autoantibodies
- Serum iron and ferritin
- Serum α-fetoprotein
- Ascitic fluid analysis
- Ultrasonography of the liver.

Why does this patient have a low serum albumin concentration?
Albumin is synthesized in the liver and in cirrhosis there is liver cell failure, causing impaired synthesis.

What are the major sequelae of cirrhosis?
- Portal hypertension (development of portosystemic collaterals)
- Variceal haemorrhages
- Hepatic encephalopathy
- Ascites and spontaneous bacterial peritonitis
- Hepatorenal syndrome
- Coagulopathy
- Hepatocellular carcinoma.

What are the important locations of the portosystemic collaterals?

- Oesophageal submucosal veins: supplied by the left gastric vein and drain into the superior vena cava via the azygous vein
- Paraumbilical veins: supplied by umbilical portion of the left portal vein and drain into abdominal wall veins near the umbilicus. These veins may form a caput medusae at the umbilicus
- Rectal submucosal veins: supplied by the inferior mesenteric vein through the superior rectal vein and drain into the internal iliac veins through the middle and inferior rectal veins
- Short gastric veins: supplied by the oesophageal submucosal veins and drain into the splenic vein
- Splenorenal shunts: spontaneous or surgically created.

ADVANCED-LEVEL QUESTIONS

What are the poor prognostic factors?

- Encephalopathy
- Low serum sodium concentration, <120 mmol/l (not caused by diuretic therapy)
- Low serum albumin level, <25 g/l
- Prolonged prothrombin time.

What is the utility of measuring serum ammonia level in patients with altered mental status?

- In patients with established hepatic encephalopathy, monitoring ammonia level during therapy is of limited value
- In patients with acute liver failure, an elevated serum ammonia is a poor prognostic sign: arterial ammonia levels >2.0 mg/l is associated with cerebral herniation in acute liver failure (Hepatology 1999;29:648–53)
- When there is no liver disease, a search for an underlying cause such as total parenteral nutrition, GI bleed, steroid use, portosystemic shunts, inborn errors of metabolism such as urea cycle disorders, drugs such as glycine, salicylates and valporates.

Remember: Altered mental status in a cirrhotic patient does not equal hepatic encephalopathy; for example in alcoholic patients with altered mental status consider Wernicke's encephalopathy

What factors can precipitate hepatic encephalopathy in a patient with previously well-compensated cirrhosis?

- Infection
- Diuretics, electrolyte imbalance
- Diarrhoea and vomiting
- Sedatives
- Upper GI haemorrhage
- Abdominal paracentesis
- Surgery.

What are the laboratory changes seen in cirrhosis?

- Aminotransferases: alanine and aspartate aminotransferases normal or moderately elevated
- Alkaline phosphatase: usually slightly elevated
- Gamma-glutamyltransferase: usually slightly elevated, high in active alcoholics
- Bilirubin: elevates later in cirrhosis; predictor of death

- Albumin: decrease in advanced cirrhosis
- Prothrombin time: increases in advanced cirrhosis since the liver synthesizes clotting factors
- Immunoglobulins: increased, mainly IgG
- Serum sodium: hyponatremia
- Thrombocytopenia: from both congestive splenomegaly and cirrhosis
- Leukopenia and neutropenia: from splenomegaly with splenic margination
- Coagulation defects: worsen with in advanced cirrhosis.

What are the diagnostic tests in cirrhosis?
- Serology for hepatitis viruses
- Serology for autoantibodies (anti-nuclear, anti-smooth muscle, anti-mitochondria)
- Ferritin and transferrin saturation: iron overload
- Copper and ceruloplasmin: copper overload
- Immunoglobulin: non-specific but may assist in distinguishing causes
- Cholesterol: primary biliary cirrhosis
- Glucose: non-alcoholic steatohepatitis
- α1-Antitrypsin.

What do you know about Childs–Pugh classification?
The Child–Turcotte–Pugh score is used to assess the prognosis of chronic liver disease. The score assesses bilirubin, albumin, INR, presence and severity of ascites and encephalopathy using 1–3 points for each depending on the severity. The point score classifies patients into three class A–C; class A has a favourable prognosis, while class C is at high risk of death.

How do you manage a patient with cirrhosis?

	Prevention	Treatment
Itching		Medication
Constipation	Diet	Laxatives (e.g. lactulose)
Variceal bleeding	Non-selective beta-blockers (e.g. propranolol), variceal band ligation	See below
Ascites	Salt restriction	See Case 115
Renal failure	Avoid hypovolaemia	Rehydration, stop diuretics, albumin infusion
Hepatic encephalopathy	Avoid precipitants	Treat precipitating factors, bleeding, electrolyte inbalance, sedatives
Spontaneous bacterial peritonitis	Treat ascites	Antibiotics

How would you manage variceal bleeding in cirrhosis?
- Blood transfusion to replace falling hematocrit
- Early endoscopy to confirm the bleeding site

- Endoscopic sclerotherapy with octreotide (N Engl J Med 1995;333:555–60)
- Intravenous antidiuretic hormone is less effective than sclerotherapy
- Endoscopic ligation (N Engl J Med 1999;340:988–93)
- Balloon tamponade is effective in temporarily stopping bleeding while awaiting more definitive therapy
- Combination of vapreotide (a somatostatin analogue) and endoscopic treatment (N Engl J Med 2001;344:23–8)
- Transjugular intrahepatic portosystemic stent shunt (N Engl J Med 1994;330:165–71)
- Combination of nadolol and isosorbide mononitrate (N Engl J Med 1996;334:1624–9).

114 JAUNDICE

INSTRUCTION

Would you like to ask this patient a few questions and perform a relevant examination?

SALIENT FEATURES

History

Take a history by asking the patient about the following:
- His or her age: hepatitis is more common in the young and carcinoma in the elderly
- Sore throat and rash: infectious mononucleosis
- Occupation: Weil's disease in sewerage and farm workers
- Contact with jaundice: hepatitis A
- Drug history: oral contraceptives, phenothiazines
- Blood transfusions, injections, arthritis, urticaria: hepatitis B
- Alcohol consumption
- Pruritus: cholestasis caused by hepatitis A, primary biliary cirrhosis
- Colour of the urine: dark, tea- or cola-coloured urine is caused by renal excretion of conjugated bilirubin
- Colour of the stools: pale stools in obstructive jaundice
- Abdominal pain: cholecystitis, gallstones, cholangitis, carcinoma of the pancreas
- Past history: recurrent jaundice, as in Dubin–Johnson syndrome
- Fever, rigors and abdominal pain: suggests cholangitis.

Examination

- Hands (clubbing, palmar erythema, Duputryen's contracture)
- Sclera (to confirm the icterus)
- Conjuctiva, for pallor
- Neck, lymph nodes
- Upper chest: spider naevi, loss of axillary hair and gynaecomastia
- Abdomen: hepatomegaly, splenomegaly, Murphy's sign, palpable gall-bladder, ascites
- Legs, for pitting oedema
- Tell the examiner that you would like to:

- examine the urine
- do a digital rectal examination.

Remember: The most important question to answer in the evaluation of any jaundiced patient is 'Will this patient require surgery to relieve biliary obstruction?'

Be prepared to discuss bilirubin metabolism.

DIAGNOSIS

This patient is markedly icteric and has spider naevi and gynaecomastia (lesions) caused by alcoholic liver disease (aetiology).

QUESTIONS

What do you understand by the term jaundice?

It is the yellowish discoloration of skin, sclera and mucous membrane caused by the accumulation of bile pigments. Scleral icterus suggests that serum biliburin of at least 51 µmol/l (30 mg/l).

How would you differentiate jaundice from carotenaemia?

The discoloration of carotenaemia is differentiated from jaundice by the absence of yellow colour in the sclera and mucuous membranes, normal urine colour and the presence of yellow–brown pigmentation of carotenoid pigment in the palms, soles and nasolabial folds.

What is Murphy's sign and what does it indicate?

It is the tenderness elicited on palpation at the midpoint of the right subcostal margin on inspiration. It is a sign of cholecystitis.

Have you heard of Courvoisier's law?

It states that in a patient with obstructive jaundice a palpable gallbladder is unlikely to be caused by chronic cholecystitis.

What is Charcot's fever?

Intermittent fever associated with jaundice and abdominal discomfort in a patient with cholangitis and biliary obstruction.

How would you investigate this patient?

- Urine for bile pigments
- FBC
- Serum haptoglobulin, reticulocyte count and Coombs' test, if you suspect haemolysis
- Liver function tests: serum albumin, bilirubin, enzymes
- Prothrombin time
- Viral studies: hepatitis antigen and antibodies, Epstein–Barr virus antibodies
- Ultrasonography of the abdomen, if you suspect cholestatic jaundice
- Special investigations: mitochondrial antibodies, endoscopic retrograde cholangiopancreatography (ERCP), CT of the abdomen, liver biopsy.

ADVANCED-LEVEL QUESTIONS

What do you know about Dubin–Johnson syndrome?

It is a rare benign condition characterized by jaundice and pigmentation secondary to a failure of excretion of conjugated bilirubin. The defect in this syndrome is mutations in the gene for multiple drug resistance protein 2. The liver is stained by melanin in the centrilobular zone. The brom-sulfthalein test shows a late secondary rise at 90 min.

What do you know about Gilbert syndrome?

Gilbert syndrome is very common, with reported incidence of 3–7% of the population and with males predominating females by a ratio of 2–7:1. It is characterized by the impaired conjugation of bilirubin caused by reduced activity of uridine diphosphate glucuronyltransferase (UDPGT). The patients typically have mild unconjugated hyperbilirubinaemia (<103 μmol/l or <30 mg/l).

Mention a few causes of postoperative jaundice

Causes of postoperative jaundice (usually occurring in the first 3 postoperative weeks) include:

- resorption of haematomas, haemoperitoneum, haemolysis of transfused erythrocytes (particularly when stored blood products are used), haemolysis in glucose-6-phosphate dehydrogenase deficiency
- impaired hepatocellular function caused by halogenated anaesthetics, sepsis, hepatic ischaemia secondary to perioperative hypotension
- extrahepatic biliary obstruction caused by biliary stones, unsuspected injury to biliary tree.

How does estimation of serum bilirubin concentration help in discerning the aetiology of jaundice?

Normal serum bilirubin concentration is usually no greater than 15 mg/l and is mainly unconjugated. If jaundice is primarily caused by haemolysis or a disorder of bilirubin conjugation, at least 85% of the bilirubin will be unconjugated. With normal liver function, haemolysis alone does not produce a serum bilirubin level >40 mg/l. A rise in serum bilirubin levels of up to 20 mg/l is compatible with extrahepatic cholestasis, but a greater rate indicates haemolysis, hepatitis or hepatic cell necrosis. The serum bilirubin in pure biliary obstruction seldom exceeds 300 mg/l; a greater value indicates that there is associated hepatocellular jaundice as well.

A Gilbert (1858–1927), Professor of Medicine at l'Hôtel Dieu in Paris.

PSA Weil (1848–1916), Professor of Medicine in Tartu, Estonia and Berlin.

JB Murphy (1857–1916), Professor of Surgery at Northwestern University in Chicago.

J Courvoisier (1843–1918), Professor of Surgery, Basel, Switzerland.

IN Dubin, Professor of Pathology, Pennsylvania, and FB Johnson, pathologist, Veterans Administration Hospital, Washington.

---

115 ASCITES

INSTRUCTION

Examine this patient's abdomen.

SALIENT FEATURES

History

- History of abdominal distension, dyspnoea
- History of pain abdomen: spontaneous bacterial peritonitis, malignancy

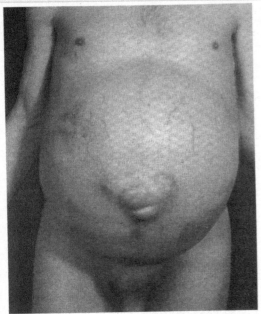

Fig. 115.1 Ascites, showing distended abdomen, dilated superficial collateral veins, haemorrhagic scratch marks and umbilical varices. (With permission from Forbes A et al. 2005.)

- History of heart failure, renal failure or liver disease
- History of TB (peritoneal TB)
- History of malignancy: mesothelioma, metastatic spread from primary tumours.

Examination

- Full flanks and umbilicus (Fig. 115.1)
- Presence of shifting dullness (always percuss with your finger parallel to the level of fluid)
- If the ascites is gross, use the 'dipping' method of palpation to feel the liver and spleen
- Look for stigmata of underlying disease (e.g. signs of cirrhosis, cardiac failure or malignancy).

Proceed as follows:

- Check for sacral oedema and swollen ankles.

DIAGNOSIS

This patient has marked ascites and leg oedema with splenomegaly (lesions) caused by portal hypertension, the underlying cause needs to be investigated (aetiology).

QUESTIONS

What are the causes of a distended abdomen?
Fat, fluid, faeces, flatus and fetus.

What do you understand by the term ascites?
It is the pathological accumulation of fluid in the peritoneal cavity.

What are the common causes of ascitic fluid?
● Portal hypertension with cirrhosis
● Abdominal malignancy
● Congestive cardiac failure.

What investigations would you do to determine the underlying cause?
Diagnostic paracentesis for proteins and malignant cells, ultrasonography of the abdomen, peritoneal biopsy or laproscopy if the cause remains unclear.

What is the difference between an exudate and a transudate?
An exudate has a protein content of >25 g/l (see Case 97).

ADVANCED-LEVEL QUESTIONS

What are the mechanisms of ascites formation in cirrhosis?
● It is caused by a combination of liver failure and portal hypertension. Liver failure decreases renal blood flow, resulting in retention of salt and water
● Secondary hyperaldosteronism caused by increased renin release and decreased metabolism of aldosterone by the liver
● Decreased metabolism of aldosterone by the liver
● Decreased metabolism of antidiuretic hormone
● Hypoalbuminaemia, which decreases colloid oncotic pressure
● Lymphatic obstruction, resulting in a 'weeping' liver
● Overproduction of nitric oxide has been proposed to be important in the pathogenesis of ascites sodium and water retention and hemodynamic abnormalities in cirrhosis (N Engl J Med 1998;339:533–41). Inhibition of nitric oxide synthesis improves sodium and water excretion in cirrhotic rats with ascites.

What is the relation between ascites and chronic liver disease?
● Ascites indicates decompensation of previously asymptomatic chronic liver disease.
● Ascites occurs in about half of the patients within 10 years of a diagnosis of compensated cirrhosis.
● The development of fluid retention in patients with chronic liver disease is a poor prognostic sign: only half of these patients survive beyond 2 years.

What do you know about the serum:ascites albumin gradient?
It is calculated by subtracting the ascitic fluid albumin concentration from the serum albumin concentration in samples obtained at the same time. This gradient correlates directly with portal pressure; those whose gradient is ≥11 g/l have portal hypertension and those with gradients of <11 g/l do not. The accuracy of such determinations is 97%.

How would you manage a patient with cirrhosis and ascites?

The most important treatments are sodium restriction and diuretics (N Engl J Med 1994;330:337–42):

- Sodium restriction to 88 mmol/day; only 15% of these patients lose weight or have a reduction in ascitic fluid with this therapy alone.
- Fluid restriction is usually not necessary unless the serum sodium concentration falls below 120 mmol/l.
- When the patient has tense ascites, 5 litres or more of ascitic fluid should be removed to relieve shortness of breath, to diminish early satiety and to prevent pressure-related leakage of fluid from the site of a previous paracentesis.
- Diuretic therapy should be initiated immediately, before which the serum sodium concentration of a random urine sample should be measured. Serial monitoring of urinary sodium concentration helps to determine the optimal dose of diuretic; doses are increased until a negative sodium balance is achieved. The most effective diuretic regimen is a combination of spironolactone and furosemide. More than 90% of patients respond to this therapy.
- Diuretic-resistant ascites:
  - Therapeutic paracentesis with infusion of salt-free albumin (reported to decrease hospital stay)
  - Peritoneovenous shunting (e.g. Le Veen shunt), limited by the high rate of infection and disseminated intravascular coagulation
  - Transjugular intrahepatic portasystemic stent shunt (TIPS) is a non-surgical side-to-side shunt consisting of a stented channel between a main branch of the portal vein and the hepatic vein. The stent shunt is associated with an operative mortality rate of 1% compared with 5–39% for surgical shunts (N Engl J Med 1995;332:1192–7)
  - Extracorporeal ultrafiltration of ascitic fluid with reinfusion
  - Liver transplantation.

In patients with cirrhosis and refractory or recurrent ascites would you prefer paracentesis or transjugular intrahepatic portasystemic stent shunt?

One study has suggested that the creation of a TIPS can improve the chance of survival without liver transplantation compared with that seen with large-volume paracentesis (N Engl J Med 2000;342:1701–7). Refractory ascites was defined as failure to respond to diuretic therapy (a daily dose of at least 300 mg spironolactone or 120 mg furosemide). The study excluded patients with hepatic encephalopathy of grade 2 or higher, a serum bilirubin concentration >86 µmol/l, portal vein thrombosis or a serum creatinine concentration of >30 mg/l (265 µmol/l). TIPS was ineffective in patients with associated intrinsic renal disease.

What are the complications of ascites?

- Respiratory embarrassment may complicate large amounts of ascites
- Spontaneous bacterial peritonitis is seen in cirrhotics: suspect when there is an ascitic fluid leukocyte count of 500×10^6 cells/l, or polymorphonuclear cell count of $>250 \times 10^6$ cells/l. Empirical therapy with a non-nephrotoxic broad-spectrum antibiotic should be initiated immediately.

Mention some uncommon causes for ascitic fluid

- Nephrotic syndrome
- Constrictive pericarditis

- Tuberculous peritonitis
- Chylous ascites
- Budd–Chiari syndrome
- Meigs syndrome.

What do you know about the pathogenesis of ascites in cirrhotics?

Two theories have been proposed (N Engl J Med 1982;307:1577).

Underfilling theory. Primary abnormality is inappropriate sequestration of fluid within the splanchnic vascular bed caused by portal hypertension, resulting in a decrease in intravascular volume. The kidney responds by retaining salt and water.

Overflow theory. Primary abnormality is inappropriate retention of salt and water by the kidney in the absence of volume depletion.

G Budd (1808–1882), Professor of Medicine at King's College, London.

H Chiari (1851–1916), Professor of Pathology at the German University in Prague.

JV Meigs (1892–1963), Professor of Gynaecology at Harvard, Massachusetts General Hospital.

Le Veen, gastroenterologist at the Veterans Administration Hospital in New York.

Sometime during the rule of Tiberius (25–50 AD), the physician Celsus wrote about oedema, describing it as a chronic malady that may develop in patients who collect water under their skin. The Greeks called this hydrops. They described three types: water is all drawn within, ascites; body is rendered uneven by swellings arising here and there, hyposrka; and a tense belly, tympanites (BMJ 1999;318:1610–13).

---

116 HAEMOCHROMATOSIS

INSTRUCTION

Examine this patient's abdomen.
Look at this patient.

SALIENT FEATURES

History

- Family history
- Skin tan
- Shortness of breath (cardiac failure)
- Diabetes (pancreatic involvement)
- Joint pain (present in 50% of cases): pseudogout usually affects the second and third metacarpophalangeal joints. Any of small joints may be involved (Fig. 116.1)
- Melaena, hematemesis (bleeding from varices).

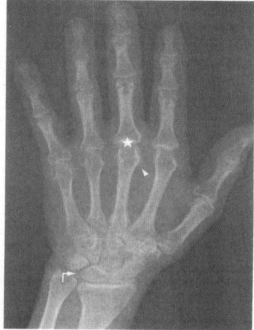

Fig. 116.1 Haemochromatosis. Hooklike osteophyte (arrowhead) at the third metacarpal head with cartilage loss at metacarpophalangeal joints (star) and chondrocalcinosis of triangular fibrocartilage (bent arrow). (With permission from Firestein et al. 2008.)

Examination

- The patient is a pigmented male over 30 years of age
- Palmar erythema, spider naevi
- Jaundice
- Ascites, hepatomegaly (firm, regular)
- Loss of secondary sexual hair.

Proceed as follows:

- Tell the examiner that you would like to investigate as follows:
  - Look for testicular atrophy (caused by iron deposition affecting hypothalamopituitary function)
  - Examine the heart for dilated cardiomyopathy, cardiac failure
  - Check urine for sugar, looking for evidence of diabetes mellitus (present in 80% of cases).

Remember: Patients with haemochromatosis develop cirrhosis and hepatocellular carcinoma.

DIAGNOSIS

This male patient has generalized hyperpigmentation, hepatomegaly and signs of liver cell disease (lesions) caused by haemochromatosis, which may be hereditary (aetiology).

ADVANCED-LEVEL QUESTIONS

Does this disease run in families?

Yes, and it is an autosomal recessive condition. At least four different genes encoding proteins involved in iron metabolism have been described: *HJV*, *HAMP*, *TfR2* and *HFE*. *HFE* is on chromosome 6. Two mutations (845A (C282Y) and 187C (H63D)) account for 90% of cases in those of European extraction. *HFE* is closely associated with *HLA-A3* and to a lesser extent with *HLA-B14*. The responsible alleles are on the short arm of chromosome 6 (Nat Genet 1996;13:399–408). Asymptomatic close relatives of patients with hereditary haemochromatosis, in particular siblings, should be advised to undergo screening (measurements of serum ferritin and iron, and saturation of iron-binding capacity). Hereditary haemochromatosis can occur in adults who do not have pathogenic mutations affecting chromosome 6 (N Engl J Med 1999;341: 718–24, 725–32). A substantial number of homozygous relatives of these patients (more commonly men) have disease-related conditions such as cirrhosis, hepatic fibrosis, elevated amiotransferase and haemochromatotic arthropathy that may not have been detected clinically (N Engl J Med 2000;343:1529–35).

However, 10% or more of the patients with clinically severe hereditary haemochromatosis do not have these mutations and this limits the value of diagnostic DNA testing. Ferroportin-associated iron overload, currently classified as hereditary haemochromatosis type 4, was clinically recognized in 1999 and was linked to *SLC40A1*, which encodes ferroportin, a protein involved in cellular iron export.

What is the mechanism of increased iron uptake?

Iron absorption is mediated by the duodenal metal transporter DMT-1 (also called NRAMP-2). It has been suggested that increased expression of mRNA for NRAMP-2 in the duodenal mucosa of patients with hereditary haemochromatosis may promote duodenal uptake of iron and result in iron overload (Lancet 1999;353:2120–23).

What is the benefit of early identification?

Early venesection has shown benefits, particularly in those who have not developed diabetes mellitus or cirrhosis. Early venesection prevents progression of hepatic disease and may consequently prevent complication of hepatocellular carcinoma.

How would you confirm your diagnosis?

- Transferrin saturation is increased
- Serum ferritin levels are raised
- Liver biopsy to measure iron stores is a definitive test
- MRI is now the modality of choice for non-invasive quantification of iron storage in the liver. It allows repeated measurements and reduces sampling errors (Fig. 116.2).

How would you manage such a patient?

- Avoidance of alcohol and Indian balti curries, which are prepared in cast iron cookware (BMJ 1995;310:1368)
- Avoidance of uncooked shellfish and marine fish, since these patients are susceptible to fatal septicaemia from the marine bacterium *Vibrio vulnificus*
- Phlebotomy: venesection prolongs life and often reverses tissue damage. Initially, weekly venesection (500 ml blood per week) for 2 years (as 50 g iron or more is removed) and then once every 3 months. Iron depletion

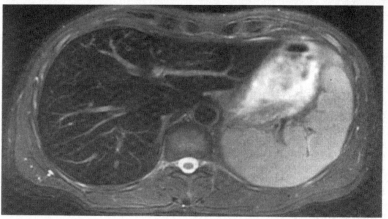

Fig. 116.2 T_2-weighted MRI image demonstrating abnormally low liver signal in haemochromatosis. (With permission from Adam et al. 2008.)

is confirmed by serum ferritin <50 µg/l and transiferrin saturation <40%. Many manifestations improve (insulin requirements often diminish) except for testicular atrophy and chrondrocalcinosis

- Deferoxamine, an iron chelating agent is used when haemodynamics do no permit venesection
- Screening of family members by measuring fasting transferring saturation and ferritin levels.

What is the commonest cause of death in patients with hereditary haemochromatosis?

The most common cause of death is hepatocellular carcinoma, for which the risk is 200-fold greater than that of the general population. Depletion of iron, and even reversal of cirrhosis, does not totally prevent the occurrence of this fatal neoplasm. Patients diagnosed in the subclinical, precirrhotic stage and treated by regular phlebotomy have a normal life expectancy (N Engl J Med 1985;313:1256–62).

Mention a few causes of generalized pigmentation

Common causes are sun tan and race.

Uncommon causes are:

- liver disease: haemochromatosis in males; primary biliary cirrhosis in females
- Addison's disease
- uraemia
- chronic debilitating conditions such as malignancy.

The term haemochromatosis was first used by von Recklinghausen (p. 279) in 1889 to describe postmortem findings in men with cirrhosis associated with massive deposition of iron in the hepatocytes (von Recklinghausen FD Ueber Hämochromatose. Tageblatt Versamml Dtsch Naturforsch Artze Heidelberg 1889;62:324–5).

The inherited nature of haemochromatosis was first recognized by Sheldon in 1935.

117   PRIMARY BILIARY CIRRHOSIS

INSTRUCTION

Examine this patient's abdomen.

SALIENT FEATURES

History

- Pruritus: affecting half of affected patients, more common in men
- Fatigue: commonest symptom
- Lethargy and right upper quadrant-pain (in 25%)
- Symptoms of hepatic decompensation (in 20%): jaundice, ascites, variceal haemorrhage
- Steatorrhoea.

Examination

- Usually occurs in middle-aged women
- Clubbing
- Generalized pigmentation
- Xanthelasma (may occur at any stage but more common in advanced disease)
- Icterus
- Scratch marks
- Hepatosplenomegaly (common in early stages).

Proceed as follows:

- Look for xanthomata over joints, skin folds and sites of trauma to the skin.

Remember: There may be clinical features of other autoimmune diseases such as rheumatoid arthritis, dry mouth of Sjögren syndrome, systemic sclerosis, CREST syndrome (p. 553), Hashimato's thyroiditis, dermatomyositis.

- Check for proximal muscle weakness from osteomalacia.
- Examine for peripheral neuropathy.
- Tell the examiner that you would like to test for high serum levels of alkaline phosphatase and anti-mitochondrial antibodies (AMA; present in 95% of the patients, with the M2 antibody being more specific; it is almost always negative in extrahepatic obstruction).

DIAGNOSIS

This middle-aged woman has generalized pigmentation, jaundice, xanthe-lasmata and pruritus with hepatosplenomegaly (lesions) caused by primary biliary cirrhosis (aetiology). She is in liver cell failure as evidenced by the hepatic flap (functional status).

ADVANCED-LEVEL QUESTIONS

How does primary biliary cirrhosis present?

Classically, it presents with itching in a middle-aged woman. However, in 50% of cases there may be no liver symptoms. There are four phases.

Asymptomatic with normal liver tests. Antibodies to pyruvate dehydrogenase complex (AMA) is detectable and about three-quarters develop symptoms of primary biliary cirrhosis (PBC) in 2 years and 83% developed abnormal liver function tests at median period of 5 years from first detection of AMA (Lancet 1996;348:1399–1402). Most patients have liver histology compatible with, or diagnostic for, PBC. In one series, none had died from liver disease 12 years after AMA detection (J Hepatol 1994;20:707–13).

Symptomless with abnormal liver tests. Circulating AMA are present. More than 50% have established fibrosis at diagnosis. Up to 80% of patients develop symptoms or signs of PBC during the first 5 years of follow-up. The median time from diagnosis to death is 8–12 years.

Symptomatic. Lethargy and pruritus is prominent and time to death or transplantation is 5 to 10 years.

Decompensated primary biliary cirrhosis. Signs include ascites, variceal haemorrhage or jaundice. The mean time to death or transplantation is 3–5 years.

What diseases are associated with primary biliary cirrhosis?

- Common (up to 80%): Sicca syndrome (p. 794)
- Frequent (~20%): arthralgia, fibrosing alveolitis, Raynaud syndrome, sclerodactyly, thyroid disease
- Rare (<5%): Addison's disease, glomerulonephritis, hypertrophic pulmonary osteoarthropathy, myasthenia gravis, SLE, thrombocytopenic purpura, vitiligo.

Is primary biliary cirrhosis associated with cancer?

It is estimated that patients with PBC have a 20-fold increased relative risk of developing hepatocellular carcinoma and increased risk of overall cancer (J Hepatol 1997(suppl 1):101).

How would you investigate this patient?

- Liver function tests are normal in the presymptomatic stage; characteristically cholestatic pattern (raised alkaline phosphatase, 5-nucleotidase and γ-glutamyltransferase) may be seen; serum aminotransferases may be slightly raised but rarely exceed five times the upper limit of normal. Serum bilirubin is normal initially but rises as diseases progresses. Once serum bilirubin is >170 μmol/l the estimated survival is <18 months (Gut 1979;20:137–140).
- Hepatic synthetic function is well preserved until late stages; a prolonged prothrombin time may indicate malabsorption of vitamin K in cholestasis.
- Serum lipids: hypercholesterolaemia is common, lipoprotein lp(a) is low, HDL cholesterol is increased in the early stages but falls as the disease progresses.
- Immunological tests: IgM and IgG are elevated; complement activation occurs although C3 levels are normal; several antibodies are elevated but antibodies to components of the nuclear pore complex and AMA are very closely elevated with PBC. AMA is found in 96% of patients with PBC but the E2 subtype is specific to PBC. Autoimmune cholangitis is a variant of PBC that has characteristic histological features of PBC but is negative for AMA in serum (Gut 1997;30:440–2). The AMA is directed against the mitochondrial pyruvate dehydrogenase complex.
- Histology identifies non-suppurative destruction cholangitis or granulomatous cholangitis.

What are the stages of primary biliary cirrhosis?

Primary biliary cirrhosis is divided into four histologic stages:

1. Defined by the localization of inflammation to the portal triads.
2. The number of normal bile ducts is reduced and inflammation extends beyond the portal triads into the surrounding parenchyma.
3. Fibrous septa link adjacent portal triads.
4. End-stage liver disease, characterized by frank cirrhosis with regenerative nodules.

Is liver biopsy necessary to confirm the diagnosis?

Athough, liver biopsy is routinely used to confirm the diagnosis, the need for this procedure for either diagnosis or prognosis is questionable (Lancet 1997;350:875–9). The very close association between histology and E2 AMA in PBC means that liver histology is not required unless clinical and serological features are equivocal. The presence of cirrhosis is of very little value in determining the prognosis, and clinically significant portal hypertension (ascites, variceal haemorrhage) may occur during the early histological stages.

What is the mechanism for itching in these patients?

The itching used to be ascribed to retention of bile acids with cholestasis, but more recent work emphasized the importance of naturally occurring opioid tone, characterized by an increase in the concentration of endogenous opioid receptors and upregulation of opioid receptors (Gut 1996;38:644–5). These findings led to the use of opioid antagonists for treatment of pruritus.

What drugs have been used to control pruritus?

Colestyramine is first line; rifampin and ursodeoxycholic acid are second line and naloxone, nalmefene and propofol are third-line agents used to treat pruritus.

What drugs have been used to treat primary biliary cirrhosis?

Ursodeoxycholic acid, corticosteroids, ciclosporin, azathioprine, tacrolimus, methotrexate and colchicines.

What is the rationale behind bile salt therapy?

Hepatocytes affected by autoimmune processes are further injured by endogenous bile acids (such as chenodeoxycholic acid and cholic acid), which accumulate as a result of associated cholestasis. Partial replacement of water-soluble bile acids such as ursodeoxycholic acid may reduce pruritus and damage to the liver cell.

Is there a cure for primary biliary cirrhosis?

Liver transplantation is the only known cure. The 5-year survival following transplantation exceeds 80%. It is associated with a rapid resolution of lethargy and itching, and bone loss slows after the first year. Although the quality of life is not normal, it is usually excellent.

When is liver transplantation indicated?

Indications for liver transplantation are either symptoms (e.g. intractable pruritus, lethargy) or signs and symptoms of end-stage liver disease: increasing jaundice with serum bilirubin >170 μmol/l, estimated survival <1 year, intractable ascites, encephalopathy, fasting serum albumin (<30 g/l), progressive muscle loss, recurrent spontaneous bacterial peritonitis, increasing osteoporosis, hepatopulmonary syndrome, early incidental hepatocellular carcinoma and unacceptable quality of life.

What factors predict survival after transplantation?

● Serum urea and albumin
● Presence of ascites
● Child's grade and United Network for Organ Sharing status (reflecting whether the patient is at home, general hospital bed or intensive care unit) (Hepatology 1997;25:672–7).

What do you understand by secondary biliary cirrhosis?

It occurs secondary to large duct obstruction and is usually caused by extrahepatic obstruction such as bile duct stricture, gallstones and sclerosing cholangitis.

Professor Peter Brunt, contemporary gastroenterologist and liver physician, Aberdeen Royal Infirmary, is also the personal physician to the Queen and is an astute clinician. He is the President of the Association of Physicians of Great Britain, a society founded by Osler.

Roger Williams, Professor at King's College, London, and Sir Roy Calne, Professor of Surgery, Cambridge, pioneered liver transplantation in the UK.

Thomas E Starzl, surgeon, Pittsburgh, USA, is an internationally known pioneer in liver transplantation.

---

118 WILSON'S DISEASE

INSTRUCTION

Look at this patient's eyes.

SALIENT FEATURES

History

● History of consanguinity
● In young adult or child: hepatitis, haemolytic anaemia, portal hypertension or neuropsychiatric abnormalities
● In adolescents: presents as liver disease
● In adults <40 years of age: consider chronic or fulminant hepatitis.

Examination

● Greenish yellow to golden-brown pigmentation at the limbus of the cornea (Kayser–Fleischer ring)
● Look for:
  • jaundice (look at the sclera)
  • sunflower cataracts
  • hepatomegaly
  • signs of liver cell failure.
● Look for neurological manifestations: tremor, chorea, mask-like facies with a vacuous smile.

DIAGNOSIS

This patient has a classical Kayser–Fleischer ring with jaundice and hepatomegaly (lesions) caused by Wilson's disease (aetiology) and does not have a hepatic flap (functional status).

ADVANCED-LEVEL QUESTIONS

What is Kayser–Fleischer ring?

Deposition of copper in Descemet's membrane (Fig. 118.1). The ring is most marked at the superior and inferior poles of the cornea. It is often apparent only on slit-lamp examination. It may be absent in patients with only hepatic manifestations, but it is present in those with neuropsychiatric disease.

Is Kayser–Fleischer ring pathognomonic of Wilson's disease?

No, it is also seen in primary biliary cirrhosis, chronic active hepatitis with cirrhosis, cryptogenic cirrhosis and long-standing intrahepatic cirrhosis of childhood.

At what age do the neurological manifestations usually manifest?

They usually appear between 12 and 30 years of age. The most frequent first neurological symptom is a difficulty in speaking or writing while in school.

What do you know about the inheritance of the disease?

Autosomal recessive inheritance with the gene *ATP7B* located on chromosome 13, often associated with a family history of consanguinity. It is caused by mutations encoding a copper-transporting P-type ATPase (Wilson's disease protein, WNDP). About 27 mutations have been reported; the most common, leading to the substitution H1069Q, is present in about a third of the patients of European extraction.

What do you know about the pathophysiology of this disease?

The precise defect is not known. The major aberration is excessive absorption of copper from the small intestine, with decreased excretion of copper by the liver, resulting in an increase in tissue deposition, particularly in the brain, cornea, liver and kidney. The animal models of this condition are the Long–Evans cinnamon rat and the toxic milk mouse.

What are the biochemical changes in Wilson's disease?

- Low serum ceruloplasmin level (ceruloplasmin is the copper-carrying protein)
- Serum copper concentration may be high, low or normal

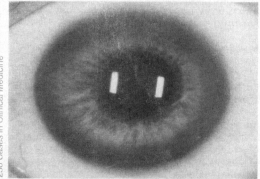

Fig. 118.1 Kayser–Fleischer ring. (With permission from Goldman L, Ausiello DA 2007.)

- Orally administered radiolabelled copper is incorporated into ceruloplasmin
- Increased urinary excretion of copper.

How is the diagnosis of a suspected case confirmed?

By the demonstration of one of the following:
- Kayser–Fleischer rings and a serum ceruloplasmin level <20 mg/l
- Serum ceruloplasmin concentration of <200 mg/l and copper concentration in a liver biopsy sample greater than 250 µg/g on a dry weight basis.

How would you treat such a patient?

- Copper-chelating agents:
  - Penicillamine, which removes and detoxifies deposits of copper; treatment is lifelong and continuous and is given with pyridoxine to minimize side effects
  - Penicillamine should never be given as initial therapy in those with neurological manifestations
  - In patients intolerant to penicillamine, trientine dihydrochloride is an acceptable alternative.
- Zinc salts
- Tetrathiomolybdate with zinc salts: treatment of choice in those with neurological symptoms.

What are the clinical stages of Wilson's disease?

Wilson's disease progresses through four clinical stages.
1. Asymptomatic accumulation of copper in the liver, which begins when the patient is born.

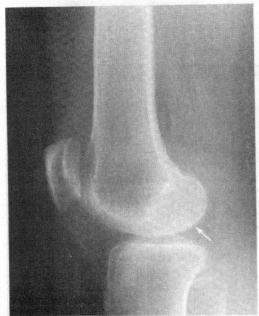

Fig. 118.2 Brushlike calcifications (arrow) along the articular surface. (With permission from Firestein et al. 2008.)

2. Patient is either asymptomatic or manifests with haemolytic anaemia or liver failure.
3. Copper accumulates in the brain.
4. Progressive neurological disease.

What are the radiographic features of Wilson's disease?

- Osteopenia: most apparent in the hands, feet, and spine
- Arthropathy
- Articular abnormalities: subchondral bone fragmentation, cyst formation and cortical irregularities, most commonly identified in the wrist, hand, foot, hip, shoulder, elbow and knee. Irregularity and indistinctness of the subchondral bone may form a characteristic 'paintbrush' appearance (Fig. 118.2)
- Osteomalacia and rickets have been reported. Radiologic signs of rickets, retardation of skeletal maturation and pseudofractures may be observed
- Additional characteristic radiographic findings are small, distinctly corticated ossicles around the affected joint and periosteal bone formation at the attachment sites of tendons and ligaments
- Chondrocalcinosis is rare, usually limited to the knees

Samuel Alexander Kinnier Wilson (1877–1937) qualified in Edinburgh and worked at the National Hospital, Queen Square, London, as a neurologist (Wilson SAK. Progressive lenticular degeneration. A familial nervous disease associated with cirrhosis. Brain 1912;34:295).

Bernard Kayser (1869–1954) and Bruno Fleischer, both German ophthalmologists, described the same condition in 1902 and 1903 respectively.

---

119 SPLENOMEGALY

INSTRUCTION

Examine this patient's abdomen.

SALIENT FEATURES

History

- Fatigue (from anaemia)
- Night sweats, low-grade fever: from hypermetabolic state caused by overproduction of white blood cells in chronic myeloid leukaemia
- Abdominal fullness: from splenomegaly
- Bleeding, bone pain: bone marrow infiltration in myeloproliferative disorders
- History of leukaemia
- History of myelofibrosis
- History of residence in endemic areas of malaria, kala-azar
- Family history of Gaucher's disease
- History of fever (infectious mononucleosis, infective endocarditis)

- Blurred vision, respiratory distress, priapism (from leukostasis in chronic myeloid leukaemia)
- Occasionally transverse myelitis (from myelopoiesis in epidural space).

Examination

- Massive spleen. There may be associated anaemia.
- Start low while examining for the spleen and be gentle during palpation. Even if you are certain it is the spleen, you must go through the motions of ruling out a palpable kidney: do a bimanual palpation and check for ballottement; feel for the splenic notch; auscultate for splenic rub.

Proceed as follows:
- Look for enlarged lymph nodes and anaemia.
- Remember that the spleen must be at least two or three times its usual size before it can be felt.
- Remember that the spleen normally does not extend beyond the anterior axillary line and lies along the 9th, 10th and 11th ribs. The spleen percussion sign is a useful diagnostic technique (Ann Intern Med 1967;67:1265).
- Comment on anaemia or facial suffusion (Fig. 119.1).

DIAGNOSIS

This patient has massive splenomegaly (lesion), probably caused by a myeloproliferative disorder (aetiology) and is short of breath because of severe anaemia (functional status).

QUESTIONS

What is your diagnosis?
- Myeloproliferative disorder
- Myelofibrosis, particularly in males
- Chronic myeloid leukaemia, particularly in females.

How would you confirm your diagnosis?
Bone marrow examination.

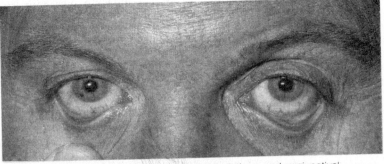

Fig. 119.1 Polycythaemia vera, showing facial plethora and conjunctival suffusion. (With permission from Hoffbrand, Pettite JE: 2000.)

ADVANCED-LEVEL QUESTIONS

In which other conditions is a massive spleen palpable?

- Malaria
- Kala-azar
- Gaucher's disease.

In which conditions can a moderately enlarged spleen (two to four finger-breadths or 4–8 cm) be felt?

- Portal hypertension secondary to cirrhosis
- Lymphoproliferative disorders such as Hodgkin's disease and chronic lymphatic leukaemia.

In which common conditions would the spleen be just palpable?

- Lymphoproliferative disorders
- Portal hypertension secondary to cirrhosis
- Infectious hepatitis
- Glandular fever (infectious mononucleosis)
- Subacute endocarditis
- Sarcoid, rheumatoid arthritis, collagen disease, idiopathic thrombocytopenia, congenital spherocytosis and polycythaemia rubra vera (95% of those with polycythaemia vera have a mutation affecting the JAK2 signalling molecule)
- Slender young women (Ann Intern Med 1967;66:301).

What do you know about the genetics of chronic myelocytic leukaemia?

The fusion of c-abl (normally present on chromosome 9) with bcr sequences on chromosome 22 is pathognomonic of the chronic phase of chronic myelocytic leukaemia (the Philadelphia chromosome). The p53 gene appears to be the culprit in myeloid blast transformation and there are structural alterations of RB1 or N-ras in <10% of those with myeloid blast crisis.

What do you understand about the terms myeloid metaplasia and extramedullary hematopoiesis?

Myeloid metaplasia and extramedullary hematopoiesis are used interchangeably. They describe the process of ectopic haematopoietic activity that may occur in any organ system but predominantly affects the liver and spleen. It may or may not be associated with bone marrow fibrosis (myelofibrosis). 'Myelofibrosis with myeloid metaplasia' is usually used to describe idiopathic myelofibrosis or agnogenic myeloid metaplasia (N Engl J Med 2000;342:1255–65). Myelofibrosis is characterized by splemomegaly, teardrop poiklocytosis in peripheral smear, leukoerythroblastic blood picture and giant abnormal platelets, hypercellular marrow with reticulin or collagen fibrosis (Fig. 119.2).

What do you understand by the term chronic myeloid disorders?

Chronic myeloid disorders include:

- chronic myeloid leukaemia: characterized by elevated white blood cell count, marked left-shift to myeloid series, but a low percentage of promyelocytes and blasts, presence of Philadelphia chromosome or bcr/abl

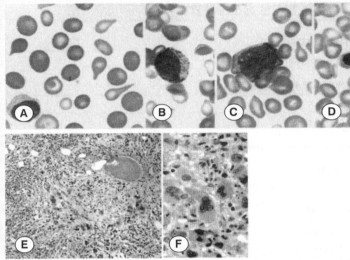

Fig. 119.2 Primary myelofibrosis. Peripheral blood: dacryocytes, or teardrop forms (A), leukoerythroblastic profile with immature granulocytic precursors (B), including blasts (C) and circulating nucleated red blood cells (D). Bone marrow biopsy is frequently hypercellular (E) with atypical megakaryocytic and granulocytic proliferation (F). (With permission from Hoffman et al. 2008.)

- myelodysplastic syndromes: characterized by cytopenias with a hyper-cellular bone marrow, morphologic abnormalities in two or more hematopoietic cell lines
- atypical chronic myeloid disorder
- chronic myeloproliferative disease: polycythaemia vera, essential thrombocythaemia, myelofibrosis with myeloid metaplasia:
  - essential thrombocythaemia, in turn, includes agnogenic myeloid metaplasia, post-polycythemic myeloid metaplasia and post-thrombocythaemic myeloid metaplasia.

What is the treatment of Gaucher's disease?

Enzyme replacement therapy with glucocerebroside (alglucerase) is ben-eficial (N Engl J Med 1991;324:1464–70, N Engl J Med 1992;327:1632–6).

PCE Gaucher (1854–1918), Professor of Dermatology in France.
    The 1902 Nobel Prize was awarded to Sir Donald Ross (1857–1932; born in Almora, India), University of Liverpool, for his work on malaria, in which he showed how the parasite enters the organism. This laid the foundation for successful research on this disease and methods of combating it.

120 FELTY'S SYNDROME

INSTRUCTION

Examine this patient's abdomen.

SALIENT FEATURES

History

- Fever, weigh loss
- Rheumatoid arthritis
- Leg ulcers, hyperpigmentation.

Examination

- Mild to moderate splenomegaly
- Rheumatoid arthritis.

Proceed as follows:

- Look for the following signs:
  - Anaemia
  - Vasculitis
  - Diffuse pigmentation
  - Leg ulcers.

DIAGNOSIS

This patient has moderate splenomegaly with rheumatoid arthritis (lesions) caused by Felty syndrome.

ADVANCED-LEVEL QUESTIONS

What is Felty syndrome?

It is a rare complication of rheumatoid arthritis in which there is leucopenia with selective neutropenia and splenomegaly. The bone marrow is typically hyperplastic. The disease typically manifests late in the course of 'burnt-out' joint disease. The prognosis is poor because of recurrent Gram-positive infections. The 'large granular lymphocyte syndrome' (Fig. 120.1), a premalignant disorder of the T lymphocyte, occurs in one-third of the patients with Felty syndrome in rheumatoid arthritis.

Note: Splenectomy does not prevent sepsis and may hasten the onset of malignancy.

What do you understand by the term hypersplenism?

It implies removal of erythrocytes, granulocytes or platelets from the circulation by the spleen. Removal of the spleen is indicated when the underlying disorder cannot be corrected.

Criteria for hypersplenism include:

- enlarged spleen
- destruction of one or more cell lines in the spleen
- normal bone marrow.

What are the indications for splenectomy?

- Hereditary spherocytosis in children
- Autoimmune thrombocytopenia or haemolytic anaemia not controlled by steroids

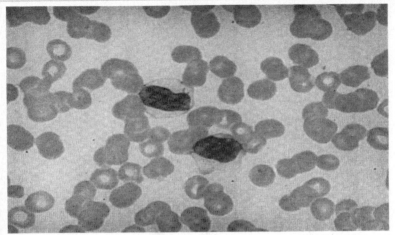

Fig. 120.1 Peripheral blood smear with large granular lymphocytes. (With permission from Firestein et al. 2008.)

- To ameliorate hypersplenism in Gaucher's disease, thalassaemia, hairy cell leukaemia
- For symptoms in massive organomegaly

What are the characteristic cells in a peripheral blood smear following splenectomy?
The presence of Howell–Jolly bodies (in all) (Fig. 120.2), siderocytes and spur cells (in 25% of patients).

What are the causes of asplenia?
- Diminished function: sickle cell disease, thalassaemia, coeliac disease, SLE, lymphoma, leukaemia, amyloidosis.
- Surgical removal: hereditary spherocytosis, thalassaemia, lymphoma, idiopathic thrombocytopenia, traumatic rupture.

To which infections is the asplenic patient susceptible?
- *Streptococcus pneumoniae, Haemophilus influenzae* B, *Neisseria meningitidis* and malaria parasites cause significant risk.
- Less common infections are babesiasis, caused by tick-borne protozoa, and infection with *Capnocytophaga canimorus* following a dog bite.

What precautions would you advise an asplenic patient in the outpatient clinic?
- Vaccination:
  - Pneumococcal vaccine: a single injection; booster doses at 5–10-year intervals
  - Hib vaccine: a single dose at the same time as pneumococcal immunization

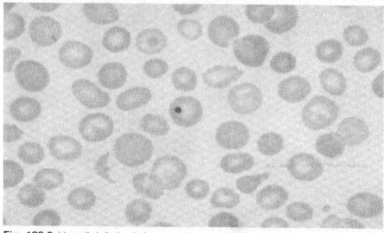

Fig. 120.2 Howell-Jolly body in an erythrocyte. (With permission from Goldman L, Ausiello DA 2007.)

- Meningococcus groups A and C vaccine (although the majority of infections are caused by group B strains for which there is no vaccine of proven efficacy).
- Antibiotic prophylaxis: phenoxymethylpenicillin or amoxicillin
- Foreign travel: antimalarial chemoprophylaxis, other precautions (insect repellants, screens at night).

Augustus R Felty (1895–1964) was a physician at Hartford Hospital, Hartford, Connecticut. He described this syndrome while he was working at the Johns Hopkins Hospital, Baltimore.

---

121 POLYCYSTIC KIDNEYS

INSTRUCTION

This patient gives a history of intermittent haematuria, obtain a brief history and examine this patient's abdomen.

SALIENT FEATURES

History

- Acute loin pain and/or haematuria (from haemorrhage in a cyst, cyst infection or urinary stone formation)
- Loin or abdominal discomfort, caused by increasing size of kidneys

- Family history of polycystic kidney disease (as the condition is autosomal dominant with nearly 100% penetrance)
- Complications of hypertension
- Stroke (as a result of ruptured berry aneurysm)
- Family history of brain aneurysm: the prevalence of intracranial aneurysms increases from 5% to 20% when there is a family history.

Examination

- Arteriovenous fistulae in the arms or subclavian dialysis catheter (remember that polycystic kidneys constitute the third most common cause for chronic renal failure in the UK after glomerulonephritis and pyelonephritis)
- Palpable kidneys: confirm by bimanual palpation and ballottement; there is a resonant note on percussion from overlying colon; the hand can get between the swelling and the costal margin.

Proceed as follows:

- Look for the following signs:
  - Enlarged liver as a result of cystic disease
  - Transplanted kidney: may be palpable in either iliac fossa
  - Third nerve palsy (berry aneurysms are associated with polycystic kidneys).
- Look for anaemia (chronic renal failure) or polycythaemia (increased erythropoiesis)
- Check the BP (hypertension develops in 75%)
- Tell the examiner that you would like to investigate as follows:
  - ECG to look for left ventricular hypertrophy (this appears to occur to a greater degree for a given rise in BP in autosomal dominant polycystic kidney disease (ADPKD) than in other renal disorders, and with essential hypertension)
  - Microscopic haematuria.

Remember: Polycystic kidney disease is a misnomer as it is a systemic disorder affecting many organs, including the liver, pancreas and, in some rare cases, the heart and brain. Polycystic kidney disease is the most common genetic, life-threatening disease, affecting an estimated 12.5 million people worldwide.

DIAGNOSIS

This patient has polycystic kidney disease (lesion and diagnosis) and is currently on dialysis as evidenced by the arteriovenous fistula in the arm (functional status).

QUESTIONS

How may polycystic disease present?

Haematuria, hypertension, urinary tract infection, pain in the lumbar region, uraemic symptoms, subarachnoid haemorrhage associated with berry aneurysm, and complications of associated liver cysts. Kidney stones (more likely to be uric acid rather than calcium oxalate stones) are twice as prevalent as the general population.

Is the kidney involvement usually unilateral or bilateral?

The disease is universally bilateral; unilateral cases reported probably represent multicystic renal dysplasia.

ADVANCED-LEVEL QUESTIONS

What do you know about the prevalence of this disease?

ADPKD is one of the most common hereditary disorders, being 10 times more common than sickle cell disease, 15 times more common than cystic fibrosis and 20 times more common than Huntington disease. It has a worldwide distribution. In the white population, the disease appears to occur in about 1 in 400 to 1 in 1000 people (Acta Med Scand 1957;328:1–255). Although the disease is rare in Africa and less common in American blacks than American whites, the incidence of end-stage renal disease caused by ADPKD is similar in blacks and whites. ADPKD is an important cause of renal failure, with 77% of patients dying or reaching end-stage renal disease by the age of 70 years (Kidney Int 1992;41:1311–19).

In which other conditions may bilateral renal cysts be observed in an ultrasonographic study?

Multiple simple cysts, autosomal recessive polycystic kidney disease in children, tuberous sclerosis and von Hippel–Lindau syndrome.

What are the criteria for diagnosis of polycystic kidney disease using ultrasonography?

- Individuals at risk and those <30 years: presence of at least 2 renal cysts (unilateral or bilateral) is sufficient to establish a diagnosis in those with a positive family history; 5 cysts bilaterally in those with no such history
- 30–60 years: at least 2 cysts in each kidney in those with a positive family history, 5 cysts bilaterally in those with no such history
- ≥60 years: at least four cysts in each kidney regardless of family history (Lancet 1994;343:824–7).

How would you like to manage this patient?

- FBC, urea and electrolytes, serum creatinine, urine microscopy, urine culture
- Ultrasonography of the kidneys to confirm the diagnosis. Ultrasound may be equivocal in subjects under the age of 20 years. Ultrasound or renal MRI can also be used to determine total kidney volume, a measure of disease progression
- Contrast-enhanced spiral CT head scan or MRI as a screening test for intracranial aneurysms in patients aged 18–40 years and with a family history of intracranial aneurysms or subarachnoid haemorrhage (N Engl J Med 1992;327:953–5).

In which other organs are cysts seen in this condition?

Liver (in 30% of cases), spleen, pancreas, lungs, ovaries, testes, epididymis, thyroid, uterus, broad ligament and bladder. Women with hepatic cysts. Women with ADPKD may have massive cystic enlargement of the liver, a complication attributed to the role of oestrogens in promoting the growth of cysts. Exogenous oestrogens and repeated pregnancies are also risk factors for this complication; therefore, oral contraceptives and hormone replacement therapy should be avoided.

What are the neurological manifestations of this condition?

Subarachnoid haemorrhage from an intracranial berry aneurysm, causing death or neurological lesions in about 9% of patients. About 8% of ADPKD have an asymptomatic intracranial aneurysm and the prevalence is twice as high with a family history of such aneurysms or of subarachanoid haemorrhage. Typically intracranial aneurysms present as a 'sentinel' or 'thunderclap' headache.

What is the pathology?

Cysts develop in Bowman's capsule and at other levels in the nephron, displacing kidney tissue. In the normal kidney, polycystin 1 is an integral membrane glycoprotein involved in cell–cell and/or cell–matrix interaction (J Am Soc Nephrol 1995;6:1125–33); polycystin 2 is similar to a subunit of voltage-activated calcium and sodium channels, which suggests a role in regulating calcium entry (Science 1996;272:1339–42). The polycystins interact through their C-terminal cytoplasmic tails, which suggests that they may function through a common signalling pathway (Bat Genet 1997;16:179–83). As activation of the intracellular calcium pathways inhibits cell proliferation, in ADPKD, with insufficient or abnormal polycystins and impaired calcium entry, the proliferative pathways dominant, resulting in cyst formation and ultimately renal failure. Renal function remains stable until kidney volumes reach a critical size.

What cardiovascular manifestations have been reported in these patients?

- Mitral valve prolapse in 26%
- Other lesions commonly seen are mitral, aortic and tricuspid valve regurgitation: adult polycysic disease of kidney with involvement of liver.

What are the renal manifestations of this disease?

- The main structural change is the formation of cysts. Cysts enlarge, lose their tubular connection and become isolated from the glomerulus, requiring transepithelial transport of solutes and fluids for further expansion. Cyst fluids have different sodium compositions, some high and others low.
- One of the earliest and most consistent functional abnormalities is a decrease in renal concentrating ability.
- There may be altered endocrine function, as reflected by increased secretion of both renin (causing increased predilection to hypertension) and erythropoietin (resulting in better maintained haematocrit in renal failure, unlike in renal failure from other causes; rarely can result in polycythaemia).

What are the causes of abdominal pain in this disease?

Infected cyst, haemorrage into cyst or diverticular perforation.

What are the complications of polycystic kidney disease?

- **Renal complications**
- Hypertension (intrarenal activation of the renin–angiotensin system is said to be the main mechanism and hence ACE inhibitors are first-line-agents to control BP; diuretics should be avoided because hypokalaemia promotes cyst formation)
- Pain: back pain or abdominal pain (cyst decompression may help to relieve pain but does not alter the rate of progression)
- Gross or microscopic haematuria
- Cyst infection (lipophilic antibiotics against Gram-negative bacteria such as co-trimoxazole, fluoroquinolones penetrate the cysts better and are preferred to standard antibacterial agents)
- Renal calculi (seen in 10–20% with ADPKD and are frequently radiolucent and composed of uric acid)
- Urinary tract infection including pyelonephritis
- Proteinuria

- Renal failure (once the glomerular filtration rate (GFR) is <50 ml/min, the rate of progression is more rapid than in other primary renal disorders and there is a reduction in GFR of about 5 ml/min every year). About one half of the patients have normal life with adequate renal function.

- **Extrarenal manifestations:**
- Cystic: cysts in the liver, ovary, pancreas, spleen and CNS. Unlike renal cyst formation, liver cysts seem to be influenced by female hormones. Whilst men and women have the same frequency of liver cysts, massive liver cysts are almost exclusively found in women
- Non-cystic:
  - Cardiac valvular abnormalities: mitral valve prolapse (seen in ~20% of ADPKD), aortic valve abnormalities
  - Intracranial saccular aneurysm or berry aneurysm: MR angiography is the most reliable technique of non-invasive screening among such patients.
- Gastrointestinal: colonic diverticula, herniae of the anterior abdominal wall.

What do you know about the genetic transmission of this disease?

Polycystic kidney disease is an autosomal dominant disorder. Mutations in at least three different genes can lead to ADPKD. The *PKD1* gene (encoding polycystin-1) is located on chromosome 16 (Cell 1994;77:881–4). The *PKD2* gene (encoding polycystin-2) is situated on chromosome 4. At least one other gene containing mutations that lead to ADPKD is known to exist; its chromosomal location is not known.

Among the European ADPKD population, *PKD1* is the cause in about 85% of families and *PKD2* the cause is about 15%. Compared with individuals affected by *PKD2*, those with *PKD1* have more severe disease with a higher prevalence of hypertension, an increased risk of progression into renal failure, and shorter life expectancy. Although *PKD2*-linked disease is clinically milder than *PKD1*-linked disease, it has a deleterious impact on overall life expectancy and cannot be regarded as a benign disorder (Lancet 1999;353:103–7).

What do you know about screening in this condition?

- The children and siblings of patients with established ADPKD should be offered screening.
- Affected individuals should have their BP checked regularly and offered genetic counselling.
- Genetic linkage analysis can be utilized in many families. Ultrasound is usually not useful before the age of 20 years.

What are the poor prognostic factors in autosomal dominant polycystic kidney disease?

Patients are liable to progress more rapidly if they are male or have *PKD1* mutations, early-onset hypertension, episodes of gross haematuria (J Am Soc Nephrol 1997;8:1560–7) or a family history of hypertension in an unaffected person (J Am Soc Nephrol 1995;6:1643–8); however, these only account for a fraction of the variability of disease progression.

What are the causes of death in these patients?

One-third of adult patients die from renal failure; another third die from the complications of hypertension (including heart disease, intracerebral haemorrhage and rupture of berry aneurysm). The remaining third die from unrelated causes.

Are there any special treatments for this condition?
Basis research suggests that patients should be advised to:
- increase their water intake to 3 litres a day (to reduce antidiuretic hormone and cyclic AMP stimulation)
- limit the sodium intake (to control hypertension or kidney cyst formation)
- avoid caffeine or methyxanthine derivatives (since they block phosphodiesterase thereby resulting in more cyclic AMP to stimulate cyst formation)
- avoid situations that could carry a high risk of abdominal trauma, such as high-impact contact sports.

Are there any clinical trials being conducted in autosomal dominant polycystic kidney disease?
- The HALT PKD (Halt Progression of Polycystic Kidney Disease) study funded by NIH is comparing the combination of ACE inhibitor and angiotensin receptor blocker with an ACE inhibitor plus placebo
- The TEMPO (Tolvaptan Efficacy and Safety in Management of Polycystic Diseases and its Outcomes) study
- Studies of mTOR inhibitors: rapamycin as pilot study, everolimus study
- Somatostatin study.

What do you know about hypertension in a pregnant woman with autosomal dominant polycystic kidney disease?
Although ACE inhibitors or an angiotensin receptor blocker are the best choice for hypertension in ADPKD, these drugs are absolutely contraindicated in pregnancy. Normotensive women with ADPKD and creatinine <12 mg/l typically have uncomplicated pregnancies, but 16% get new hypertension and are more likely to develop chronic hypertension (J Am Soc Nephrol 1994;5:1178–85). Pregnant patients with ADPKD have higher frequency of maternal complications (particularly hypertension, oedema and pre-eclampsia) than patients without ADPKD (35% vs 19%, p <0.001).

Further reading
Grantham JJ: Autosomal dominant polycystic kidney disease, *N Engl J Med* 359:1477, 2007.

Sir W Bowman (1816–1892), Surgeon at the Royal London Ophthalmic Hospital.

EL Potter (1901–), US pathologist. She also described Potter syndrome, with renal agenesis and characteristic of epicanthic folds, receding jaw and low set ears with less cartilage than usual.

OZ Dalgaard's study in 1957 clarified the autosomal dominant pattern of inheritance of the disease.

122 TRANSPLANTED KIDNEY

INSTRUCTION

Examine this patient's abdomen.

SALIENT FEATURES

History

- History of chronic renal failure: determine duration, aetiology (diabetes, hypertension, glomerulonephritis)
- History of haemodialysis
- History of arteriovenous fistula
- History of transplanted kidney.

Examination

- Laparotomy scar (comment on the scar)
- Arteriovenous fistulae in arms
- Transplanted kidney felt in either right or left iliac fossa.

Proceed as follows:

- Tell the examiner that you would like to look for other signs of uraemia (p. 785)
- Do know the differential diagnosis for masses in the right/left iliac fossa (p. 462).

DIAGNOSIS

This patient has a transplanted kidney (lesion) probably required because of diabetic nephropathy, as evidenced by the sugar-free drinks by the bedside (aetiology).

QUESTIONS

Mention a few indications for renal transplantation

End-stage renal disease: the most common diseases that result in referral of patients for transplantation include:

- diabetes mellitus with renal failure
- hypertensive renal disease
- glomerulonephritis.

ADVANCED-LEVEL QUESTIONS

Would you refer a patient for renal transplantation before instituting haemodialysis?

Referral for renal transplantation need not be delayed until the patient has begun dialysis. It is acceptable and, in fact, usually preferable to refer the patient to a renal transplant unit before dialysis is required. With judicious planning on the part of the general practitioner, renal physician and transplant surgical team, transplantation can be performed even before dialysis is required.

In which age group is transplantation preferred to dialysis?

Infants and children have a high morbidity rate on long-term haemodialysis or peritoneal dialysis. Therefore, renal transplantation from parents or siblings improves growth and allows a more normal lifestyle.

Is there any advantage to HLA-matching before transplantation?

Kidneys from living related donors who are HLA identical and also red blood cell ABO matched have a 90% survival rate at 1 year; less-identical grafts tend to have a somewhat lower survival rate. Kidney transplants from matched cadaver donors survive nearly as long, especially if the recipient does not contain antibodies to donor antigens.

There is some evidence that HLA mismatching has a greater effect on living related than it does on cadaveric donor kidney transplantation. Recent evidence has shown that HLA-matched kidneys, particularly for HLA-DR, HLA-B and HLA-A antigens, are associated with long-term survival of the patient. Complete matching of HLA-DR, HLA-B and HLA-A is associated with the best chance of success. HLA-DR matching appears to have the greatest impact on survival, followed by HLA-B and lastly HLA-A (N Engl J Med 1994;331:803–5).

Should repeated blood transfusions be avoided in a patient waiting for a renal transplant?

If the anaemia is well tolerated and is caused by the renal failure per se, blood transfusion should be avoided as it carries a risk of HLA sensitization. Pretreatment of recipients with multiple blood transfusions from the *donor* tends to increase graft survival, in contrast to the deleterious effect on bone marrow engraftment.

What other factors are known to cause sensitization to HLA antigens?

Pregnancy, previously failed transplant.

What drugs are used for post-transplant immunosuppression?

- Steroids, azathioprine and ciclosporin: used independently or in combination
- Newer drugs include tacrolimus, rapamycin, sirolimus, mycophenolate mofetil and daclizumab.

What are the contraindications for kidney transplantation?

- A positive cross-match by cytotoxicity testing between recipient serum and donor cells is considered to be a contraindication for transplantation
- Presence of HIV or other infectious agents on donor screening.

What are the complications of renal transplantation?

- Opportunistic infection, e.g. cytomegalovirus, *Pneumocystis*
- Premature coronary artery disease
- Hypertension: primarily with ciclosporin therapy
- Lymphomas and skin cancers
- De novo glomerulonephritis in the transplanted kidney
- Complications of steroid therapy, e.g. aseptic necrosis of bone.

What do you know about warm ischaemic time?

Shorter warm ischaemic time of the transplanted kidney is associated with longer survival of the recipient. However, a slight increase in the duration of cold ischaemia justifies HLA-matching before kidney transplantation because of higher rates of survival, a lower incidence of the episodes of rejection and lower risk of loss as a result of rejection (N Engl J Med 2000;343:1078–84).

What is the survival rate following kidney transplant?

The 2-year kidney graft survival rate for living related donor transplantation is 85%, whereas in cadaveric donor transplantation it is about 70%.

What do you know about rejection of the transplanted kidney?

Rejection may be acute or chronic and must be suspected when the graft is tender, the urine output is falling or the creatinine concentration is rising. It is a complex process in which both cell-mediated immunity and circulating antibodies play a role. Evaluation of a suspected rejection usually requires graft biopsy.

- Acute rejection is characterized by a lymphocytic interstitial infiltrate with destruction of epithelial cells. It usually responds to treatment, which includes high-dose methylprednisolone, anti-lymphocytic immunoglobulin and anti-T cell monoclonal antibody (OKT3).
- Chronic rejection shows histological features of interstitial fibrosis, atrophy of tubules and proliferation of the arterial intima. There is no specific treatment and general management of chronic renal failure should be reinstituted.

Is there any advantage of renal transplantation compared with long-term dialysis in end-stage renal disease?

The benefits of renal transplantation include better quality of life (Am J Kid Dis 1990;15:201–8), reduced medical expenses (Semin Nephrol 1992;12:284–9) and about a 68% reduction in the long-term risk of death (N Engl J Med 1999;341:1725–30).

What is the role of pancreas–kidney transplantation in patients with diabetes mellitus and end-stage renal failure?

Pancreas transplantation in type 1 diabetes can reverse the lesions of diabetic nephropathy but reversal requires >5 years of normoglycaemia (N Engl J Med 1998;339:69–75). Simultaneous pancreas–kidney transplantation prolongs survival in patients with diabetes and end-stage renal failure (Lancet 1999;353:1915–19).

Does acute myocardial infarction influence long-term survival among patients on long-term dialysis?

Patients on dialysis who have an acute myocardial infarction have high mortality from cardiac causes and poor long-term survival (N Engl J Med 1998;339:799–805).

In the 1920s, Alexis Carrel develop the technique of vascular anastomoses, which made possible the human allograft attempts by David Hume and Joseph Murray in the early 1950s.

Joseph E Murray (b. 1919), Professor of Surgery, Brigham and Women's Hospital and Harvard Medical School, was awarded the 1990 Nobel Prize for Medicine for his pioneering work on organ transplantation along with Thomas E Donnall (b. 1920) of the Fred Hutchinson Cancer Research Center, Seattle, Washington, USA (Murray JE et al. Prolonged survival of human-kidney homografts by immunosuppressive drug therapy N Engl J Med 1963;268:1315–23).

In 1966, Terasaki and coworkers reported the association between HLA matching and outcome in patients receiving cadaveric organs (Ann N Y Acad Sci 1966;129:500–20).

The observation by Schwartz and Damasheck that 6-mercaptopurine was effective in blocking primary but not secondary antibody response in rabbits paved the way for drug-induced immunosuppression in the late 1950s (Nature 1959;183:1682–3).

123 ABDOMINAL AORTIC ANEURYSM

INSTRUCTION

This patient presented with low-back pain; examine the abdomen.

SALIENT FEATURES

History

- Vague abdominal pain
- History of embolization
- Family history of rupture of abdominal aortic aneurysm
- History of smoking.

Remember: Three-quarters of the patients are asymptomatic.

Examination

- Large expansile pulsation along the course of the abdominal aorta (examination for a pulsatile mass should be done by bimanual palpation of the supraumbilical area)
- Auscultate for bruit over the aneurysm and over the femoral pulses
- 'Trash' foot: digital infarcts in patient with easily palpable pulses (suggests either a popliteal or abdominal aneursysmal source of emboli) (BMJ 2000;320:1193–6)
- Examine all peripheral pulses.

Proceed as follows:

- Tell the examiner that you would like to check the following:
  - Urine for sugar
  - BP
  - Serum lipid panel.

Remember:

- Popliteal artery aneurysms often coexist and, in fact, their presence should prompt the physician to look for an abdominal aortic aneurysm.
- Ninety per cent of atherosclerotic abdominal aortic aneurysms present below the origin of the renal arteries and can involve the aortic bifurcation.
- The infrarenal aorta is normally 2 cm in diameter; when it exceeds 4 cm an aneurysm is said to exist.
- True arterial aneurysms are defined as 50% increase in the normal diameter of the vessel.

- Aneursymal process may affect any medium or large artery.
- The most commonly affected vessels are the aorta and iliac arteries, followed by popiliteal, femoral and carotid vessels.

DIAGNOSIS

This patient has a large pulsatile mass in the epigastrium (lesion) caused by an aneurysm of the abdominal aorta (aetiology). The patient complains of pain over the location of the mass, suggesting inflammation and impending rupture (functional status).

QUESTIONS

Is clinical examination sensitive in the detection of abdominal aortic aneurysm?

Sensitivity of abdominal palpation for detection of abdominal aortic aneurysms increases with the diameter of the lesion: 61% for aneurysms 3·0–3·9 cm, 69% for those 4·0–4·9 cm and 82% for those ≥5·0 cm. The palpation sensitivity also depends inversely on the size of the abdominal waistline (Arch Intern Med 2000; 160:833–6).

Which investigations would you do to confirm your diagnosis?

- B mode ultrasonography of the abdomen: a simple, cheap and accurate screening test.
- Large aneurysms require angiography, but angiography may underestimate the size of lumen because of large clots.
- MRI is useful, particularly as it does not require administration of contrast.
- CT (Fig. 123.1).

Remember: Plain abdominal radiography shows a calcified aneursymal aortic wall in only half the cases (Fig. 123.2).

ADVANCED-LEVEL QUESTIONS

How would you manage an abdominal aneurysm?

<4.5 cm: follow-up with ultrasonography every 6 months

4.5–5.0 cm: follow-up with ultrasonography every 3 or 6 months

5.0–5.5 cm: surgery or follow-up

>5.5 cm: pooled data suggest there is a high risk of rupture and hence patients should be referred for surgery if there are no confounding factors that increase the risk of surgery.

The UK small aneurysm trial studied 1090 patients with an aortic aneurysm of diameter 4–5 cm and found a 30 day mortality of 5.8%, mean annual risk of rupture for small aneurysms of 1% and no difference in survival between their treatment groups at 2, 4 or 6 years (Lancet 1998;352:1649–55). Smaller aneurysms must be followed up as they enlarge at a rate of about 0.5 cm a year. In selected cases, an endovascular prosthesis is preferred.

What factors predispose to rupture of the abdominal aneurysm?

- Diameter of the aneurysm
- History of smoking
- Diastolic BP
- COAD

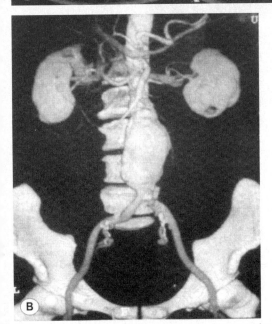

Fig. 123.1 An infrarenal abdominal aortic aneurysm by CT (A) and in three-dimensional CT reconstruction. (With permission from Bhangu, Keighley 2007.)

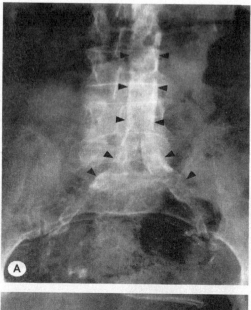

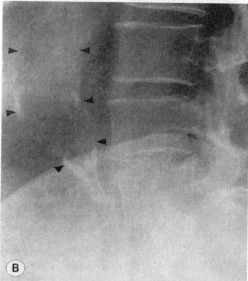

Fig. 123.2 Calcification of the abdominal aorta (arrowheads) in plain radiographs. Calcification of the abdominal aorta is usually much easier to see on the lateral view (B). (With permission from Mettler 2004.)

- Family history of ruptured aneurysm
- Rate of expansion
- Inflammatory aneurysms.

What is the prognosis of aneurysms >55 mm?
Mortality rate for a patient undergoing elective surgery is <5%, whereas that for a ruptured aneurysm is nearly 90%.

What are the sites of rupture of abdominal aortic aneurysm?
- Anterolateral free rupture in the abdominal cavity:
  - Retroperitoneal rupture
  - Rupture of retroperitoneal sac
  - Rupture into the duodenum
  - Rupture into the inferior vena cava.

What are the types of abdominal aortic aneurysm?
- Aneurysms are usually classified into true, false and dissecting aneurysms.
- The Crawford classification defines into four types by anatomic location and extent of involvement:
  - I: involve all or most of the descending thoracic aorta and the upper abdominal aorta
  - II: aneurysms involve all or most of the descending thoracic aorta and all or most of the abdominal aorta
  - III: involve the lower portion of the descending thoracic aorta and most of the abdominal aorta
  - IV: involve all or most of the abdominal aorta, including the visceral segment.
- Pathological types of abdominal aortic aneurysm include:
  - inflammatory: characterized by dense periaortic fibrosis containing abundant lymphoplasmacytic inflammation with many macrophages and often giant cells; cause unclear
  - mycotic: lesions that have become infected by the lodging of circulating microorganisms in the wall (particularly in bacteraemia from a primary *Salmonella* gastroenteritis); suppuration further destroys the media, potentiating rapid dilation and resulting in rupture.

What do you know about the pathogenesis of abdominal aortic aneurysms?
Abdominal aortic aneurysm is linked to the degradation of the elastic media of the atheromatous aorta. An inflammatory cell infiltrate, neovascularization and production and activation of various proteases and cytokines also contribute to its development Although elastin fragmentation and attenuation of the tunica media are the most important characteristics of the wall of an aneurysm, the adventitial tissue, in which collagen is predominant, is responsible for the resistance of the aorta in the absence of elastin in the tunica media. Collagen degradation is currently considered the ultimate cause of rupture.

The elastic and collagen fibres are degraded by proteolytic enzymes, mostly represented by matrix metalloproteinases (MMP) locally activated by either other MMPs or by plasmin generated by plasminogen activators. The role of MMPs and plasmin in the development of abdominal aortic aneurysms has been shown in animal models. The tissue inhibitors of matrix metalloproteinases (TIMP) are also increased in the wall of the aneurysm. The balance between proteases and anti-proteases seems to be tilted in the favour of proteolysis (Lancet 2005; 365:1577–89).

What do you understand by endovascular repair?

The technique of endovascular repair was introduced by Parodi in 1991 (Ann Vasc Surg 1991;5:491–9) and consists of the placement of a graft across the aneurysm and the fixation to the normal aortic and iliac wall with stents at both ends. The aortomonoiliac percutaneous approach consists of the insertion of a stent graft, which is a tube of conventional graft fabric containing at least two stents. A successful attachment requires a segment of non-dilated aorta (neck) between the renal arteries and the aneurysm that is at least 1.5 cm in length, and the device insertion requires that lumens of the iliac arteries be at least 7 mm in diameter. The complete exclusion of blood by the endovascular repair lowers the pressure in the aneurysm sac, which causes the graft to shrink. However, 'an endoleak' from the top or bottom (type 1) or though the graft defect (type 3) is associated with persistent risk of rupture.

In the United Kingdom Endovascular Aneurysm Repair 1 (EVAR 1), a large randomized trial, endovascular repair of large abdominal aortic aneurysm (at least 5.5 cm in diameter on CT) was associated with a significantly lower operative mortality than open surgical repair. However, no differences were seen in total mortality or aneurysm-related mortality in the long term. Endovascular repair was associated with increased rates of graft-related complications and re-interventions and was more costly (N Engl J Med 2010; 362:1863–71). In the United Kingdom Endovascular Aneurysm Repair 2 (EVAR 2) randomized trial involving patients who were ineligible for open repair, endovascular repair of abdominal aortic aneurysm was associated with a significantly lower rate of aneurysm-related mortality than no repair. However, endovascular repair was not associated with a reduction in the rate of death from any cause. The rates of graft-related complications and reinterventions were higher with endovascular repair, and it was more costly (N Engl J Med 2010; 362:1863–71).

> In 1951, C Dubost from Paris performed the first successful aortic resection for aneurysm.

124 UNILATERAL PALPABLE KIDNEY

INSTRUCTION

Examine this patient's abdomen.

SALIENT FEATURES

History

- Nephrectomy
- Congenital absence of kidney
- History of azotaemia, dialysis.

Examination

- One kidney is palpable (bimanually ballottable; there is a transverse band of colonic resonance on percussion and you will be able to insinuate your fingers between the mass and costal margin).

Proceed as follows:

- Look carefully for arteriovenous fistulae in the arms, haemodialysis catheters in the subclavian region.

DIAGNOSIS

This patient has a unilateral palpable kidney (lesion), which may be caused by either polycystic kidney disease or renal neoplasm (aetiology).

QUESTIONS

What are the common causes of a palpable kidney?

- Polycystic kidney disease
- Renal carcinoma
- Hydronephrosis
- Renal cyst
- Hypertrophy of the solitary functioning kidney.

What changes can occur in a kidney when the other is removed?

Long-term renal function remains stable in most patients with a reduction in renal mass of >50%. However, these patients are at increased risk for proteinuria, glomerulopathy and progressive renal failure. Hence it is important to monitor patients with remnant kidneys. Problems are most frequent in those in whom the amount of renal tissue removed is greatest and who have survived the longest (N Engl J Med 1991;325:1058). Survival and the risk of end-stage renal disease in carefully screened kidney donors appear to be similar to those in the general population. Most donors who were studied had a preserved glomerular filtration rate, normal albumin excretion and an excellent quality of life (N Engl J Med 2009;360:459). Renal failure has gradually developed in a small proportion of donors, and according to the United Network for Organ Sharing, 56 of >50 000 previous kidney donors have ultimately been listed for transplants themselves. Although some donors develop hypertension over time, hypertension is common in the general population. Occasionally, microalbuminuria develops in donors, and it is worth considering whether renoprotective therapy might be tailored to prevent this complication (N Engl J Med 2005;353:447).

What are the short-term risks of donation?

- The short-term physical risks are small: the death rate is 0.03%, which is similar to or lower than that for any operation involving the use of general anaesthesia
- The risk of bleeding during or after the procedure
- The risks of infection or other perioperative problems
- Donors will lose time from work. Most return to work within 4–5 weeks
- It can take a few weeks to recover fully from surgery, although the increasing use of laparoscopic donation means that a donor may now be released from the hospital in just a few days.

125 ABDOMINAL MASSES

INSTRUCTION

Examine this patient's abdomen.

SALIENT FEATURES

Examination

There is an epigastric mass.

DIAGNOSIS

Differential diagnosis:
- Carcinoma of the stomach: look for supraclavicular lymph nodes, hepatomegaly; comment on pallor and asthenia
- Carcinoma of the pancreas: look for jaundice
- Aneurysm of the abdominal aorta: look for pulsatile mass, check femoral and foot pulses, auscultate over the mass and the femoral pulses (p. 455)
- Retroperitoneal lymphadenopathy (lymphoma).

INSTRUCTION

Examine this patient's abdomen.

SALIENT FEATURES

Examination

There is a mass in the right iliac fossa.

DIAGNOSIS

Differential diagnosis:
- Crohn's disease: look for mouth ulcers; tell the examiner that you would like to look for fistulae and take a history for chronic diarrhoea (p. 778)
- Carcinoma of the caecum: look for hard mass, lymph nodes
- Enlarged lymph node: look for enlarged nodes elsewhere, feel for liver and spleen, examine the drainage area of iliac lymph nodes (such as the leg, perianal area, external genitalia) do a rectal examination)
- Transplanted kidney: comment on the laparotomy scars, stigmata of renal failure and artificial arteriovenous fistulae
- Appendicular abscess
- Iieocaecal abscess, particularly in Asians
- Ovarian tumours (must be mentioned as a differential diagnosis in female patients).

Less common causes of masses in the right iliac fossa:
- Amoebiasis
- Carcinoid (ileal)
- Actinomycosis
- Ectopic kidney.

PATIENT 3

INSTRUCTION

Examine this patient's abdomen.

SALIENT FEATURES

Examination

There is a mass in the left iliac fossa.

DIAGNOSIS

Differential diagnosis:.
- Diverticular abscess: look for tender, mobile mass
- Carcinoma of the colon: look for hepatomegaly; tell the examiner that you would like to do a per rectal examination
- Faecal mass (the mass may be moulded by pressure)
- Ovarian tumour (in females)
- Enlarged iliac lymph nodes: look for enlarged nodes elsewhere, feel for liver and spleen, examine the drainage areas
- Transplanted kidney: comment on the laparotomy scar, look for signs of renal failure, arteriovenous fistulae (p. 812).

Note: The investigation of first choice in such patients is abdominal ultrasonography.

Robin Warren, Pathologist at Royal Perth Hospital in Western Australia, and Barry J. Marshall discovered that *Helicobacter pylori* causes peptic ulcer disease (Lancet 1983;i:1273–5). In 1984, Marshall infected himself, by drinking a pure culture of *H. pylori*. After feeling fine for 5 days, he experienced nausea and vomiting. Histology confirmed acute gastritis. In 1995, he received the Albert Lasker Clinical Medical Research Award. *H. pylori* has also been implicated in the causation of gastric cancer in Japanese people. There were awarded the 2005 Nobel prize for their discovery of 'the bacterium *Helicobacter pylori* and its role in gastritis and peptic ulcer disease'.

Mr Titus Augustine, FRCS Edin, Consultant Surgeon's appointment to Manchester Royal Infirmary (MRI), led the revival and development of the pancreas transplant programme in Manchester (2001) following a short sabbatical to the University of Minnesota. Manchester is currently the second largest pancreas transplant programme in the UK. The MRI has performed the first non-heart-beating pancreas transplant, the first pancreas re-transplant and transplants in the youngest and oldest donor recipients to date in the UK. In 2002 introduced laparoscopic hand-assisted donor nephrectomy, and currently mentoring consultant colleagues in the procedure. In 2005, introduced laparoscopic adrenalectomy. In 2007 started developing a national surgical service for encapsulating peritoneal sclerosis.

126   CHRONIC LYMPHOCYTIC LEUKAEMIA

INSTRUCTION

Perform a general examination of this patient.

SALIENT FEATURES

History

- Asymptomatic in 70% of patients
- Palpable lymph nodes or left upper quadrant abdominal discomfort in a fifth of patients
- Bleeding or bruising is rare
- Symptoms of anaemia are uncommon
- Weight loss, fever and night sweats are unusual.

Examination

- Usually men over the age of 40 years (male:female ratio is 2:1)
- Symmetrical, painless, rubbery lymph nodes
- Liver or spleen may be palpable.

Proceed as follows:

- Tell the examiner that you would like to do a FBC and examine the peripheral smear (lymphocytosis >15 × 10^9 cells/l, with mature appearance of small lymphocytes) (Fig. 126.1).

Remember that chronic lymphocytic leukaemia manifests clinically with organ infiltration with lymphocytes, immunosuppression (hypogammaglobulinaemia) and bone marrow failure.

DIAGNOSIS

This elderly male patient with painless enlargement of lymph nodes probably has chronic lymphocytic leukaemia (lesion). He has severe pallor, indicating he is in Binet stage C (functional status).

QUESTIONS

What are the causes of anaemia in chronic lymphocytic leukaemia?

Bone marrow infiltration, autoimmune (Coombs' positive) haemolysis.

How may a patient with chronic lymphocytic leukaemia present?

About 25% of cases are asymptomatic; some complain of generalized malaise, weight loss and loss of appetite; others complain of bleeding.

ADVANCED-LEVEL QUESTIONS
ADVANCED-LEVEL QUESTIONS

What is the prognosis in chronic lymphocytic leukaemia?

About one-third of the patients will not require treatment and die from unrelated causes; in another third, the disease is initially indolent followed by rapid progression. In the remaining third the disease is very aggressive from the outset and needs immediate treatment.

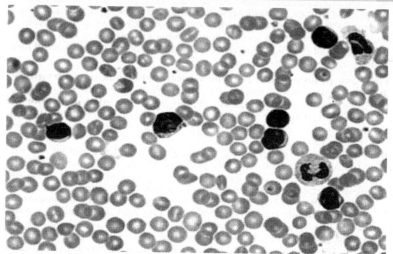

Fig. 126.1 Peripheral blood smear demonstrating lymphocytosis: small lymphocytes with condensed chromatin, imparting a 'soccer ball' pattern, and scant cytoplasm (Wright stain). (With permission from His ED. The leukemias of mature lymphocytes. Hematol/Oncol Clin North Am 2009;23:843–71.)

How is chronic lymphocytic leukaemia staged?

Binet staging (evaluates the enlargement of spleen, liver and lymph nodes in the head and neck, axillae and groin) has three stages A–C:

A: no anaemia or thrombocytopenia and less than three areas of lymphoid enlargement

B: no anaemia or thrombocytopenia, with three or more involved areas

C: anaemia and/or thrombocytopenia, regardless of the number of areas of lymphoid enlargement.

Rai staging has five stages, 0–IV:

0: lymphocytosis only (in blood and bone marrow)

I: lymphocytosis plus lymphadenopathy

II: lymphocytosis with hepatic and/or splenic enlargement

III: lymphocytosis with anaemia

IV: lymphoctyosis with thrombocytopenia.

Note: The primary role of the Rai and Binet staging systems is to help clinicians to decide when to initiate treatment. These staging systems do not predict the clinical course with precision and, therefore, are less helpful in predicting long-term prognosis. Determination of immunoglobulin variable gene (V-gene) mutation status, expression of CD38 and zeta-chain-associated protein 70 (ZAP-70) levels are emerging as promising indicators of prognosis.

What do you know about the pathogenesis of chronic lymphocytic leukaemia?

Chronic lymphocytic leukaemia is a heterogeneous disease that originates from B lymphocytes, which may differ in activation, maturation state or cellular subgroup. The B lymphocytes are antigen experienced (differ in the level of immunoglobulin *V*-gene mutations). The accumulation of leukaemic cells occurs because of survival signals delivered to a subgroup of leukaemic cells from the external environment through a variety of receptors (e.g. B cell receptors and chemokine and cytokine receptors) and their cell-bound and soluble ligands.

How are patients with chronic lymphocytic leukaemia treated?

- Stage A. Specific treatment may not be indicated until stage B or C. Patients with stage A disease should be reassured that, despite the frightening diagnosis of leukaemia, they will be able to live a normal life for many years, with a median survival of 8 years (N Engl J Med 1998;338:1506–14).
- Stage B and C. Patients will require specific and supportive therapy: correction of anaemia and folic acid deficiency, and correction of bone marrow infiltration initially with prednisolone and oxymetholone and subsequently with chemotherapeutic agents. The initial treatment of choice is the combination of the chemotherapeutic agent fludarabine plus the antibody rituximab, with or without the addition of the chemotherapeutic drug cyclophosphamide. Fludarabine is first choice for elderly patients, for whom frequent trips to the clinician's office is difficult. The monoclonal antibody alemtuzumab has been approved for treatment of refractory chronic lymphocytic leukaemia, and lenalidomide has also been shown to have effectiveness in refractory disease. The role of lenalidomide in primary therapy is being studied. The investigational agent flavopiridol has shown encouraging results in certain types of chronic lymphocytic leukaemia (such as those with deletions of 17p) that have not responded to other therapy.

What is Richter syndrome?

This is when an isolated lymph node in chronic lymphocytic leukaemia is transformed into an aggressive large cell lymphoma. There is a median survival of <1 year after its appearance.

Which lymphomas can convert to leukaemias?

- Small cell lymphoma (chronic lymphocytic leukaemia)
- Burkitt's lymphoma (B cell acute lymphoblastic leukaemia)
- Lymphoblastic lymphoma (T cell acute lymphoblastic leukaemia).

Rheumatology
General guidelines for examination of joints

History

Ask the patient whether he or she has any pain, stiffness or difficulty in dressing or walking.

Examination

- *Look* at posture, gait and joint deformity
- *Feel* for temperature, tenderness, joint fluid and crepitus of movement of the joints
- *Move*: check passive and active movements of the joints; test stability of the joints
- *Measure* muscle wasting and shortening of the limb.

- ● Examination of the hands

Figure V.1 shows patterns of peripheral joint disease and Fig. V.2 gives a useful template on which to mark joint disorders.

1. Ask the patient, 'Are your hands painful?'
2. Inspect for joint deformity:
   - Swan-neck deformity (flexion at the distal interphalangeal joints and hyperextension of the proximal interphalangeal joints)
   - Boutonnière deformity (flexion of the proximal interphalangeal joints and hyperextension of the distal interphalangeal joint)
   - Z deformity of the thumb
   - Ulnar deviation of the fingers.
3. Examine the nails:
   - Nailfold infarcts (rheumatoid arthritis).
   - Nail pitting, onycholysis, ridging, hyperkeratosis, discoloration (psoriasis).
4. Comment on the following:
   - Wasting of small muscles of the hand, in particular those on the dorsum of the hand
   - Heberden's nodes, i.e. bony nodules at the distal interphalangeal joints (osteoarthroses)
   - Bouchard's nodes, i.e. bony nodules at the proximal interphalangeal joints (osteoarthroses)
   - Spindle-shaped deformity of the fingers
   - Gouty tophi.
5. Examine the palms:
   - Wasting of the thenar or hypothenar eminence
   - Thickening of the palmar fascia: Dupuytren's contracture (rheumatoid arthritis)
   - Palmar erythema (rheumatoid arthritis)
   - Tap over the flexor retinaculum to detect median nerve entrapment (Tinel's sign, see Fig. 76.1A).
6. Get the patient to perform the following movements:
- ● Unbuttoning of clothes
- ● Pincer movements

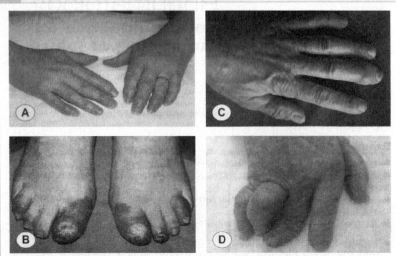

Fig. V.1 Asymmetric polyarticular disease. (A) Distal interphalangeal joint involvement and forearm lymphoedema. (B) Toe dactylitis with skin and nail change. (C) Predominant distal interphalangeal joint involvement. (D) Arthritis mutilans. (With permission from Firestein et al. 2008.)

- Hand grip
- Abduction of the thumb
- Writing.
7. Test sensation of the index and little fingers.
8. Examine the elbows for the following signs:
   - Rheumatoid arthritis.
   - Gouty tophi.
   - Psoriatic plaques.
9. Tell the examiner that you would like to examine the other joints.

Note: When asked to examine the hands, consider the possibility of arthropathy, myopathy, neuropathy, a peripheral nerve lesion or acromegaly.

- **Examination of the knees**
- Ask the patient if the joints are sore.
- Expose both knees and lower thighs fully with the patient lying supine.
- Look for:
  - quadriceps wasting
  - swelling of the joint.
- Feel for:
  - temperature
  - synovial thickening.
- Do the patellar tap (ballottement): fluid from the suprapatellar bursa is forced into the joint space by squeezing the lower part of the quadriceps and then the patella is pushed posteriorly with the fingers; this test indicates fluid in the synovial cavity (Fig. V.3).

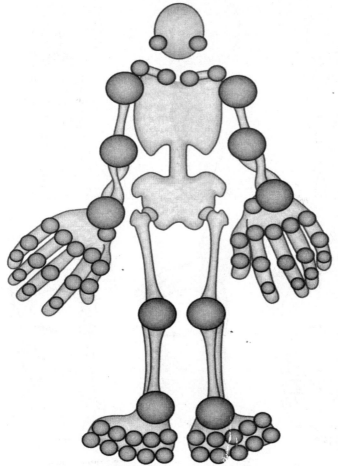

Fig. V.2 An outline sketch on which joint disease activity or destruction can be recorded at each assessment.

- Assess movement:
  - Test passive flexion and extension: make a note of the range of movements and feel for crepitus
  - Gently extend the knee and examine for fixed flexion deformity
  - Test the medial and lateral ligaments by steadying the thigh with the left hand and moving the leg with the right laterally and medially when the knee joint is slightly flexed: movement of >10 degrees is abnormal
  - Test the cruciate ligaments by steadying the foot with your elbow and moving the leg anteriorly and posteriorly with the other hand: laxity of >10 degrees is abnormal.

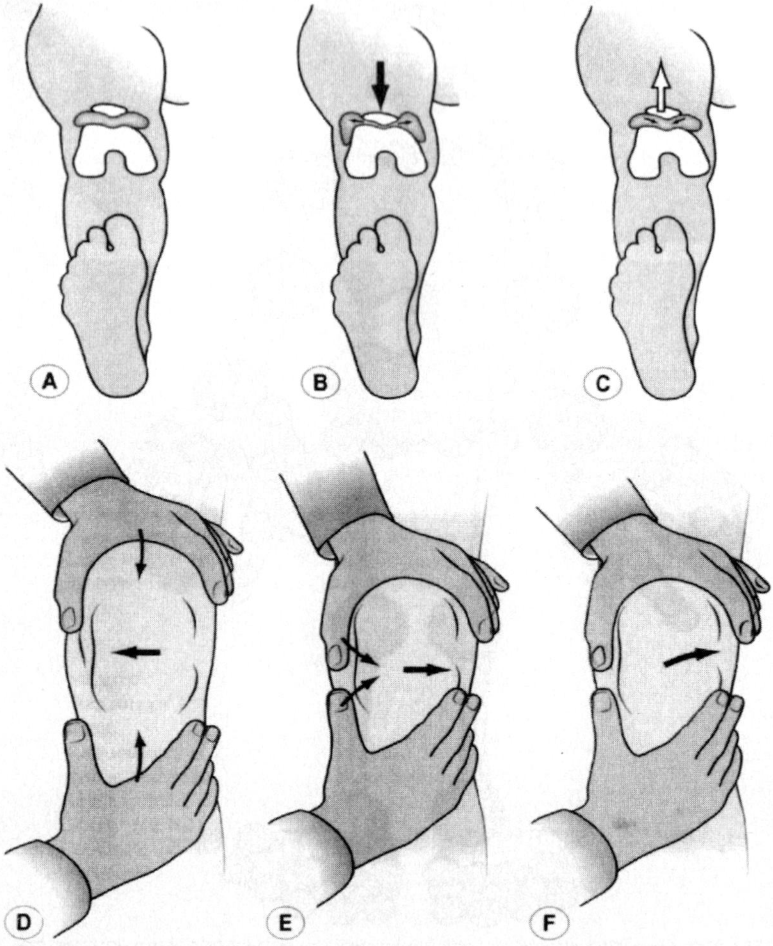

Fig. V.3 Detection of effusions. (A–C) Large effusions can be detected by 'ballotting' the patella with the knee in extension. (B) Small effusions can be identified by the 'bulge' test, where fluid is 'milked' into the suprapatellar pouch and then pressed so that it can be seen bulging below the medial edge of the patella.

- Ask the patient to lie on his or her stomach and feel the popliteal fossa when the knee is extended.

- **Examination of the feet**
- Look:
  - for skin rash, scars
  - at the nails for changes of psoriasis
  - at the forefoot for hallux valgus, clawing and crowding of the toes (rheumatoid arthritis)

- at the callus over the metatarsal heads which may occur in subluxation
- at both the arches of the foot, in particular medial and longitudinal (flat foot, pes cavus).
- Palpate:
  - ankles for synovitis, effusion, passive movements at the subtalar joints (inversion and eversion) and talar joint (dorsiflexion and plantar flexion); remember that tenderness on movement is more important than the range of movement
  - metatarsophalangeal joints for tenderness
  - individual digits, for synovial thickening
  - bottom of heel, for tenderness (plantar fasciitis), and Achilles tendon for nodules.

W Heberden, Sr (1710–1801), an English physician.
CJ Bouchard (1837–1915), a French physician.

---

127 RHEUMATOID HANDS

INSTRUCTION

Examine this patient's hands.

SALIENT FEATURES

History

- Painful swollen joints
- Morning stiffness.

Examination

- Ask the patient for permission to examine her hands and then ask whether the hands are sore.

Proceed as follows:

- Comment on deformities (Fig. 127.1) such as the following:
  - Subluxation at the metacarpophalangeal joint
  - Swan-neck deformity
  - Boutonnière deformity (hyperextension at the terminal interphalangeal joint and flexion at the proximal interphalangeal joint)
  - Z deformity of the thumb
  - Dorsal subluxation of the ulna at the carpal joint.
- Comment on the following signs:
  - Nailfold infarcts and vasculitic skin lesions
  - Palmar erythema
  - Wasting of the first dorsal interossei and other small muscles of the hand.
- Test grip and pincer movements. Quickly test for abductor pollicis brevis and interossei, and pinprick sensation over index and little fingers. The median nerve may be involved if there is associated carpal tunnel syndrome.
- Examine the elbow for rheumatoid nodules.
- Ask the patient to perform simple tasks involving hand function, such as unbuttoning clothes or writing.
- Tell the examiner that you would like to examine other joints.
- Highlight the following points:
  - Whether terminal interphalangeal joints are spared or affected
  - Whether the arthritis is active (if the joints are inflamed) or inactive
  - Be prepared to discuss the radiological features.

DIAGNOSIS

This patient has swan-neck deformity of the fingers (lesions) caused by rheumatoid arthritis (aetiology) with marked active arthritis of the interphalangeal joints, and is unable to button her clothes (functional status).

QUESTIONS

What is the significance of nodules in rheumatoid arthritis?
The presence of nodules indicates seropositive and more aggressive arthritis (Fig. 127.2).

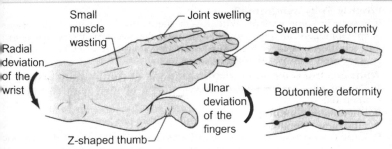

Fig. 127.1 Deformities of the hands in rheumatoid arthritis.

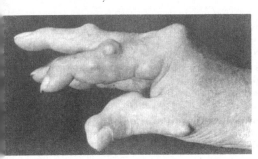

Fig. 127.2 Hand in seropositive rheumatoid arthritis, showing fixed deformities and gross rheumatoid nodules. (With permission from Canoso JJ 1997.)

Where are nodules found?
Flexor and extensor tendons of the hand, sacrum, Achilles tendon, sclera, lungs and myocardium.

What are the skin lesions in rheumatoid arthritis?
Vasculitis, nailfold infarcts.

What are the causes of anaemia in rheumatoid arthritis?
- Anaemia of chronic disease
- Megaloblastic anaemia from folate deficiency or associated pernicious anaemia
- Felty syndrome
- Drugs: NSAIDs causing iron-deficiency anaemia, gold causing bone marrow suppression.

What factors have been implicated in anaemia of chronic disease?
- Decreased production of red blood cells:
  - Inadequate iron: impaired absorption and transport, failure to release iron stores
  - Decreased concentration or marrow resistance to erythropoietin.
- Ineffective erythropoiesis
- Abnormal development of erythroid progenitor cells
- Increased destruction of red cells.

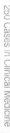

What is Felty syndrome?

It is seen in some patients with severe rheumatoid arthritis and consists of splenomegaly, anaemia, leucopenia, thrombocytopenia (hypersplenism) and leg ulcers. Splenectomy ameliorates hypersplenism. Felty syndrome is associated with positive rheumatoid factor.

What are the pulmonary manifestations of rheumatoid arthritis?

- Pleural effusion or pleurisy (seen in 25% of men with rheumatoid arthritis)
- Rheumatoid nodules
- Fibrosing alveolitis
- Caplan syndrome (rheumatoid arthritis coexisting with rounded fibrotic nodules 0.5–5.0 cm in diameter, mainly in the periphery of lung fields in coal-worker's pneumoconiosis).

What are the eye manifestations of rheumatoid arthritis?

- Episcleritis
- Scleritis
- Scleromalacia, scleromalacia perforans
- Keratoconjunctivitis sicca
- Sjögren syndrome (see above).

What precautions are necessary before upper gastrointestinal endoscopy or general anaesthesia?

It is prudent to take a cervical spine radiograph to rule out atlanto-axial subluxation.

Which joints are commonly affected in rheumatoid arthritis?

Wrists, proximal interphalangeal joints and metacarpophalangeal joints of the hands, metatarsophalangeal joints and knees.

What is palindromic rheumatoid arthritis?

Palindromic onset is seen in some patients with recurrent episodes of joint stiffness and pain in individual joints lasting only a few hours or days. Hydroxychloroquine may be of value in preventing recurrences.

ADVANCED-LEVEL QUESTIONS

How would you treat the arthritis?

Prescribe NSAIDs (ibuprofen is the safest at conventional doses) including aspirin. If, after 1 month of NSAIDs, the symptoms persist with no sign of remission then a second-line drug should be added. Second-line drugs include hydroxychloroquine, sulfasalazine and pencillamine. Low-dose methotrexate and gold salts are used to prevent disease progression. Three biologic products that inhibit the actions of tumour necrosis factor-α (TNF-α; infliximab, etanercept and adalimumab) and one that inhibits the action of interleukin-1 (anakinra) produce significant improvement in the severity of arthritis. Etanercept is a fusion protein of the ligand-binding region of the TNF receptor and the Fc portion of human IgG; infliximab is a chimeric (mouse and human) monoclonal antibody against TNF. These TNF inhibitors have surprisingly few side effects. The most common reactions are at the injection site (with etanercept) and hypersensitivity reactions (with infliximab). The TNF-α inhibitors suppress disease activity only during treatment and, consequently, relapses are inevitable once the treatment is discontinued (N Engl J Med 2000;343:1640–1). Alternative agents include lefunomide, a TNF or interleukin-1 blocker;

rituximab, an anti-CD20 chimeric monoclonal antibody; and abatacept, which blocks selective costimulation of T cells.

If the patient is known to experience gastric distress with non-steroidal anti-inflammatroy drugs, what precautions would you take while prescribing them?

Prophylaxis for NSAID-associated gastric distress may be attempted with concurrent administration of an H_2-receptor blocker (such as ranitidine), omeprazole or misoprostol. The last is a prostaglandin analogue that has been shown to protect the gastric mucosa.

What are the neurological manifestations of rheumatoid arthritis?

● Peripheral neuropathy: glove-and-stocking sensory loss
● Mononeuritis multiplex
● Entrapment neuropathy, e.g. carpal tunnel syndrome
● Cervical disease or atlanto-axial subluxation may cause cervical myelopathy.

What are the causes of proteinuria in patients with rheumatoid arthritis?

● Drug therapy: gold salts, penicillamine
● Amyloidosis.

What is Sjögren syndrome?

● The association of keratoconjunctivitis sicca (lack of lacrimal secretion) and xerostomia (dry mouth as a result of lack of salivary gland secretion) in association with a connective tissue disorder, usually rheumatoid arthritis. This syndrome may be associated with autoimmune thyroid disease, myasthenia gravis or autoimmune liver disease.
● Anti-Ro (SSA) and anti-SS-B antibodies may be seen in this syndrome.
● Treatment is symptomatic with artificial tears (hypomellose drops or 1% methylcellulose), artificial saliva and NSAIDs for the arthritis.
● The Schirmer filter paper test provides a crude measure of tear production. Filter paper is hooked over the lower eyelid and in normal people at least 15 mm is wet after 5 min, whereas in patients with keratoconjunctivitis sicca it is <5 mm.

What is the role of anti-cyclic citrullinated peptide antibodies?

The presence of autoantibodies to cyclic citrullinated peptide (CCP) is specific to rheumatoid arthritis. Their detection contributes both to the differential diagnosis and to a prediction of the severity of joint destruction, even though the mechanistic significance of these autoantibodies is unclear.

What are the criteria for rheumatoid arthritis?

Patients are definitively diagnosed with rheumatoid arthritis if they score 6 or more points on the following series of assessments:
● *Joint involvement*:
  • 1 medium–large joint: 0 points
  • 2–10 medium–large joints: 1 point
  • 1–3 small joints: 2 points
  • 4–10 small joints: 3 points
  • >10 small joints: 5 points.

- *Serology*:
  - Not positive for either rheumatoid factor or anti–citrullinated protein antibody: 0 points
  - At least one of these two tests are positive at low titre (more than the upper limit of normal but not higher than three times the upper limit of normal): 2 points
  - At least one test is positive at high titre (more than three times the upper limit of normal): 3 points.
- *Duration of synovitis*:
  - Lasting fewer than 6 weeks: 0 points
  - Lasting 6 weeks or longer: 1 point.
- *Acute phase reactants*:
  - Neither C-reactive protein nor ESR abnormal: 0 points
  - Abnormal C-reactive protein or abnormal ESR: 1 point.

Patients receive the highest point level they fulfill within each domain. For example, a patient with five small joints involved and four large joints involved scores 3 points.

What are the poor prognostic factors?

- Systemic features: weight loss, extra-articular manifestations
- Insidious onset
- Rheumatoid nodules
- Presence of rheumatoid factor >1 in 512
- Persistent activity of the disease for over 12 months
- Early bone erosions.

What are the factors leading to ulnar deviation of the hands?

In the normal grip, the fingers move to ulnar deviation; this is caused by:

- weakening of radial sides of the joint capsule and the radial insertion of the interossei ligaments
- the volar supports of the flexor tendon sheath are weakened by inflammation, allowing the tendon to bow in the direction of the ulna during gripping
- ulnar displacement of the extensor tendons in early deviation makes them slip if the dorsal metacarpophalangeal joint is taut, and this exacerbates the development of ulnar deviation by acting as a bowstring
- joint capsules of metacarpophalangeal joints are weaker on radial sides than on ulnar sides.

What is the role of cadherins in the pathogenesis of rheumatoid arthritis?

Fibroblast-like synoviocytes mediate cartilage damage in rheumatoid arthritis (rheumatoid inflammation causes damage to both articular cartilage and periarticular bone). Cadherin-11 deficiency protects mice from cartilage damage but not from bone erosion, probably because cadherin-11 seems to mediate the migration of fibroblast-like synoviocytes over the articular cartilage and its subsequent damage.

What is the role of phosphatidylinositol 3'-kinase-γ in the pathogenesis of rheumatoid arthritis?

A novel inhibitor of phosphatidylinositol 3'-kinase has been shown to be effective in blocking inflammation and joint destruction in mouse models of rheumatoid arthritis.

AB Garrod coined the term rheumatoid arthritis in 1858.

HSC Sjögren, a Swedish ophthalmologist, described this condition in 1933.

A Caplan, a British physician, was an industrial officer in the Welsh coal mines.

In 1931 Philip S Hench (1896–1965) of the Mayo Clinic observed that arthritic pain temporarily decreased in pregnant women. He then studied the phenomena for the next 8 years, finding that allergic conditions such as asthma, hay fever and food sensitivity were also lessened in the presence of jaundice or pregnancy. He reasoned that a steroid hormone may be responsible, since levels of steroid hormones are high in the blood during pregnancy. (Hench PS. A reminiscence of certain events before, during and after the discovery of cortisone. Minn Med 1953;36:705–710).

Edward Kendall (1886–1972), Chief of the Division of Biochemistry, suggested the name 'corsone' on a piece of paper but Hench amended this to 'cortisone', and thus the steroid hormone was 'baptized'. The 1950 Nobel Prize for Medicine was jointly awarded to Kendall, Hench and Tadeus Reichstein (1897–1996) of Basel University, Switzerland, for their discoveries relating to the hormones of the adrenal cortex, their structure and biological effects (Lancet 1999;353:1370).

Sir John Vane, showed that inhibition of prostaglandin synthesis was central to both the actions and side effects of aspirin (Proc R Coll Phys Edinb 2000;30:191–8).

128 ANKYLOSING SPONDYLITIS

INSTRUCTION

Examine this patient's back.
Examine this patient.

SALIENT FEATURES

History

- Back stiffness and back pain: worse in the morning, improves on exercise and worsens on rest
- Symptoms in the peripheral joints (in ~40%), particularly shoulders and knees
- Onset of symptoms is typically insidious and in the 3rd–4th decade
- Extra-articular manifestations: red eye (uveitis), diarrhoea (GI involvement), history of aortic regurgitation, pulmonary apical fibrosis (worse in smokers).

Examination

- 'Question mark' posture (as a result of loss of lumbar lordosis, fixed kyphoscoliosis of the thoracic spine with compensatory extension of the cervical spine)
- Protuberant abdomen.

Proceed as follows:

- Ask the patient to look to either side: the whole body turns when the patient does this.

- Examine the cervical, thoracic and lumbar spines (remember that cervical spine involvement occurs later in the disease and results in pain and a grating sensation on movement of the neck).
- Measure the occiput-to-wall distance (inability to make contact when heel and back are against the wall indicates upper thoracic and cervical limitation).
- Perform Schober's test. This involves marking points 10 cm above and 5 cm below a line joining the 'dimple of Venus' on the sacral promontory. An increase in the separation of <5 cm during full forward flexion indicates limited spinal mobility.
  Note: Finger–floor distance is a simple indicator but is less reliable because good hip movement may compensate for back limitation.
- Examine for distal arthritis (occurs in up to 30% of patients and may precede the onset of the back symptoms). Small joints of the hand and feet are rarely affected.
- Measure chest expansion with a tape (<5 cm suggests costovertebral involvement).
- Tell the examiner that you would like to examine the following:
  - Eyes for iritis, anterior uveitis (seen in 20% of patients)
  - Heart for aortic regurgitation (seen in 4% of patients who have had the disease for over 15 years), cardiac conduction defects
  - Lungs for mild restrictive disease, apical fibrosis, apical cavities and secondary fungal infection; look for cyanosis (patients with rigid spine syndrome often have underlying hypoventilation)
  - CNS, such as tetraplegia, etc.
  - Foot for Achilles tendinitis and plantar fasciitis.

Remember:
- The four 'A's of ankylosing spondylitis: apical fibrosis, anterior uveitis, aortic regurgitation, Achilles tendinitis
- That psoriasis and Reiter syndrome can also cause sacroiliitis.

DIAGNOSIS

This patient has fixed kyphoscoliosis of the thoracic spine with loss of lumbar lordosis (lesion) caused by ankylosing spondylitis (aetiology) on Schober's test; spinal movements are severely diminished (functional status).

QUESTIONS

What are the diagnostic criteria for ankylosing spondylitis?
Modified New York criteria 1984 for ankylosing spondylitis definite ankylosing spondylitis is present if the radiological criterion is associated with at least one clinical criterion:

Clinical criteria:
- Low-back pain and stiffness for longer than 3 months, which improve with exercise but are not relieved by rest
- Restriction of motion of the lumbar spine in both the sagittal and frontal planes
- Restriction of chest expansion relative to normal values correlated for age and sex.

Radiological criterion:
- Sacroiliitis grade ≥2 bilaterally, or grade 3–4 unilaterally

What investigations would you like to do in this patient?

Anteroposterior view of sacroiliac joints and lateral radiographs of lumbar spine (Fig. 128.1A): the earliest changes are erosions and sclerosis of the sacroiliac joints. Later in the disease syndesmophytes may be found in the lumbosacral spine. In severe disease, involvement progresses up the spine, leading to a 'bamboo spine' (Fig. 128.1B). Although the New York criteria require a combination of clinical and radiographic features, the diagnosis should be suspected on the basis of inactivity, spinal stiffness and pain, with or without additional features.

In which other seronegative arthritic disorders is low-back pain a feature?

Sacroiliitis is often seen in Reiter syndrome, psoriatic arthritis, juvenile chronic arthritis and intestinal arthropathy.

How would you manage a patient with ankylosing spondylitis?

- Encourage exercise, particularly physical therapy, to preserve back extension
- NSAIDs, in particular indomethacin. Phenylbutazone is reserved for resistant cases
- Methotrexate and sulfasalazine
- Tumour necrosis factor blockers: etanercept, adalimumab, and golimumab. Etanercept decreases stiffness and pain and improves overall function, plus showing objective findings such as an increase in chest expansion and a decrease in the ESR (N Engl J Med 2002;346:1349)

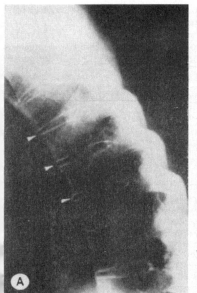
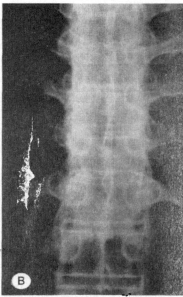

Fig. 128.1 Ankylosing spondylitis. (A) Bone erosion of dorsal aspect of thoracic spine. (B) Bamboo spine. (With permission from Kelley WN Harris ED, Ruddy S, et al. (eds) Textbook of rheumatology, 5th edn, vol. 1. Philadelphia, PA: Saunders, 1997.)

- Surgical therapy, consisting of vertebral wedge osteotomy, is occasionally indicated
- Referral to ophthalmologist when anterior uveitis occurs.

ADVANCED-LEVEL QUESTIONS

What genetic counselling would you give this patient?

In HLA-B27-positive patients, the siblings have a 30% chance of developing this disease. Hence children of such patients who develop symptoms such as joint pains or sore eyes should be referred to a rheumatologist.

What is the natural history of the disease?

About 40% go on to develop severe spinal restriction; about 20% have significant disability. Early peripheral joint disease, particularly of the hip, indicates a poor prognosis.

What is the risk in those with a 'bamboo' cervical spine when driving?

Increased susceptiblity to whiplash injury and restricted lateral vision.

What therapy may the patient have received in the past if the blood film shows a leukaemic picture?

In the past, patients were treated with irradiation of the spine. However, those treated tend to develop leukaemia several years after therapy.

What criteria predict that lower-back pain is a precursor of ankylosing spondylitis?

New criteria for inflammatory back pain in young to middle-aged adults (<50 years) with chronic back pain are:

- Morning stiffness >30 min
- Improvement in back pain with exercise but not with rest
- Awakening because of back pain during the second half of the night only
- Alternating buttock pain
- Diagnosis is confirmed if at least two of the four the parameters are present (sensitivity 70.3%, specificity 81.2%).

Further reading

Keat A: Spondyloparthropathies, *BMJ* 310:1321–1324, 1995. (classic review).

The term ankylosing spondylitis derives from the Greek words, *ankylos* (bent or crooked) and *spondylos* (vertebra). Past names have included Marie–Strümpell disease and von Bechterew's disease.

The first clinical report of ankylosing spondylitis (1831) concerned a man from the Isle of Man. Vladimir von Bechterew of St Petersburg, Russia, described a series of cases between 1857 and 1927. Adolf Strümpell (1853–1926) of Erlangen and Pierre Marie (1853–1940) of Paris independently described this condition in 1897 and 1898, respectively.

HC Reiter (1881–1969), a German physician.

Achilles is a figure from Greek mythology who was a hero of the Trojan war. His mother dipped him into the river Styx, holding him by his heel, to make him invulnerable to the attack. He slew Hector in this war, but was himself slain, wounded in his vulnerable heel by Paris.

129 PSORIATIC ARTHRITIS

INSTRUCTION

Examine this patient's hands.

SALIENT FEATURES

History

- Cutaneous psoriasis with itching in a fifth of the patients
- Joint pain, joint stiffness worse in the morning.

Examination

- Distal interphalangeal joint involvement.
- *Proceed as follows*:
- Tell the examiner that you would like to:
  - examine the nails, looking for pitting, onycholysis, discoloration, thickening (nails are involved in 80% of patients with psoriatic arthritis)
  - look for psoriatic plaques in the extensor aspects of elbows, scalp, submammary region, umbilicus and natal cleft; describe these as reddish plaques with well-defined edges and silvery white scales (Fig. 129.1).
- Comment on the fingers, which are sausage shaped because of teno-synovitis (Fig. 129.1).

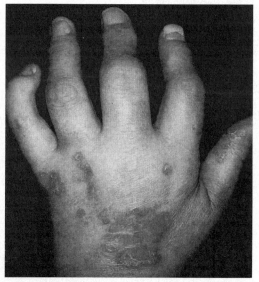

Fig. 129.1 Psoriatic arthritis, with asymmetric arthritis pattern. (With permission from Habif 2009.)

DIAGNOSIS

This patient has nail pitting, psoriatic plaques and distal interphalangeal arthropathy (lesion) caused by psoriasis (aetiology) and has good hand function (functional status).

ADVANCED-LEVEL QUESTIONS

What are the patterns of joint involvement seen in psoriasis?
The patterns include (Acta Derm Venereol 1961;41:396–403):
- asymmetrical terminal joint involvement
- symmetrical joint involvement as seen in rheumatoid arthritis
- sacroiliitis: this differs from ankylosing spondylitis, most notably in that the syndesmophytes tend to arise from the lateral and anterior surfaces of the vertebral bodies and not at the margins of the bodies
- arthritis mutilans: complicated by the 'telescoping' of digits.

What are the radiological features of psoriatic arthritis?
- 'Fluffy' periostitis
- Destruction of small joints
- 'Pencil and cup' appearance, osteolysis and ankylosis in arthritis mutilans (Fig. 129.2)
- Non-marginal syndesmophytes in spondylitis (Q J Med 1977;46:411).

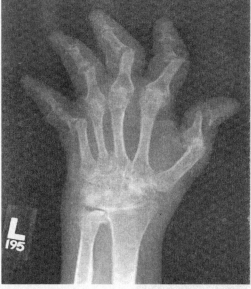

Fig. 129.2 Arthritis mutilans with destructive changes, joint deformity of the hand and pancompartmental ankylosis of the wrist. (With permission from Firestein et al. 2008.)

What is the prognosis?

Deforming and erosive arthritis is present in 40% of cases and 11% are disabled by their arthritis (Lancet 1988;ii: 375).

What are the management options?

- NSAIDs, e.g. indomethacin
- Selective cyclooxygenase 2 (COX-2) inhibitors
- Intrarticular glucocorticoids
- Disease-modifying agents: sulfasalazine, hydroxychloroquine, leflunomide, tumour necrosis factor-α (TNF-α) blockers (adalimumab, etanercept, infliximab), alefacept, efalizumab.

What do you know about pathogenesis of psoriasis and therapy to mitigate it?

T cell activation. Inhibition by drugs of molecules involved in the formation of the immunologic synapse.

Pathogenic T cells. Depletion is achieved by targeting molecules expressed specifically by activated T cells, such as the high-affinity interleukin-2 receptor or CD4.

Leukocyte recruitment to the inflamed skin. Inhibited by blocking key adhesion molecules such as selectins or certain integrins, e.g. using efalizumab, a monoclonal antibody that interferes with adhesion mediated by leukocyte-function-associated antigen 1 (LFA-1)].

Release of inflammatory cytokines (e.g. TNF-α). Targeted by several biologic agents, the monoclonal antibodies infliximab and adalimumab, and the fusion proteins etanercept and onercept

Predominance of helper T cells (Th) type 1. Induction of shift in immune balance to a milieu weighted with Th2 cells, thus alleviating psoriasis, e.g. using interleukin-10 and interleukin-4.

130   PAINFUL KNEE JOINT

INSTRUCTION

Examine this patient's leg.
Examine this patient's joints.
Examine this patient's knee joint.

SALIENT FEATURES

History

- Painful knee joint
- Take a history of trauma and fever
- History of rheumatoid arthritis, gout or haemophilia.

Examination

- Pain on movement of the joint (take care not to hurt the patient)
- Swelling of the joint (you must demonstrate fluid in the joint, see Fig. V.3)
- Check both active and passive movements
- Look for disuse atrophy of the muscles around the joint

- Tell the examiner that you would like to:
  - examine other joints
  - radiograph the knee (anteroposterior and lateral views)
  - analyse the joint fluid for cells, sugar, protein and culture.

DIAGNOSIS

This patient has a painful knee joint with restricted movement (lesion and functional status) following trauma while playing rugby (aetiology).

QUESTIONS

What are the common causes of a painful knee joint?
- Rheumatoid arthritis
- Osteoarthrosis
- Trauma
- Septic arthritis (will require emergency removal of the pus to prevent joint damage)
- Viral infection
- Gout
- Pseudogout
- Haemophilia. → Haemanthosis

ADVANCED-LEVEL QUESTIONS

What is palindromic rheumatoid arthritis?
Palindromic onset of rheumatoid arthritis refers to acute recurrent arthritis, usually affecting one joint, with symptom-free intervals of days to months between attacks. This term was introduced by PS Hench (p. 477) and EF Rosenberg.

A patient with a painful knee joint and an unilateral facial nerve palsy is seen by you in the outpatient department. Six weeks before this she developed an annular rash after a camping trip in Europe. What is your diagnosis and what confirmatory test would you carry out?
The diagnosis is Lyme disease and the confirmatory test is an antibody titre against *Borrelia burgdorferi*. The disease was first recognized in Lyme, Connecticut, USA.

What are the causes of acute monoarticular arthritis?
The causes of acute-onset monoarticular or pauciarticular arthritis includes bacterial infections (e.g. with *Staphylococcus aureus*, *Neisseria gonorrhoeae* and *Streptococcus pneumoniae*), reactive arthritis, sarcoidosis, fracture, hemarthrosis, gout, pseudogout and monoarticular rheumatoid arthritis.

What are the causes of acute polyarticular arthritis?
The causes acute polyarticular arthritis (involvement of more than just a few joints) includes endocarditis, serum sickness, acute hepatitis B infection, HIV infection, parvovirus infection, rheumatic fever, rheumatoid arthritis and SLE.

131 OSTEOARTHROSIS

INSTRUCTION

Look at this patient's hands.
Examine this patient's joints.

SALIENT FEATURES

History

- Age
- Pain in the joints
- Stiffness after a period of inactivity
- Impairment of gait as a result of joint pain
- Knees: pain on activities such as climbing stairs, getting out of a chair, and walking long distances. Morning stiffness usually lasts <30 min. Ask the patient whether their knees 'give way', a so-called instability symptom
- Hip: morning stiffness and pain (lasting <30 min) and pain at rest or at night are common. However, nocturnal hip pain may reflect inflammatory arthritis, infection, tumours or crystal diseases.

Examination

- Heberden's nodes (bony swellings) at the terminal interphalangeal joints
- Squaring of the hands as a result of subluxation of the first metacarpophalangeal joint.

Proceed as follows:

- Tell the examiner that you would like to examine the hips and knees as these joints are usually involved.
- Knee: feel for crepitus: it may be red, warm and tender, and have an effusion.
- Hip: the strongest clinical indicator of osteoarthritis of the hip is pain, exacerbated by internal or external rotation of the hip while the knee is in full extension. An assessment of the range of motion of the knee joint and lower lumbar spine may help to determine whether hip pain is referred from these other joint rather than the hip.

DIAGNOSIS

This elderly patient has Heberden's nodes and squaring of the hands with involvement of the interphalangeal joints of the hands (lesions) caused by osteoarthrosis (aetiology) and is unable to button his clothes (functional status).

QUESTIONS

Which other joints are frequently involved?
Spine, in particular cervical and lumbar spines.

Mention the types and a few causes of osteoarthrosis
- Primary
- Secondary, caused by:

- trauma: affects athletes, pneumatic drill workers, anyone doing work involving heavy lifting
- inflammatory arthropathies: rheumatoid arthritis, septic arthritis, gout
- neuropathic joints: in diabetes mellitus, syringomyelia, tabes dorsalis
- endocrine: acromegaly, hyperparathyroidism
- metabolic: chondrocalcinosis, haemochromatosis.

What are Heberden's nodes?

Bony swellings seen at the terminal interphalangeal joints in osteoarthrosis (Fig. 131.1).

What are Bouchard's nodes?

Bony swellings at the proximal interphalangeal joints in osteoarthrosis (Fig. 131.1).

ADVANCED-LEVEL QUESTIONS

What are the typical radiological features?

- Subchondral bone sclerosis and cysts
- Osteophytes (Fig. 131.2).

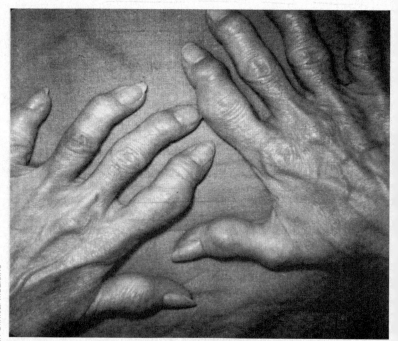

Fig. 131.1 Heberden (distal interphalangeal) and Bouchard (proximal interphalangeal) nodes on both index fingers and thumbs. Note angular changes at distal joints as result of loss of joint cartilage and instability. (With permission from Canale, Beaty 2007.)

Note: Radiological findings correlate poorly with the severity of pain.

What will the synovial aspirate show?

White blood cell count of $<100 \times 10^3$ cells/l.

What do you understand by the term nodal osteoarthrosis?

Nodal osteoarthrosis is a primary generalized osteoarthrosis with characteristic features. It occurs predominantly in middle-aged women and is autosomal dominant. It characteristically affects the terminal interphalangeal joints, with the development of Heberden's nodes. The arthritis may be acute and, although there may be marked deformity, there is little disability. It can also affect the carpometacarpal joints of the thumbs, spinal apophyseal joints, knees and hips.

How would you manage a patient with osteoarthrosis?

- Change in lifestyle: maintain optimal weight, use appropriate footwear, encourage exercise to strengthen muscles (range-of-motion exercise that does not strengthen muscles is generally ineffective). An exercise programme of water aerobics or with a physical therapist at a frequency of twice a week for at least 2 months should improve muscle strength.
- Drugs: simple analgesics, rubifacients, NSAIDs and cyclooxygenase 2 (COX-2) inhibitors for acute flare-ups; intra-articular corticosteroid injections for acute flare-ups or patients unfit for surgery.
- The combination of glucosamine and chondroitin sulfate may be effective in the subgroup of patients with moderate-to-severe knee pain (N Engl J Med 2006;354:795).
- Surgery: arthroscopic removal of loose body, arthroscopic washout or radioisotope synovectomy for persistent synovitis; joint replacement for hip and knee. A recent study suggests that arthroscopic surgery for osteoarthritis of the knee provides no additional benefit to optimized physical and medical therapy (N Engl J Med 2008;359:1097).

What is the role of aggrecan in osteoarthritis?

In osteoarthritis, the degeneration of the cartilaginous extracellular matrix far exceeds its synthesis. The extracellular matrix of cartilage wears away,

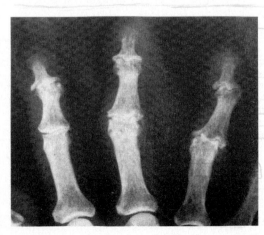

Fig. 131.2 Primary osteoarthritis of the fingers, with characteristic cartilage loss, deviations, and spurs of the proximal (Bouchard's nodes) and distal (Heberden's nodes) interphalangeal joints. (With permission from Grainger, Allison 2001.)

exposing articular cartilage and, eventually, bone. The two important components of this extracellular matrix are a type II collagen–rich collagenous network (which provides tensile strength) and a cartilage-specific proteoglycan called aggrecan (which is highly hydrated and thereby allows cartilage to resist a compressive load). Experimental studies suggest that the loss of aggrecan is the primary event leading to the destruction of cartilage. Three enzymes capable of degrading aggrecan have been identified: ADAMTS 1, ADAMTS 4, and ADAMTS 5. ADAMTS 5 is the main aggrecanase in mouse articular cartilage and is a possible pharmacologic target to prevent osteoarthritis.

William Heberden (1710–1801) was a London physician who described the nodes as 'little hard knobs' and this was first published posthumously in 1802.

JK Spender (1886), of Bath, introduced the term osteoarthritis. Archibald E Garrod from London, established the modern usage and clinical differentiation from rheumatoid arthritis in 1907.

In 1884, CJ Bouchard (1837–1915) described nodes adjacent to the proximal interphalangeal joints identical to those at the distal interphalangeal joints.

---

132 GOUT

INSTRUCTION

Examine this patient's hands or examine the feet.

SALIENT FEATURES

History

- Usually acute pain at the base of great toe, worse at night and associated with redness
- Occasionally multiple joints involved
- Systemic symptoms, e.g. low grade fever.

Examination

- Chronic tophaceous deposit with asymmetrical joint involvement.
- *Proceed as follows*:
- Tell the examiner that you would like to examine:
  - the helices of the ears
  - the elbow for olecranon bursae
  - the Achilles tendons for tophi
  - the feet or hands.

Notes

- Uric acid crystals are negatively birefringent, needle shaped and may be deposited in bursae and bone marrow. They are demonstrable in synovial fluid within leukocytes and free in the fluid during attacks of gouty arthritis. They react with nitric acid and ammonium hydroxide to give a purple colour (murexide test).

- Be prepared to discuss the differences between the clinical features of typical gout and gout in the elderly.

DIAGNOSIS

This patient has a painful great toe with swelling of the joint (lesion) caused by gout (aetiology) and is unable to walk because of the pain (functional status).

QUESTIONS

What is the basic pathophysiology of gout?

Gout is a metabolic disorder of purine metabolism. It is characterized by hyperuricaemia caused by either overproduction (75%) or underexcretion (25%) of uric acid.

What are the different clinical manifestations of gout?

- Asymptomatic hyperuricaemia
- Acute arthritis
- Chronic arthritis
- Chronic tophaceous gout (Figs 132.1 and 132.2).

How would you treat an acute attack of gout?

Prescribe an NSAID such as indomethacin. Selective cyclooxygenase-2 (COX-2) inhibitors (etoricoxib) are an alternative in patients with GI contraindications to the use of NSAIDs. Corticosteroids or subcutaneous injections of ACTH are also options. Refractory gout may require steroids.

What factors may precipitate acute gouty arthritis?

Drugs (diuretics, aspirin), copious consumption of alcohol, dehydration, surgery, fasting food high in purines (sweetbreads, liver, kidney and sardines).

ADVANCED-LEVEL QUESTIONS

Under what circumstances would you treat hyperuricaemia?

Frequent attacks of acute arthritis, renal damage and consistently raised serum uric acid levels. Before attempting to lower serum uric acid levels, it is prudent to use colchicine to treat acute attacks. Colchicine should be given within 24 h of the onset of symptoms to abort a severe attack.

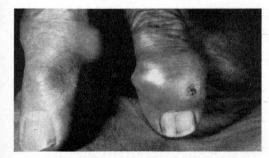

Fig. 132.1 Gouty tophi.

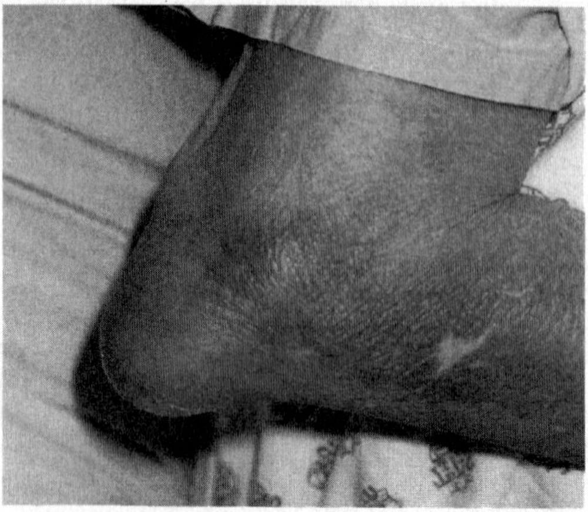

Fig. 132.2 Painful olecranon bursitis resembling septic bursitis. (With permission from Roberts, Hedges 2009.)

Remember: The incidence of gouty arthritis has been linked to serum urate level in a cohort of healthy men, the annual incidence being:
4.9% for urate of at least 90 mg/l (535 μmol/l)
0.5% for 70–89 mg/l
0.1% for <70 mg/l.

What is the drug of choice for controlling hyperuricaemia?
Allopurinol (a xanthine oxidase inhibitor). The goal of therapy is to reduce serum uric acid to <60 mg/l (350 μmol/l). At this level, monosodium urate crystals within joints and in soft tissue tophi are reabsorbed. Febuxostat, a novel non-purine xanthine oxidase inhibitor, may be a useful alternative medication in patients with renal insufficiency.

What are the diagnostic criteria for acute gout?
American Rheumatism Association diagnostic criteria (Arthritis Rheum 1977;20:895–900) for acute gout includes the presence of seven or more of the following criteria:
- More than 1 attack of acute arthritis
- Maximum inflammation developed within 1 day
- Attack of monoarthritis
- Redness observed over joints
- First metatarsophalangeal joint painful and swollen
- Unilateral attack of first metatarsophalangeal joint
- Unilateral attack of tarsal joint
- Tophus (proven or suspected)
- Hyperuricaemia
- Asymmetric swelling within a joint on radiograph
- Subcortical cysts without erosions on radiograph
- Monosodium urate monohydrate microcrystals in joint fluid during attack
- Culture of joint fluid negative for organisms during attack.

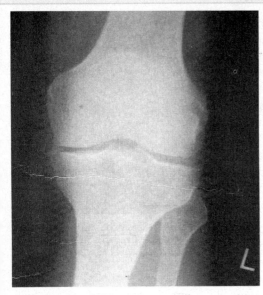

Fig. 132.3 Radiograph of knee showing typical articular chondrocalcinosis in the areas of the medial and lateral meniscus in pseudogout. (With permission from Currie, Douglas 2011.)

What drugs would you use if the patient was allergic to allopurinol?
Uricosuric drugs such as probenecid, sulfinpyrazone.

How would you determine whether a patient with elevated uric acid is an overproducer or an underexcretor?
An overproducer is one whose 24-hour urinary uric acid level >750 mg.

What is pseudogout?
Pseudogout is an acute arthritis resulting from the release of calcium pyrophosphate dihydrate crystals (deposited in the bone and cartilage) into the synovial fluid (Fig. 132.3).

Gout was recognized as early as the 4th century BC. Two concepts have prevailed: that it occurs mainly in sexually active mature men and that gastronomic and sexual excesses may precipitate acute attacks.

Antonj van Leewenhoeck (1632–1723) described the microscopic appearance of urate crystals from gouty tophus.

In 1847 Alfred Garrod, in London, identified uric acid in the serum of a gouty man.

Michelangelo's gout has been depicted in a fresco by Raphael (Lancet 1999; 354:2149–52).

133   EHLERS-DANLOS SYNDROME

INSTRUCTION

Do a general examination.
Examine this patient's joints.

SALIENT FEATURES

History

- Family history (JAMA 1997;278:1284–5)
- Hypermobile joints (Fig. 133.1)
- Fragile skin with impaired wound healing
- Bleeding diathesis.

Examination

- Skin
- The skin over the neck, axillae and groin is smooth and elastic (Fig. 133.2). It can be stretched and, when released, it returns immediately to its normal position. Late in the disease it becomes lax, wrinkled and hangs in folds.

Proceed as follows:

- Look at bony prominences for bruising, haematomas and gaping wounds. Wounds heal forming tissue-paper or papyraceous or 'cigarette-paper' scars. Haematomas heal forming pseudotumours or nodules.

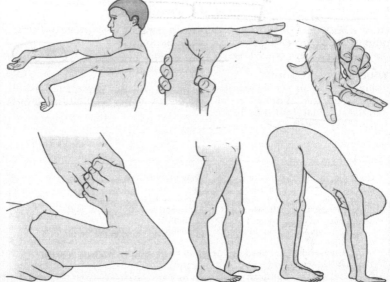

Fig. 133.1 Manoeuvres that may establish clinically significant joint laxity.

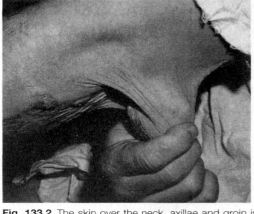

Fig. 133.2 The skin over the neck, axillae and groin is smooth and elastic; it can be stretched and, when released, it returns immediately to its normal position. Late in the disease it becomes lax, wrinkled and hangs in folds.

- Joints
- Kyphoscoliosis
- Hypermobile joints (Fig. 133.3).

Proceed as follows:
- Tell the examiner that you would like to examine the following:
    - The hernial orifices
    - The heart for mitral valve prolapse and aortic regurgitation
    - The eyes for myopia, retinal detachment.

Note: The three basic clinical criteria are: fragile skin, bleeding diathesis and hypermobile joints.

DIAGNOSIS

This patient has hypermobile joints (lesion) caused by Ehlers–Danlos syndrome (aetiology).

ADVANCED-LEVEL QUESTIONS

What are the gastrointestinal manifestations of this syndrome?
- Marked tendency to herniate
- Achalasia cardia
- Eventeration of the diaphragm
- Megacolon.

What are the cardiovascular manifestations?
- Mitral valve prolapse
- Aortic dissection.

What precautions would you take in managing skin wounds?
As the skin wounds tend to be gaping, they should be approximated with care; removable sutures are usually left in place for twice the usual time.

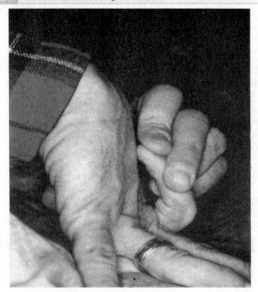

Fig. 133.3 Hypermobile joints.

What do you know about Ehlers–Danlos syndrome?

It comprises a group of heterogeneous disorders that result from defects in collagen synthesis and vary genetically and clinically from one another (Science 1973;182:298). Some molecular defects are known.

Type VI (kyphoscoliotic type). The most common and autosomal recessive form of inheritance. There is a defect in the enzyme lysyl hydroxylase, which is necessary for hydroxylation of lysyl residues during collagen synthesis. Only collagen types 1 and 3 are affected, and collagen types 2, 4 and 6 are normal. The predominant clinical features are ocular fragility with rupture of the cornea and retinal detachment. Some of these patients respond to ascorbic acid.

Type IV ('vascular type'). This is caused by a defect in the structural gene for collagen type 3 (COL3A1) and is inherited as an autosomal dominant trait. As type 3 collagen is present largely in blood vessels and intestines, the typical features of this syndrome include easy bruising; thin skin with visible veins; characteristic facial features; rupture of the large arteries, uterus or colon; and reduced life expectancy. This is the most severe form of Ehlers–Danlos syndrome (N Engl J Med 2000;342:673–80). Loeys–Dietz syndrome overlaps with this type.

Type VII. A defect in the conversion of procollagen to collagen, caused by the mutation that affects one of the two type 1 collagen genes (COL1A1 and COL1A2). Although in the single mutant allele, only 50% of type 1 collagen chains are affected, heterozygotes manifest the syndrome because these abnormal chains interfere with the formation of normal collagen helices.

Type IX. This is caused by a defect in copper metabolism, with high levels of copper in the cells but low levels of serum copper and caeruloplasmin.

Because the gene influencing copper metabolism is on the X chromosome, it is inherited as an X-linked recessive trait. This disease illustrates how copper metabolism can affect connective tissue.

Classical or types I and II. Null alleles of the *COL5A1* gene encoding type V collagen are a cause of the classical form. A single base mutation in *COL5A2* causes type II. Mutations in a gene that encodes 'tenascin-X, which is neither a collagen nor a collagen-modifying protein, can result in a variation of the classic form of the Ehlers–Danlos syndrome.

Notes

Patients with type I, II and IV disease are often investigated for bleeding diathesis before the correct diagnosis is made. Because of joint instability and laxity, many patients with types I, II, III, VI and VII disease are investigated for developmental delay before it is recognized that they have this syndrome.

Over 35 collagen genes have now been identified and these encode the chains of >20 types of collagen: types 1, 2 and 3 are the interstitial or fibrillar collagen whereas types 4, 5 and 6 are amorphous and are present in the interstitial tissue and basement membranes.

In which other condition is there a defect in collagen metabolism?

Osteogenesis imperfecta.

What are the criteria for diagnosis of joint hypermobility?

Beighton's nine-point scoring for joint hypermobility assigns two points for each of the following four paired manoeuvres (Ann Rheum Dis 1973;32:413–18):

- Hyperextension of the fifth metcarpophalangeal joint to 90 degrees
- Apposition of the thumb to the volar aspect of the forearm
- Hyperextension of the elbow beyond 10 degrees
- Hyperextension of the knee to beyond 10 degrees.

One point is assigned for the ability to place the palms of the hands on the floor with the knees extended.

It is not unusual to find extreme laxity in small joints and less laxity in large joints. Laxity decreases with age, so the dominant nature of most of these syndromes may not be appreciated when examining older family members.

Is hypermobility advantageous to musicians?

Lax fingers and wrists are good for flutists and string players, but lax knees and spines are bad for tympanists and others who stand while they play (N Engl J Med 1993;329:1079).

Further reading

Asociación Sindromes de Ehlers-Danlos e Hiperlaxitud (www.asedh.org): Spanish patient support group.

Association Francaise des Syndromes d'Ehlers-Danlos (www.afsed.com): French patient support group.

Ehlers-Danlos Foundation of New Zealand (www.edfnz.org.nz): New Zealand patient support group.

Ehlers-Danlos National Foundation (www.ednf.org): US patient support group.

Ehlers-Danlos Support Group (www.ehlers-danlos.org): UK patient support group.

Edvard Ehlers (1863–1937), a Danish dermatologist, and HA Danlos, a French dermatologist, described this condition independently in 1901 and 1908, respectively. Tschernogobow in Moscow first described this syndrome in 1892 (N Engl J Med 2000;342:730)

It is widely believed that the outstanding virtuosity of the violinist Niccolò Paganini (1782–1840) was the result of remarkable flexibility of the joints of his left hand: he could span three octaves with little effort (Arthritis Rheum 1982;25:1385–6).

Robert James Gorlin (1923–2006) described Gorlin's sign, which is the ability to touch the tip of the nose with the tongue in Ehlers–Danlos syndrome.

134 CHARCOT'S JOINT

INSTRUCTION

Examine this patient's joints.
Examine the locomotor system in this patient.

SALIENT FEATURES

History

- History of diabetes (Medicine 1972;51:191–210)
- Gait deformity
- Loss of pain threshold
- Atrophy of muscles of the joint.

" Foot, knee shoulder (handwritten)

Examination

- Enlargement of the affected joint (compare with the other side)
- Instability of the joint, in particular hypermobility of the joint
- May be warm, swollen and tender in the early stages
- Enlargement and crepitus may be present in the later stages
- Collapse of the longitudinal arch resulting in a rocker-bottom deformity.

Proceed as follows:
- Check sensation in the affected limb ✓
- Tell the examiner that you would like to investigate as follows:
  - Do a thorough neurological examination, looking for loss of proprioception, and/or pain sensation, and vibratory sensation with a 128 Hz tuning fork
  - Examine the urine for sugar (looking for evidence of diabetes mellitus).
- Ask for lancinating pains, check posterior column signs and look for Argyll Robertson pupil (tabes dorsalis)
- Check for dissociated sensory loss (syringomyelia)
- Test muscle strength.

DIAGNOSIS

This patient has Charcot's joint (lesion) caused by diabetes mellitus (aetiology) and has marked deformity of the joint with restricted movement, probably belonging to Rogers and Bevilacqua class 3C or 3D (functional status) (Fig. 134.1).

Remember: The 6Ps of prevention of neuropathic foot: podiatry, pulse examination, protective shoes, pressure reduction, prophylactic surgery, preventive education (J Am Podiatr Med Assoc 1997;87:305–12).

QUESTIONS

What do you understand by the term Charcot's joint?

It is a chronic progressive degenerative arthropathy resulting from a disturbance in the sensory innervation of the affected joint. It is a neuropathic arthropathy that is a complication of various disorders affecting the nervous system. It results in gross deformity, osteoarthrosis and new bone formation from repeated trauma.

Mention a few conditions responsible for the development of Charcot's joints

- Diabetic neuropathy: affecting tarsal joints, tarsometatarsal, metatarsophalangeal joints
- Tabes dorsalis: affecting knee, hip, ankle, lumbar and lower dorsal vertebrae

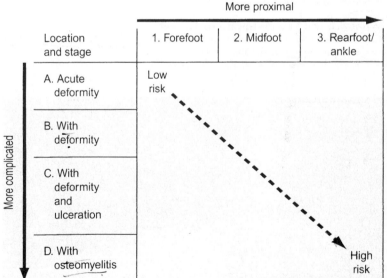

Fig. 134.1 Rogers and Bevilacqua classification. Moving towards a more complicated Charcot joint or proximally in the foot increases the risk of extremity amputation. (Adapted from Rogers, Bevilacqua 2008.)

- Syringomyelia: affecting shoulder, elbow, cervical vertebra
- Myelomeningocoele: affecting ankle, tarsus
- Miscellaneous: hereditary sensory neuropathies, peripheral nerve injury, congenital insensitivity to pain, leprosy, paraplegia (hips).

What is the advantage of measuring skin temperature in Charcot's foot?

Skin temperature difference between feet, measured with a contact or non-contact thermometer, may be significant. The average difference between the acute Charcot's foot and the unaffected side is as much as 9°F (5°C). A difference of 4°F (2°C) is considered significant.

How is Charcot's foot classified?

The Rogers and Bevilacqua classification (Fig. 134.1) combines the features of the clinical examination, radiography (Fig. 134.2) and anatomy. The graph indicates increasing risk for amputation as the Charcot foot becomes 'more complicated'.

What is the pathogenesis of acute Charcot's foot in diabetics?

It has been suggested that an initial insult triggers an inflammatory cascade through increased expression of proinflammatory cytokines (including tumour necrosis factor-α and interleukin 1β). This cascade results in increased expression of the nuclear transcription factor, NF-κB, which results in increased osteoclastogenesis. Osteoclasts cause progressive bone lysis, leading to further fracture; this, in turn, potentiates the inflammatory process (Lancet 2005; 366:2058–61).

What are the key components of gait?

Gait is classically broken into four components (heel strike, midstance, heel rise and toe push-off; see Fig. 61.1).

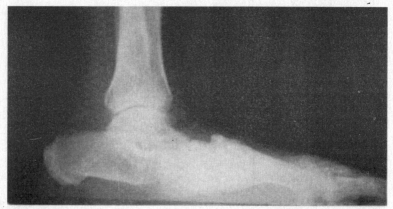

Fig. 134.2 Lateral radiograph showing equinus, tarsometatarsal subluxation and a prominent cuboid plantarly in Charcot foot. (With permission from Rogers, Bevilacqua 2008.)

Jean Martin Charcot (1825–1893) was a French neurologist. He was a
Professor of Pathology in 1872 and Professor of Nervous Diseases in 1882.
Other conditions that bear his name include Charcot's fever (intermittent fever
from cholangitis), Charcot's triad (intention tremor, nystagmus and scanning
speech in multiple sclerosis), Charcot–Leyden crystals (seen in the sputum of
asthmatics), Charcot–Marie–Tooth disease (peroneal muscular atrophy) and
Charcot-Wilbrand syndrome (visual agnosia). Charcot acknowledged that the
neuropathic arthropathy had been first reported by the American physician
John Kearsley Mitchell (1798–1858) in 1831. Mitchell's cases were secondary
to spinaldamage caused by TB, whereas Charcot's were the result of tertiary
syphilis.

135 STILL'S DISEASE

INSTRUCTION

Examine this patient's joints.
Look at this patient.

SALIENT FEATURES

History

- Maculopapular rash
- History of fever in the initial stages of the disease
- Joint pains, swelling, determine onset and course
- Sore throat.

Examination

- Micrognathia
- Joints usually involved are upper cervical apophyseal joints, carpometa-
  carpal joints and terminal interphalangeal joints (Fig. 135.1)
- Splenomegaly and lymph node enlargement
- Eyes (Fig. 135.2).

DIAGNOSIS

This patient has micrognathia, arthropathy of terminal interphalangeal
joints and a past history of maculopapular rash (lesion) caused by Still's
disease (aetiology).

Notes

- The classic triad of Still's disease is fever, oligoarticular arthritis and an
  evanescent salmon-coloured rash (which typically appears with the
  fever spikes), although the rash is persistent in up to one-third of
  patients.
- A sore throat is characteristic.
- Elevated ferritin levels, leukocyte counts, serum liver enzyme, and ESR
  are common.
- Still's disease usually occurs in patients younger than 35 years of age.

ADVANCED-LEVEL QUESTIONS

What do you know about juvenile chronic arthritis?

The diagnosis is made when a child aged <16 years has arthritis for at least 6 weeks with no other apparent cause. After 6 months of disease three major patterns are seen:

● Still's disease (10–20% of cases) is defined as arthritis associated with daily temperature spikes to 39.4°C (103°F) for at least 2 weeks with or without maculopapular rash.

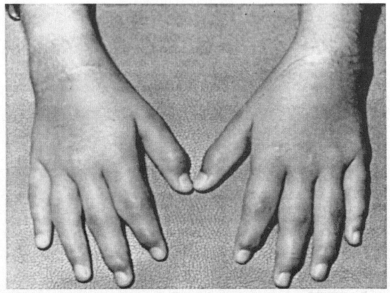

Fig. 135.1 Hands and wrists in a girl with rheumatoid factor-negative polyarticular juvenile rheumatoid arthritis. There is symmetric involvement of the metacarpophalangeal, proximal interphalangeal and distal interphalangeal joints. (With permission from Kliegman et al. 2007.)

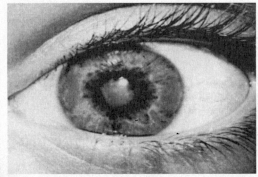

Fig. 135.2 Chronic anterior uveitis in juvenile rheumatoid arthritis, with small irregular pupil, well-developed cataract and early band keratopathy at the medial and lateral margins of the cornea. (With permission from Kliegman et al. 2007.)

- Polyarticular juvenile chronic arthritis (15–25%) in which five or more joints are affected. Early fusion of the mandible and cervical spine result in a receding chin.
- Pauciarticular juvenile chronic arthritis (60–75%), which affects four or less joints; iritis is common in girls, whereas sacroiliitis is common in boys.

What are the complications of juvenile chronic arthritis?
- Pain, lethargy, anorexia and irritability
- Joint contractures
- Anaemia
- Chronic anterior uveitis (iridocyclitis): extensive posterior synechiae result in a small, irregular pupil
- Growth disturbance
- Amyloidosis
- Joint failure

How would you treat a patient with juvenile chronic arthritis?
- Education about the disease, counselling and social support
- Physical and occupational therapy: monitoring and recording range of movement of joints, exercises to increase range of movement and muscle bulk, hydrotherapy, splinting
- NSAIDs: naproxen, ibuprofen, piroxicam, indomethacin, diclofenac
- Intra-articular steroids: triamcinolone, methylprednisolone acetate.

What is the risk of treating young children with salicylates?
Reye syndrome has been reported in children treated with aspirin for fever accompanying viral infections such as influenza. Children with juvenile chronic arthritis who are treated continuously for long periods have not been shown to have an increased incidence of this syndrome (Pediatrics 1980;66:859).

What are the poor prognostic factors?
- Chronic and polyarticular arthritis, particularly in patients with a systemic or pauciarticular onset.
- Polyarticular onset and a positive test for immunoglobulin rheumatoid factor.

Which drugs have been used in the treatment of resistant juvenile rheumatoid arthritis?
- Pencillamine
- Hydroxychloroquine
- Methotrexate (long-term therapy should be avoided as it is known to cause hepatic fibrosis)
- Etanercept, adalimumab therapy
- Leflunomide, an oral inhibitor of pyrimidine synthesis.

What do you know about the American College of Rheumatology Pedi Score?
The American College of Rheumatology Pediatric core set of disease-activity measures (ACR Pedi 30) in children with juvenile rheumatoid arthritis consists of:
- a count of swollen joints
- a count of joints with active arthritis

- global assessment of disease activity by the patient or a parent or guardian on a visual-analogue scale ranging from 0 (disease inactive) to 100 (maximal disease activity)
- physician's global assessment of disease activity
- assessment of physical function by the patient or a parent or guardian (by means of the Childhood Health Assessment Questionnaire Disability Index)
- laboratory evaluation of acute-phase reactants (ESR).

Patients with an ACR Pedi 30 response could also have worsening of 30% or more in no more than 1 of the 6 response variables. The Percent Improvement Index, a continuous variable, is calculated as the mean of the percentage changes from baseline in each core set of disease-activity measures for juvenile rheumatoid arthritis, with negative values indicating improvement and positive values set to 0, indicating no improvement.

Sir George Fredrick Still (1868–1941), a London physician, described 12 children (in 1897) who had a polyarthritis, which he stated should be distinguished from rheumatoid arthritis, and a further six children with a disease indistinguishable from adult rheumatoid arthritis. The distinctive findings in the first group included splenomegaly, lymphadenopathy, frequent occurrence of pericarditis and a predilection for cervical spine involvement. He also noted that fever and growth retardation were prominent features. (Still GF. On a form of chronic joint disease in childhood. Med Chir Trans 1897;80:47). The rash, however, was first described by Eric GL Bywaters.

RDK Reye (1912–1977), an Australian histopathologist.

Endocrinology
Examination of the thyroid

INSTRUCTION

Examine the thyroid.
Test this patient's thyroid status.
Look at this patient's neck.

SALIENT FEATURES

1. Introduce yourself to the patient and, while shaking hands, note whether the palms are warm and sweaty.
2. *The neck*:
   - Look for the JVP
   - Scars of surgery (often missed by candidates)
   - Enlarged cervical lymph nodes
   - Goitre.
3. *Palpation*:
   - Always begin by palpating from behind (Fig. VI.1)
   - Seat the patient comfortably
   - Comment first on exophthalmos
   - While palpating the gland, ensure that there is a glass of water to swallow.
   - Palpate the thyroid and note the following:
     - Size: specify the World Health Organization (WHO) grade (see below)
     - Mobility
     - Texture: simple or nodular (solitary or multiple)?
     - Tenderness.
   - Pemberton's sign: on raising the arms above the head, patients with retrosternal goitres may develop signs of compression, such as suffusion of the face, syncope or giddiness
   - Palpate cervical lymph nodes
   - Feel the carotid arteries
   - Palpate for tracheal deviation
   - Percuss for retrosternal extension
   - Auscultate over the gland for bruit, carotid bruits
   - Test sternomastoid function (this muscle may be infiltrated in thyroid malignancy).
4. *Thyroid function*:
   - Eye signs:
     - Lid lag
     - Exophthalmos
     - Lid retraction (sclera visible above the cornea)
     - Extraocular movements.
   - Hands:
     - Pulse for tachycardia or atrial fibrillation
     - Tremor
     - Acropachy or clubbing

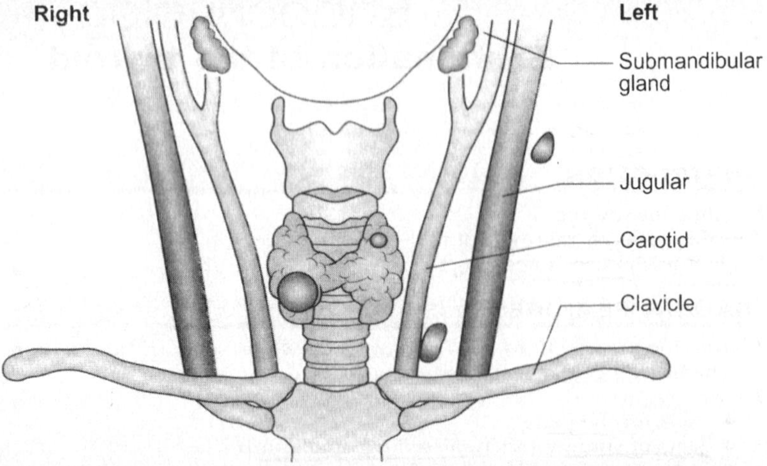

Right

Left

Submandibular gland

Jugular

Carotid

Clavicle

Fig. VI.1 Cervical map helps in communicating anatomic relationships and serves as a reference for follow-up examinations.

- Palmar erythema (thyrotoxicosis)
- Supinator jerks (inverted in hypothyroidism)
- Proximal weakness in the upper arm.
- Skin
  - Look for pretibial myxoedema.
- Elicit the ankle jerks.
5. If you are permitted to ask questions, enquire about shortness of breath, dysphagia, about iodine-containing medications and possible exposure to radiation.

QUESTIONS

How would you grade the size of the goitre?
WHO grading of goitre (Lancet 2000;355:106–110):
0: no palpable or visible goitre
1: palpable goitre (larger than terminal phalanges of examiner's thumbs)
1A: goitre detectable only on palpation
1B: goitre palpable and visible with neck extended
2: goitre visible with neck in normal position
3: large goitre visible from a distance.

What is the significance of the thyroid bruit?
The thyroid bruit is almost pathognomonic of Graves' disease and occurs only rarely in patients with colloid goitres or other thyroid disorders.

In 1915, Kendall isolated a crystalline product named thyroxine (Kendall EC. The isolation in crystalline form of the compound containing iodine which occurs in the thyroid. JAMA 1915;64:2042).

In 1927, Harrington and Barger synthesized thyroxine (Harrington CR, Barger G. Chemistry of thyroxine. Biochem J 1927;21:169).

In 1952, Gross and Pitt-Rivers identified triiodothyronine (Gross J, Pitt-Rivers R. The identification of 3,5,3'-I-triiodothyronine in human plasma. Lancet 1952;i: 439).

In 1946, HS Pemberton described the sign of the 'submerged' goitre (Pemberton HS. Sign of submerged goitre Lancet 1946;251:509). Pemberton's manoeuvre is a useful clinical sign for latent superior vena cava syndrome caused by a substernal mass (Eur J Med Res 1997;2:488–90).

136 GRAVES' DISEASE

INSTRUCTION

Look at this patient.
Determine this patient's thyroid status.

SALIENT FEATURES

- Patient is fidgety and restless.

History

- Easy irritability, nervousness, insomnia
- Fatigue
- Weight loss with increased appetite
- Frequent defaecation
- Oligomenorrhoea
- Dislike for hot weather, heat intolerance, excessive sweating
- Palpitations, dyspnoea
- Family history of thyroid disease
- Proximal muscle weakness, muscle atrophy, periodic paralysis (particularly in patients of Oriental extraction).

Examination

Proceed as follows: (Hands:)

- While shaking hands with the patient note the warm sweaty palms.
- Look for tremor, thyroid acropachy (Fig. 136.1; a hypermetabolic state leading to axial bone destruction; do not confuse it with clubbing, which is usually painless), onycholysis (Plummer's nails), vitiligo and palmar erythema.
- Check pulse for tachycardia or the irregularly irregular pulse of atrial fibrillation.

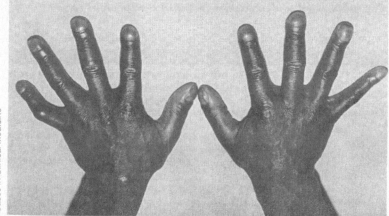

Fig. 136.1 Rare thyroid acropachy. (With permission of Kronenberg et al. 2008.)

Eyes:
- Comment on proptosis (after looking at the eyes from behind and above)
- Check for lid lag
- Check for scars of previous tarsorraphy.

Neck:
- Mention previous thyroidectomy scar if present
- Examine the neck for goitre and auscultate over the gland.

Chest:
- Gynaecomastia can occur in men as a result of increased oestrogen production.
- Examine the cardiovascular system: sinus tachycardia, widened pulse pressure, loud first heart sound, third heart sound, systolic murmur, atrial fibrillation.

Lower limbs:
- Examine the shins for pretibial myxoedema (bilateral pinkish, brown dermal plaques; see Fig. 139.1).
- Test for proximal myopathy with hyper-reflexia.

Tell the examiner:
- that you would like to check for thyroid-stimulating antibodies (TsAb): near 100% detection rate in patients with Graves' disease.

DIAGNOSIS

This patient has tremor, proptosis and lid lag (lesions) caused by autoimmune Graves' disease (aetiology), and is in fast atrial fibrillation and hyperthyroid (functional status).

QUESTIONS

How would you confirm the diagnosis in this patient?
Serum thyroxine (T_4), serum thyroid-stimulating hormone (TSH; thyrotrophin) levels and thyroid autoantibodies.

What are the causes of hyperthyroidism?
- Primary: Graves' disease, toxic nodule, multinodular goitre, Hashimato's thyroiditis, iodine-induced, excess thyroid hormone replacement, postpartum thyroiditis
- Secondary: pituitary or excess TSH hypersecretion, hydatidiform moles, struma ovarii, factitious.

What are the components of Graves' disease?
Hyperthyroidism with goitre, eye changes (see Fig. 138.1) and pretibial myxoedema: they run independent courses.

ADVANCED-LEVEL QUESTIONS

What happens to radioactive iodine uptake in Graves' disease?
Radioactive iodine uptake increases in Graves' disease.

Which is the best laboratory test to diagnose hyperthyroidism?
Serum TSH measurement is the single most reliable test to diagnose all common forms of hyperthyroidism, particularly in an outpatient setting (Arch Intern Med 2000;160:1573–5). Typically serum concentrations are <0.1 mIU/l in Graves' disease, toxic adenoma, nodular goitre, subacute and lymphocytic (silent, postpartum) thyroiditis, iodine-induced hyperthyroidism and exogenous thyroid hormone excess. To diagnose

hyperthyroidism accurately, TSH assay sensitivity, the lowest reliably measured TSH concentration, must be ≤0.02 mIU/l. Some less-sensitive TSH assays cannot reliably distinguish hyperthyroidism from euthyroidism. Free T_4 and triiodothyronine (T_3) concentrations should also be measured when less-sensitive TSH assays are utilized. In rare types of TSH-mediated hyperthyroidism (pituitary adenomas and selective pituitary resistance to thyroid hormone), serum TSH alone will not be suffice and again free T_4 and T_3 concentrations should be measured.

Remember: Although serum TSH is the best initial diagnostic test, it is useless in assessing response to therapy as it remains suppressed until after patient becomes euthyroid. Clinical assessment and free plasma T_4 is used to monitor response to therapy.

What are the causes of isolated thyroid-stimulating hormone suppression?

- Mild (subclinical) hyperthyroidism
- Recovery from overt hyperthyroidism
- Non-thyroidal illness (which can cause a low serum free T_4)
- Pregnancy during the first trimester
- Medications such as dopamine and glucocorticoids.

Mention a few causes of hyperthyroidism with reduced iodine uptake

- Thyroiditis
- Malignancy of thyroid
- Struma ovarii (ovarian tumour).

What drugs are used in the treatment of thyrotoxicosis?

- Carbimazole
- Methimazole
- Propylthiouracil.

Note: Antithyroid drug therapy is the preferred first-line therapy outside the USA, and methimazole or carbimazole are favoured over propylthiouracil because of their simple once-a-day dosing and higher adherence.

What are the disadvantages of antithyroid drugs?

- High rates of relapse once treatment is discontinued
- Occasionally complicated by troublesome hypersensitivity reaction and very rarely by life-threatening agranulocytosis and hepatitis.

What are the advantages and disadvantages of radioactive iodine compared with partial thyroidectomy for thyrotoxicosis?

Both radioactive iodine therapy and surgical thyroidectomy are extremely effective and usually result in permanent cure. Patients will require life-long thyroxine replacement. Thyroid surgery is expensive, inconvenient and occasionally complicated by injury to surrounding structures in the neck in less skilled hands; it is also complicated by the general risks of anaesthesia. In Graves' disease, the indications for surgery include:

- a large goitre
- patient preference
- drug non-compliance
- disease relapse when radioiodine is not available.

Radioactive iodine, although safe, may not be acceptable to patients who are sensitive to the calamities of Chernobyl and Hiroshima.

What are the contraindications to radioiodine therapy?

- Breastfeeding and pregnancy
- Situations where it is clear that the safety of other persons cannot be guaranteed
- Patients who are incontinent who are unwilling to have a urinary catheter
- Allergy to iodine.

What are the indications for radioiodine therapy in hyperthyroidism?

- Hyperthyroidism in Graves' disease with moderate goitre (40–50 g), with no significant eye signs and first presentation
- Toxic multinodular goitre in older persons complicated by heart failure or atrial fibrillation
- Toxic adenoma, usually with mild hyperthyroidism
- Ophthalmopathy with thyroid dysfunction with stable eye disease (note radioiodine treatment may exacerbate eye changes in Graves' disease and is not recommended in severe Graves' opthalmopathy)
- Ablation therapy in those with severe manifestations such as heart failure, atrial fibrillation or psychosis.

What advice would you give to patients who are administered radioiodine?

- Depending on the dose, they should avoid journeys on public transport, stay off work, avoid places of entertainment or close contact with other people for up to 12 days and avoid non-essential close personal contact with children and pregnant women for up to 27 days.
- Patients should be warned that in the first 14 days after administration of therapy they may experience palpitations or other exacerbations of symptoms, particularly when not euthyroid before treatment.
- The importance of regular follow-up should be emphasized and the need to report the recurrence of thyrotoxic symptoms or the development of hypothyroidism.
- Patients should be informed that atrial fibrillation often reverts to normal rhythm and that digitalis may then be discontinued.
- Patients should be reminded to avoid pregnancy for 4 months after radioiodine therapy.

Is there an increased frequency of cancer in patients with Graves' disease?

There is little evidence to suggest an increased frequency of thyroid cancer in patients with Graves' disease.

Does thyrotoxicosis affect the bone?

Yes, chronic thyrotoxicosis is associated with osteoporosis.

If a patient with thyrotoxicosis develops muscle weakness following oral carbohydrate or intravenous dextrose, which condition comes to mind?

Hypokalaemic periodic paralysis, which occurs particularly in Asian men. These attacks may last for 7–72 h.

What is the effect of iodine on thyroid status?

It may cause transient hypothyroidism (Wolff–Chaikoff effect) or hyperthyroidism (Jod–Basedow phenomenon).

What is the prevalence of hyperthyroidism?

The prevalence is 0.2% in the adult population. Mild (subclinical) hyperthyroidism (serum TSH <0.1 mIU/l, free T_4 and T_3 normal) has a prevalence of 0.1–6% of the adult population.

What is the role of monitoring thyroid-stimulating antibody in these patients?

Titres for TsAb progressively decreases over 18 months after surgery or an antithyroid drug, and ultimately disappears in most patients (Eur J Endocrinol 2008; 158:69–75).

After radioiodine ablation, TsAb levels actually increase during the first year and are less likely to disappear: over a 5-year follow-up, only 60% of patients achieed undetectable levels.

This last observation underscores the importance of TsAb monitoring in pregnant women previously treated with radioiodine, who may still harbour TsAb even though they are hypothyroid.

What do you know about the pathogenesis of Graves' opthalmopathy?

It is postulated that the TSH receptor is a target of autoimmunity within the orbit and that its recognition by a circulating TSH-like factor explains the link between hyperthyroidism and Graves' ophthalmopathy. A failure of T cells to tolerate the receptor allows autoimmunity to develop against it. The antibodies formed, in turn, stimulate the TSH receptor on thyroid follicular epithelial cells, leading to their proliferation and increased production of T_3 and T_4. The antibodies also recognize the TSH receptor on fibroblasts in the orbit and, together with the secreted interferon-γ and tumour necrosis factor, initiate the tissue changes typically occurring in Graves' ophthalmopathy (N Engl J Med 2010;362:726–38).

What is thyroid pathology in Graves' disease?

It is characterized by a non-homogeneous lymphocytic infiltration with an absence of follicular destruction.

What do you know about amiodarone-induced hyperthyroidism?

Amiodarone, which contains 37% iodine, can induce hyperthyroidism; this disorder is more common in iodine-deficient areas (Ann Intern Med 1984;101:28–34) and in patients with nodular goitres and thyroid autoantibodies.

There are two mechanisms by which amiodarone may cause hyperthyroidism: thyroid destruction through an iodine-associated increase in circulating interleukin-6 (J Clin Endocrinol Metab 1994;78:423–7) or an increase in thyroid hormone synthesis. Amiodarone-induced hyperthyroidism sometimes responds to thionamide antithyroid drugs, but it may be very resistant to treatment. A combination of potassium perchlorate and carbimazole should be tried; steroids may be effective, particularly if interleukin-6 concentrations are high, which suggests a destructive thyroiditis. In resistant disease, total thyroidectomy should be considered (Lancet 1997;349:339–43).

Which drug would you prefer in the management of a pregnant woman with thyrotoxicosis?

Propylthiouracil is preferred in the USA for pregnant hyperthyroid women because methimazole may have teratogenic effects.

Robert James Graves (1796–1853) was a Dublin physician who described this condition. In 1835, he described three patients and wrote of one patient, 'It was now observed that the eyes assumed a singular appearance for the eyeballs were apparently enlarged, so that when she slept or tried to shut her eyes her lids were incapable of closing, when the eyes were open, the white sclerotic could be seen, to a breadth of several lines all around the cornea' (Graves R. London Med Surg J 1835;7:516). Graves' disease is also termed Basedow's or Parry's disease.

137 EXOPHTHALMOS

INSTRUCTION

Examine this patient's face.
Perform a general examination of this patient.

SALIENT FEATURES

History

- Obtain history of thyrotoxicosis (see p. 516)
- History of smoking (opthalmopathy more common in cigarette smokers; Lancet 1991;338:25–7).

Examination

- Prominent eyeballs (Fig. 137.1).
- Look at the patient's eyes from behind and above for proptosis.
- Comment on lid retraction (the sclera above the upper limbus of the cornea will be seen); this is Dalrymple's sign (Fig. 137.2).
- Comment on the sclera visible between the lower eyelid and the lower limbus of the cornea (i.e. comment on the exophthalmos). Most patients have bilateral exophthalmos with unilateral prominence.
- Check for lid lag (ask the patient to follow your finger and then move it along the arc of a circle from a point above the patient's head to a point below the nose—the movement of the lid lags behind that of the globe); this is von Graefe's sign. Voluntary staring can result in a false lid lag, and the patient must be suitably relaxed before eliciting this sign.
- Check for extraocular movements and comment on the cornea.
- Look for the five important signs of exophthalmos:
  - Eyelid swelling
  - Eyelid redness
  - Conjunctival swelling (chemosis)
  - Conjunctival redness
  - Inflammation of the plica or caruncle, which both lie at the inner corner of the eye medial to the conjunctiva
- Look for:
  - signs of thyrotoxicosis: fast pulse rate, tremor and sweating
  - goitre (listen for a bruit)
  - post-thyroidectomy scar.

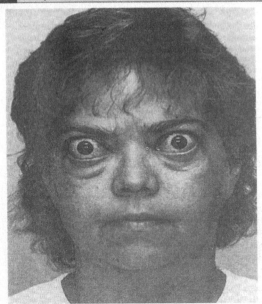

Fig. 137.1 Characteristic signs of Graves' orbitopathy: thyroid stare, asymmetry, proptosis, and periorbital oedema. (With permission from Larsen et al. 2003.)

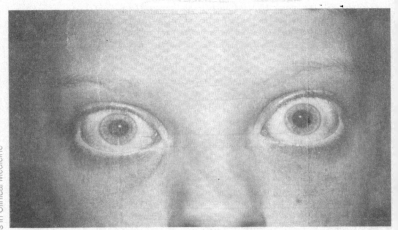

Fig. 137.2 Dalrymple sign: retraction of upper eyelids in the primary gaze. (With permission from Kanski 2001.)

DIAGNOSIS

This patient has marked exophthalmos with ophthalmoplegia (lesions) with signs of thyrotoxicosis (functional status) caused by Graves' disease (aetiology).

ADVANCED-LEVEL QUESTIONS

What eye signs of thyroid disease do you know?
Werner's mnemonic, NO SPECS (J Clin Endocrinol Metab 1977;44:203–4):
● No signs or symptoms
● Only signs of upper lid retraction and stare, with or without lid lag and exophthalmos
● Soft tissue involvement
● Proptosis
● Extraocular muscle involvement
● Corneal involvement
● Sight loss from optic nerve involvement.

How would you investigate this patient?
● History and clinical examination for signs of thyrotoxicosis and thyroid enlargement and bruit
● Serum thyroxine (T_4), triiodothyronine (T_3), thyroid-stimulating hormone (TSH)
● Thyroid antibodies.

Mention the factors implicated in the phenomenon of lid lag
● Sympathetic overstimulation, causing overaction of Müller's muscle
● Myopathy of the inferior rectus, causing overaction of superior rectus and levator muscles
● Restrictive myopathy of the levator muscle.

What is euthyroid Graves' disease?
The patient will be clinically and biochemically euthyroid but will have manifestations of Graves' ophthalmopathy. A TSH-releasing hormone (TRH) stimulation test will show a flat response curve.

What would you recommend if a patient with unilateral exophthalmos is clinically and biochemically euthyroid?
● Ophthalmological referral
● Ultrasonography of the orbit
● CT scan of the orbit.

How is proptosis quantified?
It is assessed using a Hertel's exophthalmometer. The upper limit of normal is subject to ethnic variation, and usually >20 mm is considered as proptosis.

What are the components of the clinical activity score for Graves' opthalmopathy?
The Clinical Activity Score (CAS) is calculated according to the presence or absence of the characteristics listed. The score ranges from 0 to 7, with 0 to 2 characteristics indicating inactive Graves' ophthalmopathy and 3 to 7 characteristics active Graves' ophthalmopathy:

- Spontaneous retrobulbar pain
- Pain with eye movement
- Redness of the eyelids
- Redness of the conjunctiva
- Swelling of the eyelids
- Swelling of the caruncle
- Conjunctival oedema (chemosis).

The positive predictive value for therapeutic response for a CAS of 3/7 (or 4/10) is 80%, whereas the negative predictive value is 64%. Although the CAS is extremely useful for assessment of activity, its binary scoring makes it much less useful for monitoring change over time. The European Group on Graves' Orbitopathy (EUGOGO) atlas is one tool for assessment and is freely available at www.eugogo.org

How would you manage a patient with Graves' ophthalmopathy?

The single most important aspect is a close liaison between the physician and the ophthalmologist.

Severe Graves' disease and visual loss. This should be treated immediately with high doses of corticosteroids, orbital irradiation and plasma exchange as an adjunct. If there is no improvement within 72–96 h, orbital nerve decompression by surgical removal of the floor and medial wall of the orbit is necessary.

Moderate ophthalmopathy. This improves substantially in 2–3 years in most patients. In the interim the patient is treated symptomatically:
- Pain and grittiness is treated with methylcellulose eye drops by day and a lubricating eye ointment at night
- Exposure keratitis may be relieved by lateral tarsorraphy, surgery of the lower eyelid
- Diplopia may be relieved by prisms (the Fresnel prism is stuck on to the lens of spectacle) or surgery of the extraocular muscles
- Static or worsening ophthalmopathy is an indication for steroids, orbital decompression or orbital irradiation
- Patients should be advised to stop smoking.

Mild ophthalmopathy. This can be rectified by cosmetic eyelid surgery. It is important to remember that patients can be distressed by their appearance. During the early acute phase, patients will have considerable symptomatic relief from the following measures:
- Elevating the head at night
- Diuretics to reduce oedema
- Tinted glasses for protection from the sun, wind and foreign bodies.

Note: Rituximab has been used successfully in a small number of patients with moderate-to-severe steroid-resistant Graves' ophthalmopathy.

What is the role of radioiodine in thyroid eye disease?
- Since radioiodine treatment carries a substantial risk of exacerbating pre-existing thyroid eye disease, it should be avoided as far as possible in patients with active or severe ophthalmopathy, in whom medical therapy with a thionamide drug such as carbimazole is preferable. Radioiodine may be used in patients with mild eye disease but adjuvant oral corticosteriods should be prescribed (N Engl J Med 1998;338:73–8).

- Patients without clinical evidence of thyroid disease have a small risk of developing ophthalmopathy and a very low risk of developing severe eye disease. It is prudent to warn all patients of this complication, but the risks do not justify denying most patients the benefits of·definitive treatment with radioiodine when indicated. In addition, the risks do not justify the routine use of corticosteroids in patients without ophthalmopathy (BMJ 1999;319:68–9).
- Smoking, raised serum T_3 and uncorrected hypothyroidism are also factors that can exacerbate thyroid eye disease. Therefore, to reduce the risk of thyroid eye disease, patients should be encouraged to stop smoking, be rendered euthyroid with a thionamide before radioiodine, and be monitored closely to detect and treat early hypothyroidism or persistent hyperthyroidism.

Mention the less important eponyms related to thyroid eye disease

- Infrequent blinking: Stellwag's sign
- Tremor of closed eyelids: Rosenbach's sign
- Difficulty in everting upper eyelid: Gifford's sign
- Absence of wrinkling of forehead on sudden upward gaze: Joffroy's sign
- Impaired convergence of the eyes: Möbius' sign
- Weakness of at least one of the extraocular muscles: Ballet's sign
- Paralysis of extraocular muscles: Jendrassik's sign
- Poor fixation on lateral gaze: Suker's sign .
- Dilatation of pupil with weak epinephrine solution: Loewi's sign
- Jerky pupillary contraction to consensual light: Cowen's sign
- Increased pigmentation of the margins of eyelids: Jellinek's sign
- Upper lid resistance on downward traction: Grove's sign
- Abnormal fullness of the eyelid: Enroth's sign
- Unequal pupillary dilatation: Knie's sign
- When the eyeball is turned downwards, there is arrest of the descent of the lid, spasm and continued descent: Boston's sign
- When the clinician places his or her hand on a level with the patient's eyes and then lifts it higher, the patient's upper lids spring up more quickly than the eyeball: Kocher's sign.

J Dalrymple (1804–1852), an English ophthalmologist.

Exophthalmos associated with goitre and non-organic heart disease was first described by the English physician Caleb Hillard Parry (1775–1822) in a paper published posthumously in 1825. He graduated in medicine from Edinburgh and practised in Bath. He described hyperthyroidism before Graves' disease.

In 1977, Solomon et al. presented the evidence that three independent autoimmune diseases tended to occur concomitantly in the same euthyroid Graves' ophthalmopathy: idiopathic hyperthyroidism, Hashimato's thyroiditis and Graves' ophthalmopathy.

Anthony Toft, an endocrinologist at Edinburgh Royal Infirmary, is past President of the Royal College of Physicians of Edinburgh.

250 Cases in Clinical Medicine

138 HYPOTHYROIDISM

INSTRUCTION

Obtain a history and perform relevant general examination.

SALIENT FEATURES

History

- Dryness of skin ✓
- Hair dryness or loss (Fig. 138.1)
- Cold intolerance
- Change in the voice (hoarse, husky)
- Lethargy, undue tiredness ✓
- Constipation
- Moderate weight gain in spite of loss of appetite
- Menstrual irregularity especially menorrhagia
- Infertility ✓
- Depression
- Dementia
- Muscle cramps
- Oedema

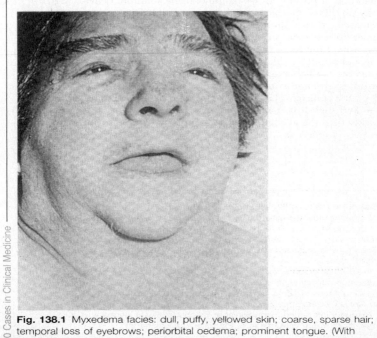

Fig. 138.1 Myxedema facies: dull, puffy, yellowed skin; coarse, sparse hair; temporal loss of eyebrows; periorbital oedema; prominent tongue. (With permission from Seidel et al. 2004.)

- Radioiodine therapy for previous Graves' disease (the patient may have associated eye signs of Graves' disease)
- Medications and other compounds such as lithium carbonate and iodine-containing compounds (e.g. amiodarone, radiocontrast agents, expectorants containing potassium iodide and kelp)
- Family history of thyroid dysfunction, pernicious anaemia, diabetes mellitus, primary adrenal insufficiency
- Obtain history of hypercholesterolaemia, angina pectoris and hypertension (remember hypertension occurs in 10% of these patients and disappears with thyroxine replacement).

Examination

- Coarse, dry skin (look for yellowish tint of carotenaemia: 'peaches and cream' complexion)
- 'Dirty elbows and knees' sign (Acta Endocrinol (Copenh) 1954;16:305)
- Puffy lower eyelids
- Loss of outer third of eyebrows (Queen Anne's sign or sign of Hertoghe)
- Xanthelasma.

Proceed as follows:
- Examine the neck for goitre and the scar of previous thyroidectomy. The typical Hashimoto gland is firm and lobulated
- Slow pulse
- Check the ankle jerks, looking for delayed relaxation
- Look for:
  - proximal muscle weakness
  - cerebellar signs
  - carpal tunnel syndrome.

DIAGNOSIS

This patient has delayed ankle jerks, puffy lower eyelids, slow pulse and hoarse husky voice (lesions), indicating that he has hypothyroidism (functional status); the cause needs to be determined (aetiology).

QUESTIONS

How is delayed relaxation best elicited in the ankle?
Get the patient to kneel on a chair with his hands holding the back of the chair and then elicit the jerks on either side.

What are the causes of goitre?
- Idiopathic (majority)
- Hashimato's thyroiditis
- Graves' disease
- Iodine deficiency (simple goitre)
- Puberty, pregnancy, subacute thyroiditis, goitrogens (lithium, phenylbutazone).

What is the thyroid status in Hashimato's disease?
Hypothyroidism (usually).

What is the single best clinical indicator for hypothyroidism?
Delayed ankle jerks.

What is the best laboratory indicator for hypothyroidism?

Elevated serum thyroid-stimulating hormone (TSH). When there is a suspicion of pituitary or hypothalamic disease, the serum free thyroxine (T_4) should be measured in addition to serum TSH. Serum triiodothyronine (T_3) is a poor indicator of hypothyroid state and should not be used.

What are the laboratory changes in hypothyroidism?

- Hypercholesterolaemia
- Hyponatraemia
- Anaemia
- Elevation of serum creatinine phosphokinase and lactate dehydrogenase
- Hyperprolactinaemia.

↑ CPK, LDH

What are the causes of isolated thyroid-stimulating hormone elevation?

- Mild (subclinical) hypothyroidism
- Recovery from hypothyroxinaemia of non-thyroidial illnesses
- Medications such as amiodarone or lithium (Arch Intern Med 2000;160:1573–5).

What are the causes of isolated thyroid-stimulating hormone suppression?

- Mild (subclinical) hyperthyroidism
- Recovery from overt hyperthyroidism
- Non-thyroidal illness, which cause low serum free T_4
- Pregnancy during first trimester
- Medications such as dopamine and glucocorticoids.

How would you investigate a simple goitre?

Estimation of serum T_4, T_3, TSH and thyroid antibodies (presence of anti-thyroid peroxidise antibodies suggests Hashimoto's thyroditis).

Remember: One does not know what free T_4 value is normal for an individual person unless the serum TSH is measured.

What is the cause for delayed relaxation in hypothyroidism?

The exact cause is not known. It is probably caused by decreased muscle metabolism.

How would you manage this patient with hypothyroidism?

Oral T_4 replacement therapy for life. The therapeutic dose varies between 100 and 200 µg/day taken as a single dose. It is taken on an empty stomach (1 h before or 2–3 h after food). Dose adjustments are made once in 3 weeks. The dose is adjusted depending on the clinical response and suppression of raised serum TSH. Lack of response to T_4 suggests:

- non-thyroid related disease
- poor compliance
- underlying psychiatric abnormalities
- presence of pernicious anaemia
- associated autoimmune disease such as Addison's disease.

In hypothyroid patients who become pregnant, T_4 requirements go up by ~50% in the first half of pregnancy.

What is the hazard in treating the elderly?

Rapid T_4 replacement may precipitate angina and myocardial infarction. The starting dose in the elderly is 25–50 µg/day.

What are the cardiovascular manifestations of hypothyroidism?
- Bradycardia
- Mild hypertension
- Pericarditis and pericardial effusion
- High LDL, low HDL levels, hypercholesterolaemia
- Diminished cardiac output and cardiac failure
- Coronary artery disease
- ECG changes: low-voltage T and P waves, prolongation of QT interval.

What are the neurological manifestations of hypothyroidism?
- Delayed deep tendon reflexes (Woltman's sign)
- Carpal tunnel syndrome, peripheral neuropathy
- Myxoedema madness
- Myxoedema coma
- Pseudodementia
- Deafness to high tones (Trotter syndrome; Br Med Bull 1960;16:92)
- In Pendred syndrome, babies are born with a goitre, deafness and mental retardation
- Cerebellar syndrome (Lancet 1960;ii: 225)
- Hoffmann syndrome (i.e. muscle aches with myotonia in myxoedema). In infants, muscle involvement may result in Kocher–Debré–Sémélaigne syndrome or 'infant Hercules'.

What do you understand by subclinical hypothyroidism?
This is a condition where there is low normal serum T_4 and there is moderately raised serum TSH (grade 1:5–10, grade 2:10.1–20, grade 3: >20 mIU/l). All these patients should be treated.

What other conditions are associated with Hashimato's thyroiditis?
- Addison's disease
- Diabetes mellitus
- Graves' disease
- Hypoparathyroidism
- Premature ovarian failure
- Pernicious anaemia
- Rheumatoid arthritis
- Sjögren syndrome
- Ulcerative colitis
- SLE
- Haemolytic anaemia.

What do you understand by the term sick euthyroid syndrome?
In severe acute non-thyroidal illness or following surgery, changes in pituitary–thyroid function result in altered thyroid indices but, despite this, patients remain euthyroid. On recovery from the illness, the indices of thyroid function return to normal (N Engl J Med 1995;333:1562–3). The changes in thyroidal indices include:
- decrease in extrathyroidal conversion of T_4 to T_3, the active form of the thyroid hormone
- a decrease in TSH secretion, which causes decreased thyroidal secretion and, in time, decreases in serum T_4 concentrations and further decreases in serum T_3 concentrations — the latter as a result of both decreased secretion of T_4 by the thyroid and diminished availability of T_4 for peripheral conversion to T_3

- decreased production or diminished affinity for thyroidal hormones of one or more major serum thyroid hormone-binding proteins: thyroxine-binding globulin, transthyretin and albumin. These decreases can result in decreased serum total T_4 levels but not in free T_4 or T_3. Serum concentrations of reverse T_3 (which is inactive) are increased because its deiodination is impaired.

What is the prevalence of hypothyroidism?

The prevalence is 2% of the adult population, whereas mild (sublinical) hypothyroidism is 5–17% (subclinical hypothyroidism is when serum TSH is elevated with a normal free T_4 concentration).

What are the components of Grover's disease?

- Hypothyroidism
- Autoimmune alopecia
- Transient acantholytic dermatosis.

Laterally truncated eyebrows came to be associated with Anne of Denmark (1574–1619), James I's Queen Consort, likely because a contemporaneous portrait of her by Paul van Somer shows a woman with fair and abbreviated brows (J Med Biogr 2007;15:97–101). The sign is named after Eugene Hertoghe of Antwerp, is a pioneer in thyroid function research.

WW Gull (1816–1890), FRS, graduated from Guy's Hospital in London and was created a Baronet when he treated the then Prince of Wales, who had typhoid. He was a good teacher and said that 'Savages explain, science investigates'. In 1873, he described several previously healthy women who acquired clinical features similar to those in cretinism. He coined the term myxoedema to describe a syndrome in five women with coarse features, mental dullness, dry skin, hypothermia and oedema (Gull WW. On a cretinoid state supervening in adult life in women. Trans Clin Soc London 1873;7: 180–185).

Ord in 1878 coined the word myxoedema when, at postmortem, he found extensive deposits of mucin in the skin of the feet (Ord WM. On myxoedema, a term proposed to be applied to an essential condition in the 'cretinoid' affection occasionally observed in middle-aged women. Med Chir Trans 1878;61:57).

Treatment for hypothyroidism with sheep thyroid extract was first reported by Murray in 1891.

Emil Theodor Kocher (1841–1917), Swiss Professor of Surgery in Berne, was awarded the Nobel Prize in 1909 for his work on the physiology, pathology and surgery of the thyroid gland. He was the first to excise the thyroid gland for goitre and described myxoedema following thyroidectomy: 'cachexia strumipriva'. His name is associated with: Kocher forceps, Kocher's transverse cervical incision for thyroidectomy, Kocher's operation for the wrist, Kocher's oblique right subcostal incision for gallbladder surgery, Kocher manoeuvre for reduction of a dislocated shoulder, and Kocher syndrome describing splenomegaly and lymphadenopathy with thyrotoxicosis.

In 1912, Hashimoto (1881–1934), a Japanese surgeon, described autoimmune thyroiditis in four women with goitres that seemed to have turned into lymphoid tissue (struma lymphomatosa).

Johann Hoffmann (1857–1919), a German neurologist.

In 1914 Thyroid hormone was crystallised by Kendall.

In 1927 Harington and Barger reported the synthesis of thyroxine; its initial physiological testing was reported in 1927.

R Debré and G Sémélaigne were both French physicians (Debré R, Sémélaigne G. Syndrome of diffuse muscular hypertrophy in infants causing athletic appearance. Its connection with congenital myxoedema. Am J Dis Child 1935;50:1351).

In 1948, HEW Roberton, a general practitioner in New Zealand, was the first to recognize postpartum thyroid disease; he successfully treated lassitude and other symptoms of hypothyroidism related to the postpartum period with thyroid extract.

In 1952, triiodothyronine was discovered by Pitt-Rivers and Gross.

In 1956, Roitt and colleagues reported the presence of circulating thyroid autoantibodies in Hashimoto thyroiditis.

In 1963, Condliffe purified thyrotrophin (TSH), and soon thereafter Odell and Utiger both reported the first immunoassays for human TSH.

In 1970, the endogenous generation of T_3 from T_4 was described by Ingbar, Sterling and Braverman.

In 1971, Mayberry and Hershman simultaneously described use of TSH immunoassays for diagnosis of hypothyroidism.

139 PRETIBIAL MYXOEDEMA

INSTRUCTION

Look at this patient's legs.

SALIENT FEATURES

History

- As in patients with thyrotoxicosis (p. 137)

Examination

- Red thickened swellings above the lateral malleoli (peau d'orange appearance), which progresses to thickened non-pitting oedema of the feet.
- Examine the following:
  - The hands for acropachy (Fig. 136.1), palmar erythema and warm, sweaty palms
  - The neck for goitre and thyroidectomy scar
  - The eyes for exophthalmos (Fig. 137.1)
  - The pulse for tachycardia and atrial fibrillation.
- Tell the examiner that you would like to know whether or not the patient has had any treatment, in particular radioactive iodine.

Remember:
- Almost all cases of thyroid dermopathy are associated with relatively severe ophthalmopathy.
- Usually ophthalmopathy appears first and dermopathy much later.

DIAGNOSIS

This patient has pretibial myxoedema (lesion) with ophthalmopathy and signs of thyrotoxicosis (functional status), which is caused by Graves' disease.

QUESTIONS

What investigations would you do?

Serum thyroxine (T_4), triiodothryonine (T_3) and thyroid-stimulating hormone (TSH).

How are these lesions treated?

- Intralesional steroids or fluorinated corticosteroids applied under polythene occlusion
- Plasmapheresis
- Cytotoxic therapy
- Octreotide.

Note: Surgical excision should be avoided because surgical scars may aggravate the dermopathy and precipitate recurrence.

ADVANCED-LEVEL QUESTIONS

What are the types of pretibial myxoedema?

Three major classes of thyroid dermopathy have been identified (Medicine 1994;73:1–7):

- Non-pitting oedema accompanied by hyperkeratosis, pigmentation and pinkish, brownish red or yellowish discoloration of the skin (Fig. 139.1);

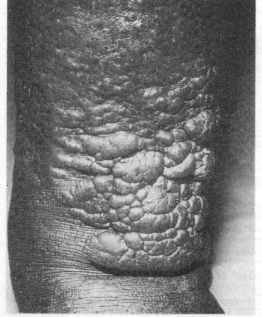

Fig. 139.1 Chronic pretibial myxoedema in a patient with Graves' disease and orbitopathy. The lesions are firm and non-pitting, with a clear edge to palpation. (With permission of Kronenberg et al. 2008.)

plaque formation and nodularity are characteristically absent in this group
- Plaque form, consisting of raised, discrete or confluent plaques
- Nodular form, characterized by nodule formation.

Less common types:
- Elephantiasic form
- Polypoid form.

Note: Almost all patients tend to have ophthalmopathy, which is usually severe.

What is the histology of pretibial myxoedema?

- Characteristic features include fraying and oedematous appearance on routine staining with haematoxylin and eosin, and increase of mucinous material staining with alcian blue–periodic acid–Schiff, with resultant connective tissue fibre separation.
- Review of pathology reports does not show any distinguishing microscopic characteristics for various clinical forms of this dermopathy.

What is the pathogenesis of pretibial myxoedema?

- All patients with localized myxoedema have high serum concentrations of TSH receptor antibodies, indicating the severity of the autoimmune condition.
- Occurrence of thyroid dermopathy in areas other than pretibial skin indicates a systemic process. ✓
- Similar to Graves' eye disease, TSH receptors in the connective tissue may be the antigen responsible for the immune process.
- Both humoral and cellular immune mechanisms are involved in the stimulation of fibroblasts and the production of large amounts of glycosaminoglycans.
- Localization in the pretibial area relates to mechanical factors and dependent position.

What are the recommendations for screening thyroid dysfunction?

It is recommended that adults be screened for thyroid dysfunction by measurement of serum TSH concentration, beginning at age of 35 years and every 5 years thereafter. The indication for screening is particularly compelling in women, but it may also be justified in men as a relatively cost-effective measure in the context of periodic health examination. Individuals with clinical manifestations potentially attributable to thyroid dysfunction and those with risk factors for its development may require more frequent serum TSH testing (Arch Intern Med 2000;1601573–5).

How can hyperthyroidism present in the elderly?

Thyrotoxicosis can present in the elderly with atrial fibrillation, and such patients may lack other common signs of thyrotoxicosis; this is known as apathetic hyperthyroidism. Also low serum TSH is a risk factor for atrial fibrillation the elderly (N Engl J Med 1994;331:1249–52).

Osteoporosis may be the result of subclinical thyrotoxicosis.

140 MULTINODULAR GOITRE

INSTRUCTION

Examine this patient's neck.

SALIENT FEATURES

History

- Stridor: trachea must be narrowed to 20–30% for this symptom
- Hoarseness of voice (caused by pressure on recurrent laryngeal nerve), suggests thyroid malignancy
- Acute painful enlargement, suggests bleeding into thyroid nodule
- Suffusion of face when the patient raises the arms above the head, suggests substernal goitre
- Dysphagia
- Deafness: if caused by eighth cranial nerve involvement suggests Pendreds syndrome (rare)
- Symptoms of thyroid hyper- or hypofunction
- Family history of thyroid cancer.

Examination

- Middle-aged or elderly patient
- Multinodular goitre (Fig. 140.1)
- Atrial fibrillation
- Signs of thyrotoxicosis (p. 516)

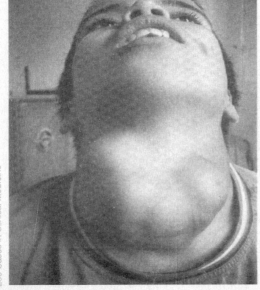

Fig. 140.1 Large nodular goitre. (With permission from Zimmermann et al. 2008.)

DIAGNOSIS

This patient has a multinodular goitre (lesion) and is hyperthyroid with atrial fibrillation (functional status).

QUESTIONS

What is the natural history of thyrotoxicosis in nodular goitre?
It is permanent and there are no spontaneous remissions; therefore, antithyroid drugs to decrease thyroid hormone secretion are not appropriate for long-term therapy.

How would you investigate a nodular goitre?
- Serum thyroid-stimulating hormone (TSH) and free thyroxine (T_4) should be measured to identify those with subclinical or overt hyperthyroidism. If the TSH is suppressed, radionuclide scanning should be performed.
- Ultrasonography of the thyroid gland indicates whether goitre is *cystic* or *solid*:
  - If *solid*, perform a radioisotope scan to indicate hot or cold nodule
  - If *cold* nodule, fine-needle aspiration.
- Patients with features of tracheal compression (inspiratory stridor and dyspnoea) should undergo CT or MRI of the neck and upper thorax, pulmonary function tests especially flow volume loop studies. When CT is used, iodinated contrast agents should not be given because of the risk of inducing hyperthyroidism.
- Antibodies against thyroglobulin (AbTG), anti-thyroperoxidase antibodies (AbTPOs) and calcitonin.
- If the patient has a family history of medullary thyroid carcinoma or multiple endocrine neoplasia type 2, the serum calcitonin level should also be checked.

How would you treat such a patient?
- Beta-blockers to control thyrotoxicosis
- Warfarin in atrial fibrillation to prevent embolic complications
- Radioiodine for hyperthyroidism
- Surgery if the patient refuses radioiodine, for large multinodular goitres or malignancy
- In patients <20 years of age, and in the case of a high clinical suspicion for cancer (e.g. follicular neoplasia as diagnosed by fine-needle aspiration and a non-functioning nodule revealed on scanning), the patient should be offered hemithyroidectomy regardless of the results of fine-needle aspiration

What are indications for treatment of patients with non-toxic multinodular goitre?
Compression of the trachea or oesophagus and venous-outflow obstruction.

Growth of the goitre, especially where there is intrathoracic extension. Neck discomfort or cosmetic issues.

What are the treatment options available for non-toxic multinodular goitre?
- Surgery is the standard therapy, especially when rapid decompression of vital structures is required. It allows pathological examination of the

thyroid. Disadvantages include postoperative tracheal obstruction, recurrent laryngeal nerve injury, hypoparathyroidism, hypothyroidism and goitre recurrence.

- Thyroxine therapy to shrink goiters is no longer recommended. Disadvantages are that it causes only a small decrease in thyroid volume; long-term efficacy is not known; it causes a decrease in bone mineral density in postmenopausal women; and there are possible cardiac side effects.

- Radioiodine is an alternative to surgery in elderly patients and in those with cardiopulmonary disease. It results in a substantial decrease in thyroid volume and improvement of compressive symptoms in most patients. Disadvantages are that it only causes a gradual decrease in thyroid volume; radiation thyroiditis (usually mild) and radiation-induced thyroid dysfunction (hyperthyroidism in 5%, hypothyroidism in 20–30%)) can occur; and there is a possible risk of radiation-induced cancer (N Engl J Med 1998;338: 1438–47).

- Treatment options depends on the nodule:
  - Functioning benign nodule: iodine-131 is generally the therapy of choice independent of concomitant hyperthyroidism
  - Non-functioning cystic nodules: aspiration and ethanol injection therapy may be considered, and ethanol injection or laser therapy if the nodules are solid; patients are followed annually with neck palpation and measurement of the serum TSH, with repeated ultrasonography and fine-needle aspiration if there is evidence of growth of the nodule.

What are the treatment options available for toxic multinodular goitre?

Treatment is always indicated when overt hyperthyroidism is present. In subclinical hyperthyroidism, treatment is advisable in elderly patients and in younger ones who are at risk for cardiac disease or osteoporosis. There are three treatment options:

- Antithyroid drugs are valuable as pretreatment for surgery and before and after radioiodine treatment in elderly patients and those with concurrent health problems. Long-term treatment is recommended only when other therapies cannot be used. The disadvantages are that the treatment is lifelong and there are potential adverse effects such as agranulocytosis.

- Surgery should be considered in large goitres when rapid relief is needed. The other advantage is that it provides tissue for a pathological diagnosis. Disadvantages include surgical mortality and morbidity; hypothyroidism and persistence or recurrence of hyperthyroidism.

- Radioiodine is an appealing option in the majority of the patients because it is highly effective for reversal of hyperthyroidism. The disadvantages include a gradual diminution of the hyperthyroid state, more than one dose may be necessary, hypothyroidism (<20%) and the theoretical risk of radiation-induced cancer (N Engl J Med 1998;338:1438–47).

ADVANCED-LEVEL QUESTIONS

How do you differentiate between Graves' disease and toxic nodular goitre?

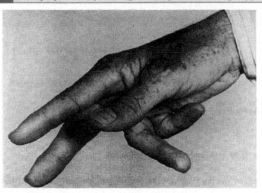

Fig. 141.1 Trousseau's sign. (With permission from Burnside, McGlynn 1987.)

- Check serum total and ionized calcium, albumin, phosphorus, magnesium and parathromone (PTH)
- ECG for prolonged QT intervals and T wave abnormalities
- Slit-lamp examination for early posterior lenticular cataract formation.

DIAGNOSIS

This patient has carpopedal spasm (lesion) caused by hypoparathyroidism as a complication of thyroidectomy (aetiology).

ADVANCED-LEVEL QUESTIONS

Mention any drugs that you would use cautiously in hypoparathyroidism

Furosemide, as it may enhance hypocalcaemia, and phenothiazine drugs, because they may precipitate extrapyramidal symptoms.

How would you manage an acute attack of hypoparathyroid tetany?

- Maintain airway
- Slow intravenous calcium gluconate and oral calcium
- Vitamin D preparations
- Magnesium (if associated hypomagnesaemia)
- Outpatient therapy with calcium carbonate three times daily and calcitriol once or twice daily adjusting the dose to maintain a target level of albumin-corrected serum calcium at the lower end of the normal range (approximately 80–85 mg/l (2.00–2.12 mmol/l)), a 24-hour urinary calcium level of <300 mg, and a calcium–phosphate product <55.

What are the causes of hypoparathyroidism?

- Damage during thyroid or neck surgery (Lancet 1960;ii: 1432)
- Idiopathic
- Destruction of the parathyroid gland caused by the following:
  - Radioactive iodine therapy
  - External neck irradiation
  - Haemochromatosis and Wilson's deficiency
  - Metastatic disease from the breast, lung, lymphoproliferative disorder.

Graves' disease	Toxic nodular goitre
Younger age group	Older individuals
Diffuse goitre	Nodular enlargement of the gland
Eye signs common	Eye signs are rare
Atrial fibrillation is uncommon	Atrial fibrillation is common (about 40% of the patients)
Other autoimmune diseases are common	Other autoimmune diseases are uncommon

What factors influence the decision to proceed to radiotherapy?

Patient's age, sex, diagnosis, severity of hyperthyroidism, presence of other medical conditions, access to radioiodine and patient and doctor preference.

141 CARPOPEDAL SPASM (POST-THYROIDECTOMY HYPOPARATHYROIDISM)

INSTRUCTION

Look at this patient's hands.

SALIENT FEATURES

History

- History of thyroid surgery
- Paraesthesias of fingers, toes and circumoral region
- Muscle cramping, carpopedal spasm, laryngeal stridor, convulsions.

Examination

- Spasm of the hands: fingers are extended, except at the metacarpophalangeal joints, and the thumb is strongly adducted.

Proceed as follows:

- Look at the feet for spasm
- Investigate as follows:
  - Tap over the facial nerve (in front of the tragus of the ear): there is contraction of the lips and facial muscles (Chvostek's sign or Chvostek–Weiss sign)
  - Inflate the BP cuff to just above the systolic pressure for 3 min; this will cause the hand to go into spasm: Trousseau's sign (Fig. 141.1)
  - Look into the mouth for candidiasis (may be seen in primary hypoparathyroidism) and defective teeth
  - Finger nails may be thin and brittle
  - Check for thyroidectomy scar
  - Look for cataracts.
- Tell the examiner that you would like to perform the following tests:
  - Do a skull radiograph (looking for basal ganglia calcification)

- Dysembryogenesis (DiGeorge syndrome)
- Polyglandular autoimmune syndrome (PGA type 1), which is also known as autoimmune polyendocrinopathy–candidiasis–ectodermal dystrophy (APECD).

How is corrected total calcium calcuated?

Albumin-corrected total calcium is calculated as follows:

$$\text{Corrected total calcium} = \text{measured total calcium} + 0.8\,(4.0 - \text{serum albumin})$$

where calcium is measured in milligrams per decilitre and albumin is measured in grams per decilitre.

What is the mechanism of hypocalcaemia?

Hypocalaemia results from PTH secretion that is inadequate to:

- mobilize calcium from bone
- reabsorb calcium from the distal nephron
- stimulate renal 1α-hydroxylase activity; as a result, insufficient 1,25-dihydroxyvitamin D (1,25-dihydrocholecalciferol) is generated for efficient intestinal absorption of calcium.

What are the biochemical features of hypoparathyroidism?

Typically it consists of low serum calcium (with intact PTH), high serum phosphate, normal alkaline phosphatase levels and reduced urine calcium excretion.

Remember: Hypomagnesaemia causes resistance to effects of PTH and when severe may decrease PTH release as well. Hypermagnesaemia may also decrease PTH release.

What do you know about pseudohypoparathyroidism?

It is a condition characterized by end-organ resistance to PTH. The biochemistry is similar to that of idiopathic hypoparathyroidism except that patients with pseudohypoparathyroidism have elevated PTH levels do not respond to injected PTH. These patients are moon-faced, short statured and mentally retarded and may have short fourth or fifth metacarpals. Patients without hypocalcaemia but who have these phenotypic abnormalities are said to have 'pseudopseudohypoparathyroidism'.

What are the main physiological effects of parathyroid hormone?

It results in a net increase of ionized calcium in the plasma through:

- increased bone osteoclastic activity, resulting in increased delivery of calcium and phosphorous to the extracellular compartment
- enhanced renal tubular absorption of calcium
- inhibited absorption of phosphate and bicarbonate by the renal tubule stimulated synthesis of 1,25-dihydrovitamin D by the kidney.

Frantisek Chvostek (1835–1884) was Professor of Medicine in Vienna, Austria.
Nathan Weiss (1851–1883), an Austrian physician.
Armand Trousseau (1801–1867), a Parisian physician, was the first to refer to adrenal insufficiency as Addison's disease.
Professor Karim Meeran, qualified from the Royal Free Hospital and trained in Endocrinology at Hammersmith Hospital and St Bartholomew's Hospital. He is Professor of Endocrinology, Imperial College Deputy Director of Medical Education and Lead Clinician for Endocrinology, Hammersmith

Hospital. He is involved with the Abu Dhabi Imperial College London Diabetes Centre. Professor Meeran's clinical focus is in all aspects of Endocrinology and Diabetes including thyroid, adrenal, hirsuitism, PCOS, prolactin and pituitary diseases, calcium and bone metabolism and neuroendocrine tumours.

142 ACROMEGALY

INSTRUCTION

Examine this patient's face.
This patient complains of excessive sweating; examine him.
Examine this patient's hands.

SALIENT FEATURES

History

- Ask the patient about old photographs of the patient for comparison
- Whether the patient has outgrown their wedding rings and shoes
- Hyperhidrosis
- Headaches, visual field defects (depends on the size of the tumour)
- Paraesthesia and symptoms of carpal tunnel syndrome (p. 296)
- Hypertension
- Acral and facial changes
- Oligomenorrhoea/amenorrhoea, galactorrhoea in females (prolactin is coproduced with growth hormone in approximately 40% of patients with acromegaly)
- Impotence in males
- Shortness of breath (cardiac failure)
- Arthritis (hands, feet, hips and knees).

Examination

Hands:
- On shaking hands there is excessive sweating: moist doughy, enveloping handshake.
- Large hands with broad palms, spatulate fingers; there is an increase in the 'volume' of the hands (Fig. 142.1).
- Look for evidence of carpal tunnel syndrome (tap over the flexor retinaculum for Tinel's sign; see Fig. 76.1A).

Face:
- Prominent supraorbital ridges
- Large nose and lips
- Protrusion of the lower jaw (prognathism); ask the patient to clench his teeth and note the malocclusion and splaying of the teeth (i.e. interdental separation)
- Ask the patient to show his tongue and look for macroglossia and for impressions of the teeth on the edges of the tongue (p. 829)

Proceed by testing:
- For bitemporal hemianopia (p. 188) and optic atrophy
- Neck for goitre

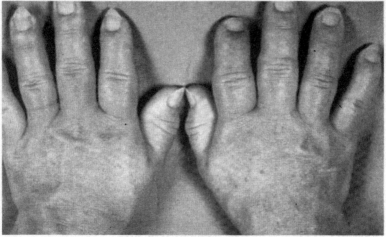

Fig. 142.1 Acromegaly: hands with sausage-shaped fingers. (With permission from Carey 2009.)

- Axillae for skin tags (molluscum fibrosum), acanthosis nigricans (black velvety papillomas)
- Chest for cardiomegaly, gynaecomastia and galactorrhoea
- Abdomen for hepatosplenomegaly
- Joints for arthropathy, i.e. osteoarthrosis, chondrocalcinosis
- Spine for kyphosis
- Blood pressure for hypertension (present in 15% of cases)
- Tell the examiner that you would like to examine the urine for sugar (impaired glucose tolerance).

DIAGNOSIS

This patient has a protruding lower jaw, splaying of teeth and large spade-like hands (lesions), which are features of acromegaly caused by a pituitary tumour (aetiology).

QUESTIONS

Would you like to ask the patient a few questions?
Ask about any increase in size of shoes, gloves and hat, and whether the wedding ring is tight to wear.

ADVANCED-LEVEL QUESTIONS

Mention some causes of macroglossia
- Acromegaly
- Amyloidosis
- Hypothyroidism
- Down syndrome.

How can this condition present?

One-third of patients notice a change in their features, one-third are noticed to have a change in their features by their GPs and the remaining third have symptoms such as excessive sweating and visual difficulties.

What are the complications of acromegaly?

- Cardiomegaly and heart failure
- Hypertension
- Impaired glucose tolerance
- Hypopituitarism
- Carpal tunnel syndrome
- Arthritis of the hip, knee and spine
- Spinal stenosis resulting in cord compression
- Visual field defects
- Increased risk of premalignant polyps and colon cancer: screening colonoscopy should be considered in all patients with growth hormone excess.

What are the indicators of disease activity?

- Symptoms such as headache, increase in size of ring, shoe or dentures
- Excessive sweating
- Skin tags
- Glycosuria
- Hypertension
- Increased loss of visual fields.

How would you investigate this patient?

- *Biochemical tests*:
  - Plasma insulin-like growth factor (IGF-1) levels (allows assessment of the efficacy of initial therapy and in the post-therapeutic period). Marked elevations establish the diagnosis
  - When IGF-1 levels are only moderately elevated, diagnosis is confirmed by non-suppressibility of growth hormone levels to <1 µg/l after oral administration of 75 g glucose
  - Serum thyroxine, prolactin, testosterone
  - Evaluate pituitary function: static and dynamic tests
  - Calcium levels (to exclude multiple endocrine neoplasia (MEN) type 1 syndrome).

  Note: Random growth hormone level measurements are not useful because of pulsatile secretion.

- *Radiography*:
  - Pituitary fossa (enlarged sella)
  - Sinuses
  - Chest (cardiomegaly)
  - Hand (terminal phalangeal 'tufting')
  - Foot (terminal phalangeal 'tufting', lateral view shows increased thickness of the heel pad)
  - MRI scan to evaluate the extent of tumour growth.

  Remember: Unlike in Cushing's disease and prolactinomas, the majority of the patients (~60%) with acromegaly have macroadenomas.

- *Other investigations*:
  - Formal perimetry
  - Obtain old photographs
  - New photographs of face, torso, hands on the chest
  - ECG
  - Triple stimulation test: if hypopituitarism is suspected.

What therapeutic options are available?

- Neurosurgical intervention, typically trans-sphenoidal, is the primary therapeutic choice for almost all patients. Diaphoresis and carpal tunnel syndrome often improve within 1 day of surgery. Although growth hormone levels fall immediately, insulin-like growth factor levels fall gradually.
- Radiation therapy is a primary treatment option for a few patients who have acromegaly but are not surgical candidates or when IGF-1 remains elevated after surgery because of residual tumour.
- The somatostatin receptor antagonist octreotide is valuable as adjunctive therapy to suppress growth hormone secretion while awaiting radiation. High doses of cabergoline (dopamine receptor antagonist) or treatment with somatostatin receptor ligands may improve the responsiveness to growth hormone in patients who otherwise have resistance to maximal doses of somatostatin receptor ligands
- Pegvisomant is a synthetic growth hormone receptor antagonist (the peptide is conjugated (pegylated) to polyethylene glycol to reduce renal clearance and immunogenicity) that lowers IGF-1 in >90% of patients, which is accompanied by clinical benefits (but no effect on tumour).

  Remember: The aim of treatment should be symptomatic control and a growth hormone concentration of <5 mU/l.

Mention four common causes of death in such patients

- Cardiac failure
- Tumour expansion (mass effect and haemorrhages)
- Effects of hypertension
- Degenerative vascular disease.

Mention other conditions with excess growth hormone secretion

- MEN type 1: parathyroid hyperplasia, pituitary tumours and gut tumours
- McCune–Albright syndrome: polyostotic fibrous dysplasia, sexual precocity and café-au-lait spots
- Carney complex is an autosomal dominant disorder that consists of multicentric tumours in many organs, including myxomas in heart, breast and testes; pigmented skin lesions; and pigmented nodular hyperplasia.

In 1886 Pierre Marie (1853–1940) used the term acromegaly in describing two patients and reviewed eight previously published papers describing patients with presumed acromegaly (Marie P (1886) Sur deux cas d'acromegalie. Hypertrophie singulière non-congénitale des extrémités supérieures, inférieures et céphaliques. Rev Med 6:297–333). He also described Charcot–Marie–Tooth disease. In 1887 Minkowski deduced that acromegaly is related to pituitary tumour (Minkowski O (1887) Uber einen Fall von Akromegalie. Berl Klin Wochenschr 24:371–374).

In 1891 the New Syndenham Society published a translation of Marie's original paper and a review by Souza-Leite of 48 patients (Marie P & de Souza-Leite JD (1891) Essays on Acromegaly. London: New Sydenham Society).

Fuller Albright, Professor of Endocrinology at Massachussetts General Hospital and Harvard Medical School, whose chief interest was calcium metabolism.

143 HYPOPITUITARISM (SIMMONDS' DISEASE)

INSTRUCTION

Look at this patient.

SALIENT FEATURES

History

- In a male, frequency of shaving, impotence
- In a female, postpartum haemorrhage, amenorrhoea
- History of radiation (e.g. proton-beam radiation): causes hypopituitarism primarily because of its effects on hypothalamic function whereas high-dose radiation can directly affect the pituitary.

Examination

- Patient is pale; the skin is soft
- Paucity of axillary and pubic hair
- Atrophy of breast (in females)
- Examine the BP for postural hypotension
- Check visual fields: bitemporal hemianopia (p. 188) may be present
- Examine the fundus for optic atrophy
- Tell the examiner that you would like to examine the external genitalia for hypogonadism (small testes).

DIAGNOSIS

This patient has pale soft skin and absence of axillary hair with atrophied breasts (lesion) caused by hypopituitarism (functional status) secondary to postpartum necrosis (aetiology).

QUESTIONS

Mention a few causes of hypopituitarism

- Iatrogenic: from surgical removal of the pituitary or irradiation
- Chromophobe adenoma (particularly in males)
- Postpartum pituitary necrosis (in females): known as Sheehan syndrome

● Lymphocytic hypophysitis, seen peripartum.

Rare causes:

● Craniopharyngioma
● Metastatic tumours (breast and lung cancers most likely), granulomas (TB, sarcoid, haemochromatosis, histiocytosis X).

How would you assess such a patient?

● FBC for normochromic normocytic anaemia
● Urea and electrolytes for hyponatraemia caused by dilution. Hyperkalaemia does not usually occur because aldosterone production is not affected
● Measurement of pituitary hormones (ACTH, thyroid-stimulating hormone (TSH), luteinizing hormone (LH), growth hormone, prolactin)
● Measurement of target organ secretion: thyroxine (T_4), triiodothyronine (T_3), plasma free T_4, 8 am serum cortisol, testosterone, oestrogen and progesterone
● Pituitary stimulation tests:
  • TSH-releasing hormone (TRH) stimulation tests
  • Tetracosactrin (synacthen) tests
  • Insulin hypoglycaemia test is considered the gold standard used to diagnose growth hormone deficiency in adults, using a diagnostic threshold of 3 mg/l
  • LH-releasing hormone (LHRH) tests.
● Skull radiography
● MRI provides the best image of parasellar lesions. The posterior pituitary usually has a high-intensity signal on sagittal MRI that is absent in central diabetes insipidus
● Assessment of visual fields (formal perimetry).

In what order do the hormone secretions generally fail?

In general growth hormone, follicle-stimulating hormone (FSH) and LH secretions become deficient early, followed by TSH and ACTH. Last of all, antidiuretic hormone secretions diminish and fail.

How would you treat such patients?

The mainstay of therapy is lifetime replacement of deficient end-organ deficiencies (thyroid, adrenal and gonads).

Does hypopituitarism affect life expectancy?

Even when hormonal replacement therapy (adrenal, gonadal and thyroid) is carried out in an adequate manner, there is a two-fold risk of death in patients with hypopituitarism (J Clin Endocrinol Metab 1996;81:1169–72). It has been suggested that this is caused by untreated growth hormone deficiency.

ADVANCED-LEVEL QUESTIONS

What is the Houssay phenomenon?

Houssay showed that diabetes of pancreatectomized dogs improved after hypophysectomy. A diminishing requirement of insulin by diabetics may be a sign of hypopituitarism with diminished secretion of growth hormone and ACTH (and thus corticosteroids). Similarly, diabetes in acromegaly may improve with pituitary surgery or octreotide therapy.

Morris Simmonds of Hamburg described this condition in 1914.

Bernado Alberto Houssay (1889–1971), an Argentinian physiologist in Buenos Aires, was awarded the Nobel Prize for his discovery of the part played by the hormone of the anterior pituitary lobe in the metabolism of sugar. The other half of the Nobel Prize was awarded to Carl and Gerty Cori of St Louis, Missouri, USA, who were awarded the prize for their discovery of the course of the catalytic conversion of glycogen.

144   ADDISON'S DISEASE

INSTRUCTION

Look at this patient, who presented with weakness, loss of appetite and weight loss.

SALIENT FEATURES

History

- Dizziness, syncope
- Skin pigmentation (ask if the patient has been sitting in the sun)
- Ask questions regarding fatigue, weakness, apathy, anorexia, nausea, vomiting, weight loss and abdominal pain
- Depression.

Examination

- The striking abnormality is hyperpigmentation.

Proceed as follows:

- Examine for hyperpigmentation, typically localized to palmar creases and knuckles:
  - Hand: compare the creases with your own
  - Mouth and lips for pigmentation
  - Areas not usually covered by clothing: nipples, areas irritated by belts, straps, collars or rings
  - Look for vitiligo.
- Tell the examiner that you would like to investigate as follows:
  - BP, in particular for postural hypotension
  - Looking for sparse axillary and pubic hair
  - The abdomen for adrenal scar (if the scar is pigmented, think of Nelson syndrome and examine field defects).
- If you suspect Addison's disease, tell the examiner that you would like to do a short tetracosactrin test (synacthen test).

DIAGNOSIS

This patient has postural hypotension, marked hyperpigmentation and sparse axillary hair (lesion) caused by autoimmune Addison's disease (aetiology). The patient has marked hypoadrenalism (functional status).

QUESTIONS

What is the size of the heart in Addison's deficiency?
The heart is small.

Mention some causes of hyperpigmentation
- Suntan
- Race
- Uraemia
- Haemochromatosis
- Primary biliary cirrhosis
- Ectopic ACTH
- Porphyria cutanea tarda
- Nelson syndrome
- Malabsorption syndromes.

Mention some causes of Addison's disease
- 80% idiopathic
- TB
- Metastasis
- HIV infection.

Which conditions may be associated with Addison's disease?
- Graves' disease
- Hashimato's thyroiditis
- Primary ovarian failure
- Pernicious anaemia
- Polyglandular syndromes.

ADVANCED-LEVEL QUESTIONS

What are the components of Schmidt syndrome?
Addison's disease and hypoparathyroidism. (In these patients cortisol should be administered before thyroxine to avoid exacerbating the hypoadrenalism.)

What do you know about polyglandular syndromes?
They are autoimmune in nature and are of two types:
I: chronic mucocutaneous candidiasis, hypoparathyroidism and Addison's disease
II: Addison's disease, insulin-dependent diabetes and thyroid disease (hyperthyroidism or hypothyroidism); syndrome is also known as 'autoimmune polyendocrinopathy–candidiasis–ectodermal dysplasia'.

What are the features of Allgrove syndrome?
Adrenal insensitivity to ACTH (resulting in cortisol deficiency), achalasia, alacrima and neurological disease.

How would you investigate this patient?
- FBC (for lymphocytosis, eosinophilia)
- Electrolytes (for hyponatraemia, hyperkalaemia, hyperchloraemic acidosis, hypercalcaemia)
- Blood glucose, looking for hypoglycaemia
- Short tetracosactrin (synacthen) test; if positive, follow-up with a prolonged ACTH stimulation test
- ACTH and cortisol levels: in Addison's disease the 9 am ACTH is elevated (>300 ng/l)

- Adrenal autoantibodies: 21-hydroxylase autoantibodies are elevated in 80%
- Chest radiography for TB
- Plain radiograph of the abdomen for adrenal calcification
- CT scan of the adrenals.

How would you manage this patient if the underlying aetiology is autoimmune?

- Immediate treatment of adrenal failure with replacement steroids: prednisolone 5 mg *in the morning* and 2.5 mg *at night*; adjust dose depending on serum levels and clinical well being
- Fludrocortisone 0.025–0.15 mg daily; adjust dose depending on postural hypotension
- Give steroid card and Medic Alert bracelet
- Stress the importance of regular therapy and increase the dose in the event of stress such as dental extraction or urinary tract infection. It is also important to tell the patient that this therapy is lifelong and that an ampoule of hydrocortisone should be kept at home
- Follow up every 6 months.

Note: In Addisonian crisis, intravenous fluids and hydrocortisone should be administered (after drawing a blood sample for cortisol determination).

Thomas Addison (1793–1860) qualified from Edinburgh and worked at Guy's Hospital, London. He wrote 'The constitutional and local effects of the disease of the suprarenal capsules'. He was one of the three 'Giants of Guy's Hospital' and all three studied in Edinburgh. The others were Richard Bright (1789–1858) and Thomas Hodgkin (1798–1866).

Armand Trosseau in Paris labelled the disease 'maladie d'Addison'. Addison also first described morphoea. The original description of the disease was reported in the following paper: Addison T. Disease of the suprarenal capsules. London Med Gaz 1855;43:517.

John F Kennedy, past president of the USA, reportedly had Addison's disease and was on replacement corticosteroid therapy.

---

145 CUSHING SYNDROME

INSTRUCTION

Examine this patient.
Look at this patient's face.

SALIENT FEATURES

History

- History of steroid therapy
- Central weight gain
- Hirsutism (p. 602)
- Easy bruising
- Acne
- Weakness of muscle

- Menstrual disturance
- Loss of libido
- Depression, sleep disturbances
- Back pain as a result of spinal osteoporosis.

Examination

- Moon-like facies (Fig. 145.1), acne, hirsutism and plethora (from telangiectasia).

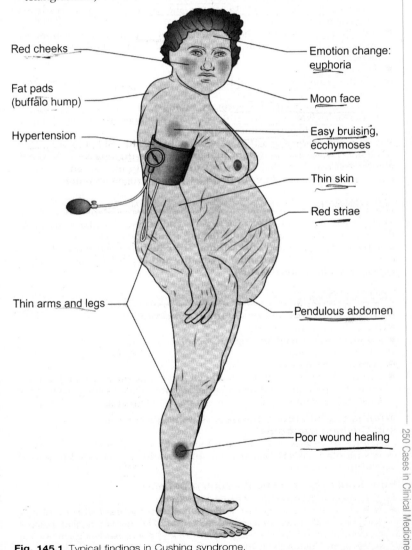

Red cheeks

Fat pads (buffalo hump)

Hypertension

Thin arms and legs

Emotion change: euphoria

Moon face

Easy bruising, ecchymoses

Thin skin

Red striae

Pendulous abdomen

Poor wound healing

Fig. 145.1 Typical findings in Cushing syndrome.

- Examine the following:
  - The mouth for superimposed thrush
  - The interscapular area for 'buffalo hump'
  - Increased fat pads and bulge above supraclavicular fossae (more specific for Cushing syndrome)
  - The abdomen for thinning of skin and purple striae (also seen over the shoulders and thighs): said to be present on almost all patients
  - The limbs for bruising, wasting of the limbs, weakness of the muscles of the shoulders and hips: get the patient to squat (proximal myopathy).
- Ask the patient whether he or she has back pain and then examine the spine, looking for evidence of osteoporosis and collapse of vertebra, kyphoscoliosis.
- Measure the BP.
- Tell the examiner you would like to:
  - test the urine for glucose
  - check visual fields (for pituitary tumour).
  - examine the fundus for optic atrophy, papilloedema, signs of hypertensive or diabetic retinopathy.
- Comment on signs of asthma, rheumatoid arthritis, SLE, fibrosing alveolitis (as these are conditions that are treated with long-term steroids).

Note: Hirsutism is not common in Cushing syndrome caused by exogenous steroids because they suppress adrenal androgen secretion.

DIAGNOSIS

This patient has moon-like facies, acne and supraclavicular pads of fat (lesions), which are features of Cushing syndrome caused by long-term steroid therapy (aetiology) for asthma. The patient is now steroid dependent and is disabled by proximal myopathy and kyphoscoliosis because of osteoporosis (functional status).

QUESTIONS

Mention some causes of Cushing syndrome

- Steroids, including ACTH
- Pituitary adenoma (Cushing's disease)
- Adrenal adenoma
- Adrenal carcinoma
- Ectopic ACTH (usually by small cell carcinoma of the lung): the presence of hyperpigmentation or hypokalaemic alkalosis suggests that the Cushing syndrome results from ectopic ACTH secretion.

What is the difference between Cushing's disease and Cushing syndrome?

Cushing's disease is increased production by the adrenals secondary to excess pituitary ACTH, whereas Cushing syndrome is caused by excess steroid from any cause.

How would you investigate such a patient?

Tests to confirm the diagnosis of hypercortisolism:

- Urinary free cortisol as 24-h collection: this is the most direct and reliable practical index of cortisol secretion. The reason is that plasma concentrations of ACTH and cortisol fall and rise episodically, in normal subjects, in Cushing syndrome and in ectopic ACTH syndrome

- Measurement of midnight salivary cortisol levels
- Overnight dexamethasone test
- Plasma cortisol.

Tests to determine the site of hormone production:

- Low-and high-dose dexamethasone test: low-dose dexamethasone fails to suppress urinary steroid secretion in Cushing's disease whereas high-dose dexamethasone (2 mg every 6 h for 2 days) suppresses at least 50% of urinary steroid secretion
- Chest radiography for carcinoma of the bronchus
- Plain radiograph of the abdomen for adrenal calcification
- Ultrasonography of the abdomen for adrenal tumours
- If Cushing's disease is suspected:
  - plasma ACTH: >10 pg per mL (2 pmol per L) suggests ACTH dependency; a level below 5 p/l (1 pmol/l) suggests an adrenal source
  - radiography of pituitary
  - MRI gadolinium enhancement: MRI can identify pituitary tumours approximately 60% of the time once ACTH dependency is established
  - bilateral measurement of ACTH in the inferior petrosal sinus; Cushing's disease is the most likely diagnosis if the sinus-to-peripheral-vein ratio of plasma ACTH is at least 2:1 before or at least 3:1 after injection of ACTH-releasing hormone (corticotrophin-releasing hormone (CRH)) during sampling from the inferior petrosal sinus
  - CRH test (helpful in distinguishing pituitary-led Cushing's disease from ectopic ACTH secretion)
  - inferior petrosal sinus sampling is used to distinguish primary and ectopic sources of ACTH when the source of the ACTH is not obvious based on clinical circumstances, biochemical evaluation and imaging studies.

(See J Clin Endocrinol Metab 1999;84:440–8.)

How would you manage Cushing syndrome?

- Cushing's disease: trans-sphenoidal microadenomectomy, pituitary irradiation, total bilateral adrenalectomy
- Adrenal tumour: surgical resection, mitotane therapy, resection of recurrent tumour
- Ectopic ACTH: surgical resection of tumour
- Taper corticosteroid therapy.

ADVANCED-LEVEL QUESTIONS

What is pseudo-Cushing syndrome?

In chronic alcoholics and patients with depression, there may be increased urinary excretion of steroids, absent diurnal variation of plasma steroids and a positive overnight dexamethasone test. All these investigations return to normal on discontinuation of alcohol or improvement of emotional status.

What do you know about Nelson syndrome?

It is a syndrome that occurs after bilateral adrenalectomy and is characterized by rapidly growing pituitary adenoma, very high ACTH levels and hyperpigmentation. As the incidence may be as high as 50%, patients with Cushing's disease who have undergone adrenalectomy should be followed by regular plasma ACTH levels and imaging for pituitary tumours.

> Harvey Williams Cushing (1869–1939) was Professor of Surgery at Harvard.
> He was awarded the Pulitzer Prize for his biography of Osler (Cushing H. The
> basophil adenomas of the pituitary body and their clinical manifestation. Bull
> Johns Hopkins Hosp 1932;1:137).

146 GYNAECOMASTIA

INSTRUCTION

Look at this patient's chest.

SALIENT FEATURES

History

- Take a drug history: oestrogens, digoxin, spironolactone, cimetidine, diazepam, alkylating agents, methyldopa, clomiphene
- Ask the patient whether it is painful.

Examination

- Unilateral or bilateral enlargement of the breasts in a male patient.
- *Proceed as follows*:
- Palpate to confirm the presence of glandular tissue (before palpation ask the patient to lie flat on his back with his hands clasped beneath his head). Using the separated thumb and forefinger, slowly bring the fingers together from either side of the breast. In patients with true gynaecomastia, a rubbery or firm mound of tissue that is concentric with the nipple–areolar complex is felt, whereas in patients with pseudogynaecomastia, no such disk of tissue is felt.
- Tell the examiner that you would like to look for stigmata of cirrhosis.

DIAGNOSIS

This patient has gynaecomastia (lesion) caused by spironolactone therapy (aetiology), which is cosmetically distressing to the patient (functional status).

QUESTIONS

Mention the physiological causes of gynaecomastia

- Newborn
- Adolescence
- Ageing.

Mention a few pathological causes

- Chronic liver disease
- Thyrotoxicosis
- Klinefelter syndrome
- Viral orchitis

- Renal failure
- Neoplasms (bronchogenic carcinoma, testicular carcinoma, hepatoma)
- Bulbospinal muscular atrophy or Kennedy syndrome (a defect in the androgen receptor alters function of motor neurons; 50% of patients have gynaecomastia)
- Drugs associated with gynaecomastia include:
  - antibiotics: isoniazid, ketoconazole, metronidazole, miconazole
  - cardiovascular drugs: atenolol, captopril, digoxin, enalapril, methyldopa, nifedipine, spironolactone, verapamil
  - antiulcer drugs: cimetidine, ranitidine, omeprazole
  - psychoactive drugs: diazepam, tricyclic antidepressants
  - anti-cancer drugs: imatinib (used in treatment of chronic myeloid leukaemia), bicalutamide.

ADVANCED-LEVEL QUESTIONS

How would you investigate such a patient?

- Chest radiography for metastatic or bronchogenic carcinoma
- Plasma β-human chorionic gonadotrophin: detectable levels implicate a testicular tumour or lung or liver neoplasm
- Plasma testosterone and luteinizing hormone in the diagnosis of hypogonadism
- Serum oestradiol (usually normal)
- Other: serum prolactin, serum thyroxine and thyroid-stimulating hormone, and chromosomal analysis for Klinefelter syndrome.

What are the causes of a feminizing state?

The pathophysiological process of gynaecomastia involves an imbalance between free oestrogen and free androgen actions in the breast tissue. Multiple processes can alter the pathways of oestrogen and androgen production and action, resulting in gynaecomastia from an enhanced oestrogen effect or a diminished androgen effect at the target-tissue level. Causes include:

- absolute increase in oestrogen formation by tumours
- increased availability of oestrogen precursors, e.g. as a result of cirrhosis
- increased extraglandular oestrogen synthesis
- relative increase in ratio of oestrogen to androgen, e.g. as a result of testicular failure
- drugs (estradiol and estrone, displaced by some drugs, resulting in an increase in free oestrogen).

How would you manage the patient?

- Acute florid stage of gynaecomastia: tamoxifen, 20 mg/day for up to 3 months, may be useful.
- When gynaecomastia has not regressed by 1 year or in patients who present with long-standing gynaecomastia who are troubled by their appearance, surgical removal of the breast glandular tissue and subareolar fat can be done for cosmetic reasons.
- Asymptomatic patients not bothered by the gynaecomastia without a suggestive history or physical examination, a more minimalist evaluation (i.e. measurements of testosterone and luteinizing hormone levels, although even the use of these tests may not be warranted): weight reduction.

Ancient Egyptian sculptures and paintings suggest that the pharaoh
Tutankhamen (1357–1339 BC) had gynaecomastia.

147 CARCINOID SYNDROME

INSTRUCTION

Look at this patient who was told by her GP that she has a 'nervous
bowel'.

SALIENT FEATURES

History

- Confirm a history of chronic intermittent diarrhoea
- Flushing attacks, which may be associated with increased lacrimation
  and periorbital oedema. Flushing may be provoked by eating, exertion,
  excitement or ethanol
- Wheeze (caused by bronchoconstriction during flushing attacks).

Examination

- Flushed face ('fire-engine' face)
- Telangiectasia.

Proceed as follows:

- Listen to the chest for wheeze (bronchial carcinoid)
- Listen to the heart (right-sided murmurs in intestinal, gastric,
  hepatic and ovarian carcinoid, left-sided murmurs in bronchial
  carcinoid)
- Look for hepatomegaly (nodular and firm from metastases, may be
  pulsatile from tricuspid regurgitation).

DIAGNOSIS

This patient has facial flushing and tricuspid regurgitation (lesion) caused
by carcinoid syndrome (aetiology) and is in cardiac failure (functional
status).

Remember

- Carcinoid tumours, now referred to as neuroendocrine tumours (NETs).
  NETs include a wide spectrum of neoplasms and clinical behaviours
  depending on their site of origin, hormonal production, and
  differentiation.
- Be prepared to discuss carcinoid biochemical pathways.

ADVANCED-LEVEL QUESTIONS

**What are the cardiac lesions seen in metastatic carcinoid
from the liver?**

- Right-sided valvular lesions, including tricuspid stenosis or regurgitation, and pulmonary stenosis or regurgitation. (**Note**: bronchial carci-
  noids metastasize to the left side of the heart.)
- Endocardial fibrosis.

Remember: Serotonin is related to the progression of carcinoid heart disease, and the risk of progressive heart disease is higher in patients who receive chemotherapy than in those who do not (N Engl J Med 2003;348:1005–15).

What are the types of gastric carcinoid?

There are three types:

Type I is associated with chronic atrophic gastritis.

Type II develops in patients with combined multiple endocrine neoplasia type 1 and the Zollinger–Ellison syndrome. (The multiple endocrine neoplasia type 1 gene locus may be involved in type II gastric carcinoid tumours.)

Type III is sporadic.

Note: Hypergastrinaemia has an important role in the development of types I and II.

How is the diagnosis confirmed?

● Raised urinary levels of 5-HIAA (hydroxyindoleacetic acid; Fig. 147.1)
● Plasma and platelet serotonin levels.

How are these tumours treated?

● Emergency treatment includes prednisolone
● Severe diarrhoea: hydration, diphenoxylate with atropine, cyproheptadine or methysergide

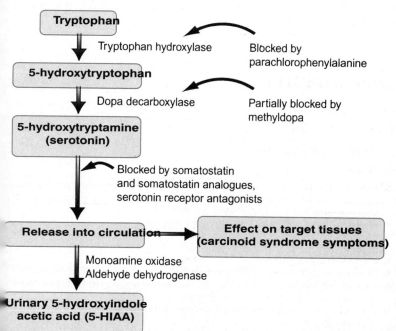

Fig. 147.1 Typical biochemical carcinoid pathway.

- Octreotide (a somatostatin analogue) is associated with a significant reduction in 5-HIAA concentration
- Surgery is useful for localized carcinoid
- Hepatic artery embolization
- Chemotherapy in advanced disease (fluorouracil, streptozocin, dacarbazine)
- Interferon-α may be useful in those who do not respond to surgery and octreotide treatment (Digestion 1994;55(suppl 3):64–9).

Further reading

Sjoerdsma A, Weissbach H, Udenfriend S: A clinical, physiologic and biochemical study of patients with malignant carcinoid (argentaffinoma). *Am J Med* 1956;20:520–32.

Carcinoid was described in 1888 by Lubarsch, the term Karznoid, or carcinoma-like, was introduced by Oberndorfer in 1907 when he described a midgut tumour that was morphologically distinct and less aggressive in behaviour than intestinal adenocarcinoma

In 1914, Gosset and Mason suggested that carcinoid tumours arose from the enterochromaffin cells of the GI tract.

Erspamer succeeded in demonstrating serotonin (5-HT) in the enterochromaffin cells and in 1953 Lembeck was able to extract 5-HT from a carcinoid tumour.

---

148 OBESITY

INSTRUCTION

Look at this patient.

SALIENT FEATURES

History

- Family history of obesity (parental obesity more than doubles the risk of adult obesity among both obese and non-obese children under 10 years of age; N Engl J Med 1997;337:869–73)
- History of sleep apnoea, snoring and insomnia
- History of hypertension, diabetes, hyperlipidaemia, cardiovascular disease
- Gastro-oesophageal reflux
- History of gallstones (cholesterol gallstones more prevalent in obesity)
- History of endometrial cancer in women (two to three times more common in obese than in lean women)
- History of breast cancer (risk increases with body mass index in post-menopausal women)
- Cancer of gallbladder and biliary system (obese women have a higher incidence)

- Cancer of colon, rectum, prostate and renal cell cancer (N Engl J Med 2000;343:1305–11) (higher in obese men)
- Medication history: antipsychotics, antidepressants, corticosteroids, oral contraceptives, beta-blockers, oral hypoglycaemic agents, insulin, anticonvulsants, antihistamines, pitzotifen.

Examination

- Patient has excessive adipose tissue.

Proceed as follows:

- Measure the height and body weight (to determine body mass index (BMI))
- Measure waist circumference
- Check BP (the prevalence of hypertension is approximately three times higher for the obese than the non-obese)
- Examine the joints to exclude osteoarthrosis
- Examine skin for intertrigo in redundant folds of skin (fungal and yeast infections of skin are also common)
- Tell the examiner that you would like to:
  - assess urine sugar (the prevalence of diabetes is three times higher in overweight than in non-overweight persons)
  - check serum lipids (these patients often have an adverse pattern of plasma lipoproteins that generally improve with weight loss)
  - assess pulmonary function (sleep apnoea)
  - exclude secondary causes (hypothyroidism, Cushing syndrome, polycystic ovarian syndrome)
  - obtain history pertaining to eating disorders.

DIAGNOSIS

This patient has gross obesity (lesion) of genetic origin, complicated by hypertension and osteoarthrosis.

ADVANCED-LEVEL QUESTIONS

Does obesity have a genetic origin?

Although many obese individuals are blamed for being obese — by their friends, physicians, family and by themselves — increasingly it has been shown that genetic influences have a substantial influence on BMI. The *ob* gene is an adipocyte-specific gene that encodes leptin, a protein that regulates body weight. Animals with mutations in *ob* are obese and lose weight when given leptin (Nature 1994;372:425–32). In humans, serum leptin concentrations correlate with the percentage of body fat, suggesting that most obese people are insensitive to endogenous leptin (leptin resistance).

What is the body mass index?

It is a measure to determine the presence of excessive adipose tissue and is calculated by dividing the body weight in kilograms by the height in metres squared. The normal spread of the BMI is from 20 to 25 kg/m^2.

What is morbid obesity?

It is relative weight greater than 200% (or BMI >40) and is associated with a 10-fold increase in the mortality rate.

Mention some adverse health consequences of obesity

They have a greater risk for diabetes mellitus (Fig. 148.1), stroke, coronary artery disease, premature mortality, thromboembolism, gallstones, reflux oesophagitis, sleep apnoea, polycythaemia and cancer of the colon, rectum, prostate, uterus, breast and ovary. The risk of death from all causes is increased and the risk is associated with a high BMI is greater for whites than black. Also higher maternal weight before pregnancy increases the risk of late fetal death, although it protects against delivery of a small-for-gestational age infant.

How common is obesity?

Obesity is becoming increasing common all over the world, particularly in the USA. About one-third of US adults ≥20 years of age are now obese. Obesity rates significantly increased between 1988–1994 and 2005–2008: by 69.3% among adults 20–39 years of age, 36.9% among those 40–59 years of age, and 44.7% among those ≥60 years. Such trends have undoubtedly helped to drive the age-adjusted prevalence of clinically diagnosed diabetes to 59 cases per 1000 population (in 2008), far above the baseline of 40 cases per 1000 (in 1997).

What patterns of obesity correlate with premature coronary artery disease?

Central obesity (abdomen and flank) and when there is excessive visceral fat within the abdominal cavity rather than subcutaneous fat around the abdomen.

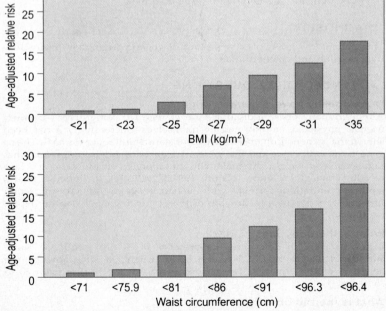

Fig. 148.1 Relative risk of developing type 2 diabetes with increasing body mass index (BMI) and waist circumference.

How would you manage such patients?

Approach is based on BMI and comorbidities such as cardiovascular disease (Fig. 148.2):

- Multidisciplinary approach to weight loss: hypocaloric diets, exercise, social support. Caloric restriction of 500 kcal daily would result in the loss of about 1 lb (0.5 kg) per week
- Behaviour modification and social support
- Drugs: Sibutramine (serotonin–norepinephrine reuptake inhibitor that reduces appetite) results in weight loss that is about 5% greater than in those taking placebo. Orlistat partially inhibits absorption of dietary fat (binds to pancreatic lipase in the GI tract; Lancet 1998;352:167–73). Side effects include oily spotting, flatus with discharge and faecal urgency. Rimonabant (a selective blocker of the cannabinoid receptor CB1) has shown to result in 5% weight loss when compared with placebo.
- Surgery:
  - Adjustable gastric banding and vertical (sleeve) gastrectomy
  - Roux-en-Y gastric bypass: a procedure that combines restriction and malabsorption and is considered by many to be the gold standard because of its high level of effectiveness and its durability
  - Biliopancreatic diversion procedures: commonly performed with a duodenal switch, in which a short, distal, common-channel length of small intestine severely limits caloric absorption; the procedure also includes a sleeve gastrectomy.

Note: Jejuno-ileal bypass is rarely used.

What are the mechanisms of obesity?

The pathophysiology of obesity is complex and poorly understood, but it includes genetic, behavioural, psychological and other factors:

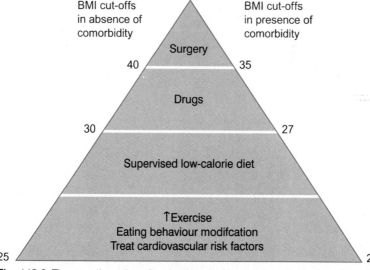

Fig. 148.2 Therapeutic options for obesity with increasing body mass index (BMI) and comorbidity.

- Insensitivity to leptin, presumably in the hypothalamus
- Neuropeptide Y-induced hyperphagia
- Deficiency of production or action of anorexigenic hypothalamic neuropeptides
- Increased secretion of insulin and glucocorticoid.

Mutation in the gene for the nuclear receptor perioxisome proliferator-activated receptor-γ accelerates differentiation of adiopocytes and may cause obesity (N Engl J Med 1998;339:953–9). The thizoladinedione class of antidiabetic drugs act at this point.

Mention some syndromes where obesity is a prominent feature

Cushing syndrome (p. 538), Laurence–Moon–Biedl syndrome (p. 724), Pickwickian syndrome (p. 410), Alstrom syndrome, Prader–Willi syndrome.

What is the link between obesity and diabetes?

Fat cells release free fatty acids and tumour necrosis factor-α, which cause insulin resistance, and leptin, which causes insulin sensitivity. A protein called resistin that is secreted by fat cells also causes insulin resistance. The antidiabetic group of drugs, the thiazoladinediones, reduce insulin resistance by suppressing the expression of resistin by the fat cells (Nature 2001;409:307–12).

Dermatology

149 SCLERODERMA

INSTRUCTION

Look at these hands.

SALIENT FEATURES

History

- Tight skin over face and joints
- Raynaud's phenomenon (Case 161, p. 587)
- Puffy hands and feet
- Fatigue
- Shortness of breath (lung involvement, cardiac fibrosis), dry cough
- GI symptoms: dysphagia, diarrhoea, bloating and indigestion
- Dry eyes
- History of renal failure.

Examination

- Thickening and tightening of the skin over fingers, sclerodactyly (finger pulp atrophy) (Fig. 149.1), beaking of nails (pseudoclubbing), atrophic nails, telangiectasia (nailfold capillaries) (Fig. 149.2)
- Raynaud's phenomenon (see Fig. 161.1)
- Subcutaneous calcification (fingers, elbows and extensor aspect of the forearms)
- Vitiligo or pigmentation.

Proceed as follows:

- Assess hand function: pincer movements, handgrip, unbuttoning of clothes, abduction of thumb and writing.
- Examine:
  - the joints for arthalgia or arthritis
  - the face for microstomia, difficulty in opening the mouth, beak-like or pinched appearance of the nose, blotchy telangiectasia
  - the abdomen for liver (primary biliary cirrhosis).

DIAGNOSIS

This patient has sclerodactyly, tightening of the skin over hands and face (lesion) caused by scleroderma (aetiology). He has difficulty in buttoning his clothes and has marked dysphagia as a result of oesophageal involvement (functional status).

QUESTIONS

What other organ systems are involved?

Skin. Raynaud's phenomenon, localized morphea, local or generalized oedema, hyperpigmentation, telangiectasia, subcutaneous calcification, ulceration, particularly at the fingertips. Ten-year survival rate is 71% with skin tightness limited to fingers but 21% with diffuse truncal skin involvement. Ilioprost, a prostacyclin analogue, helps to heal digital ulceration. Penicillamine improves the skin and prolongs survival in patients with early, rapidly progressive, systemic sclerosis.

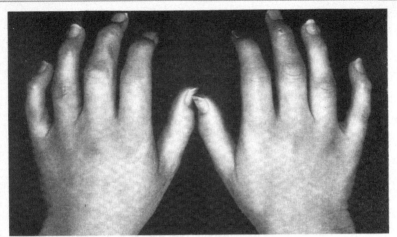

Fig. 149.1 Hands in scleroderma.

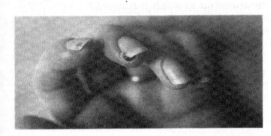

Fig. 149.2 Digital ulcers. (With permission from Charles et al. 2006.)

Musculoskeletal system. Arthritis, myositis, myopathy, bone ischaemia with resorption of the phalanges.

GI tract. Dysphagia, reflux oesophagitis, large or small bowel obstruction.

Lung. Fibrosis, atelectasis, pulmonary hypertension; pneumonia.

Kidney. Glomerulonephritis, malignant hypertension (poorest prognosis with renal involvement). ACE inhibitors dramatically improve renal crisis.

Heart. Myocardial fibrosis.

Remember: The prognosis is worse in those with renal disease and in males. Patients with skin and/or gut involvement without other organ disease have the best prognosis. Severely debilitating oesophageal dysfunction is the most common visceral complication, and lung involvement is the leading cause of death.

What are the variants of scleroderma?

CREST syndrome (see below), eosinophilic fasciitis, Thibierge–Weissenbach syndrome.

What is 'CREST' syndrome?

Calcinosis, Raynaud's phenomenon, oesophageal dysmotility, sclerodactyly and telangiectasia. It has a more favourable prognosis than systemic sclerosis and is associated with the anti-centromere antibody.

ADVANCED-LEVEL QUESTIONS

What are the criteria for diagnosis of scleroderma?

- Major criterion is proximal scleroderma (affecting metacarpophalangeals and metatarsophalangeals) (Arthritis Rheum 1980;23:581–90).
- Minor criteria are:
  - sclerodactyly
  - digital tip pitting or loss of substance of distal finger pads
  - bi-basal pulmonary fibrosis.

At least the sole criterion or two or more minor criteria are required. These proposed criteria had a 97% sensitivity for definite systemic sclerosis and 98% specificity.

What are the subsets of scleroderma?

- Limited cutaneous scleroderma: where the skin is affected only at the extremities
- Diffuse cutaneous scleroderma: skin of trunk and extremities affected
- Scleroderma sine scleroderma: skin not affected, patients present with pulmonary fibrosis, scleroderma renal crisis, cardiac failure or malabsorption and pseudo-obstruction. The presence of anti-centromere, scleroderma-70 and anti-nuclear antibodies can be helpful.

What are the causes of anaemia in such a patient?

- Iron deficiency from chronic oesophagitis
- Folate and vitamin B deficiency from malabsorption
- Anaemia of chronic disease
- Microangiopathic haemolytic anaemia.

What are the phases of skin changes in scleroderma?

- An early oedematous phase (with pitting oedema of hands and possibly forearms, legs and face)
- The dermal phase
- An atrophic phase, followed by contracture
- Other skin changes, e.g. depigmentation.

What do you know about the pathogenesis of these skin changes?

- Endothelial damage caused by a circulatory protein factor has been implicated as an early component of the 'inflammatory' phase; this endothelial damage may result in the capillary and arteriolar abnormalities seen as well as affecting local access of circulating proteins acting on fibroblast-enhancing collagen secretion.
- The profibrotic phenotype of fibroblasts in scleroderma is maintained by at least three factors:
  - Abnormal signalling by transforming growth factor-β (TGF-β) results in an increased level of platelet-derived growth factor receptor (PDGFR) (TGF-β_1 mediates fibrosis)
  - Amplification of the Ras–ERK1/2–ROS signalling loop, perhaps as a result of the upregulation of PDGFR.
  - Stimulation of autoantibodies against PDGFR that initiate and maintain the Ras–ERK1/2–ROS cascade.

How would you manage a patient with scleroderma?

- Educational and psychological support
- Treat vascular abnormalities such as Raynaud's phenomenon
- Symptomatic treatment, e.g. omeprazole for oesophagitis

- Early phase of diffuse form: immunosuppressive drugs (cyclophospha-mide, methotrexate, anti-thymocyte immunoglobulin)
- Later stages: antifibrotic drugs (penicillamine, interferon).

What is the role of prednisone in the treatment of scleroderma?

Prednisone has little or no role in the treatment of scleroderma.

What are the common fatal events in this disease?

In most cases, death results from cardiac, renal or respiratory failure.

The first reports of scleroderma were by WD Chowne in 1842 and James Startin, both from London, in 1846. The term sclerodermie was suggested by E Gintrac (1791–1877) of Bordeaux; Italian physician GB Fantonetti introduced the term sklerodermia in 1836.

Maurice Raynaud commented on the presence of Raynaud's phenomenon in scleroderma in 1863.

Heirich Auspitz (1835–1886) reported, in 1863, on death from renal failure in scleroderma; this was proved to be a more than chance association by H Moore and H Sheehan of Liverpool in 1952.

David A Isenberg is Professor of Rheumatology, University College London.

Carol Black is Professor of Rheumatology, Royal Free Hospital.

---

150 MACULOPAPULAR RASH

INSTRUCTION

Would you like to perform a general examination of this patient?
Look at this patient.

SALIENT FEATURES

History

- Ask whether or not the rash itches
- Ask where the rash started and ask the patient to describe its evolution
- Take a drug history (e.g. ampicillin, cephalosporins)
- History of fever (viral exanthems)
- Mucosal involvement.

Examination

- Reddish, blotchy maculopapular rash over the trunk (check the chest, back and axillae) and limbs (Fig. 150.1)

Proceed as follows:

- Palpate the surface of the rash to confirm your inspectory findings
- Check the mucous membranes of the mouth
- Tell the examiner that you would like to ask the patient some questions:
  - Examine for lymph nodes (glandular fever): some examiners may expect you to examine the lymph nodes as a part of the general examination. If lymph nodes are palpable, then examine all groups (cervical, supraclavicular, axillary and inguinal).

Note: Avoid waffling descriptions such as 'skin rash'.

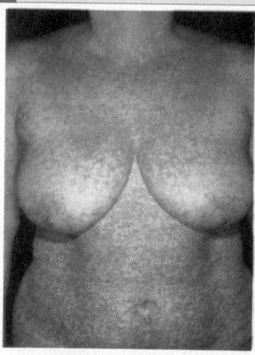

Fig. 150.1 Drug eruption (ampicillin): asymmetric, confluent maculopapular eruption. (With permission from Habif 2009.)

DIAGNOSIS

This patient has a maculopapular rash (lesion) caused by ampicillin ingestion (aetiology), which usually resolves on discontinuing the drug (functional status).

QUESTIONS

What is your differential diagnosis?
- Drug-induced rash
- Glandular fever (rash seen in only 3% of patients with infectious mononucleosis but approaches 100% when these patients take ampicillin).

Viral exanthems (measles, rubella).

What is your differential diagnosis when the rash is associated with lymphadenopathy?
- Glandular fever
- Lymphoproliferative disorders such as Hodgkin's disease
- HIV infection.

151 PURPURA

INSTRUCTION

Examine this patient's skin.

SALIENT FEATURES

History

- Take a drug history: steroids, anticoagulants, carbimazole, phenylbutazone, chloramphenicol, gold salts
- Age (senile purpura)
- History of chronic liver disease
- History of mouth ulcers (severe neutropenia).

Examination

- Small circumscribed bleeding into the skin, purpura, or larger lesions, bruises or ecchymoses (Fig. 151.1). Lesions begin as 1–3 mm papules, which increase in size and become palpable. They may coalesce to form plaques; in some instances, they may ulcerate.

Proceed as follows:

- Look for an underlying cause
- Comment on the patient's age: consider senile purpura
- Comment on the distribution: Henoch-Schönlein purpura is seen over the buttocks and lower limbs (p. 566)
- Look for the following signs:
  - Rheumatoid arthritis where purpura is drug induced (steroids, gold)
  - Anaemia (leukaemia, marrow aplasia or infiltration)
  - Chronic liver disease
  - Ulcers in the mouth (severe neutropenia)
  - Bleeding gums, corkscrew hair and perifollicular haemorrhages of scurvy (particularly in the elderly)
  - Stigmata of Ehlers–Danlos syndrome.
  - Bleeding from multiple venepuncture sites (disseminated intravascular coagulation).
- Tell the examiner that you would like toexamine spleen, liver and lymph nodes.

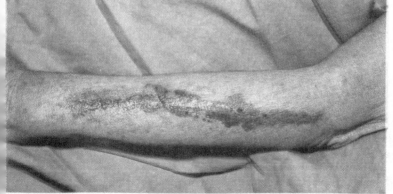

Fig. 151.1 Purpura.

DIAGNOSIS

This patient has purpura (lesion) that is caused by ingestion of steroids (aetiology) and is cosmetically unacceptable to the patient (functional status).

QUESTIONS

What are the common causes of purpura?
- Senile purpura, as a result of senile changes in the vessel walls
- Purpura induced by steroids or anticoagulants
- Thrombocytopenia as a result of leukaemia and marrow aplasia.

What are causes of bruising?
- Thrombocytopenia: idiopathic thrombocytopenic purpura, marrow replacement by leukaemia or secondary infiltration
- Vascular defects: senile purpura, steroid-induced purpura, Henoch–Schönlein purpura, scurvy, von Willebrand's disease, uraemia
- Coagulation defects: haemophilia, anticoagulants, Christmas disease
- Drugs: thiazides, sulphonamides, phenylbutazone, sulphonylureas, sulindac, barbiturates.

ADVANCED-LEVEL QUESTIONS

What do you know about Moschcowitz syndrome?
Moschcowitz syndrome or thrombotic thrombocytopenic purpura is an acute disorder characterized by thrombocytopenic purpura, microangiopathic haemolytic anaemia, transient and fluctuating neurological features, fever and renal impairment.

> E Moschcowitz (1879–1964), New York physician.
> In 1951 William Harrington, then a trainee in haematology at the Barnes Hospital in St Louis, Missouri, had severe thrombocytopenia immediately after voluntarily receiving plasma from a patient with the disease, establishing beyond doubt that a plasma factor causes the destruction of platelets in chronic idiopathic thrombocytopenic purpura.

152 PSORIASIS

INSTRUCTION

Look at this patient.
Do a general examination.

SALIENT FEATURES

History

- Symptoms (itching, pain, flexural intertrigo, limitation of manual dexterity), cosmetic problems or both
- Joint pains (psoriatic arthropathy (p. 481); psoriatic arthritis may be found in 10–15% of patients)
- Family history (30% of patients have family history)

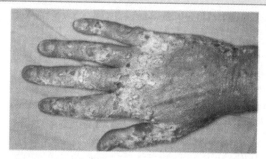

Fig. 152.1 Psoriasis.

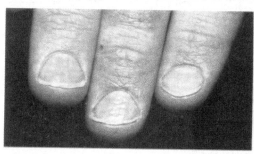

Fig. 152.2 Nail pitting.

- Aggravating factors (emotional stress, overuse of alcohol, streptococcal infections, drugs such as beta-blockers, lithium or tumour necrosis factor-α therapies).

Examination

- Well-demarcated salmon pink plaques with silvery white scales (Fig. 152.1) over extensor surfaces, scalp, naval and natal cleft. They often tend to have a pink or red line in the intergluteal fold
- A white blanching ring, known as *Woronoff's ring*, may be observed in the skin surrounding a psoriatic plaque.

Proceed as follows:

- Look at the nails for pitting (Fig. 152.2) and onycholysis (separation of the nail plate from the bed; p. 675)

DIAGNOSIS

This patient has silvery white scales and nail pitting (lesion) caused by psoriasis (aetiology), with considerable itching (functional status).

QUESTIONS

What are the characteristics of psoriasis?

Psoriasis is a papulosquamous disease with variable morphology, distribution, severity and course. Papulosquamous diseases are characterized by scaling papules (raised lesions <1 cm in diameter) and plaques (raised lesions >1 cm in diameter).

Other papulosquamous diseases include tinea infections, pityriasis rosea and lichen planus.

The lesions of psoriasis are distinct and are classically very well circum-scribed, circular, red papules or plaques with a grey or silvery-white, dry scale. In addition, the lesions are typically distributed symmetrically on the scalp, elbows, knees, lumbosacral area and in the body folds.

How common is this condition?
It affects 1–2% of the population of the UK.

What are the typical features of psoriatic plaques?
Distinguishing features include:
- silvery colour of the scaling
- the moist red surface on removal of the scales (*Bulkeley's membrane*)
- capillary bleeding when the individual silvery scales are plucked from the plaque (*Auspitz's sign*)
- new skin lesions at the site of trauma (*Koebner's phenomenon*).

ADVANCED-LEVEL QUESTIONS

How is the severity of involvement usually estimated?
- The patient's own perception of the disability
- Objective assessment of disability.

It is usually estimated by using the *Psoriasis Area and Severity Index* (PASI), which takes into consideration the area of involvement, thickness, redness and scaling. The maximal score on this index is 72, with mild, moderate and severe having scores of <10, 10–50 and >50, respectively.

What are the types of psoriasis?
- **Depending on the natural history**
- Type 1: young patients with a strong family history, has a more aggressive disorder
- Type 2: older patients with no family history, has a more indolent course.

- **Depending on the nature of skin lesion**
- *Chronic plaque psoriasis*
- With gradual peripheral extension, plaques may develop different configurations including:
  - psoriasis gyrata, in which curved linear patterns predominate
  - annular psoriasis, in which ring-like lesions develop secondary to central clearing
  - psoriasis follicularis, in which minute scaly papules are present at the openings of pilosebaceous follicles.
- *Rupioid and ostraceous,* which relate to distinct morphological subtypes of plaque psoriasis:
  - Rupioid plaques are small (2–5 cm in diameter) and highly hyperkeratotic, resembling limpet shells
  - Ostraceous psoriasis are hyperkeratotic plaques with relatively concave centres, similar in shape to oyster shells.
- *Inverse psoriasis:* plaques evolve in the intertriginous areas and, therefore, lack the typical silver scale appearance because of moisture and maceration
- *Guttate psoriasis:* numerous small popular lesions with silvery scaling evolve suddenly over the body surface
- *Pustular psoriasis:* can be localized or generalized; superficial pustules may stud the plaques

- *Erythrodermic psoriasis:* generalized erythema and scaling; can be life threatening.

What do you know about the genetics of psoriasis?

- Clear identification of the causative gene has been difficult because of the extensive linkage disequilibrium (i.e. genes on one chromosome are inherited together and are not easily separable by recombination events) observed within the major histocompatibility complex (MHC).
- The major genetic determinant of psoriasis is *PSORS1*, which probably accounts for 35–50% of the heritability of the disease in multiple genomewide studies. *PSORS1* is located within the MHC on chromosome 6p. Guttate psoriasis (an acute-onset form usually occurring in adolescents) is strongly associated with *PSORS1*, whereas late-onset cases of psoriasis vulgaris (usually in persons >50 years of age) and palmoplantar pustulosis are not associated with *PSORS1*.
- In a genomewide association study, polymorphisms in the genes for interleukin-12 (*IL12B*) and interleukin-23 (*IL23R*) are associated with psoriasis. These interleukins are cytokines that induce naive CD4 T cells to differentiate into type 1 helper T cells (Th1 cells) and type 17 helper T cells (Th17 cells), respectively; they have been identified as key mediators of psoriasis.

What do you know about the pathology of plaque psoriasis?

- Hyperproliferation of the epidermis
- Inflammation of the epidermis and dermis.

What do you understand by the term Koebner's phenomenon?

Injury or irritation of psoriatic skin tends to provoke lesions of psoriasis in the site of trauma in some patients: this is known as the Koebner's phenomenon.

Mention a few exacerbating factors?

- Drugs: beta-blockers, ACE inhibitors, lithium, indomethacin, antimalarials, alcohol
- Psychological factors
- Infection: β-haemolytic streptococci, HIV (pre-existing psoriasis may become more refractory to therapy and plaque psoriasis may change to the guttate form in HIV-positive patients)
- Injury to the skin: mechanical injury, sunburn.

How would you manage a patient with psoriasis?

- Educate the patient that there is no cure and that only suppression of the disease is possible
- Indications for treatment include symptoms (itching, pain, flexural intertrigo, limitation of manual dexterity), cosmetic problems or both
- Weight loss and smoking cessation may lower the risk or severity of psoriasis
- Initial treatment is topical when <20% of the body is involved
- Topical therapy in some form is usually the mainstay of treatment and includes:
  - emollients (soft yellow paraffin or aqueous cream)
  - keratolytic agents (salicylic acid)

- coal tar, which is usually used in combination with ultraviolet B phototherapy: *Goeckerman treatment*
- anthralin (often used according to the Ingram regimen: a daily coal tar bath, ultraviolet B phototherapy and 24 h application of an anthralin paste containing salicylic acid)
- topical steroids, such as betamethasone ointment
- calcipotriol (vitamin D), which is known to act locally to increase extracellular calcium concentrations, which leads to increased keratinocyte differentiation and decreased proliferation and scaling; it is an excellent alternative to steroids.
- Systemic therapy:
  - Phototherapy (ultraviolet B radiation): narrowband ultraviolet B has replaced broadband ultraviolet B as it induces longer remissions and fewer burns (BMJ 2000;320:850–3).
  - Photochemotherapy (methotrexate with ultraviolet a therapy)
  - Methotrexate
  - Etretinate and acitretin (vitamin A derivatives), retinoids
  - Systemic steroids
  - Ciclosporin, tacrolimus or mycophenolate mofetil.
- Novel approach:
  - Anti-CD4 monoclonal antibody
  - Biologic agents that block both interleukin-12 and interleukin-23, e.g. ustekinumab
  - Agents that selectively block tumour necrosis factor-α, e.g. etanercept, adalimumab, infliximab.

What are the indications for systemic treatment?

- Failure of topical therapy
- Repeated hospital admissions for topical treatment
- Extensive plaque psoriasis in the elderly
- Generalized pustular or erythrodermic psoriasis
- Severe psoriatic arthropathy.

What underlying condition would you suspect when psoriasiform lesions are seen on the nose, ears, fingers and toes?

Such lesions are paraneoplastic eruptions associated with squamous cell carcinoma of the oropharynx, tracheobronchial tree and oesophagus: this is known as *Bazex syndrome.*

Further reading

Russell B: Lepra, psoriasis, or the Willan–Plumbe syndrome, *Br J Dermatol Syphilis* 62:359–361, 1950.

B Russell, in 1950, proposed that psoriasis be known by the eponym Willan–Plumbe syndrome. The first clear descriptions were by Willan (1808) and Plumbe (1824) and ended hundreds of years of confusion and laid the foundation for establishing psoriasis as a disease entity that is separate from leprosy.

153 BULLOUS ERUPTION

INSTRUCTION

Look at this patient.

SALIENT FEATURES

History

- Onset and blisters
- History of mucosal involvement (mouth ulcers)
- Drug history: thiols (e.g. benzylpenicillin), ACE inhibitors, aspirin, NSAIDs, rifampin. levodopa, phenobarbital, interferon, propanolol, nifedipine.

Examination

- Bullous eruption (Fig. 153.1)
- Crusts or superficial erosions (these suggest a preceding fluid-filled lesion).

Proceed as follows:

- Comment on the distribution: knee, thighs, forearms and umbilicus in the elderly (pemphigoid).
- Look in the mouth for ulceration; if the blisters break easily leaving denuded skin, it is more likely to be pemphigus.
- Tell the examiner that a biopsy of the skin is essential to confirm the diagnosis.

DIAGNOSIS

This patient has a bullous eruption (lesion) caused by sulphonamides (aetiology); it is widespread with involvement of mucous membrane and mild dehydration (functional status).

QUESTIONS

What do you understand by the term bulla?
It is a circumscribed elevation of the skin, larger than 0.5 cm and containing fluid.

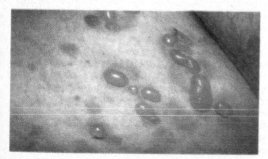

Fig. 153.1 Bullous eruption.

How would you confirm the diagnosis?

A biopsy of a fresh blister (<12 h old) with a portion of perilesional skin for histology and immunofluorescent studies.

ADVANCED-LEVEL QUESTIONS

Mention a few blistering conditions

- Common: friction, insect bites, drugs, burns, impetigo, contact dermatitis
- Uncommon:
  - Autoimmune bullous diseases (pemphigoid, pemphigus vulgaris, dermatitis herpetiformis, immunoglobulin-A-mediated diseases, bullous erythema multiforme, epidermolysis bullosa acquisita)
  - Porphyria cutanea tarda
  - Paraneoplastic pemphigus.

How would you manage a patient with pemphigus vulgaris?

Barrier nursing, antibiotics, intravenous fluids, large doses of systemic steroids, usually with immunosuppressive drugs (azathioprine, cyclophosphamide or methotrexate), which act as steroid-sparing agents. Other drugs used include dapsone, nicotinamide, gold and ciclosporin.

What are the forms of pemphigus?

There are two main forms; both occur commonly in middle age:

- Pemphigus vulgaris and its variant pemphigus vegetans; the vulgaris form begins in the mouth in over 50% of cases
- Pemphigus foliaceus and its variant pemphigus erythematosus, which are more superficially blistering conditions; the foliaceus form may be drug induced (e.g. penicillamine toxicity) or is associated with autoimmune disease.

What are the characteristics of pemphigus vulgaris?

Pemphigus vulgaris is characterized by bullae in the epidermis. It is often preceded by bullae in the mucous membrane. Superficial separation of the skin after pressure, trauma or on rubbing the thumb laterally on the surface of uninvolved skin may cause easy separation of the epidermis (Nikolsky's sign), indicating acantholysis. Biopsy shows disruption of epidermal intercellular connections (acanthocytolysis). Immunofluorescence shows intercellular deposition of immunoglobulin G in the epidermis.

What are the characteristics of bullous pemphigoid?

It is a relatively benign condition with remissions and exacerbations. Characteristically, tense blisters are present in non-mucosal surfaces such as flexural areas and trunk, typically in the elderly. The blisters are tense and do not rupture easily. The bullae are subepidermal and rich in eosinophils; immunoelectron microscopy shows deposits of immunoglobulin G and complement 3 (C3) in the lamina lucida of the basement membrane. It has a chronic course marked by exacerbation and remission.

Although clinical findings often lead to a correct diagnosis, positive histopathological studies represent the usual diagnostic standard, particularly direct immunofluorescence studies of perilesional skin demonstrating deposition of C3 and immunoglobulins (IgG) in a linear pattern at the epidermal basement membrane.

Therapy involves systemic glucocorticoids and/or immunosuppressives such as azathioprine, methotrexate, mycophenolate mofetil, rituximab and intravenous immunoglobulin.

What do you know about herpes gestationis?

It is a self-limiting disease with the initial appearance of bullae in the periumbilical region, trunk and extremities, usually in the fifth or sixth month of pregnancy. Pruritus is typically severe. It may recur in subsequent pregnancies. Menses and oestrogen are known to precipitate flare-ups. The blisters are eosinophil-rich and subepidermal, with ·C3 in the basement membrane and serum complement-fixing immunoglobulin antibody. Corticosteroids, usually systemic, are the treatment of choice.

What do you know about the pathogenesis of pemphigus?

In pemphigus vulgaris, autoantibodies are directed against desmoglein 3 on the surface of the keratinocytes (J Clin Invest 1997;99:31–40). In pemphigus foliaceus the antibodies are directed against desmoglein 1 on keratinocytes in the subcorneal region (J Clin Invest 2000;105:207–13). The desmogleins are desmosomal glycoproteins in the cadherin family of cell adhesion molecules. There is strong evidence that the endemic form of pemphigus foliaceus is initiated by an environmental vector, whose antigens mimic those of desmoglein. The quantitative levels of desmoglein 1 or 3 are used to guide treatment because changes in antibody titre correlates with disease activity: disappearance of the antibody from serum often precedes clinical remission.

How would you manage generalized forms of autoimmune bullous disease?

- The treatment of patients with autoimmune blistering diseases is grounded in clinical experience rather than randomized controlled trials.
- Systemic steroid therapy is usually chosen first to treat patients with generalized forms of any autoimmune bullous disease except those mediated by immunoglobulin A. Topical steroids have little, if any, value in the treatment of such patients, although they are sometimes effective in patients with localized disease.
- Other immunosuppressive drugs: many patients with moderate to severe pemphigus, bullous pemphigoid, cicatricial pemphigoid or epidermolysis bullosa acquisita require a second immunosuppressive drug (such as azathioprine or cyclophosphamide), either for its corticosteroid-sparing effect or to achieve complete remission. The specific choice is a matter of personal experience, concern over the relative toxic effects and possible contraindications. Some patients have been treated successfully with prednisone and ciclosporin, but the latter alone is not beneficial. Low-dose methotrexate plus prednisone may benefit patients with pemphigus or bullous pemphigoid.
- Azathiprine is usually as used as steroid-sparing agent. Alternatives include methotrexate, intravenous chlorambucil, cyclophosphamide and mycophenolate mofetil.
- Dapsone and related drugs: dapsone is the drug of choice for patients with dermatitis herpetiformis or linear immunoglobulin A dermatosis who are not allergic to sulphonamides. It inhibits the chemotaxis of neutrophils, reducing their accumulation in the upper dermis and thus diminishing tissue inflammation. The response is rapid, with most lesions resolving within 48–72 h. Alternatives to dapsone include sulfapyridine, sulfoxone sodium and sulfamethoxypyridazine. Dapsone is effective as monotherapy in only a minority of patients with bullous pemphigoid.

- Chrysotherapy: systemic gold is rarely used as an alternative or adjunct to prednisone therapy in patients with pemphigus because it is efficacious in only a subgroup of patients and carries the potential risk of side effects on prolonged administration.
- Intravenous immunoglobulin therapy, intravenous rituximab, is usually reserved for patients with recalcitrant disease.
- Plasmapheresis: is used in patients with severe pemphigus unresponsive to conventional therapy and high titres of pemphigus autoantibodies. Plasmapheresis may also be beneficial in patients with bullous pemphigoid even in the absence of detectable autoantibodies, although its mechanism of action in such patients is not known.
- Gluten-free diets are advised in dermatitis herpetiformis.
- Other therapies: extracorporeal absorption of antibodies for pemphigus, combination tetracycline and nicotinamide in bullous pemphigoid, colchicine in immunoglobulin A dermatosis.

PV Nikolsky (b. 1858), Professor of Dermatology, first in Warsaw and later in Rostov.

Pemphigus (from the Greek *pemphix*, meaning blister or bubble).

---

154 HENOCH–SCHÖNLEIN PURPURA

INSTRUCTION

Look at this patient's legs.

SALIENT FEATURES

History

- Ask the patient about the following:
  - Upper respiratory tract infection
  - Joint pains (knees and ankles are commonly involved)
  - Abdominal pain
  - The rash: its onset and evolution
  - Recent drug ingestion.

Examination

- Purpuric rash over the legs (Fig. 154.1) and buttocks.
Remember: Palpable purpura implies an inflammatory process, most classically cutaneous small cell vasculitis.
Proceed as follows:
- Tell the examiner that you would like to examine the rest of the body — including arms, body, scalp and behind the ears — for distribution of rash.
- Examine the mouth to confirm or rule out involvement of mucous membranes.
- Tell the examiner that you would like to examine the urine for haematuria.

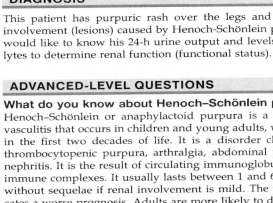

Fig. 154.1 Henoch–Schönlein purpura: palpable purpuric lesions.

DIAGNOSIS

This patient has purpuric rash over the legs and buttocks with renal involvement (lesions) caused by Henoch-Schönlein purpura (aetiology). I would like to know his 24-h urine output and levels of urea and electrolytes to determine renal function (functional status).

ADVANCED-LEVEL QUESTIONS

What do you know about Henoch–Schönlein purpura?

Henoch–Schönlein or anaphylactoid purpura is a distinct, self-limiting vasculitis that occurs in children and young adults, with a peak incidence in the first two decades of life. It is a disorder characterized by non-thrombocytopenic purpura, arthralgia, abdominal pain and glomerular nephritis. It is the result of circulating immunoglobulin (Ig) A-containing immune complexes. It usually lasts between 1 and 6 weeks and subsides without sequelae if renal involvement is mild. The presence of IgG indicates a worse prognosis. Adults are more likely to develop renal involvement (Lancet 1992;339:280). In biopsy specimens obtained from the skin of patients with Schönlein–Henoch purpura, the dermal vessels frequently contain IgA deposits.

What investigations would you like to do?

- Examine the urine for haematuria and proteinuria
- Antinuclear factor
- Venereal Disease Research Laboratory Test
- Skin biopsy to detect arteriolar and capillary vasculitis.

250 Cases in Clinical Medicine

What is the differential diagnosis?
- Drug-induced purpura
- SLE
- Gonococcal arthralgia
- Keratoderma blenorrhagicum
- Secondary syphilis.

How would you classify vasculitis clinically?
- Purpuric disorders: Henoch–Schönlein purpura, leukocytic vasculitis
- Microscopic polyarteritis: polyarteritis nodosa
- Aortic type: Takayasu disease, polyarteritis nodosa (in the latter, the subclavian artery is spared)
- Pulmonary type: Wegener's granulomatosus, Churg–Strauss syndrome.

How would you treat this patient?
- First line: rest, reduced activity and leg elevation
- First-line oral therapy: antihistamines and NSAIDS
- Second-line therapy: colchicine dapson
- Chronic or severe disease may require systemic immunosuppressants
- Patients with IgA nephropathy with protein excretion >500 mg/day, should be treated with an ACE inhibitor and/or an angiotensin receptor blocker. Patients with IgA nephropathy, increased urinary protein excretion (1.0–3.5 g daily) and plasma creatinine concentrations of ≤133 μmol/l (≤15 mg/l) may benefit from a 6-month course of steroid treatment (Lancet 1999;353:883–7). Steroids, plasma exchange, immunoglobulins and cytotoxic agents have all been used in complicated cases and there are no data from controlled trials (Lancet 2000;356:562).

What is the prognosis of Ig A nephropathy?
IgA nephropathy tends to progress slowly and only about half the patients develop end-stage renal disease within 25 years. Factors that predict an accelerated course are persistent proteinura, persistent microscopic haematuria, elevated serum creatinine at the time of diagnosis, poorly controlled hypertension and extensive glomerulosclerosis or interstitial fibrosis on renal biopsy.

What is the the difference between primary Ig A nephropathy and Henoch–Schönlein purpura?
IgA nephropathy (or Bergers disease) was first described by Berger and Hinglais as recently as 1968 (J Urol Nephrol (Paris) 1968;74:694–5) and is now generally accepted to be the most common form of primary glomerulonephritis (N Eng J Med 2002;347:738–48). There are two conditions that should be distinguished from primary IgA nephropathy: Henoch–Schönlein purpura and thin glomerular basement membrane disease. Thin glomerular basement membrane disease is a common condition that occurs more often in female patients and has a benign clinical course in that end-stage renal disease does not develop. Its diagnosis is established by electron microscopy, where glomerular capillary loops can be shown to have diffusely attenuated basement membranes.

What are the other cutaneous manifestations of immune complex-mediated small vasculitis?
Vesicles, pustules, superficial ulcerations, urticaria, splinter haemorrhages, hyperpigmentation (Fig. 154.2).

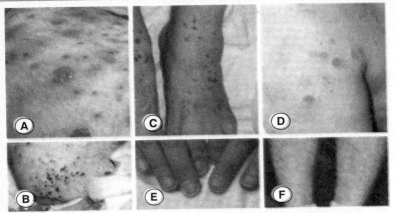

Fig. 154.2 Immune complex-mediated small vessel vasculitis. (A) Vesicles. (B) Pustules. (C) Superficial ulcerations. (D) Urticaria. (E) Splinter hemorrhages. (F) Hyperpigmentation. (With permission from Firestein et al. 2008.)

What are the different types of immune complex-mediated vasculitis?
- Henoch–Schönlein purpura
- Cutaneous leukocytoclastic angiitis
- Mixed cryoglobulinaemia
- Connective tissue disease/rheumatoid vasculitis.

This disorder was first reported in the English literature by Willan in 1808.

Eduard Heinrich Henoch (1820–1910) qualified in Berlin, where he ran the neurology department; he studied under Schönlein and eventually became a paediatrician. In 1874 he reported the coexistence of purpura and GI haemorrhage.

Johannes Lucas Schönlein (1793–1864) was initially Professor of Medicine in Würzburg but, because of his liberal views, he was dismissed; he eventually became Professor of Medicine, first in Zurich and then in Berlin. In 1837 he reported the coexistence of purpura and arthritis.

Anthony Fauci is contemporary Director of the National Institute of Allergy and Infectious Diseases and Director of AIDS Research, NIH, Bethesda; his chief interests include immunological disorders including AIDS.

155 ICHTHYOSIS

INSTRUCTION

Look at this patient.
Examine this patient's skin.
Perform a general examination on this patient.

SALIENT FEATURES

History

- Take a family history of the disorder.
- Ask whether or not it is of recent onset (underlying malignancy).

Examination

- Rough, dry skin with fish-like scales (Fig. 155.1).

Proceed as follows:

- Examine the palms for dry skin and hyperkeratotic creases.

Note: Although ichthyosis is said not to be increased in frequency in HIV/AIDS, it may be more severe when associated with this condition.

DIAGNOSIS

This patient has rough, dry skin with fish-like scales (lesion) caused by ichthyosis (aetiology), which causes severe itching and may be cosmetically unacceptable (functional status).

ADVANCED-LEVEL QUESTIONS

What do you know about ichthyosis?

Ichthyosis is a disorder of keratinization characterized by the development of dry, rectangular scales. It can be classified as inherited, metabolic or malignant.

- Inherited ichthyosis
- *Inherited ichthyosis* is present from birth or childhood and may be apparent only in winter.
- *Ichthyosis vulgaris* (Fig. 155.2A) is autosomal dominant and present from childhood. It has white, translucent, quadrangular scales on the extensor aspects of the arms and legs, sparing flexural areas, and is associated with atopy.

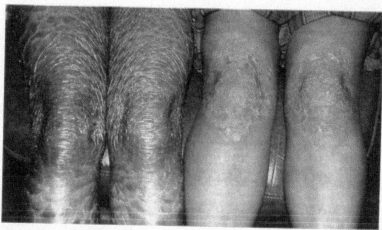

Fig. 155.1 Icthyosis.

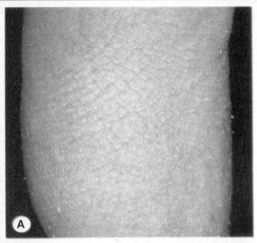

Fig. 155.2 Inherited icthyosis. (A) Dominant ichthyosis vulgaris. (B) X-linked ichthyosis vulgaris. (With permission from Habif 2009.)

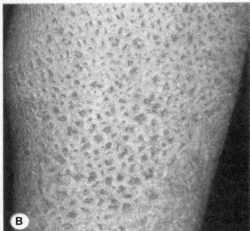

- *X-linked ichthyosis* (Fig. 155.2B) is present from birth. It occurs all over the trunk with large, brown, quadrangular scales that may encroach on the antecubital and popliteal fossae; it is associated with corneal opacities. Affected individuals have a deficiency of steroid sulfatase, an enzyme important for the removal of proadhesive cholesterol sulfate secreted into the intercellular spaces. The desquamation process is impaired by the accumulation of cholesterol sulfate, which results in persistent cell-to-cell adhesion within the stratum corneum.
- *Lamellar ichthyosis* is autosomal recessive and present from birth. It is seen over the body, palms and soles and is associated with ectropion.
- *Epidermolytic hyperkeratosis* is autosomal dominant and present since birth. There is predominant flexural involvement.

Note: Filaggrin is a key protein involved in skin barrier function. Mutations of the gene for filaggrin has been reported in patients with ichthyosis.

- **Metabolic ichthyosis**
- *Refsum's disease:* a metabolic disorder of lipid metabolism.

- **Malignancy**
- Ichthyosis is a cutaneous marker in:
  - Hodgkin's disease
  - multiple myeloma
  - breast cancer.

How would you manage such patients?
Regular use of emollients and moisturizing creams. Creams containing urea are useful.

S Refsum, a Norwegian physician.

---

156 HEREDITARY HAEMORRHAGIC TELANGIECTASIA (RENDU–OSLER–WEBER DISEASE)

INSTRUCTION

Examine the patient's face and obtain a relevant history.
Perform a general examination.
Look at this patient's face.

SALIENT FEATURES

History

- Does it run in the family (autosomal dominant)?
- Is there a history of GI bleeding?
- Is there a history of epistaxis?
- Is there a history of repeated blood transfusions?
- Is there a history of dyspnoea, fatigue, cyanosis or polycythaemia (pulmonary arteriovenous malformations)?
- Is there a history of headaches, subarachnoid haemorrhage (cerebral arteriovenous malformations)?

Examination

- Punctiform lesions and dilated small vessels present on the face, in particular around the mouth (Fig. 156.1).
- The patient may be pale (as a result of iron-deficiency anaemia).
Proceed as follows:
- Look into the patient's mouth and inspect the tongue and palate for telangiectasia.
- Examine the nail beds, arms, trunk for telangiectasia.

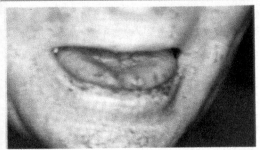

Fig. 156.1 Hereditary haemorrhagic telangiectasia. (A) Lesions are commonly on or close to mucous membranes. (B) Lesions may occur anywhere on the body, such as on the fingers. The lesions are dilated capillaries, and they blanch if pressure is applied with a glass slide. (With permission from Forbes, Jackson 2003.)

- Examine the chest for bruits (pulmonary arteriovenous malformations with a predilection·for lower lobes).
- Look for signs of cardiac failure caused by left-to-right shunting and hepatic bruits (both from hepatic arteriovenous malformations) (N Engl J Med 2000;343:938–52).

DIAGNOSIS

This patient has multiple telangiectasia around the mouth and on the tongue and lips (lesion), probably hereditary in nature (aetiology). The patient is severely anaemic, probably as a result of upper GI bleeding, and is currently receiving a blood transfusion (functional status).

QUESTIONS

What do you understand by the term telangiectasia?

Telangiectasia is a cluster of dilated capillaries and venules. The lesions blanch if pressure is applied with a glass slide. In hereditary haemorrhagic telangiectasia (HHT), the telangiectases consist of focal dilatations of postcapillary venules. Lesions are commonly on or close to mucous membranes but may occur anywhere on the body, such as on the fingers.

Mention a few conditions in which telangiectasia are seen

- Face:
  - Those who work outdoors in a temperate or cold climate (e.g. farmers)
  - In mitral stenosis
  - Myxoedema
  - Transitory phenomenon during pregnancy.
- Other sites:
  - Secondary to irradiation
  - Scleroderma (CREST syndrome)
  - Dermatomyositis
  - SLE
  - Acne rosacea
  - Lupus pernio
  - Polycythaemia
  - Necrobiosis lipoidica diabeticorum.

ADVANCED-LEVEL QUESTIONS

What do you know about the genetics of hereditary telangiectasia?

Mutations have been identified in two genes encoding proteins expressed on vascular endothelial cells and involved in signalling by members of the transforming growth factor (TGF)-β superfamily: endoglin-β (chromosome 9q3; Nat Genet 1994;6:205–9) and activin receptor–like kinase 1 (ALK-1; Nat Genet 1996;13:189–95). Interestingly heterozygote endoglin knockout mice develop a phenotype (J Clin Invest 1999;104:1343–51) similar to that of humans who are heterozygous for a null mutation in the gene for endoglin-β. These heterozygous mice develop nose bleeds and cutaneous telangiectasia, and curiously the ears are more commonly affected than in human beings. In patients with this condition and juvenile polyposis there may be mutations in one gene — the *MADH4* gene (also known as *SMAD4*). Pulmonary hypertension in association with hereditary haemorrhagic telangiectasia can involve mutations in *ALK1* (N Engl J Med 2001;345:325).

What do you know about the pathology of the condition?

- Skin
- The small telangiectasias are focal dilatations of postcapillary venules with prominent stress fibres in the pericytes along the luminal border.
- In fully developed telengiectasia, there is marked dilatation of the venules, which are also convoluted. They extend along the entire dermis, with excessive layers of smooth muscle devoid of elastic fibres. These often are directly connected to dilated arterioles.
- Mononuclear cells, predominantly lymphocytes, accumulate in the perivascular space.

- Lungs, liver and brain Arteriovenous malformations lack capillaries and consist of direct connections between arteries and veins.

What are the clinical criteria for diagnosing hereditary haemorrhagic telangiectasia?

Shovlin criteria:

- Recurrent epistaxis
- Telangiectasia at a site other than in the nasal mucosa
- Evidence of autosomal dominant inheritance
- Visceral involvement.

The HHT diagnosis is definite if three criteria are present. A diagnosis of HHT cannot be established in patients with only two criteria, but should be recorded as possible or suspected to maintain a high index of clinical suspicion. If fewer than two criteria are present, HHT is unlikely, although children of affected individuals should be considered at risk in view of age-related penetrance in this disorder (Am J Med Genet 2000;91:66–7).

What are the complications of hereditary telangiectasia?

- Epistaxis (usually begins by the age of 10 years and by age 21 in most; it becomes more severe in later decades in about two-thirds of affected patients) (N Engl J Med 1995;333:918–24)
- GI haemorrhage (usually does not manifest until the fifth or sixth decade). Arteriovenous malformations, angiodysplasias and telangiectasias are present in the stomach, duodenum, small bowel, colon and liver

- Symptomatic liver involvement: the typical clinical presentations include high-output heart failure, portal hypertension and biliary disease (N Engl J Med 2000;343:931)
- Iron-deficiency anaemia
- Haemoptysis, cyanosis, clubbing, cerebral abscess and embolic stroke from the pulmonary arteriovenous malformations
- Headache and subarachnoid haemorrhage
- High-output cardiac failure is almost always associated with shunts from the hepatic artery to the hepatic veins (N Engl J Med 2000;343: 931–6).

How would you manage such patients?

- Anaemia: ferrous sulfate, multiple blood transfusions
- Epistaxis: oestrogen, cauterization, septal dermatoplasty, laser ablation and transcatheter embolotherapy of arteries leading to the nasal mucosa
- Cutaneous telangiectasia: cosmetic therapy with topical agents, laser ablation
- Pulmonary arteriovenous malformations: embolotherapy, surgical resection or ligation of arterial supply
- GI telangiectasia: blood transfusions, photocoagulation, oestrogen–progestogen therapy
- Brain and spinal cord arteriovenous malformations: embolotherapy, neurosurgery, stereotactic surgery
- Active bleeding: ε-aminocaproic acid (N Engl J Med 1994;330:1789, N Engl J Med 1994;330:j1822)
- Anti-vascular endothelial growth factor antibody, bevacizumab (N Engl J Med 2009;360:2143).

This condition was described by HJLM Rendu, a French physician, in 1896, by Sir William Osler in 1901 and by F Parkes Weber, a London physician, in 1936. Dr Claire Shovlin is a Senior Lecturer in NHLI Cardiovascular Sciences, and Honorary Consultant in Respiratory Medicine for Imperial College Healthcare NHS Trust (Hammersmith Hospital campus) research focus on gene identification of this condition.

---

157 HERPES LABIALIS

INSTRUCTION

Look at this patient's mouth.

SALIENT FEATURES

History

- Pain, itching, burning lasting several hours
- Vesicles
- Sore mouth
- Fever
- Gum swelling
- Mouth ulcers.

Examination

- Small vesicles with an erythematous base on the lips and around the mouth (Fig. 157.1)
- Look for:
  - vesicles in the mouth (gingiva, tongue, soft and hard palate) and pharynx
  - tender anterior cervical lymph nodes.

DIAGNOSIS

This patient has small vesicles around the mouth (lesion) from herpes labialis (aetiology), which is causing severe itching (functional status).

QUESTIONS

What usually causes a 'cold sore'?

Skin manifestations include vesicular lesions on an erythematous base. Only 10–30% of new infections are symptomatic.

Herpes simplex virus (HSV) type 1 causes an asymptomatic gingivostomatitis in children.

In adults, there may be severe stomatitis with mouth ulcers, local lymph node enlargement and systemic features.

What do you know about herpes simplex virus type 2?

HSV-2 causes a genital infection called vulvovaginitis. Women with genital herpes should have cervical screening as a link is suspected with carcinoma of the cervix.

ADVANCED-LEVEL QUESTIONS

What are the complications of herpes infections?

- Erythema multiforme
- Disseminated infection in the immunocompromised individual
- Herpes keratitis, scarring and visual impairment
- Herpes simplex encephalitis (propensity for the temporal lobe)
- Herpetic whitlow (infection of the finger) (Fig. 157.2)
- Herpes gladiatorum (infection of the skin, described among wrestlers)
- Visceral infections, especially in viraemia in HIV (oesophagitis, pneumonitis, hepatitis)

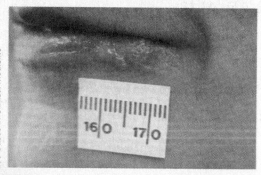

Fig. 157.1 Clustered intact vesicles at the skin-vermilion junction. (With permission from DeLee et al. 2009.)

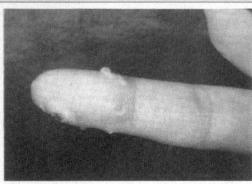

Fig. 157.2 Herpetic whitlow.

- Neonatal HSV infection (neonates <6 weeks of age); usually visceral and/or CNS infection
- CNS complicatiosn: aseptic meningitis, sacral radiculopathy, transverse myelitis and benign recurrent lymphocytic meningitis (Mollaret's meningitis).

How would you confirm your clinical diagnosis?
- Scrapings of the base of the lesions stained with Wright, Giemsa (Tzanck preparation) or Papanicolaou's stain will demonstrate characteristic giant cells or intranuclear inclusions of herpes infection (does not differentiate from zoster infection)
- Isolation of virus in tissue culture
- Demonstration of HSV antigens in scrapings from lesions
- HerpeSelect HSV-1 and HSV-2 enzyme-linked immunosorbent assays and HSV-1 and HSV-2 immunoblot tests.

How would you treat herpes labialis?
Aciclovir cream applied locally.

What drugs are available for herpes simplex infections?
- Mucocutaneous herpes: topical aciclovir, valaciclovir, famciclovir, foscarnet
- Eye infections: idoxuridine, trifluorothymidine, topical vidarabine. Prophylactic use of aciclovir can prevent recurrent ocular HSV disease (N Engl J Med 1998;339:300–6)
- Encephalitis: intravenous aciclovir
- Neonatal infections: high-dose intravenous vidarabine and aciclovir.

In a patient suspected of herpes encephalitis, which test allows early detection?
PCR of CSF to detect HSV DNA.

What is the interaction between human immunodeficiency virus and herpes simplex virus infections?
It has been argued that HSV-2 and HIV infections are synergistic, since suppression of HSV-2 decreases HIV load, while others insist that interactions between HSV-2 and HIV-1 are more complex and that HSV-2 coinfection might, in certain cases, be associated with elevated CD4 T cell counts.

What do you know about the pathogenesis of herpes simplex mucocutaneous infections?

In the initial infection, HSV enters through breaks in the skin or mucosa; it then attaches to and enters epithelial cells to replicate. It is taken up by free sensory nerve endings found at the dermis, and the nucleocapsid containing the viral genome is transported by retrograde axonal flow to the nucleus in the sensory ganglion.

After recovery from the initial infection, the virus remains latent in the sensory ganglion for the life of the host. Periodically, the virus reactivates from the latent state and travels back down the sensory nerves to the skin or mucosal surface.

Viral shedding from mucosal surfaces occurs from lesions (clinical reactivation) obut can occur with very mild or no symptoms (subclinical reactivation). Shedding leads to transmission to other sexual partners and in some cases HSV can be transmitted from mother to infant at delivery (Lancet 2007; 370:2127–37).

158 HERPES ZOSTER SYNDROME (SHINGLES)

INSTRUCTION

Look at this patient.

SALIENT FEATURES

History

- Pain, particularly in the ophthalmic branch of the trigeminal nerve (Fig. 158.1), and in the lower thoracic dermatomes (postherpetic neuralgia occurs in about 50% of patients with zoster over the age of 60 years)
- Past history of chickenpox
- Presence of an underlying immunocompromised state (e.g. recurrent zoster indicates a poorer prognosis in patients with established AIDS). Zoster occurs at least seven times more frequently in homosexual men with HIV infection than in HIV-negative controls.

Examination

- Vesicular rash along a dermatome (usually affects thoracic and lumbar dermatomes)
- Enlargement of a draining lymph node.

Remember: The virus affects both the posterior horn of the spinal cord and the skin supplied by sensory fibres that pass through the diseased root ganglion (Fig. 158.2).

DIAGNOSIS

This patient has a vesicular rash along the sixth thoracic dermatome (lesion) caused by herpes zoster (aetiology), and has severe local pain (functional status).

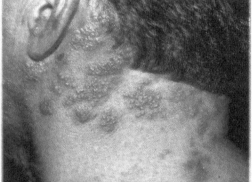

Fig. 158.1 Vesicular rash and pain in the ophthalmic branch of the trigeminal nerve.

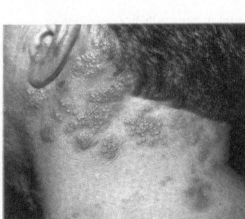

Fig. 158.2 Rash in skin supplied by sensory fibres of the nerve.

ADVANCED-LEVEL QUESTIONS

In which layer of the skin are the vesicles formed?
They are formed in the prickle-cell layer of the epidermis as a result of the 'balloon degeneration' of cells and serous exudation from the corium.

How does this condition present?

Pain in the distribution of the dermatome; malaise; fever, followed a few days later by a rash in the same distribution as the pain. Starts as macules then forms vesicles and then pustules.

Which nerve is affected when the lesions are present on the tip of the nose?

The ophthalmic division of the trigeminal nerve.

How would you confirm the diagnosis?

The diagnosis is usually clinical. It is confirmed by rising viral titres and isolation of the virus from the blister. The Tzanck smear demonstrates a multinucleated giant cell and virual inclusions when material scraped from the floor of a vesicle is stained with the Wright's stain. The Tzanck test can be positive in infections with herpes simplex, herpes zoster and varicella.

How would you manage such a patient?

- Pain relief, including gabapentin, pregabalin, lidocaine patch, topical casaicin and amitriptyline in severe cases
- Antiviral therapy (aciclovir, valaciclovir or famciclovir) results in faster healing, lessening of acute pain and reduced incidence and intensity of post-herpetic neuralgia
- Interferon appears to be effective in limiting zoster in patients with cancer.

What is the role of vaccination?

There is waning cell-mediated immunity to the virus in the elderly. Therefore, vaccination in patients >60 years reduces the incidence of herpes zoster by 50% and lessens the severity and chance of complications (N Engl J Med 2005;352:2271–84).

Is varicella-zoster immunoglobulin useful in preventing zoster eruptions?

There are no known means of effectively preventing zoster eruptions; however, results on the effectiveness of the recently developed live attenuated varicella vaccine are awaited. Although there is considerable controversy, with arguments for and against universal vaccination, the American Academy of Pediatrics has recently adopted a position in support of universal vaccination of healthy non-immune children and adults.

What are the complications of herpes zoster?

- Corneal ulcerations
- Gangrene of the affected area
- Phrenic nerve palsy
- Meningoencephalitis
- Ramsay Hunt syndrome
- Postherpetic neuralgia: intrathecal methyl prednisolone is an effective treatment for post-herpetic neuralgia (N Engl J Med 2000;343: 1514–19)
- Disseminated zoster including pneumonia.

What are the features of herpes zoster in patients with human immunodeficiency virus infection?

It is usually unidermatomal and uneventful. However, it may be multidermatomal, disseminated recurrent, or chronically persistent as a hyperkeratotic nodular lesion.

How does the varicella zoster virus affect the central nevous system in such co-infected patients?

In AIDS, the virus may cause the following:

- Multifocal encephalitis
- Ventriculitis
- Acute haemorrhagic meningomyeloradiculitis
- Focal necrotizing myelitis
- Vasculitis of the leptomeningeal arteries.

J Ramsay Hunt (1874–1937), a US neurologist.
Shingles, from the Latin *cingulum* or 'girdle.'

---

159 LICHEN PLANUS

INSTRUCTION

Look at this patient's skin.

SALIENT FEATURES

History

- Itching
- Medication history: thiazides, furosemide, beta-blockers, ACE inhibitors, phenothiazines, gold, organic mercurials, chloroquine, mepacrine, methyldopa, quinine, chlorpropamide, tolbutamide, proton pump inhibitors
- Occupational history: (whether the patient is in contact with colour film developer
- Hepatitis C infection: erosive-lichen planus is more common.

Examination

- Papular, purplish, flat-topped eruption with fine white streaks lace-like pattern (Wickham's striae) (Fig. 159.1) over the anterior wrists and forearms, sacral region, ankles, legs and penis.
- Involvement of the skin is characterized by the '4Ps': purple, polygonal, pruritic papules.

Proceed as follows:

- Look into the mouth (buccal mucosa, tongue, gum or lips) for a lace-like pattern of white lines and papules (Fig. 159.2). (Remember that oral lichen planus must be differentiated from leukoplakia.)
- Examine the scalp for cicatricial alopecia.
- Examine the nails for longitudinal ridging, pterygium formation from the cuticle (Fig. 159.3), 20-nail dystrophy dystrophy (roughened nail surface and brittle free nail edge) and total nail loss.
- Comment on eruptions that present along linear scratch marks (Koebner's phenomenon).

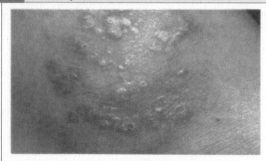

Fig. 159.1 Flat-topped, purple polygonal papules of lichen planus. (With permission from Kliegman et al. 2007.)

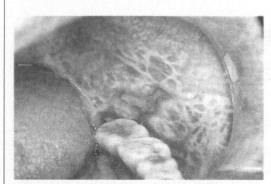

Fig. 159.2 Lace-like keratoses, erythema and ulceration of the buccal mucosa. (With permission from Goldman, Ausiello 2007.)

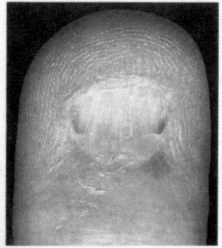

Fig. 159.3 Adhesion of the proximal nailfold to the scarred matrix throws the nail plate into folds, pterygium. (With permission from Habif 2009.)

- Comment on the residual hyperpigmented macules that lichen planus leaves in their wake.

Note: The three cardinal features of lichen planus are the typical skin lesions, histopathological features of T cell infiltration of the dermis in a band pattern, and IgG and C3 immunofluorescence at the basement membrane of the dermis.

DIAGNOSIS

This patient has violaceous, flat-topped eruptions (lesion) caused by lichen planus (aetiology), with several scratch marks indicating moderately severe pruritus (functional status).

ADVANCED-LEVEL QUESTIONS

Mention a few conditions that present as white lesions in the mouth

- Leukoplakia
- Candidiasis
- Aphthous stomatitis
- Squamous papilloma
- Verruca vulgaris
- Secondary syphilis.

Mention a few conditions in which ulcers can be found in the mouth

- Erosive lichen planus
- Pemphigus vulgaris
- Recurrent aphthous ulcers
- Behçet's disease
- Stevens–Johnson syndrome
- Recurrent herpes simplex.

What is the prognosis in lichen planus?

Lichen planus is a benign condition that lasts for months to years. It may be recurrent. Oral lesions may be persistent.

How would you manage these lesions?

- Local measures: local steroid creams or intralesional steroids
- General measures: psoralen plus ultraviolet A (PUVA), isotretinoin, dapsone
- Ultraviolet light to control pruritus
- Mucous membrane lesions: corticosteroids or 'swish and spit' ciclosporin.

LF Wickham (1860–1913), a French dermatologist.
H Koebner (1838–1904), a German dermatologist.

160 VITILIGO

INSTRUCTION

Look at this patient.

SALIENT FEATURES

History

- Age of onset (about half the patients present before the age of 20)
- Whether or not it runs in the family (familial in 36% of cases)
- About other autoimmune disorders (hypothyroidism, hyperthyroidism, thyroiditis, Addison's disease, diabetes mellitus, pernicious anaemia).

Examination

- Hypopigmented patches (Fig. 160.1) that are distributed symmetrically; sometimes the border may be hyperpigmented. The distribution often includes wrists, axillae, perioral, periorbital and anogenital skin
- White hairs in the vitiliginous area
- Some spontaneous re-pigmentation in the sun exposed regions (in a third of cases).

Proceed as follows:

- Look at the scalp for alopecia and white hair.

Note: Scratching when the disease is active may induce lesions along the scratch marks; this is termed isomorphic response or Koebner's phenomenon. It is also seen in response to the friction or pressure resulting from such common activities as brushing hair, drying skin with a towel and wearing a belt or watch.

DIAGNOSIS

This patient has vitiligo (lesion), which is of autoimmune origin (aetiology) and can be cosmetically distressing to the patient (functional status).

ADVANCED-LEVEL QUESTIONS

Mention some associated conditions

Organ-specific autoimmune conditions:

- Thyroid disease: Graves' disease, myxoedema, Hashimato's disease
- Pernicious anaemia
- Diabetes mellitus
- Alopecia areata
- Addison's disease.

What are the types of vitiligo?

Non-segmental vitiligo. White patches that are often symmetric and that usually increase in size over time, corresponding to a substantial loss of functioning epidermal melanocytes and sometimes hair-follicle melanocytes. The key precipitating factors include immunologic factors, oxidative stress or a sympathetic neurogenic disturbance. Accounts for 85–90% all cases of vitiligo.

Segmental vitiligo. Unilateral distribution that may completely or partially match a dermatome. In most patients there is one unique segment of depigmentation. Rarely, two or more segments with ipsilateral or

Fig. 160.1 Vitiligo.

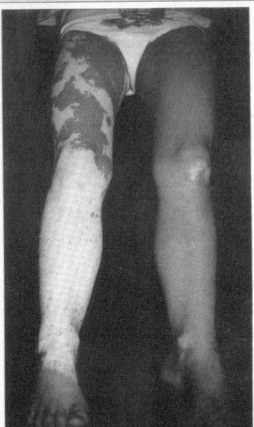

contralateral distribution may occur. A neurogenic sympathetic disturbance is considered a key precipitating factor. Seen in autoimmune
diseases.

Which fungal condition can be mistaken for vitiligo?

Pityriasis versicolor (caused by the fungus *Malassezia furfur*).

How would you confirm the diagnosis?

Examination with a Wood's lamp in a completely dark room after the
examiner's eyes have adapted to the darkness (it is less useful in patients
with darker skin types). It is a hand-held ultraviolet A (UVA) irradiation
device that emits at approximately 365 nm. Wood's lamp provides bright
reflection of white patches and enhanced details on intermediate pigment
tones. Lamps that incorporate a magnifying lens are useful in evaluating
terminal and vellus pigmentation of hair. A complete examination should
include inspection of the genitalia and areas of skin folds as these areas
can be easily overlooked.

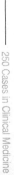

How would you manage such patients?

- Cosmetics are useful for concealing disfiguring patches.
- When <20% of the skin is involved: topical methoxsalen with long-wavelength UVA is used, followed by thorough washing and application of an SPF 15 sunscreen.
- When >20% of the skin is affected: oral methoxsalen with UVA.
- Non-segmental vitiligo: phototherapy, preferably narrow-band UVB. Acral lesions and lesions with depigmented hairs will hardly or not react.
- When extensive: good cosmetic results may be obtained when normal skin is 'de-pigmented' with a bleaching agent such as hydroquinone.
- New lesions of vitiligo: may benefit from topical steroids.
- Segmental vitiligo or stable non-segmental vitiligo in a limited area (<200 cm^2): epidermal autografts and cultured epidermis combined with PUVA (split-thickness skin grafting, punch-grafting, suction blister epidermal grafting, non-cultured epidermal cell suspension grafting).

Note: On the whole, treatment of vitiligo remains unsatisfactory.

Mention a few conditions in which hypopigmentation is common

- Hypopituitarism
- Albinism
- Phenylketonuria
- Leprosy
- Burns
- Radiodermatitis
- Piebaldism (an autosomal dominant condition manifested by a white forelock)
- Ash leaf spots (tuberous sclerosis)
- Leukoderma (occurs as a complicaton of lichen planus, lichen simplex chronicus, atopic dermatitis and discoid lupus erythematosus).

What is the histology of vitiligo?

Characteristically there is partial or complete loss of pigment-producing melanocytes in the epidermis. In contrast, some forms of albinism have melanocytes but no melanin pigment is produced because of lack of, or a defect in, the tyrosinase enzyme.

Why are melanocytes progressively lost in this condition?

The various theories of pathogenesis include:

- autoimmune destruction from circulating antibodies against the melanocytes and impaired cell-mediated immunity
- self-destruction by toxic intermediates of melanin production
- neurohumoral factors.

Further reading

Gawkrodger DJ, Ormerod AD, Shaw L, et al: Guideline for the diagnosis and management of vitiligo, *Br J Dermatol* 159:1051–1076, 2008.

Parsad D, Gupta S: Standard guidelines of care for vitiligo surgery, *Ind J Dermatol Venereol Leprol* 74(Suppl):S37–S45, 2008.

161 RAYNAUD'S PHENOMENON

INSTRUCTION

Examine this patient's hands.

SALIENT FEATURES

History

- Ask the patient about the following:
  - Whether precipitated by cold, emotion and relieved by heat
  - The different phases change: in idiopathic Raynaud's disease, the cold dead-white hands (ischaemia) become blue (stasis) and finally red (reactive hyperaemia) and painful
  - Sensory changes secondary to vasospasm (numbness, stiffness, aching pain)
  - Occupation (polishing tools, vibrating tools)
  - Dysphagia (CREST syndrome)
  - Butterfly rash, arthralgia, xerostomia (SLE, collagen vascular disorder)
  - Use of electrically heated gloves.

Examination

- Hands may be painful: ask the patient.
- The hands and fingers are cyanosed and cold, or may be warm and red or blue (Fig. 161.1). The thumbs are rarely affected.

Proceed as follows:

- Examine the hands carefully for signs of scleroderma (tightening of skin, telangiectasia).
- Examine the face for tightening of skin around the mouth (scleroderma), butterfly rash (SLE).
- Tell the examiner that you would like to examine upper limb pulses and BP in both upper limbs (useful in the detection of cervical rib).

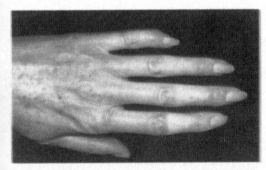

Fig. 161.1 Scleroderma showing Raynaud's phenomenon: pallor, cyanosis, and often rubor of the skin, in response to cold or emotional stimuli.

250 Cases in Clinical Medicine

DIAGNOSIS

This patient has cold, blue hands (lesion) caused by Raynaud's phenomenon (aetiology) and is unable to continue her occupation, which requires using a vibratory hand drill (functional status).

ADVANCED-LEVEL QUESTIONS

How is primary Raynaud's differentiated from secondary Raynaud's phenomenon?

- Primary:
  - Attacks are symmetric
  - No tissue necrosis, ulceration, or gangrene
  - No secondary cause on the basis of a patient's history and general physical examination
  - Normal nailfold capillaries
  - Negative result when tested for anti-nuclear antibody
  - Normal ESR.
- Secondary:
  - Age at onset of >30 years
  - Episodes are intense, painful, asymmetric, or associated with ischaemic skin lesions
  - Clinical features suggestive of a connective-tissue disease (e.g. arthritis and abnormal lung function)
  - Specific autoantibodies
  - Evidence of microvascular disease on microscopy of nailfold capillaries.

What are the causes of Raynaud's phenomenon?

- Immunological and connective tissue disorders:
  - Scleroderma
  - SLE
  - Dermatomyositis
  - Rheumatoid arthritis.
  - Mixed connective tissue disorders.
- Obliterative arterial disease:
  - Atherosclerosis
  - Thoracic outlet syndrome, cervical rib.
- Occupational:
  - Vibration, causing white fingers
  - Cold injury, e.g. from handling frozen commodities
  - Vinyl chloride.
- Drugs:
  - Beta-blockers
  - Bromocriptine
  - Sulphasalazine
  - Ergot alkaloids.
  - Combination of bleomycin and vincristine (as for testicular cancer).
- Miscellaneous:
  - Cold agglutinins
  - Cryoglobulins
  - Idiopathic.

Note: Raynaud's disease is diagnosed if the phenomenon persists for greater than 3 years without evidence of associated disease.

What investigations would you do to look for autoimmune rheumatic disease in a patient with Raynaud's phenomenon?

- FBC, ESR
- Total immunoglobulin and electrophoresis strip
- Urine analysis
- Nail-fold capillaroscopy
- Chest radiography
- Renal and liver function tests
- Test for anti-nuclear antibody
- *Helicobacter pylori* (one paper suggested that eradication of *H. pylori* ameliorates Raynaud's phenomenon; Dig Dis Sci 1998;43:1641)
- Hand radiography.

What drugs have been used to treat Raynaud syndrome?

Nifedipine, nitrates, stanazolol, inositol nicotinate, naftidrofuryl oxalate, prostaglandin 12, thymoxamine, guanethidine, prazosin.

What is the role of surgery in treating Raynaud's disease?

In patients resistant to medical therapy with severe, frequent attacks and if trophic changes have occurred interfering with work, dorsal sympathectomy may be indicated.

Do you know of any other vasospastic conditions?

- White finger syndrome
- Livedo reticularis
- Erythromelalgia
- Chilblains.

Further reading

Raynaud M: Selected monographs, vol 121, 'On local and symmetrical gangrene of the extremities (Barlow T trans). London, 1888, New Sydenham Society.

Auguste-Maurice Raynaud (1834–1881) described the sign in 1862. He was a physician at Hôpital Lariboisière, Paris. He died from an attack of angina pectoris.

---

162 SYSTEMIC LUPUS ERYTHEMATOSUS

INSTRUCTION

Examine this patient's face (usually a young woman).

SALIENT FEATURES

History

- Fatiguability and tiredness: suggests anaemia
- Joint symptoms: particularly small joints (90% of patients)
- Gangrene of the digits: vasculitis

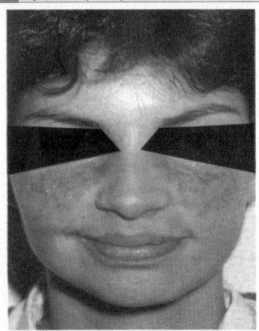

Fig. 162.1 Malar rash in a patient with systemic lupus erythematosus. Note that the rash does not cross the nasolabial fold. (With permission from Klippel, Dieppe 1998.)

- Skin rash (butterfly rash on face; Fig. 162.1) in sun-exposed areas, livedo reticularis, alopecia, Raynaud's phenomenon
- Mouth ulcers
- Hypertension, oedema (suggesting renal involvement)
- Fever, enlargement of lymph nodes
- Bleeding from gums excessive menstrual bleeding, purpura (caused by thrombocytopenia)
- Neuropsychiatric symptoms, seizures
- History of remissions and exacerbations
- Drug history (hydralazine, procainamide, minocycline).

Examination

- Butterfly rash: follicular plugging, scales, telangiectasia and scarring affecting the bridge of the nose and cheeks (the patient may be cushingoid because of steroids)
- Examine the following:
  - Conjunctiva for anaemia (often Coombs' test positive)
  - Mouth ulcers (seen in one-third of cases; Fig. 162.2)
  - Scalp for alopecia
  - Sun-exposed areas and elbows for vasculitic rash, subcutaneous nodules
  - Nails for splinter haemorrhages, nailfold capillaries and periungal infarcts
  - Hands for palmar erythema, Raynaud's phenomenon (Fig. 161.1), arthritis

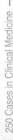

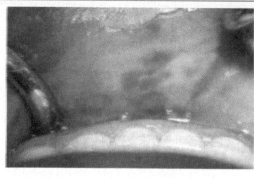

Fig. 162.2 Oral mucosal ulcerations: generally painless and can present on other cutaneous tissues. (With permission from Powers 2008.)

- Knees for vasculitic rash
- Feet for secondary oedema (secondary to nephrotic syndrome).
- Tell the examiner that you would like to examine the urine for proteinuria.

Note: SLE principally affects skin, joints, kidney and serosal membranes.

DIAGNOSIS

This patient has a butterfly rash of the face with telangiectasia (lesion) caused by systemic lupus erythematosus (aetiology) and has renal failure, probably caused by lupus nephritis as evidenced by the haemodialysis catheter (functional status).

ADVANCED-LEVEL QUESTIONS

What is the histology of the skin rash in systemic lupus erythematosus?

- Liquefactive degeneration of the basal layer of the epidermis together with oedema at the dermoepidermal junction. Immunofluorescence microscopy shows deposition of immunoglobulin and complement along the dermoepidermal junction.
- Oedema of the dermis accompanied by infiltrates of perivascular mono-nuclear cells.
- Vasculitis with fibrinoid necrosis of the vessels.

What are the skin manifestations of systemic lupus erythematosus?

Butterfly rash, periungal erythema, nailfold telangiectasia, alopecia, livedo reticularis, hyperpigmentation, urticaria, purpura, scarring eruption of discoid lupus.

What are the criteria for diagnosis of systemic lupus erythematosus?

Any four of the following 11 criteria are required to make a diagnosis:

- Malar rash
- Discoid rash
- Photosensitivity
- Oral ulcers
- Arthritis: non-erosive arthritis
- Serositis: pleuritis, pericarditis

- Renal involvement: proteinuria, cellular casts (nephritis is more common in patients with anti-native DNA)
- Neurological involvement: seizures, psychosis
- Haematological involvement: haemolytic anaemias, leukopenia, thrombocytopenia
- Anti-nuclear antibody (ANA): seen in over 95% of patients
- Immunological disorder: positive for LE cell (a specific type of cell found in SLE), anti-DNA antibody, false-positive syphilitic serology.

Note: American Rheumatic Association criteria are intended to provide a degree of diagnostic certainty primarily for research purposes. It is often possible to be reasonably confident about a diagnosis of SLE on less-strict clinical grounds. A diagnosis of SLE is usually made when patients have three or four typical manifestations, such as a characteristic skin rash, thrombocytopenia, serositis or nephritis and ANA. Polyarthritis and dermatitis are the most common manifestations. It should be noted that antibodies to double-stranded DNA and the so-called Smith antigen (Sm) are virtually diagnostic of SLE.

What do you know about systemic lupus erythematosus in older patients?

The initial presentation of idiopathic SLE usually occurs between the first and fourth decades of life. However, about 10% may first occur in patients >60 years of age. Patients with SLE after the age of 50 years less often present with malar rash, arthritis and nephritis.

Diagnosis of SLE in older patients must be one of exclusion. The frequency of low titres on ANA tests increases with advancing age, and a positive test may be associated with malignant disease or chronic infection.

What do you know about drug-induced lupus erythematosus?

- Procainamide is responsible for the majority of the cases. Other causes include hydralazine, quinidine, isoniazid.
- Drugs causing lupus-like syndrome do not seem to aggravate primary SLE.
- Patients with drug-induced lupus usually present with skin and joint manifestations.
- Although multiple organs are affected, nephritis and CNS features are not ordinarily present.
- Anti-histone antibodies are characteristic of drug-induced lupus but are not specific for this syndrome; anti-native DNA is almost never detected.
- Clinical manifestations and many laboratory features return to normal after the offending drug is withdrawn.

How useful is the detection of anti-nuclear antibodies in the diagnosis of systemic lupus erythematosus?

The detection of ANA is a sensitive screening test for SLE. Since ANA occurs in 95% of the patients, it is hard to be certain of the diagnosis in their absence. The degree of positivity is diagnostically important. Serum dilutions below which normal serum may be positive for these antibodies vary in different laboratories. Titres that are less than two times higher than the normal limit in any laboratory ought to be viewed sceptically. The positive predictive value of the test increases with higher titres.

What are the patterns of lupus nephritis?

The WHO's morphological classification of lupus nephritis describes five patterns:

- Normal by light, electron and immunofluoroscence microscopy (rare)
- Mesangial lupus glomerulonephritis
- Focal proliferative glomerulonephritis
- Diffuse proliferative glomerulonephritis
- Membranous glomerulonephritis.

Note: None of these patterns is specific for lupus.

How would you manage a patient with systemic lupus erythematosus?

- Avoidance of sunlight provocation. In Britain, patients should avoid being outside from 11 am to 3 pm from March to September and should wear protective clothing, including hats; patients should holiday in temperate latitudes or during the winter. In addition, sun block creams such as titanium dioxide (rather than barrier cream) are essential
- Avoidance of drug provocation: penicillin, sulphonamides
- Encourage the patient to join the Lupus Society
- Educate the patient that no therapy is curative and that medical treatment is largely empirical, selected on the basis of specific manifestations:

Disease manifestation	Treatment
Serological abnormalities and minor cytopenia unaccompanied by symptoms	No treatment
Rash and mild systemic symptoms	Antimalarial drugs
Mild or moderate arthritis, fever, pleuropericarditis	NSAIDs or low-dose prednisolone
Malaise, weight loss and lymphadenopathy	Low-dose steroids
High fever, active inflammatory glomerulonephritis, severe thrombocytopenia, severe haemolytic anaemia and most neurological disturbances	High-dose prednisolone (>60 mg per day for 4–6 weeks)
Rapidly progressive renal disease	Intravenous administration of bolus doses of 1000 mg methylprednisolone
Lupus nephritis with high histological activity score	Oral or intravenous cyclophosphamide or mycophenolate mofetil with high-dose steroids (N Engl J Med 2000;343: 1156–62)
Thromboembolism with antiphospholipid antibody	Long-term anticoagulation
Severe disease	Experimental treatments

Experimental treatments include apharesis, intravenous gammaglobulin, ciclosporin, immunoadsorption, photochemotherapy, nodal irradiation, various monoclonal antibodies and autologous haemopoietic stem-cell infusion (Lancet 2000;356:701–7).

What are the common causes of death in systemic lupus erythematosus?

The most common causes of death are renal failure and intercurrent infections followed by diffuse CNS disease.

What do you know about the pathogenesis of systemic lupus erythematosus?

- *Pathogenic autoantibodies* are the primary cause of tissue damage in patients with lupus including:
  - anti-double-stranded DNA, anti-nucleosome and anti–α-actinin antibodies contribute to lupus nephritis (anti-double–stranded DNA antibodies also occur, however, in 23–64% of patients with type 1 autoimmune hepatitis, depending on the assay used)
  - anti-Ro antibodies, anti-La antibodies, or both in pregnancy confers a 1–2% risk of fetal heart block
  - antibodies against the N-methyl-D-aspartate (NMDA) receptor may be important in CNS lupus (NMDA is an excitatory amino acid released by neurons)
  - anti-Ro and anti-nucleosome antibodies may play a role in cutaneous lupus.
  - autoantibody-mediated destruction of red cells is important in the haemolytic anaemia that can occur in patients with lupus
  - anti-platelet antibodies are important in the pathogenesis of thrombocytopenia that can occur in patients with lupus
- *T lymphocyte help* is critical in the pathogenesis of lupus. The effect on the T cell depends on the interaction between molecules on the surface of the cell with the antigen presented on the surface of the antigen-presenting cell.
- *B cells* acting as an antigen-presenting cells also interact with T cells, costimulation requiring interaction between CD40 and the CD40 ligand. The interaction stimulates the T cell to produce cytokines, some of which act on the B cell to promote antibody formation, to stimulate cell division, to switch antibody production from IgM to IgG, and to promote changes in the secreted antibody so that it binds more strongly to the driving antigen. (**Note**: CD20 and CD22 are present on B cells and interleukin-10 is produced by B cells).
- Plasmacytoid dendritic cells (producing interferon) have been found in the inflamed skin of lupus. They can internalize immune complexes in SLE, which, in turn, triggers the cells to secrete interferon-α through activation of toll-like receptor (TLR).

Promising therapies base on these pathlogical changes include:
- rituximab: antibody against CD20 on the surface of all mature B cells; non-specific
- abetimus sodium: depletes only B lymphocytes that produce anti-double-stranded DNA antibodies and forms complexes with anti-double-stranded DNA antibodies, which can then be cleared from the circulation; more specific.

Further reading

Cervaera R, the European Working Party on SLE: Systemic lupus erythematosus: clinical and immunologic patterns of disease expression in a cohort of 1000 patients, *Medicine* 72:113, 1993.

Hay EM, Snaith ML: Systemic lupus erythematosus and lupus-like syndromes, *BMJ* 310:1257–1261, 1995.

Mills JA: Systemic lupus erythematosus, *N Engl J Med* 330:187, 1994.

Tan EM, Cohen AS, Fries JF, et al: The 1982 criteria for classification of SLE, *Arthritis Rheum* 25:1271, 1982.

Ferdinand von Hebra (1816–1880) from Vienna described an eruption that occurs 'mainly on the face, on the cheeks and nose in a distribution not dissimilar to a butterfly' in 1845.

Pierre Louis Alphée Cazenave (1795–1877) from Paris first used the term lupus érythémateux in 1851.

Sir William Osler (1849–1919) first described the systemic manifestations of SLE under the name exudative erythema between 1895 and 1904.

RRA Coombs (1921–2006), Professor of Immunology at Cambridge, is reported to have said 'red blood cells were primarily designed by God as tools for the immunologist and only secondarily as carriers of haemoglobin'.

---

163 PHLEBITIS MIGRANS

INSTRUCTION

Look at this patient's leg: he has had similar such lesions at different sites at intervals.

SALIENT FEATURES

History

- Time course, pain and tenderness of skin lesions
- Ask the patient about:
  - local trauma (including intravenous infusions)
  - gastrointestinal malignancies (pancreatic or gastric cancer)
  - history of oral contraceptives.

Examination

- Inflamed superficial leg veins.

Proceed as follows:

Tell the examiner that you would like to investigate for the underlying malignancy, usually carcinoma of the pancreas or stomach (Trousseau's sign; Fig. 142.1) (N Engl J Med 1992;327:1128–33, N Engl J Med 1994;327: 1163–4).

DIAGNOSIS

This patient has migratory phlebitis (lesion) and I would like to investigate for an underlying pancreatic or gastric malignancy (aetiology).

ADVANCED-LEVEL QUESTIONS

In which other condition is superficial phlebitis a prominent sign?
Thromboangiitis obliterans (N Engl J Med 2000;343:864).

Is superficial thrombophlebitis associated with deep vein thrombosis?
It may be associated with occult deep vein thrombosis in about 20% of cases, although pulmonary emboli are rare.

Is phlebitis more frequently associated with plastic venous catheters or with steel intravenous needles?
It is more likely to be associated with plastic catheters, but this may be caused by the catheter remaining in the vein for longer periods (Fig. 163.1).

How is superficial phlebitis treated?
- Local heat, elevation of the leg and NSAIDs
- When very extensive or in proximity to the saphenofemoral junction, ligation and division of the saphenous vein at the saphenofemoral junction (as pulmonary embolism may result if the phlebitis of the saphenous vein extends into the deep vein)
- Septic thrombophlebitis, which is usually caused by *Staphylococcus aureus*, requires excision of the involved vein up to its junction with an uninvolved vein in order to control infection.

What other dermatoses complicate pancreatic disease?
- Panniculitis
- 'Bronze' pigmentation of haemochromatosis
- 'Necrolytic migratory erythema' of glucagonoma syndrome
- Cutaneous haemorrhage of acute pancreatitis: 'bruising' of the left flank (Grey Turner's sign) or umbilicus (Cullen's sign) (see Fig. IV.1).

What is relationship between venous thromboembolism and cancer?
Cancer risk is increased in patients with venous thromboembolism. Several reports have shown an increase over rates in the general population during

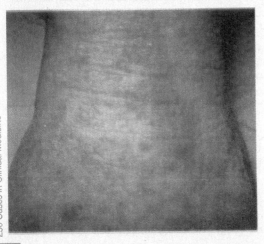

Fig. 163.1 Venous flare reaction overlying access vein of the forearm. (With permission from Abeloff et al. 2008.)

the first 1 or 2 years after admission for venous thromboembolism: a four-fold increase in the first year, particularly for cancers of the brain, liver, pancreas and ovary, Hodgkins's disease and polycythaemia vera (Lancet 1998;351:1077–80); an advanced stage and poor prognosis for cancer diagnosed at the same time or in the following year (N Engl J Med 2000;343:1846–50). The risk seems to be lower among patients treated with oral anticoagulants for 6 months than those treated for 6 weeks (N Engl J Med 2000;342:1953–8).

A long-term risk has also been identified: a 30% increased overall incidence of malignancy over a 10-year period (Lancet 1998;351:1077–80).

Armand Trousseau (1801–1867), physician at the Hôtel-Dieu in Paris, noted the sign as his death warrant, confirming his suspicion of an underlying malignancy in 1865. (Trousseau A. Phlegmasia albia dolens. In Lectures on clinical medicine, delivered at the Hôtel-Dieu, Paris, London: New Wydenham Society, 1872, pp. 281–295).

G Grey Turner (1877–1951), Professor of Surgery, Hammersmith Hospital, London.

TS Cullen (1868–1953), Canadian born, Professor of Gynaecology, Johns Hopkins Hospital, Baltimore, USA.

---

164 ERYTHEMA MULTIFORME

INSTRUCTION

Perform a general examination.

SALIENT FEATURES

History

- History of preceding sore throat or cold
- Low-grade fever
- Drug history: barbiturates, sulphonamides, phenytoin, penicillins
- Blister-like skin rash with intense itching
- Mouth ulcers: mucosal involvement suggests Stevens–Johnson syndrome
- History of recurrent episodes: suggests herpes simplex infection.

Examination

- Target-shaped lesions (Fig. 164.1), usually over the palms, soles and skin. A classical target lesion consists of three concentric zones of colour change: typically there is a central, dark, purple area or blister surrounded by a pale, oedematous round zone; this, in turn, is surrounded by a peripheral rim of erythema
- Pleomorphic eruption with macules, papules and bullae.

Proceed as follows:

- Look at the mucous membranes of the mouth (cutaneous and mucosal lips, gingival sulcus, sides of tongue), nares and conjuctiva (Stevens–Johnson syndrome).

250 Cases in Clinical Medicine

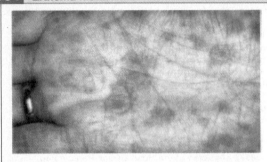

Fig. 164.1 Erythema multiforme with 'target' or 'iris' lesions.

- Tell the examiner that you would like to examine the external genitalia for ulcers.

Note: Erythema multiforme is a cell-mediated hypersensitivity reaction to many different immunological insults, including drugs and infectious agents such as viruses (most notably herpes simplex). In its so-called 'minor' form, it is manifested by heterogeneous cutaneous eruption, at times bullous.

DIAGNOSIS

This patient has target-shaped lesions (lesion) caused by sulphonamides (aetiology), which usually resolve on discontinuing the drug (functional status).

QUESTIONS

What is the underlying aetiology?

- Infections (herpes simplex, mycoplasma, streptococcal)
- Drug hypersensitivity (sulphonamides, penicillin, barbiturates, salicylates, antimalarials)
- Collagen vascular disorder (SLE, dermatomyositis, periarteritis nodosa)
- Malignancy (carcinomas and lymphomas)
- Multiple myeloma
- Idiopathic: in 50% no cause may be found.

ADVANCED-LEVEL QUESTIONS

How would you investigate this patient?

- Viral titres, in particular for herpes simplex type 1
- Complement fixation test for mycoplasma
- Antistreptolysin O (ASO) titres

If the above are negative:

- Serum(s) antibodies
- Protein electrophoresis, urine for Bence-Jones proteins.

What is the histology of erythema multiforme?

Early lesions. Superficial perivascular lymphocytic infiltrate with oedema of the dermis, accompanied by degeneration and necrosis of keratinocytes and margination of lymphocytes at the dermoepidermal junction.

Late lesions. Upward migration of lymphocytes into the epidermis; discrete and confluent portions of the epidermis necrose, resulting in blister formation and subsequently erosions (as a result of sloughing of the epidermis).

Target lesions. Characterized by central necrosis surrounded by perivenular inflammation.

What do you understand by Stevens–Johnson syndrome?

Stevens–Johnson syndrome, also referred to as erythema multiforme major, is characterized by fever and mucous membrane involvement (usually oral cavity, eye and genital) in addition to the eruptions of erythema multiforme.

How would you manage a patient with erythema multiforme and Stevens–Johnson syndrome?

Erythema multiforme is a self-limiting condition, but Stevens–Johnson syndrome may be fatal:

- Symptomatic treatment with antipyretics, intravenous fluids and antibiotics.
- Systemic corticosteroids, although the role of steroids is controversial.
- Other immunosuppressive drugs used in recurrent erythema multiforme and Stevens–Johnson syndrome include levamisole, azathioprine, dapsone, thalidomide, high-dose intravenous immunoglobulin and ciclosporin.
- Aciclovir is recommended by some authors as a therapeutic trial in any patient with severe recurrent erythema multiforme, even if no preceding herpes simplex infection has been documented.
- Other therapeutic options:
  - Localized care including use of antibiotic creams, ointments, sterile dressing, special beds containing beads, amnion dressings on denuded skin
  - Ophthalmological care including use of artificial tears and topical vitamin A
  - Extensive denudation of the skin is best treated in a burns unit.

FC Johnson (1894–1934) and AM Stevens (1884–1945), both American paediatricians, described this condition in 1922 (Stevens AM, Johnson FC. A new eruptive fever associated with stomatitis and ophthalmia: report of two cases in children. Am J Dis Child 1922;24:526–33).

H Bence-Jones (1814–1873), English physician, St George's Hospital, London.

---

165 ERYTHEMA AB IGNE

INSTRUCTION

Examine this patient's legs.
Examine this patient's abdomen.

SALIENT FEATURES

History

- Ask the patient whether she exposed the affected area to heat.

Examination

- Reticular erythematous or pigmented rash, usually on the forelegs (or abdomen), known as 'Granny's tartan'

Proceed as follows:

- Look for features of hypothyroidism (pulse, ankle jerks).
- Tell the examiner that you would like to proceed as follows:
  - measure serum thyroxine and thyroid-stimulating hormone
  - investigate for chronic pancreatitis and intra-abdominal malignancy.

Note: If the rash is present over the anterior abdominal wall or lumbar region, it is very likely that there is an intra-abdominal malignancy or chronic pancreatitis.

DIAGNOSIS

This patient has a reticular pigmented rash (lesion) on the abdomen caused by local heat from a hot-water bag (aetiology); I would like to exclude an underlying intra-abdominal malignancy.

ADVANCED-LEVEL QUESTIONS

What do you know about erythema ab igne?

It is dusky discolouration of the skin that is associated with repeated exposure to heat. Typically the heat is not painful (<45°C) and does not burn the skin but produces a net-like reticulated pigmentation. It is usually found on the front of the lower legs of the elderly who sit in front of open fireplaces (Fig. 165.1) or and on the abdomen or back of patients with

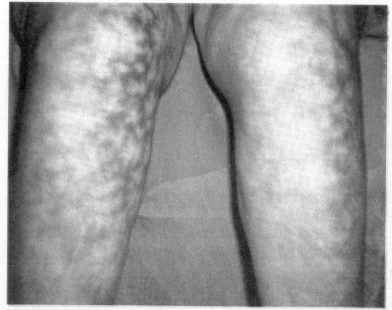

Fig. 165.1 Erythema ab igne.

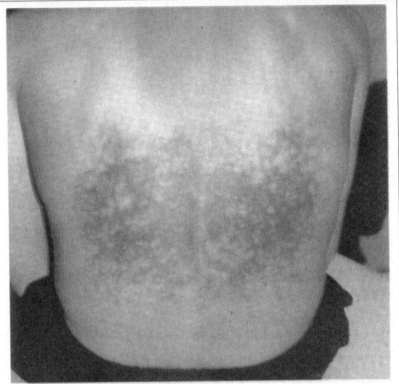

Fig. 165.2 Erythema ab igne produced by applying a heating pad to a painful back. (With permission from Townsend et al. 2007.)

chronic conditions who seek relief of pain by the long-term application of hot-water bottles or heating pads (Fig. 165.2).

How may erythema ab igne be complicated?

Epitheliomas may develop in keratoses, which form in later stages of this condition.

What other reticulated rashes do you know?

- Livedo reticularis (Fig. 165.3), seen in the following conditions:
  - Polyarteritis nodosa
  - SLE
  - Occult malignant neoplasm
  - Atherosclerotic microemboli to the skin
  - Physiological in young women (it is most apparent on the thighs of young females playing outdoor sports on a cold day).
- Cutaneous marmota seen in children.

Mention some skin abnormalities related to heat or cold

- Erythema ab igne
- Livedo reticularis (as a result of cold in young women)
- Raynaud's phenomenon
- Chilblains.

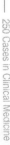

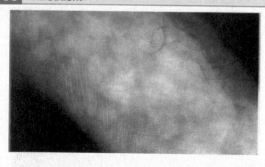

Fig. 165.3 Livedo reticularis.

166 HIRSUTISM

INSTRUCTION

Examine this patient.

SALIENT FEATURES

History

- Age of onset
- Rate of progression of hirsutism
- History of thinning of scalp hair, or deepening of voice
- History of obesity
- Drug history: corticosteroids, androgen, phenytoin, minoxidil, diazoxide, ciclosporin
- Take a menstrual history: oligomenorrhoea, infertility, acne, seborrhoea or voice change suggest polycystic ovaries
- Family history (familial).

Examination

- Excessive hair growth, particularly over the face (Fig. 166.1) and upper and lower limbs.
  Note: The amount and distribution of hair is an index of androgen effect. Terminal hairs on the face, around the areolae or on the lower abdomen or lower back may be normal, but hair on the upper back, shoulders and upper abdomen suggests a more marked increase in androgen production.

Proceed as follows:
- Tell the examiner that you would like to:
  - check the BP and urine for sugar
  - look for signs of virilization (receding hairline, muscular development, breast atrophy, clitoromegaly).
- Comment on cushingoid features, if any.

DIAGNOSIS

This patient has hirsutism (lesion) caused by polycystic ovarian disease (etiology) that is cosmetically unacceptable (functional status).

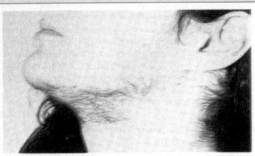

Fig. 166.1 Hirusutism.

QUESTIONS

What do you understand by the term hirsutism?

Hirsutism is the male pattern of hair growth in women and consists of excessive *terminal* hair (androgen-sensitive hair). It is abnormal, particularly on the chin, sternum, upper abdomen and upper back in women. Terminal hair may normally occur on the arms, legs, upper lips, linea alba and periareolar area in women. To be active in hair follicles, testosterone has to be converted locally to dihydrotestosterone by 5α-reductase. The sensitivity of the hair follicle to androgens is governed largely by cutaneous 5α-reductase activity. Consequently, similar androgen production profiles may produce different hair growth patterns in different women. Even in hirsute women, hair growth may have greatly variable patterns.

The degree of hirsutism can be assessed by the Ferriman–Gallwey Score, which records distribution and severity of excess body hair on a scale of 1–4 for nine regions (J Clin Endocrinol Metab 1961;21:1440–7).

Why do you want to take a menstrual history?

If menstruation is normal, it indicates that there is no increase in testosterone production. However, if menstruation is abnormal, the commonest cause is polycystic ovary disease (POCD or Stein–Leventhal syndrome), which is the underlying cause in 92% of the women with hirsutism (the popular belief that most cases of hirsutism are idiopathic is untrue).

ADVANCED-LEVEL QUESTIONS

What other causes of hirsutism are there?

- Cushing syndrome
- Adrenal or ovarian tumours
- Acromegaly
- Drugs:
  - those that increase *vellus* growth: phenytoin, minoxidil, diazoxide, ciclosporin
  - those that increase *terminal* hair growth: androgens.
- Familial
- Ethnic: a 'male-pattern' of hirsutism is common in women whose ancestors hail from southern Europe.

What is the relationship between body weight and hirsutism?

Hirsute women are more likely to be obese than non-hirsute women. Therefore, weight loss must be a priority in treating overweight women with hirsutism.

What is the role of testosterone in hirsutism?

Testosterone is the most potent androgen and is derived directly from ovarian secretion (60%) and from peripheral conversion of androstenedione (40%). About 65% of testosterone is strongly bound to sex hormone-binding globulin (SHBG) and 33% is weakly bound to albumin. The remaining 2% is free testosterone and can enter target cells to exert its androgenic effect. Other androgens include androstenedione (secreted in equal amounts by adrenals and ovaries) and dehydroepiandrosterone (derived exclusively from the adrenals).

What is the pathophysiology of polycystic ovary disease?

It is caused by an abnormality of pulsatile secretion of gonadotrophin-releasing hormone (GnRH), which causes increased secretion of luteinizing hormone (LH) and follicle-stimulating hormone (FSH). This results in hyperplasia of the ovarian thecal cell leading to multiple follicular cysts and excessive androgen synthesis and anovulation.

Remember: POCD is the association of hyperandrogenism with chronic anovulation in women without specific underlying diseases of adrenals or pituitary glands.

How would you investigate suspected polycystic ovary disease?

- Ovarian ultrasonography is the most accurate investigation; typically it shows thickened capsules, multiple cysts of 3–5 mm diameter and a hyperechogenic stroma (Fig. 166.2).
- Biochemistry:
  - Total testosterone levels may be normal, but free androgens are raised
  - SHBG is low
  - LH:FSH ratio is raised, usually greater than 2:1, but FSH level is low or normal
  - Mild hyperprolactinaemia is common and rarely exceeds 1500 mU/l.

Is glucose metabolism affected in polycystic ovary disease?

POCD is associated with hyperinsulinaemia and insulin resistance, and consequently patients may have impaired glucose tolerance. The site of insulin resistance is skeletal muscle and fatty tissue, not the liver (as in

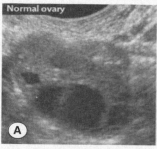
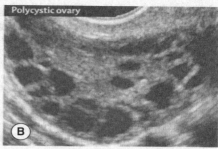

Fig. 166.2 Transvaginal ultrasonography during the follicular phase of a menstrual cycle, showing the fluid-filled antrum of a developing follicle (dark circle); the polycystic ovary is typically enlarged and contains an abnormally increased number of developing follicles (With permission from Mitani et al. 2007.)

non-insulin-dependent diabetes mellitus). It is believed that full expression of POCD requires both the insulin abnormality and the disorder of androgen biosynthesis.

How would you treat hirsutism?

- Treatment is directed towards the underlying cause of hyperandrogenism
- Mild hyperandrogenism that is idiopathic or mild POCD: oral contraceptives
- Severe hirsutism: anti-androgens (spironolactone, cyproterone acetate, flutamide) and finasteride (5α-reductase inhibitor) prevent the cutaneous conversion of testosterone to active dihydrotestosterone; GnRH analogues (leuprolide, nafarelin)
- Local treatment: shaving, epilation, laser-assisted epilation (phototricholysis), waxing, electrolysis or bleaching.

IF Stein (1887–1976), a US gynaecologist, and ML Leventhal (1901–1971), a US obstetrician (Stein IF, Leventhal ML. Amenorrhea associated with bilateral polycystic ovaries. Am J Obstet Gynecol 1935;29:181–191).

---

167 ACANTHOSIS NIGRICANS

INSTRUCTION

Perform a general examination.

SALIENT FEATURES

History

- Age (>40 years of age more likely to be associated with malignancy; in younger individuals more likely to be associated with endocrinopathies)
- Carcinoma stomach or other neoplasms (in 80% the cancer is abdominal and in 60% the cancer is in the stomach): symptoms of weight loss, asthenia and decreased appetite
- Diabetes mellitus (insulin-resistant diabetes)
- Endocrinopathies: acromegaly, Cushing's disease, polycystic ovaries, hypothyroidism, hyperthyroidism.

Examination

- Black, velvety overgrowth seen in the axillae (Fig. 167.1), neck, umbilicus, nipples, groins or facial skin
- Acrochordons or skin tags may accompany acanthosis nigricans and occur in similar areas.

Proceed as follows:

- Look for the following signs:
  - Tripe palms (roughness of the palmar and plantar skin; Fig. 167.2)
  - Filiform growths around the face and mouth, and over the tongue (when mouth and tongue are involved it is highly suggestive of an underlying neoplasm) (Fig. 167.3).

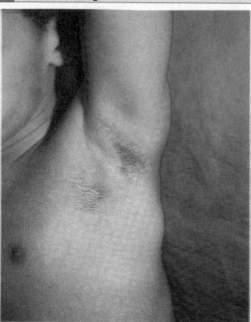

Fig. 167.1 Acanthosis nigricans in the axilla.

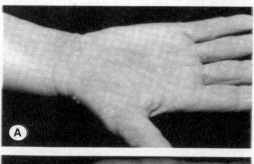

Fig. 167.2 Tripe palms. (With permission from Moore, Devere 2008.)

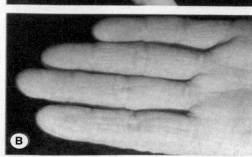

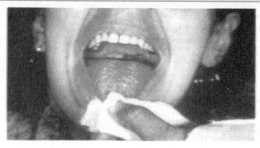

Fig. 167.3 Malignant acanthosis nigricans in the mouth. (With permission from Moore, Devere 2008.)

- Tell the examiner that you would like to investigate for:
  - underlying malignancy, in particular adenocarcinoma of the stomach
  - for endocrine disorders (diabetes, Cushing syndrome, acromegaly).
- Comment if the patient is obese or non-obese (when pigmented verrucous areas develop in the body folds of non-obese individuals, about 80–90% have an underlying gastric cancer).

DIAGNOSIS

This patient has a velvety black overgrowth in the axillae (lesion) and I would like to exclude an underlying adenocarcinoma, particularly of the stomach (aetiology).

ADVANCED-LEVEL QUESTIONS

What are the types of acanthosis nigricans?
(1) Benign, (2) obesity-associated, (3) syndromic, (4) malignant, (5) acral, (6) unilateral, (7) medication-induced, and (8) mixed type.

What is the histology of acanthosis nigricans?
- Undulating epidermis with numerous sharp peaks and valleys
- Variable amount of hyperplasia, hyperkeratosis and slight pigmentation of the basal cell layer (but no melanocytic hyperplasia).

With which conditions is acanthosis nigricans associated?
- Benign conditions:
  - Diabetes, associated with marked insulin resistance
  - Cushing syndrome
  - Acromegaly
  - Stein–Leventhal syndrome
  - Obesity: nearly 75% of these patients develop acanthosis nigricans.
- Malignant conditions (caused by abnormal production of epidermal growth factors):
  - Adenocarcinomas (usually stomach, GI tract, and uterus; less commonly lung, ovary, breast and prostate)
  - Lymphomas (rarely).

What is the relationship between the course of the skin lesion and the underlying malignancy?
Acanthosis nigricans may precede the neoplasm by >5 years. In about two-thirds of cases, the course parallels that of the tumour, including remission with cure.

Mention some cutaneous manifestations of visceral malignancy

- Dermatomyositis (in individuals >40 years, the prevalence of internal malignancy particularly lung and breast cancer is increased)
- Migratory thrombophlebitis
- Ichthyosis (when acquired suggests GI leiomyosarcoma, lymphoma, multiple myeloma)
- Paget's disease of the nipple
- Tylosis or palmar hyperkeratosis (suggests oesophageal cancer)
- Lesar-Trelat sign, which is the sudden appearance of multiple seborrheic keratosis and suggests underlying cancer in the elderly
- Necrotic migratory erythema suggests tumours of the alpha cells of the pancreas, which secrete glucagon
- Bazex syndrome or acrokeratosis paraneoplastica suggests malignancy of the upper respiratory tract, particularly squamous cell carcinomas of the mouth, pharynx, larynx, oesophagus and bronchus
- Lymphamatoid papulosis is cutaneous lymphoid infiltration associated with T cell lymphomas or Hodgkin's disease.

What is the therapy for acanthosis nigricans?

Some patients have benefited from medications such as metformin, oral isotretinoin, topical retinoic acid, topical salicylic acid and oral fish oil. Successes have been reported with the CO laser and the long-pulsed Alexandrite laser.

Note: Acanthosis is hyperplasia of the stratum spinosum of the epidermis.

168 LIPOATROPHY

INSTRUCTION

Look at this patient.
Look here (examiner pointing at the patient's thighs).

SALIENT FEATURES

History

- Ask whether the patient is taking insulin for diabetes.
- Is there a past history of renal disease (mesangiocapillary glomerulonephritis)?
- History of HIV and whether patient is receiving antiretroviral agents
- Family history.

Examination

- Atrophy of the subcutaneous fat leading to disfiguring excavations and depressed areas (Figs 168.1 and 168.2).

DIAGNOSIS

This patient has atrophy of subcutaneous fat or lipoatrophy (lesion) caused by local injection of subcutaneous insulin (aetiology).

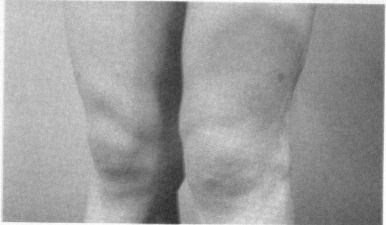

Fig. 168.1 Lipoatrophy.

ADVANCED-LEVEL QUESTIONS

With which conditions is lipoatrophy associated?

- Mesangiocapillary glomerulonephritis
- Localized scleroderma
- Morphea
- Chronic relapsing panniculitis
- HIV.

What advice would you give this patient on insulin?

The insulin should be changed to a more purified form. The purified form should be injected directly into the atrophic area, which often results in the restoration of the local contours.

What is the mechanism of lipoatrophy?

It results from an immune reaction.

Can lipohypertrophy occur with insulin injections?

Yes, as a consequence of insulin being deposited in the same location repeatedly; it has an estimated prevalence of 3.6%. The condition can be unsightly clinically and theoretically could lead to erratic insulin absorption. The precise pathogenesis remains unclear, but possible mechanisms include immune reaction to insulin or excipients of the injection solution, injury from cold insulin, or trauma from repeated local injections. Rotation of injection sites can prevent this complication. It can occur with purified insulins and responds best to liposuction.

What is relationship between lipoatrophy and human immunodeficiency virus?

HIV-1-infected patients receiving antiretroviral therapy have been reported to have abnormal fat distribution including (a) lipoatrophy or loss of subcutaneous fat and (b) central or visceral fat accumulation. Typically these patients have wasting of face and limbs along with adipose tissue

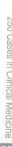

250 Cases in Clinical Medicine

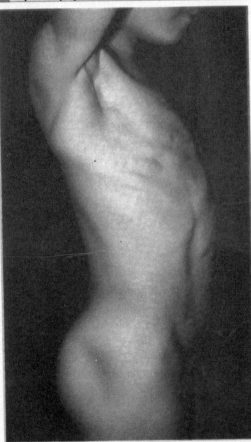

Fig. 168.2 Lipoatrophy.

accumulations in the abdomen and back of the neck, the latter giving a 'buffalo hump' appearance. It was initially considered to be only caused by HIV-1 protease inhibitors but subsequently this has not been substantiated. It has also been associated with nucleoside reverse transcriptase inhibitors (NRTI), via mitochondrial toxicity and interference with lipid metabolism (Lancet 2001;357:592–8). Stavudine-based regimens have a higher cumulative prevalence of lipoatrophy than regimens based on zidovudine, abacavir or tenofovir. Regimens based on nelfinavir are associated with more rapid fat loss than efavirenz. In general, thymidine-based nucleoside analogues have been most associated with lipoatrophy and protease inhibitor drugs most associated with the metabolic syndrome. Leptin deficiency contributes to the insulin resistance and other metabolic abnormalities associated with severe lipodystrophy. Leptin-replacement therapy improves glycaemic control and decreased triglyceride levels in patients with lipodystrophy and leptin deficiency.

What are genes implicated in familial lipoatrophy?

● Familial partial lipodystrophy of the Dunnigan variety. Genes encoding lamins A and C
● Congenital generalized lipodystrophy *(Berardinelli–Seip syndrome)*. Two molecularly distinct forms have been defined:
  ● Type 1: mutations in *AGPAT2*, the gene for 1-acylglycerol-3-phosphate *O*-acyltransferase
  ● Type 2: mutation in Bscl2, the gene encoding seipin gene.
● Some patients have neither type, so that additional genes are most likely involved, possibly mutation affecting the gene for the peroxisome-proliferator–activated receptor-γ.

The 1923 Nobel Prize in Medicine was awarded for the discovery of insulin to a Canadian surgeon, Sir Fredrick G Banting (1891–1941), and a Scottish physiologist, John JR Macleod (1876–1935) working in Toronto. Banting shared his monetary prize with Charles Best whereas Macleod shared his prize with JJ Collip (the latter purified insulin to the point that it could be used in humans). Macleod corrected Banting's deficiencies on carbohydrate metabolism and provided him with laboratory support including the services of a graduate student in physiology viz., Charles Best. Macleod was from Aberdeen.

---

169 LUPUS PERNIO

INSTRUCTION

Look at this patient's face.

SALIENT FEATURES

History

● Shortness of breath, cough, chest discomfort
● Fatigue, weight loss, malaise, anorexia
● History of therapy with interferon-alfa (particularly in patients with hepatitis C; interferon-alfa increases interferon-γ and interleukin-2, thus promoting granuloma formation).

Examination

● Reddish blue or violaceous plaques on the nose (Fig. 169.1), cheeks, ears and fingers, with telangiectasia over and around the plaques (Fig. 169.2).
Proceed as follows:
● Tell the examiner that you would like to do radiography for hilar adenopathy and examine the eyes for ocular manifestations

DIAGNOSIS

This patient has violaceous plaques on his face (lesion) caused by sarcoidosis (aetiology), which is cosmetically disfiguring (functional status).

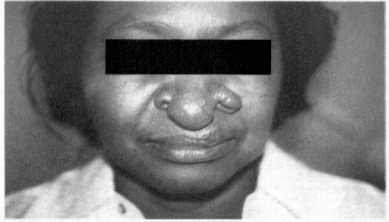

Fig. 169.1 Lupus pernio plaques on the nose.

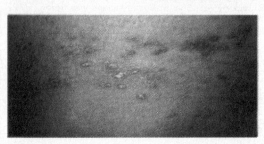

Fig. 169.2 Telangiectasia over and around the plaques.

ADVANCED-LEVEL QUESTIONS

What is the differential diagnosis of such a lesion?
- Rhinophyma (p. 633)
- Lupus vulgaris
- Leprosy.

What are the cutaneous manifestations of sarcoid?
- Erythema nodosum (p. 665)
- Micropapular sarcoid
- Scar infiltration
- Sarcoid plaques of limbs, shoulders, buttocks and thighs.

How may sarcoid present?
- Acute sarcoidosis usually presents in the third decade, characterized by erythema nodosum, parotid enlargement and hilar lymphadenopathy.
- Chronic sarcoidosis usually presents in the fifth decade with an insidious onset characterized by fatigue, dyspnoea, arthralgia and lupus pernio. Bone cysts are another feature.

How would you investigate such a patient?
- FBC and ESR: leukopenia, eosinophilia and raised ESR

- Chest radiography. Three stages of sarcoidosis are defined depending on radiographic findings, although these stages do not indicate chronology of disease:
  - I: bilateral hilar adenopathy alone
  - II: both hilar adenopathy and lung parenchymal involvement
  - III: parenchymal involvement alone.
- Slit-lamp examination of the eyes
- Kviem's test: the antigen is cultured in human spleen and thus, increasingly, it is recommended that this test should not be performed because of the risk of transmitting viral infections
- Mantoux test: skin anergy is present in 70%
- Serum ACE levels: raised in 40–80% with active disease, although this finding is neither sensitive nor specific enough to have diagnostic significance
- Lung function tests: usually restrictive changes with decreased lung volumes and diffusing capacity; occasionally airflow obstruction
- Serum calcium levels: hypercalcaemia in 10% of patients
- Gallium-67 scan
- Bronchoalveolar lavage: usually characterized by an increase in lymphocytes and a high CD4:CD8 T cell ratio
- Histological confirmation is by the presence of non-caseating granulomas with typical manifestations (fibrotic response develops over time) in biopsy of lung (transbronchial), lymph node, skin, liver, gums or minor salivary glands.

What is the prognosis and treatment of sarcoidosis?

- Acute sarcoidosis usually regresses spontaneously within 2 years and does not recur; it may not require treatment.
- Chronic sarcoidosis may require systemic cortiocosteroids in order to prevent serious disability and even death from respiratory failure.

What is the treatment of cutaneous sarcoid?

Monthly intralesional triamcinolone injections, topical and systemic steroids, hydroxychloroquine, allopurinol, thalidomide and tranilast (N Engl J Med 1997;336:1224–34).

What are the specific indications for systemic steroids in sarcoidosis?

- Progressive deterioration in lung function, particularly transfer factor and vital capacity. Serial evaluation should be performed every 2 months initially, gradually increasing the intervals between follow-up to about 4–5 months; patients should be followed for at least 2 years after steroids are stopped
- CNS involvement
- Hypercalcaemia
- Severe ocular disease
- Hepatitis
- Cutaneous lesions
- Constitutional symptoms
- Symptomatic pulmonary lesions.

What are the ocular manifestations of sarcoidosis?

- Anterior uveitis, seen in about 5% of all cases and either acute or chronic: mutton fat keratic precipitates, iris nodules

- Retinal vasculitis, neovascularization
- Vitreous opacities
- Choroidal granulomata
- Optic nerve granuloma.

What is Löfgren syndrome?

Erythema nodosum, hilar adenopathy and polyarthralgias in a patient with sarcoidosis.

What is the source of the raised serum angiotensin converting enzyme in sarcoidosis?

It is derived from the cell membranes of epithelioid cells in the sarcoid granuloma and its synthesis is controlled by epithelioid cells.

What is Blau syndrome?

It is a multisystem granulomatous disorder of the skin, eyes and joints that resembles childhood sarcoidosis; it was described by Edward Blau, a Wisconsin pediatrician (Lancet 1999;354:1035).

Is there any relationship between viral infections and sarcoid?

Variant human herpesvirus type 8 DNA sequences have been found in sarcoid tissue. Also mycobacteria-like 16S ribosomal RNA are more frequently found in sarcoid tissue but this does not indicate infection by a particular mycobacterial species (Lancet 1997;350:655–61).

What is the cardinal feature in the pathogenesis?

The cardinal feature of sarcoidosis is the presence of CD4 T cells that interact with antigen-presenting cells to initiate the formation and maintenance of granulomas.

What are the diagnostic features of cardiac sarcoidosis?

- *Histologic diagnosis group*: cardiac sarcoidosis is confirmed when histologic analysis of operative or endomyocardial biopsy specimens demonstrates epithelioid granuloma without caseating granuloma (Dis Mon 2009;55:675–92).
- *Clinical diagnosis group*: in patients with a histologic diagnosis of extracardiac sarcoidosis, cardiac sarcoidosis is suspected when item (a) and one or more of items (b) to (e) are present:
  (a) ECG: complete right bundle branch block, left axis deviation, atrioventricular block, ventricular tachycardia, premature ventricular contraction or abnormal Q or ST–T change
  (b) Abnormal wall motion, regional wall thinning or dilatation of the LV
  (c) Myocardial scintigraphy: perfusion defect detected by thallium-201 or abnormal accumulation of gallium-67 or technetium-99m
  (d) Abnormal intracardiac pressure: low cardiac output, abnormal wall motion or depressed ejection fraction of the LV
  (e) Interstitial fibrosis or cellular infiltration over moderate grade even if the findings are non-specific.

Further reading

James DG, Jones Williams W: *Sarcoidosis and other graulomatous disorders*, Philadelphia, PA, 1984, Saunders.
Spalton DJ, Saunders MD: Fundus changes in histologically confirmed sarcoidosis, *Br J Ophthalmol* 65:348–358, 1981.

MA Kviem (b. 1892), a Norwegian pathologist.

C Mantoux (1877–1947), a French physician from Cannes, who showed that his intradermal test was more sensitive than the older Pirquet subcutaneous tests using tuberculin.

Norwegian dermatologist Caesar P.M. Boeck (1845–1917) from Olso, Norway, coined the term to describe skin nodules characterized by compact, sharply defined foci of 'epithelioid cells with large pale nuclei and also a few giant cells'. Thinking this resembled sarcoma, he called the condition 'multiple benign sarcoid of the skin'.

S Löfgren, a Swedish physician.

D Geraint James, contemporary Professor of Medicine, Royal Free Hospital, London; his chief interest is sarcoidosis. His wife, Dame Sheila Sherlock, is a renowned hepatologist.

170 XANTHELASMA

INSTRUCTION

Examine this patient's eyes.

SALIENT FEATURES

History

- Jaundice, generalized pigmentation, itching (primary biliary cirrhosis)
- Family history of hyperlipidaemia
- History of diabetes, hypertension.
- Symptoms of hypothyroidism (p. 516)
- History of oral contraceptives.

Examination

- Xanthelasmata (flat yellow nodules or plaques) seen on eyelids and around both eyes, particularly on the inner canthus (Fig. 170.1)
- Look for the following signs:
  - Corneal arcus
  - Jaundice, generalized pigmentation, scratch marks (primary biliary cirrhosis)

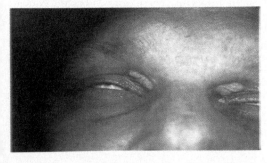

Fig. 170.1 Xanthelasma. Multiple, soft, yellow plaques involving the eyelid.

- Tendon xanthomata
- Palmar xanthomata.
- Tell the examiner that you would like to check the following:
  - Urine sugar
  - Blood pressure
  - Pulse and ankle jerks (hypothyroidism).

Remember: Blood lipids can often be normal.

DIAGNOSIS

This patient has xanthelasmata on the eyelids (lesions) and I would like to test serum lipids to exclude an underlying lipid disorder (aetiology).

ADVANCED-LEVEL QUESTIONS

In which conditions are xanthelasmata seen?
Those in which there is an increase in serum cholesterol (see Fig. 173.1C–E):

- Type IIb hyperlipidaemia: increased cholesterol and triglycerides
- Type IIa hyperlipidaemia: increased cholesterol only
- Type III hyperlipidaemia: equal increase in cholesterol and triglycerides.

Mention a few secondary causes of hyperlipidaemia
Diabetes mellitus, hypothyroidism, nephrotic syndrome, cholestatic jaundice, excess alcohol intake, oral contraceptives.

How would you manage a patient with hyperlipidaemia?
- Lifestyle advice
- Dietary modification (usually adequate for those whose cholesterol level is in the range 6.5–8 mmol/l)
- Avoidance of alcohol, smoking, oestrogens and thiazides
- Exercise
- Control of hypertension and diabetes
- Lipid-lowering drugs.

Mention a few lipid-lowering drugs
- Ion exchange resin: colestyramine
- Fibrates: bezafibrate, gemfibrozil
- Sitostanol-ester margarine (a plant sterol that reduces serum cholesterol concentration by inhibiting cholesterol absorption)
- Hydroxymethylglutaryl (HMG) coenzyme A (CoA) reductase inhibitors: simvastatin, pravastatin, lovastatin. These drugs block the endogenous synthesis of cholesterol and reduce levels of LDL cholesterol
- Nicotinic acid derivatives: nicotinic acid, probucol.

Are HMG CoA reductase inhibitors useful in patients with hypercholesterolaemia and coronary heart disease?
Yes, the Scandinavian Simvastatin Survival Study (the 4S trial) demonstrated a survival benefit from lowering cholesterol with simvastatin in patients with coronary disease (Lancet 1994;344:1383–9). In the LIPID study (Long-Term Intervention with Pravastatin in Ischemic Heart Disease), a major secondary prevention trial, pravastatin administered to 9000 patients with unstable angina or acute myocardial infarction significantly reduced total mortality by 23%, coronary heart disease

mortality by 24%, the need for coronary revascularization, the number of admissions to hospitals (Lancet 2000;355:1871–5) and the risk of stroke by 20% (N Engl J Med 2000;343:317–26). The Lescol in Severe Atherosclerosis (LISA) study evaluated fluvastatin in patients with coronary artery disease and hypercholesterolaemia and found that it reduced cardiac events by 71%.

What is the role of HMG CoA reductase inhibitors in patients with hypercholesterolaemia and no signs of coronary heart disease?

A study from Scotland showed that treatment with pravastatin significantly reduced the incidence of myocardial infarction (30% reduction) and death from cardiovascular causes (33% reduction) without adversely affecting the risk of death from non-cardiovascular causes in men with moderate hypercholesterolaemia and without a history of myocardial infarction (N Engl J Med 1995;333:1301–1307).

What is the role of HMG CoA reductase inhibitors in patients with coronary artery disease and 'average' cholesterol levels?

The CARE study (Cholesterol and Recurrent Events Trials Investigators) found that pravastatin lowered rates of coronary events (including fatal events and non-fatal myocardial infarction) in majority of the patients with coronary disease who have average cholesterol levels (N Engl J Med 1996;335:1001–9).

What is the effect of statins on elevated triglyceride concentrations?

Serum triglyceride concentrations are reduced by all statins with atovastatin and simvastatin having the greatest effect. Higher the baseline concentration of triglycerides, greater is the reduction induced by statin therapy.

Mention some adverse effects of statins?

- Common: GI upset, myalgias and hepatitis
- Rare: rash, myopathy, peripheral neuropathy, insomnia, bad dreams, difficulty in sleeping or concentrating.

What is the effect of meals on statin absorption?

Lovastatin is better absorbed when taken with food whereas pravastatin is best taken on an empty stomach or at bedtime. Food has less of an effect on the absorption of other statins.

Why are all statins best given in the evening?

Because the rate of endogenous cholesterol synthesis is higher at night.

In a patient with hypercholesterolaemia on treatment with statins who requires further lowering of LDL cholesterol, what second drug would you add if the patient's serum HDL is low?

Nicotinic acid is the preferred second drug. Nicotinic acid usually increases serum HDL concentrations by 30%, fibrates by 10–15%, statins by 5–10% and bile acid resins by 1–2% (N Engl J Med 1999;341:498–511). The ARBITER 6–HALTS (Arterial Biology for the Investigation of the Treatment Effects of Reducing Cholesterol 6–HDL and LDL Treatment Strategies) trial compared the effects of two combination therapies — either niacin or ezetimibe added to long-term statin therapy — on carotid intima–media thickness over a 14-month period. Addition of extended-release niacin caused significant regression in thickness that was superior to that seen with ezetimibe (N Engl J Med 2009; 361:2113–22). The two much-anticipated outcome studies for niacin are AIM-HIGH, due out in 2011, and HPS2-THRIVE, which is expected to be completed in 2013.

What is the role of statins in patients with elevated low density lipoproteins and LDL and high-sensitivity C-reactive protein?

In the JUPITER trial (Justification for the Use of Statins in Primary Prevention: an Intervention Trial Evaluating Rosuvastatin), rosuvastatin significantly reduced the primary end-point (a composite of non-fatal myocardial infarction, non-fatal stroke, hospitalization for unstable angina, arterial revascularization, or confirmed death from cardiovascular causes) in apparently healthy people with LDL cholesterol levels of <1.3 g/l (3.4 mmol/l) but with elevated high-sensitivity C-reactive protein levels of ≥2.0 mg/l (N Engl J Med 2008;359:2195–207).

James Scott, FRS contemporary Professor and Chairman of the Department of Medicine at Hammersmith Hospital, London, is a physician, biochemist and molecular biologist. He has made a considerable contribution to lipid and cardiovascular research.

---

171 NECROBIOSIS LIPOIDICA DIABETICORUM

INSTRUCTION

Look at this patient's legs.
Examine this patient's back.

SALIENT FEATURES

History

- History of diabetes (according to a recent study from Ireland only a minority of the patients have diabetes; Br J Dermatol 1999;40:283–6).

Examination

- Usually seen in females (two to four times more frequently than in men)
- Sharply demarcated oval plaques seen on the shin (Fig. 171.1), arms or back
- The plaques have a shiny surface with yellow waxy atrophic centres and brownish red margins with surrounding telangiectasia.

Proceed as follows:

- Tell the examiner that you would like to check the urine for sugar.

DIAGNOSIS

This patient has plaques with yellow waxy centres on the shins (lesions) caused by diabetes mellitus (aetiology); the lesions are cosmetically disfiguring (functional status).

Remember: In necrobiosis lipoidica diabeticorum, although the shins, ankles and feet are typically affected, 15% of patients may have lesions elsewhere.

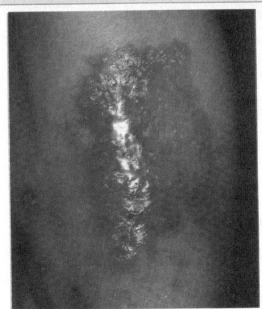

Fig. 171.1 Necrobiosis lipoidica diabeticorum. Well-demarcated, waxy erythematous plaques with prominent telangiectasias.

ADVANCED-LEVEL QUESTIONS

What is the histology of these lesions?

Microscopical studies have shown that it is a disorder of collagen degeneration characterized by a granulomatous response (surrounded by epithelioid and giant cells), thickening of the walls of blood vessels and fat deposition. The exact cause is unknown. Necrobiosis lipoidica diabeticorum may be an antibody-mediated vasculitis with secondary collagen degeneration or the microangiopathy of diabetes (but it is not correlated with the extent of glucose control).

What may complicate it?

Ulceration of the plaque.

What treatment is available for such lesions?

- Good diabetic control
- Whirlpool therapy, occlusive dressings, aspirin, pentoxifylline
- Local steroids.
- Excision and skin grafting
- Hyperbaric oxygen (Diabetes Metab 1998;24:156–9).

Flare-ups are frequent. No treatment is completely effective.

What other skin lesions are usually seen on the shins?

- Erythema nodosum (p. 665)
- Pretibial myxoedema (p. 521)
- Diabetic dermopathy
- Erythema ab igne (p. 599)
- Livedo reticularis.

What are the other skin lesions seen in diabetes?

- Granuloma annulare
- Chronic pyogenic infections and carbuncles (indicating poor control)
- Eruptive xanthomata (from hypertriglyceridaemia associated with poor glycaemic control) (p. 625)
- Xanthelasmata (p. 615)
- Lipoatrophy and lipohypertrophy (p. 609)
- Leg ulcers and gangrene
- Acanthosis nigricans (p. 605)
- 'Pebbles' on the dorsal aspect of the fingers (Postgrad Med 2000;107:207–10)
- Peripheral anhydriosis (from autonomic neuropathy)
- Vulval candidiasis.

172 RADIOTHERAPY MARKS

INSTRUCTION

Look at this patient's chest.

PATIENT 1

SALIENT FEATURES

History

- History of breast cancer
- Ask about chemotherapy and schedule of radiotherapy.

Examination

- Telangiectasia over the chest wall
- There may be a unilateral mastectomy.

DIAGNOSIS

This patient has telangiectasia and a unilateral mastectomy (lesion), indicating that she has had radiotherapy (aetiology) for breast cancer in the past.

PATIENT 2

SALIENT FEATURES

Examination

- India-ink marks over the chest (Fig. 172.1)
- Localized erythema in the same region.

DIAGNOSIS

This patient has India-ink marks over the chest with localized erythema (lesion) indicating that she is currently undergoing radiotherapy treatment (aetiology).

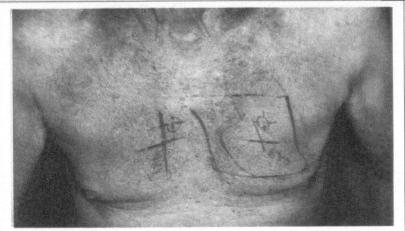

Fig. 172.1 Radiation therapy marks

ADVANCED-LEVEL QUESTIONS

Which other normal tissues, apart from the skin, are affected by radiation therapy?

Tissues that exhibit early or late damage from radiation therapy include mucosa, spinal cord, bone marrow and lymphoid system. To minimize these effects, radiation is normally delivered in a fractionated manner allowing recovery of normal host tissues (but not of tumour).

The most serious potential late complications of radiation therapy to the breast are injury to the lungs and heart and the risk of inducing secondary cancers, such as sarcoma, lung cancer and contralateral breast cancer. Early studies of radiation therapy in patients with breast cancer demonstrated that inclusion of the LV in the high-dose region increased the long-term risk of death from cardiovascular disease.

Radiation treatments for breast cancer are now given from linear accelerators and typically use medial and lateral opposed tangential fields that obliquely cross the anterior chest wall. CT planning of therapy ensures that the heart is outside the radiation field and the included lung volume is minimal.

What modalities may be used to minimize the side effects of radiation?

- Fractionation of dose
- Rendering the tumour more sensitive to radiotherapy by prior chemotherapy, thereby reducing the dose
- Regional hypothermia (40–42°C), particularly in superficial tumours and relatively bulky non-vascular tumours
- Radiolabelled antibodies, which deliver high levels of radiation locally to the tumour bed.

How is radiotherapy usually delivered?

It is usually delivered either as brachytherapy (where the radiation source is close to the tumour) or as teletherapy (where supervoltage radiotherapy is usually delivered with a linear acclerator).

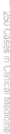

250 Cases in Clinical Medicine

In which conditions is radiotherapy beneficial?
- **Malignant conditions**
- Radiotherapy as the sole agent with a curative intent in Hodgkin's disease, some neoplasms of brain and spinal cord, oral cavity, pharynx, oesophagus, laryngeal tumours (permitting cure without loss of voice), tumours of cervix and vagina cavity
- Radiation with surgery in cancers of lung, breast, urinary bladder, seminomas, ovary, uterus, sarcomas of soft tissue and testicular seminomas
- Radiation as adjuvant to chemotherapy in lymphomas, lung cancers and childhood cancers
- Radiation as palliative therapy for pain and or dysfunction in superior vena caval obstruction, dysphagia of terminal illness, upper airway obstruction, spinal cord compression and pericardial tamponade secondary to malignant pericardial tumours.

- **Non-malignant conditions**
- Exophthalmos
- Rheumatoid arthritis (total lymphoid irradiation is an experimental therapeutic procedure)
- Ankylosing spondylitis, where local external irradiation of an involved peripheral joint or injected radiation synovectomy can be valuable in ameliorating pain and allowing mobility. Spinal irradiation is no longer used because of the risk of haematological malignancy.

What are the side effects of radiotherapy?
- Acute toxicity: systemic symptoms including malaise, fatigue, anorexia, nausea and vomiting, diarrhoea and local skin and mucosal changes. Bone marrow suppression may occur following irradiation to the pelvis and long bones
- Long-term toxicity: cutaneous hyperpigmentation, impaired function of irradiated viscera, bone necrosis, myelopathy and secondary malignancies.

What is the difference between the units gray and sievert, and which is the unit of radiation dose?
Sievert (Sv) is a measure of the biological effect of a dose, whereas gray (Gy) measures the absorbed dose.

What do you know about the inverse square law?
The inverse square law states that radiation intensity decreases with the square of the distance away from a point source of radiation. The intensity of radiation at any given radius is given by the source strength divided by the area of the sphere. For example, the energy intensity three times as far from a point source is spread over nine times the area, hence one ninth the intensity.

The use of radiation began shortly after the discovery of X-rays by Roentgen in 1895 (Lancet 1997;349(suppl II):1–3).

RAGE (Radiotherapy Action Group Exposure) is a pressure group formed by patients who suffered the side effects of radiotherapy including brachial plexus neuropathy, often resulting in severe pain and the loss of use of the arm.

173 TENDON XANTHOMATA

INSTRUCTION

Look at this patient's hands.

SALIENT FEATURES

History

- Family history of hyperlipidaemia
- History of premature coronary artery disease.

Examination

- Tendon xanthomata seen on the extensor tendons and becoming more prominent when the patient clenches his fist (Fig. 173.1B)

Proceed as follows:

- Look at other tendons, particularly the patellar and Achilles tendon (Fig. 173.1A)
- Look at the eyes for xanthelasmata (see Fig. 170.1) and corneal arcus
- Tell the examiner that you would like to:
  - check fasting lipids, in particular for an increase in cholesterol level
  - screen family members for hypercholesterolaemia
  - examine the heart for aortic valve stenosis caused by lipid deposition (N Engl J Med 2003;349:717).

DIAGNOSIS

This patient has tendon xanthomata (lesion) caused by hypercholestero-laemia (aetiology).

QUESTIONS

In which condition are these seen?

Familial hypercholesterolaemia, an autosomal dominant trait with an excess of LDL or β-lipoprotein in the blood. It occurs in 1 in 200–500 of the population.

ADVANCED-LEVEL QUESTIONS

What is the basic defect?

Autosomal dominant familial hypercholesterolaemia is caused by muta-tions either in the gene encoding the LDL receptor or in the gene encoding apolipoprotein B (the protein in LDL cholesterol that is recognized by the LDL receptor).

Recessive familial hypercholesterolaemia arises from mutations in the gene encoding an adapter protein involved in the internalization of the LDL receptor.

Another variant of familial hypercholesterolaemia with dominant inheritance and an identical phenotype to the other forms is associated with missense mutations in *PCSK9*, encoding protease proprotein conver-ase subtilisin/kexin type 9.

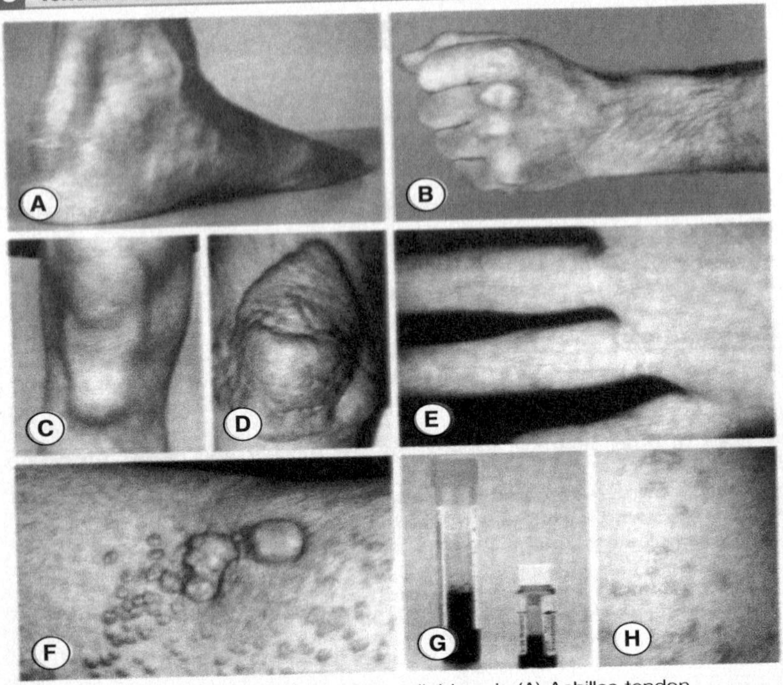

Fig. 173.1 Clinical manifestations of hyperlipidaemia (A) Achilles tendon xanthoma (heterozygous familial hypercholesterolaemia). (B) Tendon xanthomata on dorsum of hand (heterozygous familial hypercholesterolaemia). (C) Subperiosteal xanthomata (heterozygous familial hypercholesterolaemia). (D) Planar xanthoma in antecubital fossa (homozygous familial hypercholesterolaemia). (E) Striate palmar xanthomata (type III hyperlipoproteinaemia). (F) Tuberoeruptive xanthomata on elbow and extensor surface of arm (type III hyperlipoproteinaemia). (G) Milky plasma from patient with acute abdominal pain (severe hypertriglyceridaemia). (H) Eruptive xanthomata on extensor surface of forearm (severe hypertriglyceridaemia). (With permission from Durrington 2003.)

At what age do these patients manifest the condition?

Homozygotes usually have xanthomata at birth or as children. They have a predisposition to ischaemic heart disease, which usually results in death before the age of 30 years. About 50% of heterozygotes also present by the same age.

What are xanthomata?

Xanthomata are tumour-like collections of foamy histiocytes within the dermis. There are five types of xanthoma:

- Eruptive xanthoma (seen in types I, IIb, III, IV, V)
- Tuberous xanthoma (types IIa, III, rarely IIb, IV)
- Tendon xanthoma (types IIa, III, rarely IIIb)
- Palmar xanthoma (types III, IIa, associated with primary biliary cirrhosis)
- Xanthelasma (types IIa, III; also without lipid abnormalities).

Is there any treatment for familial hypercholesterolaemia?

One view is that statin treatment should be started in these patients when boys are in their late teens and women from their late twenties. However, if the family history is particularly adverse then there is an increasing tendency for pediatricians to commence treatment (Lancet 2001;357:574). The Simvastatin in Children Study Group reported that, in such children, LDL cholesterol was reduced by 41% after 48 weeks of treatment with simvastatin and no safety issues were evident. With the exception of small decreases in dehydroepiandrosterone sulfate, there were 'no significant changes from baseline in adrenal, gonadal or pituitary hormones in the children given simvastatin. There are no adverse effects on growth or pubertal development.' Inhibition of apolipoprotein B synthesis by mipomersen represents a novel, effective therapy to reduce LDL cholesterol concentrations in patients with homozygous familial hypercholesterolaemia who are already receiving lipid-lowering drugs, including high-dose statins (Lancet 2010;375:998–1006).

What do you know about phytosterolaemia?

Phytosterolaemia is caused by increased intestinal absorption of dietary sterols (not only cholesterol, but also plant sterols) and decreased biliary excretion of sterols. As a consequence, large amounts of plant sterols accumulate in most tissues, and xanthomas and premature cardiovascular disease develop. It is an autosomal recessive condition caused by mutations in the genes encoding the family of ATP-binding cassette transporters (ABCG5 and ABCG8), which pump sterols out of intestinal cells in the lumen of the gut.

Michael S Brown (b. 1941) and Joseph L Goldstein (b. 1940), both of the University of Texas Health Science Centre in Dallas, were awarded the 1983 Nobel Prize for their discoveries concerning the regulation of cholesterol metabolism.

174 ERUPTIVE XANTHOMATA

INSTRUCTION

Examine this patient's skin.
This uncontrolled diabetic has developed a profuse eruption; what are these lesions?

SALIENT FEATURES

History

Duration and treatment of diabetes
History of hyperlipidaemia
Rash: duration, onset and evolution and associated symptoms such as itching.

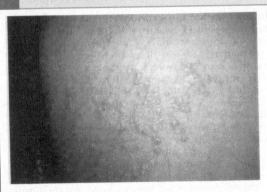

Fig. 174.1 Eruptive xanthomata.

Examination

- Multiple, itchy, red–yellow vesicles or nodules seen over extensor surfaces, i.e. buttocks, back, knees and elbows (Fig. 174.1 and see Fig. 173.1F,H).

Proceed as follows:

- Tell the examiner that would like to:
  - examine the fundus for lipaemia retinalis
  - check the urine for sugar
  - do a lipid profile (remember that eruptive xanthomata signify triglyceridaemia).

DIAGNOSIS

This patient has eruptive xanthomata (lesion) caused by hypertriglyceridaemia (aetiology).

ADVANCED-LEVEL QUESTIONS

In which conditions are eruptive xanthomata seen?
- Type IV hyperlipidaemia
- Familial hypertriglyceridaemia
- Lipoprotein lipase deficiency
- Apolipoprotein CII deficiency
- Type I hyperlipidaemia: chylomicronaemia
- Type V hyperlipidaemia: increased levels of triglycerides and chylomicrons.

Mention some other causes of hypertriglyceridaemia
- Primary hypertriglyceridaemia (usually >5.0 mg/l): familial hypertriglyceridaemia, familial combined hyperlipidaemia.
- Secondary hypertriglyceridaemia: diet, obesity, excess alcohol intake, diabetes mellitus, hypothyroidism, uraemia, dysproteinaemias, drugs (beta-blockers, oral contraceptives and oestrogens, retinoids).

What is the relationship between hypertriglyceridaemia and coronary artery disease?
Triglycerides are an independent risk factor for coronary artery disease, irrespective of LDL cholesterol. For every increase in serum triglyceride of 890 mg/l, the risk increases by ~30% in men and ~75% in women.

What is the particular risks for patients with serum triglycerides markedly raised (>10.0 mg/l)?

They are more susceptible to acute pancreatitis and hyperchylomicronaemia.

How would you manage a patient with raised levels of serum triglycerides?

- Diet: restrict dietary fat, decrease intake of alcohol and simple sugars
- Weight loss if the patient is overweight
- Exercise
- Discontinuation of drugs, e.g. beta-blockers
- Control secondary causes
- Niacin, gemfibrozil or omega-3 fatty acids may be used to treat elevated triglycerides (>5.0 mg/l) regardless of LDL or HDL cholesterol.

175 PALMAR XANTHOMATA

INSTRUCTION

Examine this patient's hands.

SALIENT FEATURES

History

- Family history of hyperlipidaemia and coronary artery disease.

Examination

- Yellowish-orange discolorations over the palmar and digital creases (Fig. 175.1 and see Fig. 173.1E)
- Look for the following signs:
  - Xanthelasmata around the eyes (Fig. 170.1)
  - Tuboeruptive xanthomata around the elbows and knees (Fig. 173.1F)
  - Signs of primary biliary cirrhosis (p. 434)
- Tell the examiner that this patient probably has a type III hyperlipidaemia.

Note: A more generalized form may be associated with monoclonal gammopathy of myeloma or lymphoma.

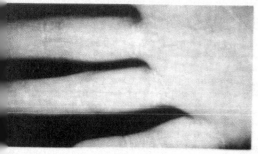

Fig. 175.1 Striate palmar xanthomata. (With permission from Durrington 2003.)

Remember: Xanthomas are usually not present in mild-to-moderate hypertriglyceridaemia; when present, they do not help to distinguish the various hypertriglyceridaemic disorders

ADVANCED-LEVEL QUESTIONS

How would you classify hyperlipidaemia?

Fredrickson classification, depending on laboratory findings (see Fig. 173.1 for clinical correlates):

- Type I: raised levels of chylomicrons and triglycerides, normal cholesterol concentration (pancreatitis, eruptive xanthomata and lipaemia retinalis)
- Type IIa: raised LDL and cholesterol levels, normal concentration of triglycerides (premature coronary artery disease, tendon xanthomata and arcus corneae)
- Type IIb: raised levels of LDL, VLDL, cholesterol and triglycerides (premature coronary artery disease)
- Type III: raised β-VLDL (cholesterol-rich) remnants, cholesterol and triglycerides (premature coronary artery disease, peripheral vascular disease, palmar and tuberous xanthomata)
- Type IV: raised VLDL and triglycerides, normal cholesterol (premature coronary artery disease: in some forms, risk of developing chylomicronaemia syndrome)
- Type V: raised chylomicrons, VLDL, cholesterol and triglycerides (pancreatitis, eruptive xanthoma, lipaemia retinalis).

What are the causes of hypercholesterolaemia?

- Primary hypercholesterolaemia: familial hypercholesterolaemia, familial combined hyperlipidaemia, polygenic hypercholesterolaemia
- Secondary hypercholesterolaemia: biliary cirrhosis, hypothyroidism, nephrotic syndrome, diet, drugs (thiazides, beta-blockers, oestrogens).

What is the histology of xanthomas?

Xanthomas are collections of foamy histiocytes within the dermis. These cells have abundant and finely vaculated cytoplasm giving it a foamy appearance. Cholesterol (both free and esterified), triglycerides and phospholipids are present within the cell. Often the cells are surrounded by inflammatory cells and fibrosis about the central zone of lipid-laden cells.

176 PSEUDOXANTHOMA ELASTICUM

PATIENT 1

INSTRUCTION

Look at this patient's fundus.

SALIENT FEATURES

History

- Family history (either autosomal recessive, which is most common, or autosomal dominant; the gene for both forms has been mapped to chromosome 16, Human Mol Genet 1997;6:1823)

- Upper GI haemorrhage, myocardial infarction, stroke and intermittent claudication, visual loss
- Hypertension (from involvement of renal vasculature)
- Intracranial haemorrhage.

Examination

- Fundus shows angioid streaks: linear grey or dark red streaks with irregular edges lying beneath the retinal vessels (Fig. 176.1) (roughly 50% of patients with angioid streaks have pseudoxanthoma elasticum, whereas 85% of those with pseudoxanthoma have angioid streaks).

Proceed as follows:

- Look at the neck (Fig. 176.2), antecubital fossae, axillae (Fig. 176.3), groin and periumbilical region for loose 'chicken skin' appearance of skin
- Examine peripheral pulses: absent pulses from peripheral arterial involvement but acral ischaemia is uncommon because of development of collaterals.

DIAGNOSIS

This patient has angioid streaks on fundoscopy and 'chicken-skin' appearance in the neck and axillae (lesions) caused by pseudoxanthoma elasticum (aetiology).

PATIENT 2

INSTRUCTION

Look at this patient.

SALIENT FEATURES

Examination

- Small yellow papules arranged in a linear or reticular pattern in plaques on the neck, axillae, cubital fossae, periumbilical region and groin

Proceed as follows:

- Tell the examiner that you would like to examine the fundus.

DIAGNOSIS

This patient has 'chicken-skin' appearance in the neck and axillae (lesions) caused by pseudoxanthoma elasticum (aetiology).

ADVANCED-LEVEL QUESTIONS

In which other conditions are angioid streaks seen?

- Regularly seen in Paget's disease, sickle cell disease
- Occasionally seen in Ehlers–Danlos syndrome, hyperphosphataemia, lead poisoning, trauma, pituitary disorders and intracranial disorders.

What are angioid streaks caused by?

They are caused by abnormal elastic tissue in the Bruch's membrane of the retina.

Which fundal finding is virtually pathognomonic of pseudoxanthoma elasticum?

'Leopard skin spotting' changes, which consist of yellowish mottling of the posterior pole temporal to the macula. These may antedate angioid streaks.

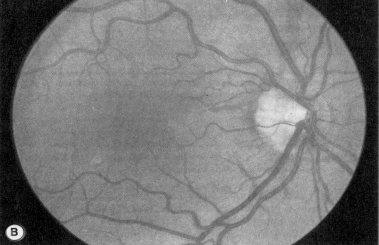

Fig. 176.1 Fundus showing angioid streaks.

What is the triad of pseudoxanthoma elasticum, angioid streaks and vascular abnormalities known as?
Groenblad–Strandberg syndrome.

What are the cardiovascular manifestations of this condition?
- Mitral valve prolapse
- Restrictive cardiomyopathy

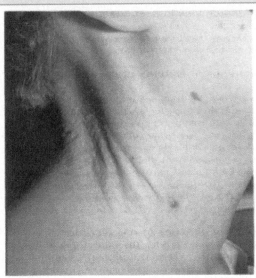

Fig. 176.2 'Chicken skin' appearance of neck.

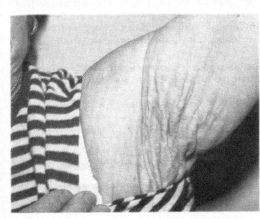

Fig. 176.3 Thickened sagging skin of the axilla with peau d'orange appearance.

- Renovascular hypertension
- Premature coronary artery disease resembling accelerated atherosclerosis from calcification of the internal elastic laminae of arteries. Arterial grafts should not be used for coronary artery bypass surgery in these patients because of possible calcification of the internal elastic laminae of the internal mammary artery
- Peripheral vascular disease.

What are the gastrointestinal manifestations of this disease?
GI haemorrhage, particularly during the first decade. Bleeding complications can be prevented by avoiding aspirin in patients with pseudoxanthoma elasticum.

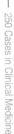

What are the causes of visual loss in pseudoxanthoma elasticum?

Macular involvement by a streak, disciform scarring secondary to choroidal haemorrhage or traumatic macular haemorrhage.

What are cutaneous histological features of pseudoxanthoma elasticum?

The histological diagnosis is made by doing a 4 mm punch biopy of scars or flexural skin of the neck or axillae in patients who have angioid streaks on fundoscopy but no visible skin lesions. The Verhoeff–van Gieson stain (for elastic tissue) reveals characteristic fragmentation and clumping of elastic tissue in middle and deep dermis. The von Kossa stain (for calcium) shows staining of calcified elastic tissue in the middle and deep dermis. Calcified elastic tissue is the hallmark of pseudoxanthoma elasticum. An arteriorlar sclerosis develops in the media of muscular arteries and arterioles and, as a result, the lumen may become progressively and concentrically narrowed.

What do you know about the genetics of this disorder?

A mutation affecting *ABCC6*, which encodes the multidrug resistance-associated protein MRP6 is the cause in 80%. This protein is a homologue of the cellular export pumps of the adenosine triphosphatase-binding cassette transporter superfamily. *ABCC6* is primarily expressed in the liver and kidneys, suggesting that pseudoxanthoma elasticum may be a metabolic disorder. However, the normal function of MRP6 and its role in the mineralization of connective tissues in pseudoxanthoma elasticum-affected organs remain unclear.

Which heritable connective-tissue disorders are associated with the presence of intracranial aneurysm and subarachnoid haemorrhage?

Polycystic kidney disease, Ehlers–Danlos syndrome (type IV), pseudoxanthoma elasticum and fibromuscular dysplasia.

KWL Bruch (1819–1884), Professor of Anatomy at Giessen, Germany.
   EE Groenblad, Swedish ophthalmologist and J Strandberg, Swedish dermatologist.
   TL Terry (1899–1946), Head of Ophthalmology at Harvard University, described angioid streaks in Paget's disease.

---

177 ROSACEA

INSTRUCTION

Look at this patient.

SALIENT FEATURES

History

- Age (typically occurs between the ages of 30 and 50 years)
- Intermittent facial flushing

- Blushing of the face with caffeine, alcohol or spicy foods
- History of unilateral headaches (an increased incidence of migranous headaches accompanying rosacea has been reported).

Examination

- Red patch with telangiectasia, acneiform papules and pustules overlying the flush areas of the face: cheeks, chin and nose (Fig. 177.1). (The papules and pustules distinguish it from the rash of SLE.)
- Comment on the following:
  - Rhinophyma or 'whiskey nose' or 'rum blossom' (Fig. 177.2) (irregular thickening of the skin of the nose with enlarged follicular orifices caused by hyperplasia of the sebaceous glands and hyperplasia of connective tissue); although rhinophyma is often referred to as 'end-stage rosacea', it may occur in patients with few or no other features of rosacea
  - Blepharitis, conjunctivitis.
- Tell the examiner that you would like to obtain an opthalmological evaluation for chalazion and progressive keratitis, which can lead to scarring and blindness.

Remember: The common misconception that both the facial redness and the rhinophyma associated with rosacea are caused by excessive alcohol consumption makes rosacea a socially stigmatizing condition for many patients.

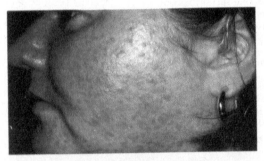

Fig. 177.1 Papulopustular rosacea.

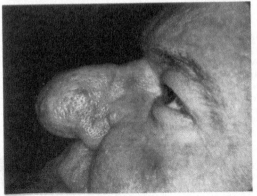

Fig. 177.2 Rhinopyma.

DIAGNOSIS

This patient has a red patch on the face with papules and pustules (lesion) caused by rosacea (aetiology), which is cosmetically disfiguring (functional status).

ADVANCED-LEVEL QUESTIONS

How many types of rosacea have been described?

There are four subtypes of rosacea, with the severity of each subtype graded as 1 (mild), 2 (moderate), or 3 (severe):
1: Erythemato telangiectatic
2: Papulopustular
3: Phymatous rosacea, e.g. rhinophyma
4: Ocular.

How would you distinguish rosacea from acne?

Rosacea is distinguished from acne by age (middle-aged and older people), the presence of a vascular component (i.e. rosy hue, erythema and telangiectasia) and the absence of comedones.

Remember: The diagnosis of rosacea is a clinical one. There is no confirmatory laboratory test. Biopsy is warranted only to rule out alternative diagnoses, since histopathological findings are not diagnostic.

How would you manage such a patient?

- Avoid factors that provoke facial flushing
- Avoid sun; sunscreens to limit photodamage
- Topical therapy: metronidazole, sodium sulfacetamide, azelaic acid; these are usually effective in eliminating erythematous papules and pustules
- Oral tetracycline in those who fail to respond to topical therapy. Also useful in ameliorating nodular lesions and eye symptoms
- Hydrocortisone cream
- Retinoids: in resistant disease
- Yellow light laser for telangiectasia
- Surgical removal for rhinophyma.

What are the causes of red face in an adult?

- Malar rash of SLE
- Heliotrope rash of dermatomyositis
- Seborrheic dermatitis
- Perioral dermatitis.

What is the role of vascular endothelial growth factor in rosacea?

Vascular endothelial growth factor (VEGF) receptor–ligand binding may contribute to the vascular changes and cellular infiltration that occurs in rosacea. Expression of receptors for VEGF on both vascular endothelium and infiltrating mononuclear cells is observed in rosacea. Although not produced by endothelium, VEGF is present in epidermis and epithelium and is released from infiltrating cells (Br J Ophthalmol 2007;91:226–9).

It has been suggested that the painter Rembrandt had rosacea, which he depicted in his self portrait (Lancet 1997;350:1835–7).

178 DERMATITIS HERPETIFORMIS

INSTRUCTION

Look at this patient's skin, who in the past had chronic diarrhoea.

SALIENT FEATURES

History

- History of diarrhoea
- History of gluten intolerance (although these patients rarely have gross malabsorption)
- Ask the patient whether the rash itches.

Examination

- Dry, itchy vesicles and urticarial plaques (Fig. 178.1) occurring bilaterally and symmetrically over the extensor surfaces, elbows, knees, posterior neck, back and buttocks.

Proceed as follows:

- Look for similar lesions on the scalp, face, neck, shoulders, buttocks, knees and calves.

DIAGNOSIS

This patient has itchy vesicles on the elbows (lesion) caused by dermatitis herpetiformis (functional status).

ADVANCED-LEVEL QUESTIONS

From which other itchy skin disorder should dermatitis herpetiformis be differentiated?

Scabies.

What are the extracutaneous manifestations of dermatitis herpetiformis?

- Gluten-sensitive enteropathy (frequent, asymptomatic)
- Thyroid dysfunction (especially hypothyroidism)
- Lymphoma (especially GI).

How would you investigate such a patient?

- Skin biopsy: fibrin and neutrophils accumulate selectively at the *tips of dermal papillae*, forming small microabscesses. Subepidermal vesicles have a neutrophilic infiltrate. Immunofluorescence demonstrates granular dermal papillary immunoglobulin A deposits
- Circulating anti-endomysium antibodies are present in all cases
- Jejunal biopsy: patchy abnormality showing subtotal villous atrophy with increased lymphocyte infiltration in the epithelium
- Therapeutic test: dapsone dramatically reduces itching in 72 h, often providing confirmation before the biopsy result is available
- HLA-B8 and HLA-DRw3 are positive in >80% of patients.

How would you treat such a patient?

- Gluten restriction (Br J Dermatol 1994;131:541)
- Dapsone or sulfapyridine: neither drug should be given to a patient with glucose-6-phosphate dehydrogenase deficiency. Treatment is lifelong; there is usually a rapid relapse if the drug is stopped.

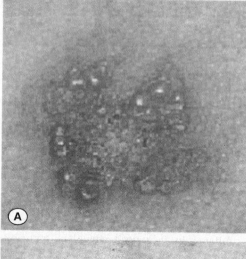

Fig. 178.1 Dermatitis herpetiformis. (A) Pruritic, urticarial papules and small blisters. (B) Occurrence in the lumbosacral area. (With permission from Habif 2009.)

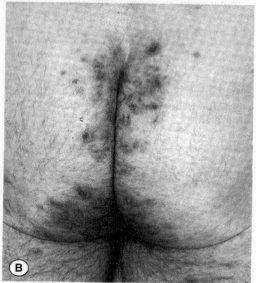

In which foods is gluten found?

Wheat, barely and rye (rice and maize are permitted in these patients).

Is it advisable for these patients to add oats to their gluten-free diets?

Moderate amounts of oats can be ingested without harmful effects in coeliac disease (N Engl J Med 1995;333:1033–7, BMJ 1996;313:1300–1) and in dermatitis herpetiformis (N Engl J Med 1997;337:1884–7, Gut 1998;43:490–3). Oats do not contain gliadin but do have avenin. However, as avenin makes up only 5–15% of the total protein content, even if it were as toxic as gliadin (a fact that is not universally conceded), a large amount of oats would need to be ingested to bring about an equivalent effect, in terms of the amount of protein ingested.

What do you know about gluten?

Gluten is the protein component that persists following the removal of water and starch from defatted flour. Gliadin is a class of protein found in the gluten fraction of flour. There are four gliadin fractions (α, β, γ and ω). α-Gliadin is injurious to the small intestinal mucosa, although there is some disagreement about the toxicity of other peptides. Patients with dermatitis herpetiformis develop IgA and IgG antibodies to gliadin and reticulin (the latter a component of the anchoring fibrils that tether the epidermal basement membrane to the upper dermis).

What are the benefits of a gluten-free diet?

It gradually improves skin lesions, improves any associated manifestations of malabsorptive enteropathy and may reduce the late risk of intestinal lymphoma. It also normalizes histological abnormalities.

Note: An elemental diet lacking protein has been reported to benefit patients with dermatitis herpetiformis even in the presence of a gluten challenge.

Dermatitis herpetiformis was first described in 1884 by LA Duhring (1845–1913), Professor of Diseases of the Skin at the University of Pennsylvania. He studied dermatology in Paris, London and Vienna, and wrote the first American textbook of dermatology. Others believe that dermatitis herpetiformis was first described by F von Hebra, who also wrote a textbook of dermatology.

Samuel J Gee (1839–1911) of St Bartholomew's Hospital, London, provided the first thorough description of coeliac sprue in 1888 (Gee S On the coeliac affection. St Barth Hosp Rep 1888;24:17–20).

Dutch paediatrician WK Dicke astutely observed that wheat and rye were harmful in children with this disease (Dicke WK Coeliac disease: investigation of the harmful effects of certain types of cereal on patients with coeliac disease. Doctoral thesis, University of Utrecht, The Netherlands, 1950; N Engl J Med 1995;333:1075–6).

---

179 HAIRY LEUKOPLAK

INSTRUCTION

Look at this patient's tongue.

SALIENT FEATURES

History

- Usually asymptomatic
- Patients may complain of pain or voice changes
- Tell the examiner that you would like to know whether the patient is immunocompromised (caused by HIV or immnosuppressive treatment particularly in kidney transplant recipients).

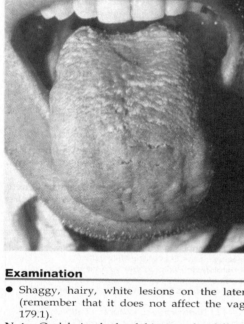

Fig. 179.1 Hairy leukoplakia.

Examination

- Shaggy, hairy, white lesions on the lateral margins of the tongue (remember that it does not affect the vaginal or anal mucosa) (Fig. 179.1).

Note: Oral hairy leukoplakia may be difficult to distinguish from oral candidiasis, but, in contrast to oral candidiasis, it does not rub off, does not respond to antifungal therapy and may change its appearance daily.

DIAGNOSIS

This patient has whitish hairy lesions on the lateral edges of the tongue (lesions), which is oral hairy leukoplakia caused by the Epstein–Barr virus (aetiology).

QUESTIONS

What is the cause of this lesion?
Hairy leukoplakia is caused by the Epstein–Barr virus (N Engl J Med 1985;313:1564–71)

ADVANCED-LEVEL QUESTIONS

What is the significance of this lesion?
In HIV-seropositive subjects, usually it is a harbinger of rapid progression to AIDS. It is rarely seen in non-HIV immunosuppressed patients.

What are the histological features of this condition?
- Hyperkeratosis
- Hyperplasia and ballooning of prickle cells (acanthosis)
- Depletion of Langherhans cells.

Why is the tongue dark colored?

The dark colour is secondary to porphyrin pigment deposition by bacterial metabolism.

How would you treat this condition?

Treatment is seldom indicated, but ganciclovir or aciclovir may be helpful if the patient has discomfort. Also podophyllin and retinoin has been used (Lancet 1996;348:729–33).

P Langerhans (1847–1888), German pathologist and dermatologist.
    Oral 'hairy' leukoplakia was initially reported in the Lancet in 1984 (Lancet 1984;ii:831–34).

---

180 KAPOSI'S SARCOMA

INSTRUCTION

Look at this skin lesion.

SALIENT FEATURES

History

- Determine whether the patient is immunocompromised (from HIV or from therapy following organ transplantation).
- If the lesion is in the mouth, ask patient whether there is any difficulty in eating (the gingival margin may cause oral hygiene difficult because of secondary infection and pain).

Examination

- Plum-coloured violet plaques, either solitary or in crops, on the limbs, mouth, tip of the nose and palate (Fig. 180.1).

Proceed as follows:

- Tell the examiner that you would like to check HIV antibody titres (Kaposi's sarcoma has an estimated prevalence of 10–20% in HIV-positive patients and was one of the first diseases to define AIDS in 1981).

DIAGNOSIS

This patient has Kaposi's sarcoma (lesion), which has been shown to be caused by human herpesvirus 8 (aetiology) in patients with AIDS.

ADVANCED-LEVEL QUESTIONS

What are the varieties of Kaposi's sarcoma?

- *Classic Kaposi's sarcoma or epidemic type* (Fig. 108.1B): initially described in Jews; indolent; found on the legs of elderly men; confined to the skin and may be present for decades; not fatal.
- *African variety or endemic type* (Fig. 180.2): violaceous skin plaques, black under Negroid skin; this is an aggressive invasive tumour that is

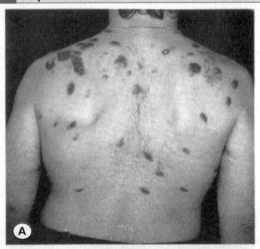

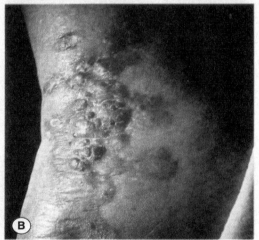

Fig. 180.1 Kaposi sarcoma. (A) Violet plaques. (B) Nodules and infiltrated plaques.

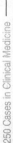

ultimately fatal. It occurs in children and younger men. In the former it is often associated with generalized lymphadenopathy.

- *AIDS-associated Kaposi's sarcoma* (Fig. 180.3): found in approximately one-third of patients with AIDS and more common in homosexuals. The cutaneous lesions respond to interferon-alfa and cytotoxic chemotherapy. About one-third develop a second malignancy such as lymphoma, myeloma or leukaemia. Patients eventually die from a secondary infection seen in AIDS rather than as a direct consequence of Kaposi's sarcoma.
- *Transplantation-associated Kaposi's sarcoma*, particularly in patients on high-dose immunosuppressive therapy; these often regress when therapy is stopped. Transmission of human herpesvirus 8 infection

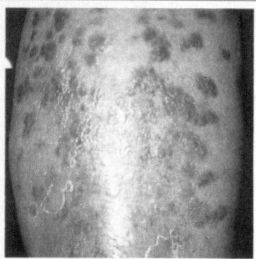

Fig. 180.2 African variety.

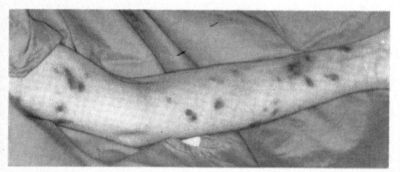

Fig. 180.3 Kaposi's sarcoma associated with AIDS.

occurs from renal transplant donors to recipients and is a risk factor for Kaposi's sarcoma (N Engl J Med 1998;339:1358–63).

What is the aetiology of Kaposi's sarcoma?

The aetiology is not known but epidemiological data support a viral infection (N Engl J Med 1995;332:1181–5, N Engl J Med 1998;332:1186–91). Reports have implicated a herpes-like virus (human herpesvirus 8). This has been detected in all forms of Kaposi's sarcoma. Between 70% and 100% of patients with Kaposi's sarcoma have antibodies to human herpesvirus 8 (compared with 1–5% of the general population). Seroconversion may occur several months before the appearance of the lesions.

What is the histology of Kaposi's sarcoma?

Histologically all varieties are similar:

- Early or 'patch' stage: similar to granulation tissue and characterized by jagged, thin-walled, dilated vascular spaces in the epidermis with interstitial inflammatory cells and extravasated red cells (with haemosiderin deposition)
- Plaque stage
- Later or 'nodular' lesions: features are more characteristic at this stage and comprise spindle-shaped stromal cells with irregular slit-like spaces filled with red blood cells and lined by recognizable endothelium, intertwined with normal vascular channels.

Is there any difference in the prognosis of AIDS depending on whether the patient has oral or cutaneous Kaposi's sarcoma?

It has been reported that there is a greater mortality risk with oral (median 72 months) compared with cutaneous (median 24 months) KS independent of the CD4 cell count (Lancet 2000;356:2160).

How would you manage Kaposi's sarcoma in patients with HIV infection?

- Baseline treatment includes a retroviral agent such as zidovudine, which has no direct effect on Kaposi's sarcoma but diminishes the degree of immunosuppression (note: eczema, xerosis, warts and Kaposi's sarcoma are associated with HIV infection but do not improve with antiretroviral therapy). Retinoic acid is a promising alternative.
- Localized mucocutaneous lesions respond well to liquid nitrogen, radiotherapy, cryotherapy, surgical excision, intralesional vinblastine or sclerosing solutions, bleomycin or interferon-alfa.
- Interferon-alfa as systemic treatment is effective in 40–50% of patients with indolent Kaposi's sarcoma, a CD4 cell count >400×10^6 cells/l, few systemic symptoms and no opportunistic infections.
- Radiation therapy.
- Combination therapy of surgery, chemotherapy and radiation or with chemotherapy alone.
- Relatively marrow-sparing chemotherapy (bleomycin, vincristine or low-dose liposomal doxorubicin) is used when other treatment fails in patients with aggressive Kaposi's sarcoma (Lancet 1997;350:1363). Complete or partial remission may be obtained in >75% of those with Kaposi's sarcoma; shorter survival is associated with low CD4 cell count.

What do you know about the pathogenesis of Kaposi's sarcoma?

Lymphatic endothelial cells achieve the Kaposi's sarcoma phenotype probably caused by upregulation of lymphangiogenic molecules such as angiopoietin-2, vascular endothelial growth factor (VEGF) and VEGF-D. Thus neutralizing antibodies to angiopoietin-2, VEGF and VEGF-D may provide a suitable tool for anti-lymphangiogenic therapies (Nat Genet 2004;36:687–93). New data suggest that vasculotropic virus human herpesvirus may also have a pathogenetic role in primary pulmonary hypertension.

Mortiz Kaposi (1837–1902) a Hungarian dermatologist in 1872 described five men with 'idiopathic multiple pigmented sarcoma'. He also described in the rash in SLE as 'butterfly rash' in 1875 (Kaposi M Idiopathisches multiples Pigmentsarkom der Haut. Arch Dermatol Syph 1872;4:265–73).

181 PEUTZ–JEGHERS SYNDROME

INSTRUCTION

Look at this patient's face.

SALIENT FEATURES

History

- Pain in the abdomen as a result of intestinal intussusception
- Haemorrhage in the upper GI tract or rectal bleeding
- Family involvement (autosomal dominant).

Examination

- Pigmented freckles around the lips (Fig. 181.1A).
Proceed as follows:
- Look in the mouth for similar pigmentation (Fig. 181.1B) and anaemia.

DIAGNOSIS

This patient has pigmented freckles arounds the lips (lesions) caused by Peutz–Jeghers syndrome (aetiology).

ADVANCED-LEVEL QUESTIONS

What are the types of colonic polyp?

- *Tubular adenomas*: over 60% are in the rectosigmoid colon and may cause bleeding or obstruction. The risk of malignancy correlates with size. The

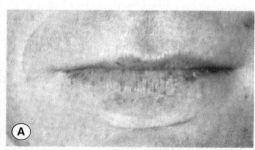

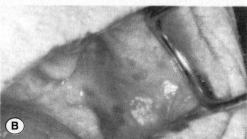

Fig. 181.1 Peutz–Jeghers syndrome. (A) Cutaneous pigmentation on the lips. (B) Pigment changes in the buccal mucosa. (With permission from Winship, Dudding 2008.)

tubular adenoma is removed endoscopically. Follow-up surveillance is by colonoscopy every 2 years.

- *Villous adenomas* are usually found in the left colon and have a high risk of malignancy. Polyps larger than 2 cm have a 50% risk of malignancy. They may present with hypokalaemia as a result of potassium loss in the stools. They are removed by colonoscopic resection.
- *Hyperplastic polyps* are benign and rarely undergo malignant change. They are usually detected as an incidental finding at colonoscopy.

What is the histology of polyps in Peutz–Jeghers syndrome?

The polyps, which are large and pedunculated, histologically show an arborizing network of connective tissue and well-developed smooth muscle that extends into the polyp and surrounds; normal abundant glands are lined by normal intestinal epithelium rich in goblet cells. Polyps are distributed in the small bowel (100%), stomach (25%) and colon (30%).

What do you know about the genetics of Peutz-Jeghers syndrome?

The gene has been identified and encodes the serine threonine kinase LKB1 (STK11). Studies of the original kindred described by Peutz found an inactivating germline mutation in *LKB1*. The clinical features included GI polyposis, mucocutaneous pigmentation, nasal polyps and rectal polyps. Family longevity was reduced by intestinal obstruction and malignant transformation (Lancet 1999;353:1211–15).

What polyposis syndromes do you know?

- *Familial adenomatous polyposis and variants*:
  - *Familial* adenomatous polyposis (FAP) is an autosomal dominant condition with the defect localized to *APC* on chromosome 5q21 (N Engl J Med 1993;329:1982). There are several thousand polyps in the colon, which start to appear between the ages of 10 and 35 years. The potential malignant change is 100% by the age of 40 years. Hence all relatives should be screened annually from the age of 12 years and all patients should have prophylactic colectomy by the age of 30. A protein assay can diagnose the genetic defect in 87% of such families, and 150 mg sulindac twice daily has been shown to reduce the number and size of the adenomatous polyps in the rectum (N Engl J Med 1993;328:1313). Another promising drug is celecoxib, a cyclooxygenase-2 inhibitor (N Engl J Med 2000;342:1946–52), which significantly reduces the number of colorectal polyps. Calcium supplementation has been shown to reduce the risk of recurrent colorectal adenomas (N Engl J Med 1999;340:101–7).
  - *Gardner syndrome.* This is a variant of FAP in which affected members develop extraintestinal soft tissue tumours (osteomas, lipomas, dermoid tumours) and pigmentation of fundi.
  - *Turcot syndrome.* In this varient, CNS gliomas may also develop. Disruption of any of three genes — *APC, hMLH1* or *hPMS2* — can lead to Turcot syndrome (N Engl J Med 1995;332:839–47).

- **Other polyposis syndromes**
- *Familial juvenile polyposis* is an autosomal dominant condition occurring in children and teenagers. It causes GI bleeds, abdominal pain, diarrhoea and intussusception. There is an increased incidence of malignant

change in the interspersed adenomatous polyps. The affected genes are *Smad4 (DPC4), BMPRIA, PTEN.*

- *Peutz–Jeghers syndrome* is an autosomal dominant condition character-ized by mucocutaneous melanosis with GI hamartomas. The intestinal polyps may give rise to haematemeis, melaena or rectal bleeding, anaemia or intussusception depending on their location. These polyps are usually found in the ileum and jejunum and they rarely undergo malignant change. However, affected people tend to have an increased incidence of other malignancies, both of GI tract (stomach and duode-num) and other viscera (lung, breasts, pancreas and gonads).

- *Cronkhite–Canada syndrome* comprises sporadic, colonic, small bowel or gastric polyps associated with ectodermal changes such as hyperpig-mentation, nail atrophy and alopecia.

- *Cowden's disease* is is an autosomal dominant condition characterized by multiple GI hamartomas with warty papules on the mucosa, and skin malformations. The affected genes are *PTEN (MMAC1, DEP1).*

- *Bannayan–Ruvalcaba–Riley syndrome* comprises microcephaly, hamar-toatous polyps, fibromatosis, speckled penis and haemangiomas. The affected gene is *PTEN.*

What do you know about the genetics of colorectal cancer?

Three separate research groups have reported a gene on chromosome 2 seen in familial colonic cancer that, it is claimed, may predispose to up to 15% of colorectal cancer. Screening in colorectal cancer should include colonoscopy, and in women pelvic ultrasonography. Those who develop colorectal cancer should be treated by subtotal colectomy.

Further reading

Morrison PJ, Nevin NC: Peutz–Jeghers syndrome, *N Engl J Med* 329:774, 1993 (classical picture of a patient with Peutz–Jeghers syndrome).

This condition was originally described by JL Peutz of Holland in 1921 and rediscovered by HJ Jeghers et al. of the USA in 1949 (N Engl J Med 1949;241:993–1005, 1031–6).

EJ Gardner (1909–1989), US geneticist and Professor of Zoology at Utah University.

J Turcot, Canadian surgeon, J-P Després and F St Pierre first described Turcot syndrome in 1959. In 1949, HW Crail had described a similar syndrome (US Naval Medical Bull 1949;49:123–8).

LW Cronkhite, physician, Massachusetts General Hospital.

Wilma J Canada, US radiologist.

---

182 PYODERMA GANGRENOSUM

INSTRUCTION

Look at this patient's skin.

SALIENT FEATURES

History

- Diarrhoea (inflammatory bowel disease)
- Joint pains (rheumatoid arthritis)
- Leukaemia, multiple myeloma.

Examination

- Necrotic ulcer with purplish overhanging edges, usually seen on the lower limbs or trunk (Fig. 182.1).

DIAGNOSIS

These are necrotic ulcers (lesions), which are a feature of pyoderma gangrenosum (aetiology); I would like to investigate for underlying inflammatory bowel disease.

QUESTIONS

What are the variants of this condition?

Variants have been described based on the location of the lesion or the associated process, the skin lesion being similar to the classical pyoderma gangrenosum:

- Peristomal pyoderma gangrenosum at site of ileostomy (Fig. 182.2) or colostomy in ulcerative colitis or Crohn's disease
- Vulvar pyoderma gangrenosum
- Penile or scrotal in adolescent adults
- Associated with preleukaemic state (the ulcer is shallow with bullous blue-grey border)
- Pyostomatitis vegetans is an oral variant with chronic pustular and eventually vegetative lesions in the mucous membrane of the mouth.

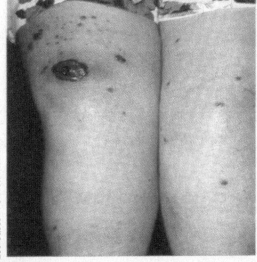

Fig. 182.1 Pyoderma gangrenosum.

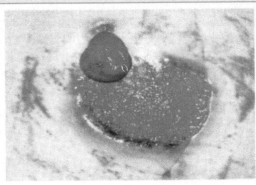

Fig. 182.2 Pyoderma gangrenosum at ileostomy site. (With permission from Ennis et al. 2001 pp. 533.)

What is the histology in this condition?
Non-specific features including massive neutrophilic infiltration, haemorrhage and necrosis of the epidermis.

How would you evaluate these patients?
- Detailed history and physical examination
- Skin biopsy (with cultures for bacteria, fungus and viral)
- GI studies
- Serology for anti-neutrophil cytoplasmic antibodies (ANCA), anti-nuclear antibodies (ANA), anti-phospholipid antibody and serum protein electrophoresis
- Complete blood count, peripheral smear and bone marrow examination.

In which conditions can pyoderma gangrenosum be seen?
- Ulcerative colitis
- Crohn's disease
- Chronic active hepatitis
- Rheumatoid arthritis, seronegative arthritis associated with GI symptoms
- Acute and chronic myeloid leukaemia, myelocytic leukaemia, hairy cell leukaemia
- Polycythaemia rubra vera
- Multiple myeloma
- IgA monoclonal gammopathy.

ADVANCED-LEVEL QUESTIONS

How would you manage these lesions?
- High-dose steroids
- Intralesional steroids
- Topical therapy including dressings, limb elevation rest
- Systemic therapy with dapsone
- Some regress with treatment of the underlying cause.

What conditions can be mistaken for pyoderma gangrenosum?
Six broad disease categories may simulate pyoderma gangrenosum (N Engl J Med 2002;347:1412–8.):

- Vascular occlusive or venous disease: anti-phospholipid antibody syndrome, livedoid vasculopathy, venous stasis ulceration, small-vessel occlusive arterial disease, type I cryoglobulinaemia, Klippel–Trénaunay–Weber syndrome
- Vasculitis: Wegener's granulomatosis, polyarteritis nodosa, cryoglobulinemic (mixed) vasculitis, Takayasu's arteritis, leukocytoclastic vasculitis plus secondary
- Infection: herpes simplex virus, cutaneous TB, *Entamoeba histolytica* (amoeba cutis), deep fungal infections such as *Penicillium marneffei*, *Sporotrichosis*, *Aspergillosis*, *Cryptococcosis*, *Zygomycosis* spp.
- Malignancy: lymphoma, Langerhans cell histiocytosis, leukaemia cutis
- Exogenous tissue injury: drug induced or direct injury
- Other inflammatory disorders.

How would you exclude these lesions?

- History. Markedly painful ulcer, rapid progression of ulceration, type of skin lesion preceding the ulcer (papule, pustule, or vesicle), minor trauma (pathergy) preceding development of the ulcer, symptoms of an associated disease (e.g. inflammatory bowel disease or arthritis)
- Medication history (e.g. bromides, iodide, hydroxyurea, or granulocyte–macrophage colony-stimulating factor)
- Examination. Characteristic features of ulcer: tenderness, necrosis, irregular violaceous border, undermined, rolled edges
- Skin biopsy. Elliptical incisional biopsy preferable to punch biopsy (include inflamed border and ulcer edge at a depth that includes subcutaneous fat). The inflamed border is examined for routine histology (haematoxylin and eosin) and microorganisms (Gram, methenamine silver and Fite stains). The edge of ulcer is cultured in appropriate media to detect bacteria, fungi and atypical myobacteria
- Laboratory investigations. Complete blood count, ESR, blood chemistry (liver and kidney function tests), protein electrophoresis, coagulation panel (including anti-phospholipid antibody screening), ANCA, cryoglobulins
- Venous and arterial function studies
- Chest radiography
- Colonoscopy.

(See N Engl J Med 2002;347:1412–18.)

Pyoderma gangrenosum was first described in 1930 by Brunsting, Goeckerman and O'Leary, with five cases (Arch Dermatol Syphiol 1930;22:655–80).

---

183 STURGE–WEBER SYNDROME (ENCEPHALOTRIGEMINAL ANGIOMATOSIS)

INSTRUCTION

Look at this patient's face.

SALIENT FEATURES

History

- Obtain history of seizures (focal or generalized)
- Hemiparesis, hemisensory disturbance
- Ipsilateral glaucoma
- Mental subnormality.

Examination

- A port-wine stain is present on the face in the distribution of the first and second division of the trigeminal nerve (Fig. 183.1)
- Hypertrophy of the involved area of the face.

Proceed as follows:

- Look for haemangiomas of episclera and iris
- Tell the examiner that you would like to:
  - examine the fundus for unilateral choroidal haemangiomata: the so-called haemangioma is in almost all cases on the side of the facial naevus flammeus and is so diffuse that the colour change it causes is commonly called a *'tomato ketchup'* fundus (Fig. 183.2)
  - do a skull radiograph or cranial CT (Fig. 183.3) for intracranial 'tram-line' calcification, particularly in the parieto-occipital lobe (caused by mineral deposition in the cortex beneath the intracranial angioma)
  - check BP: may be associated with phaeochromocytoma.

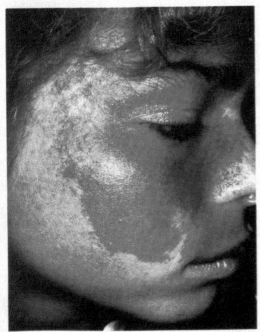

Fig. 183.1 Sturge–Weber syndrome.

250 Cases in Clinical Medicine

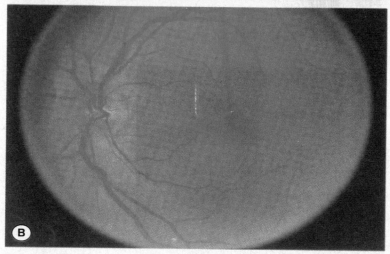

Fig. 183.2 Diffuse choroidal hemangioma. (A) The affected right fundus has saturated red colour and a large deep cup of optic disc. (B) The uninvolved left fundus, with more orange coloured choroid and a normal optic disc. (With permission from Yanoff, Duker 2008.)

DIAGNOSIS

This patient has a port-wine stain on the face in the distribution of the first two divisions of the trigeminal nerve (lesion), which is probably caused by Sturge–Weber syndrome (aetiology); these lesions may be cosmetically unacceptable (functional status).

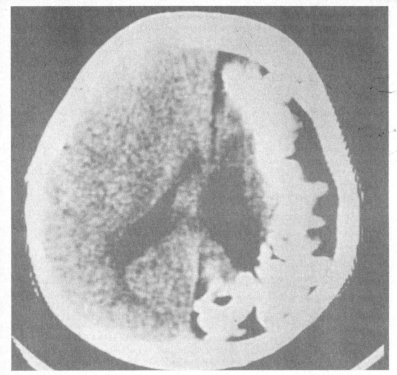

Fig. 183.3 CT scan showing unilateral calcification and underlying atrophy of a cerebral hemisphere. (With permission from Kliegman et al. 2007.)

ADVANCED-LEVEL QUESTIONS

What is the inheritance in such patients?

This is the only syndrome of the phacomatoses that does not have a hereditary tendency. It occurs sporadically and has no sexual predilection.

What are the neurological manifestations in such patients?

Jacksonian epilepsy, contralateral hemianopia, hemisensory disturbance, hemiparesis and hemianopia, low IQ.

What other ocular manifestations do you know?

Choroidal angioma, glaucoma (in 30%), buphthalmos (large eye), optic atrophy.

What is the histology of port-wine stains?

They are composed of networks of ectatic vessels in the outer dermis, under a normal dermis.

Does the location of the port-wine stain predict Sturge–Weber syndrome?

Patients who do not have port-wine stain in the distribution of the first two branches of trigeminal nerve are unlikely to have neuro-opthalmological manifestations of the syndrome.

How would you treat such a patient?

- Treatment is aimed at the pharmacological control of seizures.
- The patient should be referred to the ophthalmologist for management of increased intraocular pressure or choroidal angioma.
- Photothermolysis to treat the port-wine stains. If this occurs in early childhood, the psychological burden on the family and child may be alleviated. The pulsed dye laser provides individual pulses of 0.35 ms at 585 nm. It is the treatment of choice for most port-wine stains, particularly in children. Wavelengths of 577–590 nm are optimal as they are minimally attenuated by epidermis and dermis, and strongly absorbed by blood. Pulse durations of 0.5–5.0 ms produce only transmural injury to the vessel wall, by heat conduction from hot red cells, and hence prevent non-specific dermal injury. One study reported that there was no efficacy in treating port-wine stains with flash-lamp-pumped dye laser in early childhood compared with at a later age (N Engl J Med 1998;338:1028–33).

William A Sturge (1850–1919), a London physician, described this condition in 1879. He was attached to the The Royal Free Hospital, London, and founded the Society of Prehistoric Archaeology in East Anglia.

Otto Kalischer, a German pathologist, described postmortem findings in a case as early as 1901.

Frederick Parkes Weber (1863–1962), a London physician, was the first to describe the radiological appearances in this condition. Two other syndromes to which Weber's name is attached are Weber–Christian disease (relapsing, febrile, nodular, non-suppurative panniculitis) and Osler–Rendu–Weber syndrome (hereditary haemorrhagic telangiectasia).

---

184 ACNE VULGARIS

INSTRUCTION

Look at this patient.

SALIENT FEATURES

History

- Steroid ingestion
- Isoniazid ingestion
- Occupational exposure to oils (oil-induced acne).

Examination

- Comedones or blackheads (Fig. 184.1), caused by plugging of hair follicles by keratin; these are hallmarks of acne.
- Generally found over the chin, face, neck, chest, upper back and upper arms (areas which have the most and the largest sebaceous glands)
- Whiteheads (i.e. distended sebaceous glands without a pore)
- Cysts (larger, deeper masses of retained sebum)
- Greasy skin
- There may be associated scarring: ice-pick scars.

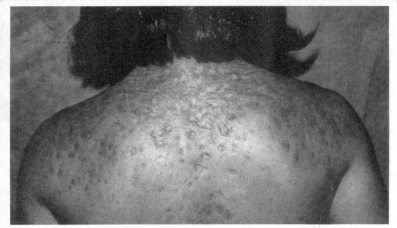

Fig. 184.1 Acne vulgaris.

Remember: Acne vulgaris is a multifactorial disease affecting the pilose-baceous follicle and characterized by open and closed comedones, papules, pustules, nodules and scars.

DIAGNOSIS

This patient has blackheads on the face with greasy skin (lesions), which is acne vulgaris caused by *Propionibacterium acnes* (aetiology); it may be cosmetically unacceptable to the patient (functional status).

ADVANCED-LEVEL QUESTIONS

What do you know about the pathogenesis of acne?

Follicular keratinization, seborrhoea and colonization of the pilosebaceous unit with *P. acnes* are central to the development of these lesions. Genetic and hormonal factors also play a role, possibly by optimizing the follicular environment suitable for the growth of *P. acnes* or by influencing the inflammatory response and thus the nature of these lesions.

How is the severity of acne graded?

Lesions can be inflammatory or non-inflammatory and are graded by severity (Fig. 184.2):

- Mild disease: open and closed comedones and some papules and pustules
- Moderate: more frequent papules and pustules with mild scarring
- Severe disease: all of the above plus nodular abscesses; leads to more extensive scarring, which may be keloidal in some instances.

What factors may exacerbate acne?

- Cosmetics, oils
- Clothing (turtlenecks, bra straps, sports helmets)
- Trauma
- Excessive sweating.

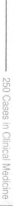

250 Cases in Clinical Medicine

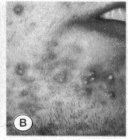
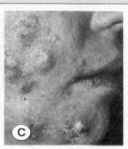

Fig. 184.2 Acne classification. (A) Mild, open and closed comedones and some papules/pustules. (B) Moderate, many papules/pustules plus some nodules. (C) Severe, with multiple papules/pustules and nodules, leading to scarring. (With permission from Habif 2009.)

How would you manage acne?

The aims of treatment are to prevent scarring, limit the disease duration and reduce the impact of the psychological stress, which may affect over half of sufferers:

- Wash affected parts with soap not more than twice a day
- Avoid steaming: saunas, Turkish baths
- Dietary restriction has no role in therapy (N Engl J Med 1997;336:1156).
- Reduce *P. acnes* proliferation:
  - Topical therapy: sulfur, benzyl peroxide, retinoic acid, azaleic acid, erythromycin, tetracycline
  - Systemic therapy: tetracycline, erythromycin, doxycycline, minocycline, co-trimoxazole, clindamycin, isotretinoin.
- Reduce sebum overproduction with systemic agents: oestrogens, antiandrogens, spironolactone, isotretinoin
- Reduce inflammation:
  - Systemic agents: corticosteroids, isotretinoin
  - Topical agents: metronidazole, intralesional steroids.
- Reduce abnormal desquamation of follicular epithelium:
  - Systemic agents: isotretinoin, antibiotics by indirect effect
  - Topical agents: tretinoin (most effective), salicyclic acid, adapalene, tazarotene, isotretinoin, antibiotics.
- Physical or surgical methods: comedo extraction, dermabrasion, chemical peeling, laser resurfacing, pulsed-dye laser treatment and punch grafts.

Randomized, controlled trials are needed to define the relative efficacies of various therapies outlined above.

Have you heard of acne fulminans?

It is a rare but severe variant seen exclusively in adolescent boys. It is caused by an immune complex reaction to *P. acnes*. The lesions eventually become necrotic and form haemorrhagic crusts, causing disfigurement and scarring. There may be associated systemic features such as fever, malaise, arthralgia, arthritis and vasculitis. Osteolytic bone lesions can arise. Inpatient treatment with systemic steroids is necessary.

What do you know about acne conglobata?

It is seen in tall Caucasian males with cystic skin lesions and multiple abscess formation. It rarely regresses.

185 ALOPECIA AREATA

INSTRUCTION

Examine this patient's scalp.

SALIENT FEATURES

History

- Young adult (75% of patients are below the age of 40 years)
- History of atopy
- Ask whether there is a family history (25% give a family history)
- Ask the patient whether there are any local symptoms and if the hair loss is cosmetically unacceptable.

Examination

- Well-defined patch of hair loss (Fig. 185.1); short, fractured, exclamation-point hairs may be seen at periphery.
- Regrowing hair in the patch appears as a fine, depigmented downy growth.

Proceed as follows:

- Look for patches of hair loss over the eyebrows and beard area
- Examine the nails for fine pitting, transverse lines, dystrophy, fragmentation (anonychorrhexis) and ridging and 20-nail dystrophy (roughened nail surface and brittle free nail edge) (Fig. 185.2)
- Tell the examiner that you would like to:
  - look for atopy
  - look for other autoimmune conditions including vitiligo (see below).

DIAGNOSIS

This patient has alopecia areata (lesion), which is suspected to be of autoimmune aetiology; it may be cosmetically unacceptable to the patient (functional status).

ADVANCED-LEVEL QUESTIONS

What are the signs of disease activity?

At the advancing edge, broken hairs that look like exclamation marks indicate active disease. These are very short hairs, tapering and becoming

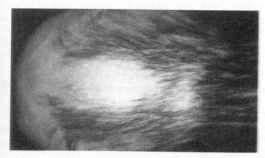

Fig. 185.1 Alopecia areata.

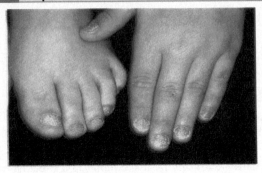

Fig. 185.2 Nail dystrophy.

depigmented as the scalp is approached. Plucking reveals such hair to be in the telogen phase.

Mention some associated disorders

- Autoimmune conditions (vitiligo, thyrotoxicosis, Addison's disease, pernicious anaemia)
- Down syndrome
- Hypogammaglobulinaemia.

What is the difference between alopecia totalis and alopecia universalis?

Both of these conditions can occur in alopecia areata. Alopecia totalis is the loss of all scalp hair and alopecia universalis is the loss of hair from all body sites.

Is alopecia areata associated with scarring?

No.

Mention the causes of hair loss associated with scarring

Discoid lupus erythematosus, lichen planus.

What is the treatment for alopecia areata?

- Steroids (both topical and systemic) (N Engl J Med 1999;341:964)
- Psoralen plus ultraviolet A (PUVA), but alopecia often returns after discontinuation of PUVA (Lancet 1997;349:222)
- Anthralin left on the scalp for 20–60 min
- Topical minoxidil
- Topical immunotherapy: dinitrochlorobenzene, squaric acid dibutylester and diphencyprone have been used for contact sensitization
- Antibodies to tumour necrosis factor-α.

Cessation of treatment may be associated with recurrent hair loss.

Mention some causes of drug-induced alopecia

Anticoagulants, retinoids, vitamin A, antithyroid drugs, oral contraceptives, anticancer drugs (invariably reversible).

What do you understand by the term trichotillomania?

It is the self-inflicted pulling out of one's own hair and can be differentiated from alopecia areata as the hair loss is irregular and there is always growing hair, since these cannot be pulled out till they are long enough. These patches are unilateral and are usually on the same side as the patient's dominant hand. The patient may be unaware of this habit.

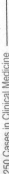

What do you know about the growth of the hair follicle?
Each follicle has cyclical growth controlled by a constitutional 'time clock'. It has three phases of growth (anagen) with >90% of hair in this phase, a short involutional phase (catagen) and a resting (telogen) phase. The anagen phase is 3–5 years, catagen is 2–3 weeks and the telogen phase is 2–4 months. Anagen hairs are anchored deeply into the subcutaneous fat and cannot be pulled out easily. Each hair shaft may persist on the scalp for 3 to 7 years before falling out and being replaced by a new hair. Compared with anagen hair, telogen hair is located higher in the skin and can be pulled out relatively easily. Hair found on the pillow and hairbrush is telogen hair and can be recognized by the fact that the club is depigmented as well as expanded; anagen hair obtained by traction is fully melanized.

How much hair is usually lost by a normal person?
About 70–100 hairs/day. The human scalp contains about 100 000 follicles, 5–10% are in telogen at any time, i.e. 5000–10 000. As telogen lasts for about 100 days, the number of telogen hairs pushed out each day is 70–100.

What is telogen effluvium?
It is a transitory (about 2–4 months) increase in the number of hairs in the resting (telogen) phase of the hair growth cycle. There is a sudden increase in shedding of hairs, with white bulbs about 3–5 months after a period of stress. The amount of hair loss exceeds 150/day. It is associated with high fever, stress, crash dieting, malnutrition, surgery, termination of pregnancy or oral contraceptives. The prognosis is good.

What do you know about male pattern baldness?
On the scalps of men who have a predisposition for this pattern of baldness, androgens cause a switch from terminal to vellus or vellus-like follicles and a reduction in the duration of anagen. In these individuals, androgen receptors and 5α-reductase activity (converts testosterone to 5-dihydrotestosterone) are greater in frontal hair follicles than occipital follicles; higher activites of aromatase (involved in conversion of testosterone to oestrodiol) are found in occipital follicles. This is one explanation for frontal baldness in men. Finasteride, a 5α-reductase inhibitor which does not affect the androgen receptor results in some regrowth of hair in about 70% of men after 2 years of continuous use. If treatment is successful, the drug is continued indefinitely because the balding process continues when it is stopped.

What do you understand by the term trichorrhexis nodosa?
It is the fracture of the hair shaft and is common in black patients who straighten their hair. Usually the hair regrows healthily if gentle hair-care practices are adopted.

186 ATOPIC DERMATITIS (ECZEMA)

INSTRUCTION
Look at this patient's skin.

SALIENT FEATURES

History

- Pruritus: this an important symptom because it affects the quality of life
- Tell the examiner that you would like to know whether there is a personal or family history of atopy (asthma, allergic rhinitis, atopic dermatitis) or food allergy.

Examination

- Scratch marks
- Hyperpigmented or hypopigmented lichenified lesions in flexures (including face, neck, upper trunk, wrists, hand, in the antecubital and popliteal folds) (Fig. 186.1).

DIAGNOSIS

This patient has atopic dermatitis (lesion), which is caused by atopy as supported by a history of asthma (aetiology); it is causing the patient severe itching (functional status).

QUESTIONS

What are the stages of atopic dermatitis?

There are three age-related stages, which are separated by remission.

Infantile stage (up to 2 years of age). Red, scaly, itchy crusted rash on both cheeks and extensors of the extremities. The napkin area is generally spared. Eczema of the scalp may also be seen

Childhood stage (2–12 years). There is papulation (rather than exudation) in the flexural areas including neck, cubital fossa, popliteal fossa and volar aspect of wrists and ankles. The plaques show both excoriation and lichenification. In black children, there may be hypopigmentation

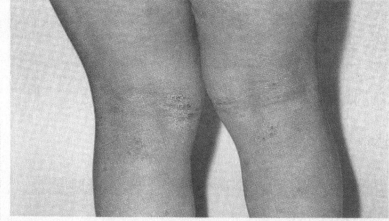

Fig. 186.1 Flexural atopic dermatitis. (With permission from Kumar, Clark 2005.)

Adults (puberty onwards). The face is commonly involved and there is lichenification of flexures including wrists, hands, fingers, ankles, toes and feet, head and neck.

What are the criteria for diagnosis?

Hanifin and Rajka's major criteria require three or more of the following:
- Pruritus
- Typical morphology and distribution: flexural lichenification in adults, facial or extensor involvement in children
- Chronic or chronically relapsing dermatitis
- Family or personal history of atopy (asthma, allergic rhinitis, atopic dermatitis).

Many of the minor criteria are under dispute and include ichthyosis, nipple eczema, food intolerance, keratoconus, subcaspular anterior cataracts, cheilitis, pityriasis alba and anterior neck folds. Fissuring below the auricles of the ear and diffuse scaling of the scalp may be seen in severe disease.

How would you treat such patients?

- Foods (typically dairy products, peanuts, eggs and wheat) which cause itching should be avoided
- Patient should be instructed about skin care including avoiding frequent baths and scratchy fabrics, and regular use of emollients
- Adequate cutaneous hydration
- Treatment of infected skin
- Antihistamines to control itching
- Corticosteroid lotion, cream or ointment: topical steroids are first-line drug therapy
- Phototherapy with psoralen plus ultraviolet A (PUVA) in those unresponsive to topical treatment
- Severe recalcitrant disease: ciclosporin, azathioprine, tacrolimus, mycophenolate, mofetil, pimecrolimus, Grenz-rays
- Investigational treatment: phosphodiesterase inhibitors, interleukin-2 and thymopentin.

What are the potential complications of atopic dermatitis?

- Staphylococcal superinfection; a deficiency in the expression of antimicrobial peptides may account for the susceptibility of patients with atopic dermatitis to skin infection with *Staphylococcus aureus* (N Engl J Med 2002;347:1151–60).
- Eczema herpeticum.

What do you know about natural history of atopic dermatitis?

- Non-atopic dermatitis is the first manifestation of atopic dermatitis (as a result of genetically determined epidermal barrier dysfunction and the effect of environmental factors).
- Sensitization occurs subsequently (because of the genetic predisposition for IgE-mediated sensitization). This phenomenon is favoured by *S. aureus* enterotoxin products.
- Tissue damage and the release of structural proteins occurs finally (from scratching), which triggers an IgE response in patients with atopic dermatitis. This sensitization to self-proteins can be the result of the homology of allergen-derived epitopes and human proteins in the context of molecular mimicry.

What is known about the genetic aspects of atopic dermatitis?
Atopic dermatitis is a complex genetic disease that emerges in the context of two major groups of genes:
- Genes encoding epidermal or other epithelial structural proteins
- Genes encoding major elements of the immune system.

What are the proposed mechanisms of atopic dermatitis?
One mechanism proposes that the primary defect resides in an immunologic disturbance that causes IgE-mediated sensitization, with epithelial barrier dysfunction as a consequence of local inflammation.

Another proposal is that an intrinsic defect in the epithelial cells leads to the barrier dysfunction and that the immunologic aspects are an epiphenomenon.

187 VENOUS ULCER

INSTRUCTION

Look at this patient's leg.

SALIENT FEATURES

History

- Varicose veins; ask about duration
- Past history of venous thromboembolism
- Duration of ulceration and whether this is the first episode or recurrent
- Pain (lack of pain suggests neuropathic aetiology)
- Rheumatoid arthritis (remember up to half the patients with rheumatoid arthritis have venous leg ulcers rather than the result of rheumatoid arthritis).

Examination

- Ulcer located on the medial aspect of leg (around the ankles) with pigmentation
- Surrounding dermatitis and excoriation from pruritus (stasis dermatitis)
- White atrophy with scars in the overlying skin
- The ulcer may be secondarily infected (cellulitis or thrombophlebitis)
- Look for varicose veins (Fig. 187.1)
- The range of hip, knee and ankle movement should be determined
- Sensation should be tested with a monofilament to exclude peripheral neuropathy (neuropathic arthritis or Charcot's joints, see p. 496).

DIAGNOSIS

This patient has a venous ulcer (lesion) caused by varicose veins (aetiology), which has caused severe pigmentation and dermatitis around the ankles (functional status).

ADVANCED-LEVEL QUESTIONS

What causes the surrounding pigmentation?
It results from extravasation of red blood cells and haemosiderin deposition.

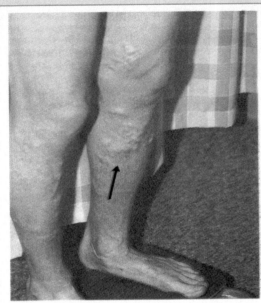

Fig. 187.1 Varicose veins of the leg (arrow). (With permission from Kumar et al. 2009.)

What causes the white atrophy (atrophie blanche)?
It results from hyalization of skin vessels, leading to scars in the overlying skin.

What is the pathogenesis of venous ulcer?
Disturbed venous flow patterns and chronic inflammation probably underlie all the clinical manifestations of the disease.

How is the diagnosis confirmed?
- When the diagnosis is in doubt, a punch biopsy from the border (not the base) of the lesion is helpful.
- Color duplex scanning to define underlying venous abnormality: 60% of patients have normal deep veins with isolated superficial venous competence.

How would you manage such an ulcer?
- Reduction of venous hypertension and oedema. Elevation of the limbs, wearing support bandages, weight reduction in the obese. The mainstay of community management of venous ulcers is graduated compression bandaging (in these patients the ankle brachial pressure index must be at least 0.8). The healing rate depends on the initial size of the ulcer, but 65–70% of venous ulcers heal within 6 months
- Control surrounding inflammation. Wet compresses, topical steroids
- Infection: antibiotics for cellulitis
- Dermatitis: zinc and salicylic acid paste
- Skin on the lower leg must be kept moist: emollient such as simple aqueous cream or 50:50 liquid paraffin
- Ulcers: cleaning with potassium permanganate, debridement, skin grafting

- Treatment of varicose veins. Long saphenous or short saphenous incompetence in the presence of normal deep veins may benefit from surgery to correct venous abnormality in the leg and allow ulcer healing. Patients with refluxing deep veins would benefit from compression bandaging.

Is recurrence common?

The 5-year recurrence rate of healed venous ulcers is about 40%; it is about 69% in non-compliant patients compared with 19% in patients wearing class 2 compression hosiery.

Are varicose veins in the absence of skin changes indicative of chronic venous insufficiency?

Varicose veins in the absence of skin changes are not indicative of chronic venous insufficiency. Chronic venous disease encompasses the full spectrum of signs and symptoms associated with all the CEAP (clinical, aetiologic, anatomical and pathophysiological classification; used to grade chronic venous disease) classes, whereas the term 'chronic venous insufficiency' is generally restricted to disease of greater severity (i.e. classes C4 to C6).

The CEAP uses clinical signs in the affected legs to place the venous disease into seven classes, C0 to C6. Leg symptoms associated with chronic venous disease include aching, heaviness, a sensation of swelling and skin irritation; limbs categorized in any clinical class may be symptomatic (S) or asymptomatic (A).

What are the factors that influence venous pressure in the legs?

Pressure in the veins of the leg is determined by three components.

- *Hydrostatic component* related to the weight of the column of blood from the right atrium to the foot (during standing without skeletal muscle activity, venous pressures in the legs are determined by the hydrostatic component and capillary flow, and they may reach 80–90 mmHg)
- *Hydrodynamic component* related to pressures generated by contractions of the skeletal muscles of the leg and the pressure in the capillary network (skeletal muscle contractions, as during ambulation, transiently increase pressure within the deep leg veins)
- *Venous valve component,* if effective, ensures that venous blood flows toward the heart, thereby emptying the deep and superficial venous systems and reducing venous pressure, usually to <30 mmHg. Both hydrostatic and hydrodynamic effects are profoundly influenced by the action of the venous valves. Even very small leg movements can provide important pumping action. In the absence of competent valves, the decrease in venous pressure with leg movements is attenuated. If valves in the perforator veins are incompetent, the high pressures generated in the deep veins by calf muscle contraction can be transmitted to the superficial system and to the microcirculation in skin.

Note: The clinical signs of chronic venous disease probably reflect venous pressures in the leg reaching higher than normal values and remaining elevated for prolonged periods.

What are the causes of lower extremity ulcers?

- Cardiovascular disease
- Diabetic nephropathy
- Arterial insufficiency

- Trauma
- Vasculitis
- Sickle cell anaemia
- Malignancy infection
- Pyoderma ganagrenosum.

What factors are associated with poorly healing ulcers?

- Large initial size (>20 cm^2)
- Duration of time before compression treatment (>1 year)
- Combined arterial insufficiency
- Poor improvement in first 4 weeks of compression treatment
- Age
- Venous refill time on plethsymography of <20 s.

Further reading

Bergan JJ, Schmid-Schönbein GW, Coleridge Smith PD, et al: Mechanisms of disease: chronic venous disease, *N Engl J Med* 355:488–498, 2006.

London NJM, Donnelly R: ABC of arterial and venous disease: ulcerated lower limb, *BMJ* 320:1589–1591, 2000 (review).

188 ARTERIAL LEG ULCER

INSTRUCTION

Look at this patient's leg.

SALIENT FEATURES

History

- Intermittent claudication
- History of underlying cardiovascular or cerebrovascular disease
- Pain in the distal foot when the patient is supine ('rest pain' syndrome)
- Impotence
- Absence of bleeding from the ulcer
- History of precipitating trauma or underlying deformity
- History of diabetes, chronic renal failure.

Examination

- Tender, punched-out ulcers on leg (usually away from the ankle region) (Fig. 188.1)
- The ulcer is usually in the plantar surface over the heads of first and fifth metatarsals (uncommon on the dorsum of the foot because the pressure is less sustained and perfusion is better)
- Cold atrophic skin
- Loss of hair
- Thickened nails
- Peripheral pulses are not palpable or diminished (in diabetics and in chronic renal failure the arteries may be calcified, making the results of pulse examination less reliable)
- Pallor on elevation

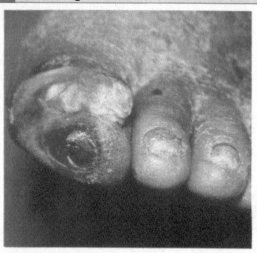

Fig. 188.1 Circumscribed necrotic arterial ulcer. (With permission from Zipes DP et al. 2007.)

- Redness of foot on lowering the leg (dependent rubor)
- Sluggish filling of toe capillaries.

DIAGNOSIS

This patient has an arterial ulcer (lesion) caused by vascular insufficiency, as evidenced by the absence of popliteal pulses (aetiology).
Remember: An ankle–brachial index <0.6 suggests arterial compromise.

QUESTIONS

How would you investigate such a patient?
- Radiographs may show calcification of the arteries of the leg
- Doppler ultrasonography to define the severity of arterial involvement
- Measurement of segmental limb pressures
- Pulse–volume waveform and transcutaneous oxygen are particularly useful in evaluating perfusion of the diabetic foot because they are not affected by vessel calcification
- Aortography shows narrowing and stenosis of the leg arteries.

How would you manage arterial ulcers?
- General: stop smoking; control diabetes, obesity and hypertension
- Limbs: should be kept warm (but avoid local heat)
- Feet: chiropodist and foot care, appropriate foot-wear
- Regular exercise to promote development of anastomotic collateral vessels
- Low-dose aspirin
- Surgery: balloon dilatation for local iliac or femoral stenoses, aortoiliac bypass, amputation when complicated by gangrene
- Flow-limiting arterial lesions should be evaluated and reconstructed or bypassed: prosthetic vascular grafts or autologous vein grafts may be used.

Mention other causes of leg ulcers

- Venous ulcers (Case 187)
- Neuropathic: diabetes mellitus, leprosy
- Vasculitis: rheumatoid arthritis, SLE, pyoderma gangrenosum
- Haematological disorders: sickle cell anaemia, spherocytosis
- Neoplastic: basal cell carcinoma, Kaposi's sarcoma (Case 180)
- Trauma or artefact
- Infection: postcellulitis, fungal.

Further reading

London NJM, Donnelly R: ABC of arterial and venous disease: ulcerated lower limb, *BMJ* 320:1589–1591, 2000 (review).
Sumpio BE: Foot ulcers, *N Engl J Med* 343:787–793, 2000.

189 ERYTHEMA NODOSUM

INSTRUCTION

Look at this patient's shins.

SALIENT FEATURES

History

- Elicit a history of:
  - fever (may precede the skin lesions by 1–7 days)
  - painful nodules
  - arthalgias
  - sore throat (β-haemolytic streptococcal infection)
  - drugs (sulphonamides, penicillins, oral contraceptives)
  - GI symptoms (*Yersinia enterocolitica* infections)
  - infections (TB, leprosy, coccidiomycosis, histoplasmosis)
  - sarcoidosis.

Remember:

- about half the cases are idiopathic
- lesions can be less intense in coloration, like large pink hives
- lesions appears in crops; consequently, there may lesions in different stages of evolution.

Examination

- Poorly defined, exquisitely tender, erythematous nodules (which are better felt than seen) (Fig. 189.1).

DIAGNOSIS

This patient has tender erythema nodosum (lesions) on the shins caused by the use of oral contraceptives (aetiology).

QUESTIONS

How can a definitive diagnosis be obtained?
By a deep wedge biopsy of the tissue.

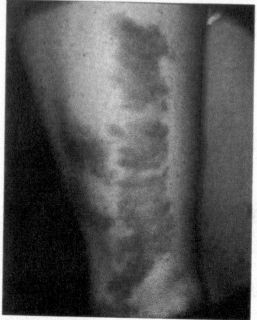

Fig. 189.1 Erythema nodosum lesions.

ADVANCED-LEVEL QUESTIONS

What is the histology?

Erythema nodosum is a panniculitis, which is an inflammatory reaction in the subcutaneous fat:

- In early lesions, there is widening of the connective tissue septa owing to oedema, fibrin exudation and infiltration by neutrophils
- Later, there is infiltration by lymphocytes, histiocytes, multinucleated giant cells and occasionally eosinophils, associated with septal fibrosis.

Note: Vasculitis is absent.

Mention some examples of panniculitis

- Erythema induratum (associated vasculitis)
- Weber–Christian disease (relapsing febrile nodular panniculitis)
- Factitial panniculitis.

How would you treat these patients?

Local: hot or cold compresses

Systemic: NSAIDs, saturated solution of potassium iodide, corticosteroid therapy, salicylates.

FP Weber (1863–1962), a British physcian who graduated from St Bartholomew's Hospital, London, and was a keen collector of coins and vases. He was an alpinist, like his father Sir HD Weber (1823–1918), who described Weber syndrome.

Henry A Christian (1876–1951), Professor of Medicine and the first Physician-in-Chief of the Peter Bent Brigham Hospital. He also described histiocytosis X (Hand–Schüller–Christian disease).

190 FUNGAL NAIL DISEASE

INSTRUCTION

Look at this patient's toenails.

SALIENT FEATURES

History

- Embarrassment from a cosmetic perspective
- Mechanical problems including the fact that nails get snagged in clothing, etc.
- History of diabetes.

Examination

- Nails are white, green or, occasionally, black when the infection is superficial or proximal (Fig. 190.1A,B).
- When the infection is distal there may be onycholysis (Fig. 190.1C,D; see Case 193).

Proceed as follows:

- Look at the fingernails: thickened, yellow or white nail with scaling under the elevated distal free edge of the nail plate
- Tell the examiner that you would like to look for underlying immunodeficiency states such as HIV and circulatory disorders (Raynaud syndrome).

DIAGNOSIS

This patient has fungal nail disease (lesion), which is usually caused by *Trichophyton* or *Candida* (aetiology), and it is cosmetically unacceptable to the patient (functional status).

ADVANCED-LEVEL QUESTIONS

What do you understand by the term onychomycosis?

It refers to a fungal infection of nails. Diagnostic criteria (J Am Acad Dermatol 2007;56:939–44) include:

- Clinical primary criteria:
  - White/yellow or orange/brown patches or streaks
- Clinical secondary criteria:
  - Onycholysis
  - Subungual hyperkeratosis/debris
  - Nail-plate thickening.
  - **Note**: Tinea pedis often occurs concomitantly with pedal onychomycosis, and tinea manuum with infected fingernails.

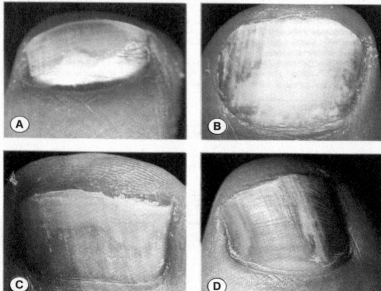

Fig. 190.1 Onychomycosis. (A) Proximal subungal onychomycosis. (B) Superficial onychomycosis with a dry, white, powdery surface that can be easily scraped away. (C) Distal onychomycosis: early changes. (D) Distal onychomycosis: late changes where the infection has progressed along a linear channel. (With permission from Habif 2009.)

- Laboratory criteria:
  - Positive microscopic evidence
  - positive culture of dermatophyte.

What are the different causative organisms?

- Dermatophytes (ringworm, tinea unguium): *Trichophyton rubrum, T. interdigitale* (toenails are more commonly affected than fingernails). *T. rubrum* infection is associated with distal or lateral involvement of the nail plate that spreads proximally, eventually affecting the whole nail; this may be associated with proximal subungual nail dystrophy associated with separation of the nail from the bed. *T. interdigitale* infection, characteristically seen in patients with AIDS, produces superficial white onychomycosis with crumbly white areas on the nail surface.
- Yeasts: *Candida albicans, C. parapsilosis* (fingernails are more commonly affected than toenails).
- Non-dermatophytes (moulds): *Fusarium, Scopulariopsis brevicaulis* (toenails are more commonly affected than fingernails).

Does the clinical picture vary according to the nature of the infecting organism?

Yes, as follows:

- Dermatophytes: distal or lateral nail involvement spreading proximally, proximal subungual dystrophy, superficial white dystrophy, white or yellow thickened nails, crumbling of nail plate, adjacent web or skin involvement may be present.
- *Candida*: chronic paronychia, shiny red bolstered nailfold, almost exclusively affects finger nailfolds, loss of cuticle, pus exuding from under nailfold, usually proximal nail involvement, distal nail dystrophy (associated with circulatory disorders), total dystrophic onychomycosis, nails white, green or occasionally black.
- Non-dermatophyte: superficial white onychomycosis, solitary nail involvement, colour of the nail may be influenced by the nature of infecting mould (e.g. the nails are white with *Fusarium*, white, yellow, brown or green with *S. brevicaulis*).

What are the patterns of fungal nail involvement?
Distal lateral subungual onychomycosis.
Superficial white onychomycosis.
Proximal white subungual onychomycosis.
Total dystrophic onychomycosis (i.e. all the previous three sites are affected).

Is laboratory diagnosis essential before starting treatment?
Yes, for the following reasons:
- Antifungal treatment is prolonged and the causative organism may be non-fungal
- To identify contacts of the patient
- To exclude mixed infection
- To optimize treatment as certain fungi are less responsive to treatment.

What are the poor prognosis factors?
- Areas of nail involvement >50%
- Significant lateral disease
- Subungual hyperkeratosis >2 mm
- White/yellow or orange/brown streaks in the nail
- Total dystrophic onychomycosis (with matrix involvement)
- Non-responsive organisms (e.g. *Scytalidium* mold)
- Immunosuppression
- Diminished peripheral circulation.

Mention some non-fungal nail infections
Bacterial nail infection, e.g. *Pseudomonas aeruginosa* (green or blackish discoloration of the nails), *Staphylococcus aureus* (causes acute paronychia or whitlow).

How are specimens obtained for mycological diagnosis?
Scrapings are taken with a blunt scalpel as proximally as possible in the nail:
- In distal and lateral onychomycosis, specimens are taken from the proximal part of the diseased portion of the nail and subungual material
- In superficial white onychomycosis, the scrapings are taken from the diseased nail surface
- In proximal white mycosis, the scrapings are taken from the nail surface.
In the laboratory, 20–30% potassium hydroxide is added to part of the specimen to macerate nail keratin before direct microscopy and the rest of the specimen is inoculated on different media.

What is the recommended treatment for onychomycosis?

- Dermatophyte infections (BMJ 1995;311:1277–81):
  - Localized distal nail disease: tioconazole with undecylenic acid paint, amorolfine paint weekly and 40% urea paste for dissolution
  - Proximal or extensive nail disease: terbinafine, itraconazole, fluconazole, griseofulvin and amorolfine nail paint. Data have suggested that terbinfaine is the treatment of choice for onychomycosis (Lancet 1998;351:541, BMJ 1999;318:1031–5).
- Candidal infections:
  - Chronic paronychia (localized): imidazole creams or paints, nystatin ointment, terbinafine cream; there is insufficient evidence on the effects of topical antifungal agents in people with frequently infected toenails (BMJ 2001;322:288–9)
  - Distal infection: tioconazole with undecylenic acid paint, amorolfine nail paint
  - Severe infection or severe chronic paronychia: itraconazole.
- Non-dermatophyte (mould) onychomycosis:
  - Localized disease: tioconazole with undecylenic acid paint, amorolfine paint weekly, 40% urea paste for dissolution or even avulsion of the nail
  - Persistent disease: itraconazole.

Mention some fungal infections that do not respond to oral treatment

Scopulariopsis, Scytalidium, Fusarium and *Acremonium* spp.

What is the definition of cure in fungal nail infections?

Cure in fungal nail infections is defined by the absence of clinical signs or the presence of negative nail culture and/or microscopy results with one or more of the following minor clinical signs (J Am Acad Dermatol 2007;56:939–44):

- Minimal distal subungual hyperkeratosis
- Nail-plate thickening.

Persistent onychomycosis is suggested at the end of the observation period by:

- White/yellow or orange/brown streaks or patches in or beneath the nail plate
- Lateral onycholysis with subungual debris.

Although nail appearance will usually continue to improve after therapy is stopped, the nails may have a persistent abnormal appearance even where therapy has been effective.

What information is available about the genetic susceptibility to fungal nail infections?

One study reported an autosomal recessive form of susceptibility to chronic mucocutaneous candidiasis that was associated with homozygous mutations in *CARD9* – the gene encoding the caspase recruitment domain containing protein 9. The patients had low numbers of Th17 cells (helper T cells that produce interleukin 17) (N Engl Med Med 2009;361:1727).

Another study reported a mutation leading to replacement of Tyr-238 in the β-glucan receptor dectin-1 in a family in which four women had either recurrent vulvovaginal candidiasis or onychomycosis. This Tyr-238 polymorphism hampered the recognition of *Candida* β-glucan and was associated with an impaired cytokine response by monocytes and macrophages. The mutation did not, however, impair killing of *Candida* by neutrophils, which seems to prevent invasive fungal infections (N Engl Med Med 2009;361:1760).

Further reading

Denning DW, Evans EGV, Kibbler CC, et al: Fungal nail disease: a guide to good practice (report of a Working Group of the British Society for Medical Mycology), *BMJ* 311:1277–1281, 1995.

191 LICHEN SIMPLEX CHRONICUS (NEURODERMATITIS)

INSTRUCTION

Look at this patient's skin.

SALIENT FEATURES

History

- Itching (self-perpetuating scratch-itch cycle).

Examination

- Several scratch marks (from pruritus)
- Well-circumscribed plaque with lichenified or dry, thickened, leathery skin (Fig. 191.1)
- Look for similar plaques in common areas, including the posterior nuchal region, wrists, perineum, dorsum of the feet or ankles (Fig. 191.2).

DIAGNOSIS

This patient has lichen simplex chronicus (lesion), which is caused by chronic itching and scratching (aetiology) and is cosmetically disturbing to the patient.

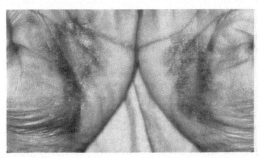

Fig. 191.1 Lichen simplex chronicus.

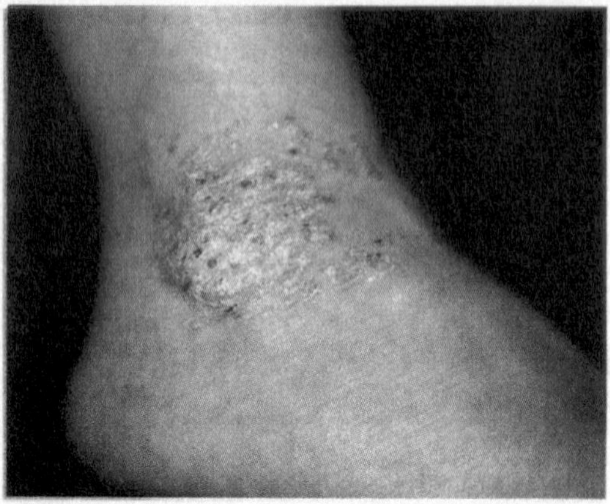

Fig. 191.2 Lichen simplex chronicus. (With permission from Habif 2009.)

ADVANCED-LEVEL QUESTIONS

How would you treat such a patient?

- Break the scratch–itch–scratch cycle by adminstering antipruritic agents
- High-potency topical steroids (under occlusion or intralesional injection)
- The area should be protected
- Patient should be made aware of when he or she is scratching.

What is the prognosis?

The disease tends to remit during treatment; however, it may recur or develop at another site.

What is the classification of itch?

Twycross (Q J Med 2003;96:7–26) classification of itch is based on peripheral and central origins of itch:

- *Pruritoceptive itch* is itch that originates in the skin, from inflammation, dryness or other skin damage, and is transmitted by nerve C-fibres, e.g. itch caused by reactions to insect bite, scabies, urticaria.
- *Neuropathic itch* is itch that arises because of disease located at any point along the afferent pathway, e.g. post-herpes zoster neuropathy, the itch occasionally associated with multiple sclerosis and brain tumours.
- *Neurogenic itch* is itch that originates centrally but without evidence of neural pathology, e.g. itch of cholestasis, which is the result of the action of opioid neuropeptides on opioid μ-receptors.
- *Psychogenic itch*, as in the delusional state of parasitophobia.

Often one type of itch can coexist with another, for example in the itch of atopic eczema, neurogenic as well as pruritoceptive itches seem to arise in the same patient.

Which spinal tracts conduct itch and pain information?

Information on itch and pain is conveyed centrally in two separate systems that both use the lateral spinothalamic tract.

192 NAIL CHANGES

INSTRUCTION

Look at these nails.

SALIENT FEATURES

- Disorders of the nail bed:
  - Terry's nail (Fig. 192.1): brownish-red distal transverse band; occurs normally in the elderly, also seen in cirrhosis and congestive cardiac failure
  - Lindsay's half-and-half nail (Fig. 192.2): distal brown band occupying about 25–50% of the nail bed, and seen in chronic renal failure
  - Muehrcke's nail: pale transverse bands resulting from oedema of the nail bed; seen in hypoalbuminaemia
  - Onycholysis (see Figs 190.1 and 193.1).

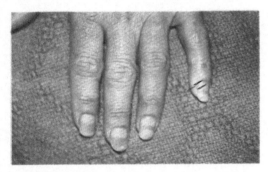

Fig. 192.1 Terry's nail.

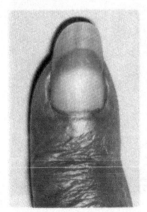

Fig. 192.2 Lindsay's half and half nail.

- Disorders of the lunula:
  - Blue lunula: in Wilson's disease the normally white lunula becomes blue (p. 437); the lunula has the largest area in the fingers closest to the thumb; in the elderly it becomes smaller or absent.
- Disorders of the nail plate:
  - Clubbing (p. 756)
  - Leukonychia (Fig. 192.3): whitish discoloration, which may be diffuse (liver disease, congenital, fungal), punctate or linear (Mees' lines (Fig. 192.4) seen in arsenical poisoning) or vasculitic
  - Koilonychia (spoon-shaped nails) seen in iron-deficiency anaemia, thyrotoxicosis
  - Onychogryphosis: hypertrophy and thickening of the nail
  - Onychomycosis: dystrophy, destruction of the nail caused by fungal or yeast infections (see Case 191)

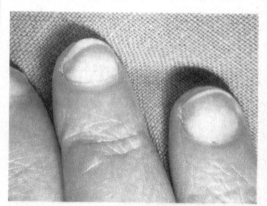

Fig. 192.3 Leukonychia.

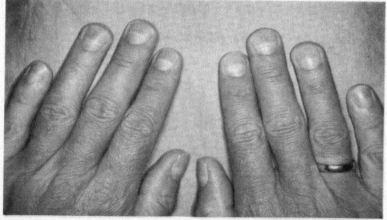

Fig. 192.4 Mees' lines.

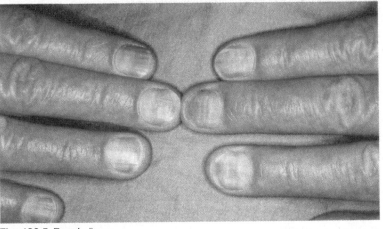

Fig. 192.5 Beau's lines.

- Pitting: seen in psoriasis (p. 558), alopecia areata
- Pterygium formation: growth of the cuticle onto the nail plate
- Longitudinal brown streaks: junctional naevi seen in black patients
- Beau's lines (Fig. 192.5): transverse depression occuring in severe systemic illness; it allows estimation of the date of the illness (normal nail grows at the rate of 0.1 mm/day and it takes approximately 3–4 months for the nail plate to grow out completely).
- Disorders of the nailfold:
  - Nailfold telangiectasia: seen in dermatomyositis, scleroderma, collagen vascular disease
  - Paronychia: may be acute or chronic, and includes the swelling and inflammation of the proximal or lateral nailfolds.
- Disorder of the hyponychium:
  - Koenen's subungual angiofibromas (p. 692) seen in tuberous sclerosis (p. 690)
  - Warts.

Note: The hyponychium is the most distal region of the nail bed and marks the transition to normal skin.

193 ONYCHOLYSIS

INSTRUCTION

Examine this patient's hands.

SALIENT FEATURES

History

- Take a history for excessive exposure to detergents, alkalis and keratolytic agents, and demeclocycline-induced photolysis
- History of psoriasis (p. 558)

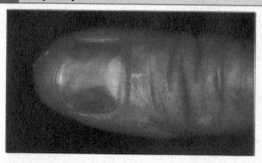

Fig. 193.1 Onycholysis.

- History of thyrotoxicosis (p. 506)
- History of diabetes (fungal infection).

Examination

- Distal separation of the nail plate from the nail bed (Fig. 193.1 and see Fig. 190.1C).

Proceed as follows:

- Look for nail pitting and silvery white plaques (psoriasis)
- Glance at the neck for goitre and tell the examiner that you would like to exclude thyrotoxicosis, hypothyroidism and diabetes mellitus
- Tell the examiner that you would like to exclude a fungal infection (Case 190).

DIAGNOSIS

This patient has onycholysis (lesion), probably caused by thyrotoxicosis, as evidenced by tachycardia, exophthalmos and goitre (aetiology).

QUESTIONS

What nail changes are associated with psoriasis?

Yellow, friable nails with pitting and onycholysis (lifting of nail from the bed), distal subungual hyperkeratosis.

How would you manage these nail lesions?

- Manicure and careful debridement
- Reduction of exposure to irritants (detergents, bleaches, alkalis)
- Intradermal steroids in the area of nail matrix (these are very painful injections)
- Non-surgical removal of dystrophic nails using urea ointments.

What are Plummer's nails?

This term refers to the onycholysis that occurs in hyperthyroidism and typically occurs in the fourth finger.

Further reading

DeNicola P, Morsiani M: Nail diseases in internal medicine, *J Am Acad Dermatol* 12:552–560, 1985. (review).

S Plummer (1874–1936), physician at the Mayo Clinic, Rochester, Minnesota, also described Plummer–Vinson syndrome (iron-deficiency anaemia and dysphagia).

194 MALIGNANT MELANOMA

INSTRUCTION

Look at this skin lesion.

SALIENT FEATURES

History

- Age (<50 and location on trunk has better prognosis)
- Family history (a patient with a dysplastic naevus with two relatives having malignant melanoma has a 300 time increased chance of having a malignant melanoma)
- Ask the patient:
  - has the mole has changed in colour?
  - does the mole itch?
  - has it changed in shape/morphology?
  - does your skin have freckles or tendency to freckling?
  - how may moles does your skin have, greater than 20?
  - how may times in your life have you had bad sunburn (with peeling of your skin)?
- Remember MacKie's four independent risk factors for melanoma: freckles, moles (Fig. 194.1), atypical naevi (Fig. 194.2) and a history of severe sunburn.

Examination

- Irregular and asymmetrical, with a fuzzy border where the pigment appears to be leaking into the surrounding skin (Fig. 194.3). (The American Cancer Society mnemonic to suspect malignancy in a mole is ABCDE: **a**symmetry, **b**order irregular, **c**olour variegation and **d**iameter >6 mm; **e**levated lesions are more suspicious.)

Proceed as follows:

- Comment if the mole stands out from the patient's other moles.
- Comment if bleeding and ulceration are present (these are ominous signs).
- Examine regional lymph nodes and the liver (for metastatic spread).

DIAGNOSIS

This patient has a malignant melanoma (lesion) as evidenced by its irregular border and, without delay, biopsy and histological examination must be performed to exclude or confirm the diagnosis.

Fig. 194.1 Mole.

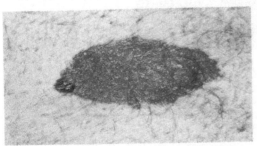

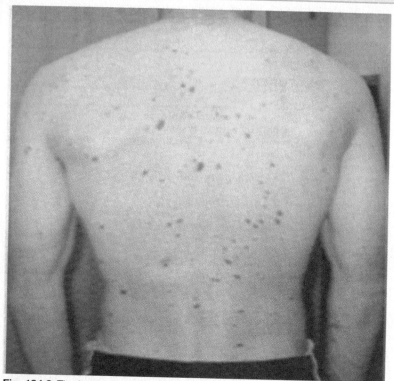

Fig. 194.2 The back of an individual with multiple atypical naevi.

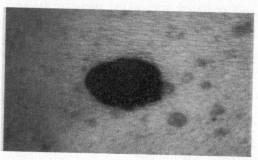

Fig. 194.3 Mole with pigment that appears to be leaking into surrounding skin.

QUESTIONS

What are the different types of malignant melanoma?

Depending on the clinical picture and histological findings these include:

- superficially spreading malignant melanoma (commonest type)
- nodular malignant melanoma
- acral lentiginous melanomas (arising on the palms, soles and nail beds)

- malignant melanoma on mucous membranes
- lentigo maligna melanoma (arising in lentigines in older individuals)
- amelanotic (non-pigmented) melanoma
- miscellaneous: melanoma arising from blue naevi, congenital and giant nevocytic naevi.

ADVANCED-LEVEL QUESTIONS

What are the patterns of growth of malignant melanoma?
- Radial growth: where the growth is horizontal within the epidermis and superficial dermal layers (e.g. lentigo maligna, acral/mucosal lentiginous, superficial spreading types). During this stage of growth, the tumour does not have the capacity to metastasize.
- Vertical growth: occurs with time, and the melanoma grows downward into the deeper dermal layers as an expansile mass lacking cellular maturation; this correlates with the emergence of a clone of cells with metastatic potential. The nature and extent of this vertical growth phase determines the biological behaviour of malignant melanoma.

What are the predisposing factors?
These include sunlight, the presence of a pre-existing naevus (e.g. dysplastic naevus), hereditary factors.

What is the treatment of such lesions?
Surgery remains the mainstay of treatment and the extent of surgery depends on the thickness of the primary melanoma:
- Excision: following histological examination the area is usually re-excised with margins dictated by the thickness of the tumour
- Elective lymph node dissection is controversial; in general, it is indicated only in melanomas of intermediate thickness with one draining chain of lymph nodes
- Intralesional injection of avirulent herpes simplex virus (but capable of replication) may be of therapeutic benefit in malignant melanoma; this is an experimental therapy (Lancet 2001;357:525)
- Interferon-alfa and vaccine therapy may reduce recurrences.

What are the prognostic factors in these patients?
- Tumour thickness: the deeper the melanoma the more likely is metastasis. Thin melanomas (<0.76 mm) approach 100% cure rate whereas only 20–30% survive for 5 years if the lesion has a depth >1.6 mm
- Level of invasion
- Sex of the patient
- Anatomical location: melanomas in the TANS areas (thorax, upper arms, neck and scalp) show a higher relative risk.

What are melanoma-associated genes?
Candidate genes include:
- the gene for growth regulator p16 on chromosome 9
- CMM1 on chromosome 1p36
- CDK4 on chromosome 12q14, encoding a cyclin-dependent kinase
- rarely, melanoma susceptibility is increased >10-fold by heritable mutations in the genes for the cell cycle regulators CDKN2A and CDK4.

Further reading

N Engl J Med 331:163, 1994.

Rona Mackie is contemporary professor of dermatology in Glasgow.

195 SEBORRHOEIC DERMATITIS

INSTRUCTION

Comment on this patient's skin.

SALIENT FEATURES

History

- History of itching
- History of Parkinson's disease, strokes and HIV.

Examination

- Greasy scales overlying erythematous plaques or patches affecting the face (eyebrows, eyelids, glabella, nasolabial folds or ears; Fig. 195.1), submammary folds, gluteal clefts. Occasionally it is generalized.
- Severe dandruff on the scalp.

Proceed as follows:

- Tell the examiner that you would like to look for the underlying disorder (Parkinson's disease, HIV and strokes).

Remember:

- The name is misleading and the condition is unrelated to seborrhoea (excess sebum production).
- Distinguishing severe seborrheic dermatitis from early facial psoriasis can be particularly difficult.

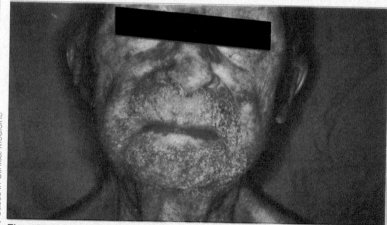

Fig. 195.1 Seborrhoeic dermatitis.

DIAGNOSIS

This patient has seborrhoeic dermatitis (lesion) with Parkinson's disease, and finds the lesion cosmetically unacceptable (functional status).

ADVANCED-LEVEL QUESTIONS

What is the aetiology of this disorder?

It is based on a genetic predisposition mediated by several factors including nutritional status, infection and hormones. Its response to antifungal agents has suggested that it represents an inflammatory reaction to *Pityrosporum ovale* yeasts present in the scalp of humans.

Mention some clinical variants?

- *Adult variants*:
  - Pityriasis capitis (dandruff)
  - Blepharitis
  - Pityriasiform seborrheic dermatitis: rare form involving the trunk and limbs
  - Flexural seborrheic dermatitis: involves any body folds, especially the retroauricular areas, the inner thighs, the genitalia and the breast folds, with intertriginous, sometimes oozing, lesions
  - Pitirosporum (malassezia) folliculitis: itchy, erythematous follicular papules, sometimes pustules, typically in sites rich in sebaceous glands; often occurs in immunocompromised hosts
  - Erythroderma (exfoliative dermatitis): generalized redness and scaling of the skin with systemic manifestations.
- *Infantile variants:*
  - Scalp seborrheic dermatitis (cradle cap): red-yellow plaques covered by scales on the scalp of infants; develops after a few weeks of age
  - Leiner's disease: poorly defined entity that includes a primary immunodeficiency syndrome not related to seborrheic dermatitis
  - Pityriasis amiantacea: thick, asbestos-like scales adhering to tufts of scalp hairs; may be associated with psoriasis, atopic dermatitis, or tinea capitis.
- *HIV-related seborrheic dermatitis:*
  - Occurs particularly in those with CD4 cell counts $<400 \times 10^6$ cells/l
  - Is usually more severe, diffuse and inflammatory than in otherwise healthy persons.
- *Drug-related seborrheic-like dermatitis:*
  - Common in patients treated with erlotinib or sorafenib
  - Also reported in patients treated with recombinant interleukin-2, psoralen plus ultraviolet (PUVA).

How would you treat these skin lesions?

- Topical antifungals are the mainstain in treatment, including ketoconazole, bifonazole and ciclopirox olamine (ciclopiroxolamine), which are available in different formulations such as creams, gels, foams and shampoos
- Topical glucocorticoids (avoid fluorinated preparations on the face)
- Shampoos containing coal tar and salicylic acid
- Selenium sulfide shampoos for the scalp
- Eyelid margins respond to gentle cleaning of lid margins with undiluted Johnson and Johnson baby shampoo using a cotton swab

- Oral ketoconazole is invaluable in the persistent seborrhoeic dermatitis of AIDS but should rarely be used otherwise
- Topical lithium succinate and lithium gluconate are effective alternatives for the treatment of seborrheic dermatitis in areas other than the scalp
- Topical 1% pimecrolimus.

What is the prognosis of this condition?
There is a tendency to lifelong recurrences.

Further reading

Naldi L, Rebora A: Seborrheic dermatitis, *N Engl J Med* 360:387–396, 2009.

196 MOLLUSCUM CONTAGIOSUM

INSTRUCTION

Look at these skin lesions.

SALIENT FEATURES

History

- Ask the patient whether there are similar lesions elsewhere (particularly genitals).

Examination

- Multiple rounded, dome-shaped, waxy papules that are 2–5 mm in diameter and contain central umbilication with a caseous plug (Fig. 196.1)
- The common sites are face, hands, lower abdomen and genitals.
Proceed as follows:
- Tell the examiner that you would like to investigate for an underlying HIV infection.

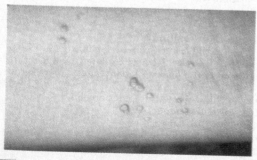

Fig. 196.1 Molluscum contagiosum. Multiple raised nodules, with areas of confluent lesions. (With permission from Rakel 2007.)

DIAGNOSIS

This patient has molluscum contagiosum (lesion), which is of viral aetiology; you would like to rule out an underlying HIV infection as the lesions are extensive and widely distributed on the face, neck and other parts of the body.

QUESTIONS

How do these lesions spread from one part of the body to another?
Probably by autoinoculation.

How is the infection spread from one patient to another?
By direct contact.

What is the histology of these lesions?
Microscopically they show cup-like verrucous epidermal hyperplasia. Large inclusion bodies called 'molluscum bodies' are present in the cells of the stratum corneum and granulosum. These bodies are also seen in the curd-like material that can be expressed from the central umbilication. Numerous virions are present within the molluscum bodies.

What is the aetiology of these lesions?
It is caused by a pox virus that is characteristically brick shaped and has a central dumb-bell-shaped DNA core.

How are these lesions treated?
- Curettage or cryotherapy (applications of liquid nitrogen to freeze the lesions)
- Physical expression by squeezing
- Phenol ablation (causes more scarring than squeezing; BMJ 1999;319: 1540)
- Light electrosurgery with a needle
- Imiquimod cream (50%) applied three times per week eradicates about 50% of anogenital warts (Arch Dermatol 1998;134:25–30). Imiquimod is an immune-enhancing agent with antiviral and anti-tumour effects
- Anecdotal reports suggest that topical cidofovir may be useful in severe molluscum contagiousm particularly in immunodeficient individuals (Lancet 1999;353:2042).

Note: In children these lesions tend to resolve spontaneously.

197 URTICARIA

INSTRUCTION

Look at the skin of this patient, who has recurrent lesions.

SALIENT FEATURES

History

- Determine physical causes that could have precipitated this response: cold urticaria, dermatographism (Fig. 197.1), pressure, sunlight, exercise, hot shower
- Drug history: aspirin, NSAIDs, morphine, codeine, penicillin, sulphonamides

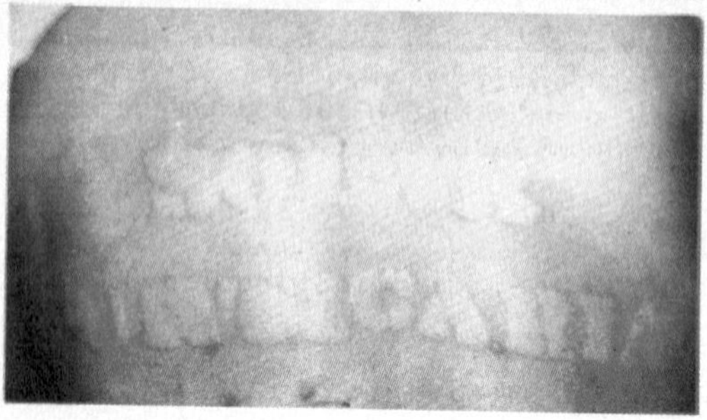

Fig. 197.1 Urticaria.

- Whether any foods precipitate the rash such as strawberries, seafood, nuts, chocolate
- Blood products causing these lesions.
- Wasp or bee stings
- Viral infections and febrile illnesses
- Know whether the patient has recurrent angioedema
- Obtain a history of atopy.

Examination

- Wheals that are smooth, oedematous, pin or red, and surrounded by a bright red flare. Clearing of the central area may leave an annular pattern.
- Associated scratch marks, indicating the wheals are itchy.

Proceed as follows:

- Tell the examiner that you would like to exclude infections (hepatitis, chronic sinusitis) and connective tissue disorders.

DIAGNOSIS

This patient has wheals (lesion) caused by chronic urticaria and dermatographism (aetiology), complicated by severe itching (functional status). Tell the examiner that you would like to exclude urticarial vasculitis before making a firm diagnosis.

Notes

- SLE and Sjögren's sydrome may present with urticarial lesions, which are usually urticarial vasculitis.
- Chronic urticaria is the occurrence of daily or almost daily widespread itchy wheals for at least six weeks (N Engl J Med 1995;332:1767–72). This includes urticarial vaculitis and physical urticaria.

ADVANCED-LEVEL QUESTIONS

What do you understand by the term dermatographism?

It is the presence of itchy, linear wheals with a surrounding bright red flare at sites of scratching or rubbing.

Which systemic disorder is associated with urticaria?

- Hashimoto's disease is the only systemic disorder with a clear and common association with chronic urticaria and angioedema.
- Less common is an association with Graves' disease.

How would you investigate a patient with chronic urticaria?

- FBC and white count; if eosinophilia is present
- Examination of the stool for ova and parasites
- Physical urticaria must be assessed by appropriate challenge testing
- Peanut-specific Ig-E when peanut allergy is suspected
- Serum complement C4 when there is a history of repeated cutaneous or mucosal angioedema
- Thyroid function tests because of diagnostic overlap between chronic urticaria and thyroid disease. The percentage of patients with chronic urticaria who have antithyroglobulin antibody, antimicrosomal antibody or both is 27%; 19% have abnormal thyroid function.

How would you manage patients with chronic urticaria?

- Identify avoidable cause such as food additives. Challenge testing for food additives should be avoided in patients with a history of severe angioedema, asthma or episodes of anaphylaxis.
- Antihistamines: about 85% of cutaneous histamine receptors are of the H_1 subtype, and the remaining 15% are H_2 receptors. The addition of an H_2-receptor antagonist to an H_1-receptor antagonist augments the inhibition of a histamine-induced wheal-and-flare reaction once H_1-receptor blockade has been maximized. H_1 antihistamines (terfenadine, doxepin) with a low potential for sedation are first-line treatment; 2% ephedrine spray is useful for oropharyngeal oedema. Non-sedating antihistamines such as loratadine, fexofenadine and cetirizine alleviate pruritus and decrease the incidence of hives.
- Leukotriene antagonists (zafirlukast and montelukast) have been shown to be superior to placebo.
- Calcium channel blockers can be used.
- A tepid shower temporarily alleviates itching.
- Corticosteroids merits consideration in patients who have little response to even a combination of H_1-receptor blockers, H_2-receptor blockers, and leukotriene-receptor blockade.
- Ciclosporin is the best studied immunosuppressive therapy for chronic urticaria.
- All patients should be advised to avoid aspirin and other NSAIDs, ACE inhibitors, macrolide antibiotics and imidazole antifungal agents.

198 MYCOSIS FUNGOIDES (CUTANEOUS T-CELL LYMPHOMA)

INSTRUCTION

Look at this patient's skin.

SALIENT FEATURES

History

- Age (usually fifth and seventh decade)
- Pruritus.

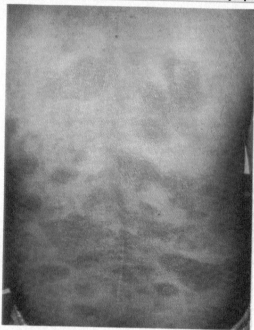

Fig. 198.1 Patch-stage mycosis fungoides: itchy, brownish-red plaques.

Examination

- Itchy, brownish-red plaques on the hips, buttocks and interscapular region (Fig. 198.1).

Proceed as follows:

- Tell the examiner that it may also involve the lymph nodes and viscera.

DIAGNOSIS

This patient has itchy brownish-red plaques with lymph node involvement (lesions), indicating mycosis fungoides (aetiology).

ADVANCED-LEVEL QUESTIONS

How would you confirm the diagnosis?

Skin biopsy to detect *Pautrier's microabscesses*, atypical cells in the nests in the epidermis, atypical mononuclear cell infiltrates, large hyperchromic cells with irregular nuclei — the 'mycosis cells'. The hallmark of mycosis fungoides is the identification of the *Sézary–Lautner cells*. These are T helper cells (CD4 positive) that characteristically form band-like aggregates within the superficial dermis and invade the dermis as single cells and small clusters (Pautrier's microabscesses).

What is the prognosis?

Very slow progression of skin lesions with eventual tumour formation and systemic dissemination of lymphoma. In most patients this process takes several weeks.

What is the differential diagnosis?
Psoriasis.

How would you treat this patient?
Treatment is palliative with steroids, chemotherapeutic agents and electron-beam therapy.

What are the stages of cutaneous T-cell lymphoma?
- Stage I: eczematoid or psoriasiform erythematous lesions
- Stage II: infiltrated plaques
- Stage III: nodules (Fig. 198.2), ulcers, tumours
- Stage IV: lymph node involvement with or without systemic dissemination.

Prognosis is good for early mycosis fungoides (Arch Dermatol 1996;132: 1309–13).

Staging is by a tumour/node/metastases/blood system or by the WHO indolent versus aggressive clinical behaviour system (Lancet 2008; 371: 945–57).

What is the treatment of mycosis fungoides?
- Various superficial treatments: topical steroids and chemotherapeutic agents (mechlorethamine and carmustine), psoralen plus ultraviolet A (PUVA) and electron-beam radiotherapy improve skin disease, but none has been shown to alter the natural history of the disease.
- Novel approaches being explored include aciclovir, interferons, retinoids, pentostatin, monoclonal antibodies directed to T-cell antigens, extracorporeal photopheresis and interferon-alfa (Lancet 1997;350: 32–3).

Have you heard of Sézary syndrome?
It is a rare leukaemic, erythrodermic variant of mycosis fungoides characterized by lymphadenopathy and large mononuclear cells (*Sézary cells*) in the skin and blood. It is often resistant to traditional treatment and has a poor prognosis. Extracorporeal photopheresis (which consists of oral

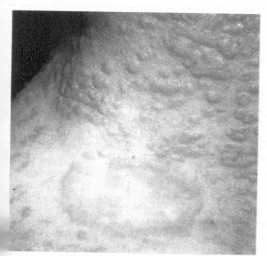

Fig. 198.2 Mycosis fungoides. Tumour stage III with nodules.

administration of methoxsalen, exposure of a lymphocyte-enriched blood fraction to ultraviolet A light and reinfusion of the cells into the patient) has recently shown promise.

Further reading

Hwang ST, Janik JE, Jaffe ES, Wilson WH: Mycosis fungoides and Sézary syndrome, *Lancet* 371:945–957, 2008. (review).

> Jean Louis M Alibert, a French dermatologist, first described this condition in 1806.
> A Sézary (1880–1956), a French dermatologist.

199 URTICARIA PIGMENTOSA

INSTRUCTION

Look at this patient's skin.

SALIENT FEATURES

History

- Urticaria with pruritus on trauma, rubbing or heat: *Darier's sign*
- Headache
- Diarrhoea
- Itching.

Examination

- Itchy reddish-brown macules and papules (Fig. 199.1)
- Telangiectasia.
Proceed as follows:
- Look for hepatosplenomegaly.

DIAGNOSIS

This patient has itchy reddish-brown macules with telangiectasia and Darier's sign (lesions) indicating urticaria pigmentosa (aetiology).

ADVANCED-LEVEL QUESTIONS

What do you know about urticaria pigmentosa?
It is the cutaneous manifestation of systemic mastocytosis.

What is the histology of urticaria pigmentosa?
It varies from an increase in the number of spindle-shaped and stellate mast cells about the superficial dermal vessels to large numbers of tightly packed round-to-oval mast cells in the upper and mid dermis. Variable fibrosis, oedema and a small number of eosinophils may also be present.

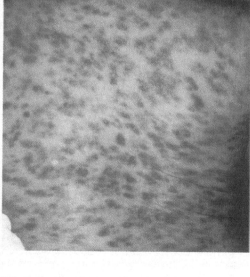

Fig. 199.1 Urticaria pigmentosa: reddish-brown macules and papules.

What do you know about systemic mastocytosis?

It is a condition characterized by mast cell hyperplasia that, in most cases, is neither clonal nor neoplastic. It can occur at any age and is slightly more common in men. Four forms have been recognized:

- Indolent form: does not alter life expectancy and constitutes the majority of cases
- Associated with frank leukaemia or dysmyelopoiesis: the prognosis is determined by the underlying haematological disorder
- Aggressive form: the prognosis is determined by the extent of organ involvement
- Mast cell leukaemia: rare, invariably fatal.

What diagnostic tests would you order?

- Urinary histamine is elevated in most cases (an elevated urinary histamine level is not a required finding for a diagnosis of mastocytosis; there is poor correlation between the urinary histamine content and the severity of symptoms in mastocytosis).
- Serum tryptase is elevated in most cases (the tryptase level is elevated in >83% of patients and is highly specific for this disease).
- Coagulation defects may occur as a result of the release of mast-cell heparin.
- Bone marrow biopsy is often diagnostic (revealing the focal infiltration of mast cells).
- Immunohistochemical analysis with monoclonal antibodies against the mast-cell markers tryptase and CD117 is used to confirm the diagnosis.

How would you manage such patients?

Treatment is based on blocking mast cell products, including histamine, prostaglandin D_2 and leukotrienes:

- H$_1$ blocker: for flushing and itch (e.g. chlormethiazole)
- H$_2$ blocker: for gastric and duodenal manifestations (e.g. ranitidine, cimetidine)
- Oral sodium cromoglycate for diarrhoea and abdominal pain
- NSAID for flushing not responsive to antihistamines
- High-dose aspirin
- Interferon-alfa has been used for patients with aggressive disease
- Imatinib, an inhibitor of c-Kit tyrosine kinase, also shows promise
- Intravenous cladribine.

FJ Darier (1856–1938), a French dermatologist.

200 TUBEROUS SCLEROSIS (BOURBEVILLE'S OR PRINGLE'S DISEASE)

INSTRUCTION

Look at this patient who has a history of seizures and mental retardation.

SALIENT FEATURES

History

- Family history (autosomal dominant inheritance with variable penetrance)
- Seizures
- Psychomotor retardation in childhood
- Reddened nodules (adenoma sebaceum) on the face since childhood.

Examination

- Angiofibromas (adenoma sebaceum) distributed in a butterfly pattern over the cheeks (Fig. 200.1), chin and forehead
- Shagreen patches: leathery thickenings in localized patches over the lumbosacral region
- Ash-leaf patches: hypopigmented areas (Fig. 200.2)
- Subungual fibromas (Fig. 200.3)
- Examine the fundus (retinal glial hamartomas).

DIAGNOSIS

This patient has adenoma sebaceum (lesions) caused by tuberous sclerosis. I would like to know his IQ and elicit a history of seizures to determine his functional status.

ADVANCED-LEVEL QUESTIONS

What other lesions may be present?

- Hamartomas within the CNS occurring as cortical tubers and subependymal hamartomas
- Renal angiomyolipomas

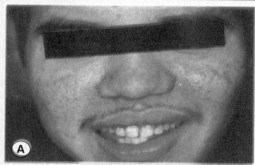

Fig. 200.1 Tuberous sclerosis: angiofibromas in a butterfly pattern over the cheeks, chin and forehead.

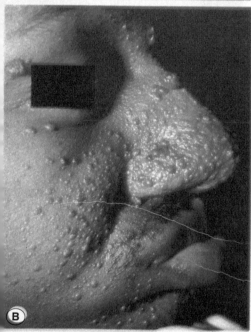

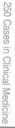

Fig. 200.2 Hypopigmented macules (ash-leaf pattern).

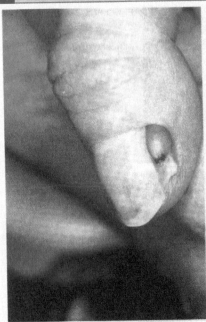

Fig. 200.3 Subungual fibromas.

- Cardiac rhabdomyomas and pulmonary myomas
- Cysts in the liver, kidney and pancreas.

Give some examples of the appearance of clinical manifestations at distinct developmental points

- Hypopigmented macules (formerly known as ash-leaf spots) are usually detected in infancy or early childhood.
- Shagreen patch is identified with increasing frequency after the age of 5 years.
- Ungual fibromas characteristically appear after puberty and may develop in adulthood.
- Facial angiofibromas (formerly called adenoma sebaceum) may be detected at any age but are generally more common in late childhood or adolescence.
- Cortical tubers and cardiac rhabdomyomas form are typical findings in infancy because they form during embryogenesis.
- A subependymal giant cell tumour of the brain may develop in childhood or adolescence.
- Renal cysts can be detected in infancy or early childhood.
- Angiomyolipomas develop in childhood, adolescence or adulthood.
- Pulmonary lymphangiomyomatosis is found in adolescent girls or women

What is the prevalence of tuberous sclerosis?

Population-based studies in UK estimate a frequency of 1 in 12 000 to 1 in 14 000 in children <10 years of age. Improved methods of determination have detected individuals who are not severely affected by tuberous sclerosis, increasing the estimates of its frequency: the disorder has a birth rate of 1 in 6000. It is estimated to be at 8 per 10 000 in Wessex UK (Lancet 1998;351:1490).

What are the diagnostic criteria for tuberous sclerosis?

Major and minor criteria exist to diagnose tuberous sclerosis (J Child Neurol 1998; 13:624–8). The diagnosis is made when two major features, or one major and two minor ones, can be shown. In one series of patients >90% had skin lesions, about 90% had symptoms of cerebral pathology, 70–90% had renal abnormalities and about 50% had retinal hamartomas.

- *Major features*:
  - Facial angiofibromas or forehead plaque pits in dental enamel
  - Non-traumatic ungula or periungual fibroma
  - Hypomelanotic macules (three or more)
  - Shagreen patch (connective tissue nevus) migration lines
  - Multiple retinal nodular hamartomas
  - Cortical tuber
  - Subependymal nodule
  - Subependymal giant cell astrocytoma
  - Cardiac rhabdomyoma, single or multiple
  - Lymphangiomyomatosis, renal angiomyolipoma, or both.
- *Minor features*:
  - Multiple, randomly distributed lesions
  - Hamartomatous rectal polyps
  - Bone cysts
  - Cerebral white matter radial
  - Gingival fibromas
  - Non-renal hamartoma
  - Retinal achromic patch
  - Confetti-like skin lesions
  - Multiple renal cysts.

How would you manage such patients?

- Symptomatically, with anticonvulsant therapy for seizures and genetic counselling. When severe epilepsy and mental retardation is present, the prognosis for life beyond the third decade is poor. Death is usually from seizures, associated neoplasms or intercurrent illness.
- Long-term follow-up includes the monitoring of lesion growth. No conclusive guidelines for surveillance have been established. The growth of angiomyolipomas or subependymal giant cell tumours requires regular follow-up. Periodic imaging of the brain and abdomen to monitor the growth of lesions in the brain and kidney should occur at least every 3 years and more often in patients with lesions that have progressive growth. Annual MRI of the brain is suggested until patients are at least 21 years of age, and then MRI should be done every 2 to 3 years both to diagnose and to monitor subependymal giant cell tumours. Annual ultrasonography, MRI or CT is indicated in patients with multiple angiomyolipomas or a single lesion that is progressive.
- Lymphangiomyomatosis: yearly pulmonary function testing may be useful to monitor lung function; some patients may require more frequent assessments.

- Electroencephalography can determine background cerebral activity and characterize patterns such as hypsarrhythmia in infantile spasms.
- Regular dermatologic evaluation is required since facial angiofibromas can cause cosmetic disfiguration and ultimately the lesions will require laser therapy or surgical removal.

Are you aware of any therapies currently being evaluated?

- The discovery of upregulation of the 'mammalian target of rapamycin' (mTOR) pathway in tumours associated with tuberous sclerosis presents new possibilities for therapy. Interferon-γ and interferon-α interact with mTOR, leading to deactivation of the translational repressor 4E-BP1, which could be beneficial for therapy.
- Sirolimus therapy causes the dysregulated mTOR pathway to return to normal in cells that lack hamartin or tuberin (encoded by the genes TSC1 or TSC2, respectively). Sirolimus is effective in diminishing the volume of lesions in patients with renal angiomyolipomas, subependymal giant cell astrocytomas and sporadic lymphangio leiomyomatosis. However, angiomyolipomas increased in volume after the sirolimus was discontinued, and some patients taking sirolimus experienced serious adverse events. Another concern is that sirolimus therapy may restore the cell's ability to activate AKT, suggesting that long-term treatment may increase the risk of malignant tumours in these patients.
- Genetic counselling should be recommended to patients to aid with family planning. It is an autosomal dominant disorder; therefore, those affected should be advised that the risk of having an affected child is approximately 50%

Do you know on which chromosome the gene is localized?

Tuberous sclerosis is an autosomal dominant disorder, although two-thirds of patients have sporadic mutations. The genes in which abnormalities are found are called TSC1 and TSC2. Both have been studied by multigenerational linkage analysis and have been localized to chromosome 9 (TSC1) (Science 1997;277:805–8) and chromosome 16 (TSC2) (Cell 1993;75:1305–15).

What do you know about the benign metastasis hypothesis?

The 'benign metastasis' hypothesis for the pathogenesis of lymphangiomyomatosis proposes that histologically benign cells with mutations in TSC1 or TSC2 may have the ability to travel to the lungs from angiomyolipomas in the kidney.

What do you know about the pathogenesis of tuberous sclerosis?

Several downstream protein cascades from tuberin and hamartin might be affected, for example the mTOR pathway, which detects signals of nutrient availability, hypoxia or growth factor stimulation. The mTOR pathway is stimulated by a small G-protein of the Ras superfamily RHEB (Ras homologue enriched in brain). Rheb is active when bound to GTP. Tuberin and hamartin form intracellular complexes that activate GTPase, thus reducing the stimulation of mTOR. Whether Rheb is the sole downstream effector or whether mTOR is the only clinically relevant target of Rheb remains to be characterized.

DM Bourneville (1840–1909), a French neurologist described tuberous sclerosis in 1880 (Bourneville, DM. Sclérose tubéreuse des circonvolutions cérébrales. Arch Neurol 1880;1:81–91).

JJ Pringle (1855–1922), an English dermatologist who was also the editor of the British Journal of Dermatology.

The Eker rat is an animal model of tuberous sclerosis.

Examination

1. Tell the patient, 'Look straight ahead with your right or left (R/L) eye while I look into your L/R eye'. (The candidate need not remove his or her spectacles while the fundus is being examined.) The candidate should use his or her own R/L eye to examine the patient's R/L eye.
2. Look at the eye from a distance of at least 50 cm and check for the red reflex. The presence of a red reflex indicates that the media in front of the retina is transparent and that the retina is firmly in apposition with the underlying choroid. Red reflex may be absent when there is a lens opacity, vitreous haemorrhage or retinal detachment.
3. Look systematically at the following:
   - The optic discs (comment on the colour, contour, cup and lamina cribrosa)
   - The macula (one or two disc diameters away from and a little below the temporal margin of the optic disc); it appears darker than the surrounding retina, and in young individuals has a central yellow point called the fovea centralis (Fig. VIII.1)
   - The nasal and temporal halves of the fundus
   - The retinal vessels (remember that the retinal artery has four main branches and the normal ratio of the artery to the vein is 2:3); assess the transparency of the vessels (the arteries usually have a shiny central reflex stripe), the presence of pressure effects such as AV nicking, the presence of focal narrowing of arteries as well as the tortuosity of the venule.

Note:
- Lesions in the fundus are measured using the disc diameter as the reference size.
- Elevation of any lesion is measured by noting the difference between lens powers that focus clearly on the top of the lesion and an adjacent normal area of the fundus. Elevation of 3-dioptres lens changes is approximately equal to 1 mm in actual elevation.

CLINICOPATHOLOGIC CORRELATIONS OF RETINAL HAEMORRHAGES AMD EXUDATES

The location of the haemorrhage within the retina determines its appearance by ophthalmoscopy. The retinal nerve fibre layer is oriented parallel to the internal limiting membrane. Haemorrhages here appear to be flame shaped. The deeper retinal layers are oriented perpendicular to the internal limiting membrane and haemorrhages here appear as 'dots'.

Exudates from leaky retinal vessels accumulate in the outer plexiform layer.

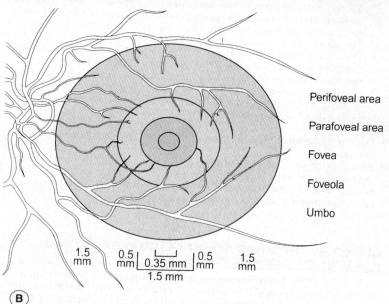

Fig. VIII.1 (A) Normal fundus with macula encompassed by major vascular arcades. (B) The components, from centre to periphery, of the macula. (With permission from Yanoff, Duker 2008.)

201 DIABETIC RETINOPATHY

INSTRUCTION

Examine the fundus in these patients.

- You will be expected to comment on whether it is background (Fig. 201.1) or proliferative (Fig. 201.2) retinopathy.
- You may have a clue about the underlying diabetes, either from a diabetic chart or from the presence of diabetic fruit juices at the bedside.

SALIENT FEATURES

History

- Gradual or acute loss of vision
- History of floaters
- History of diabetes, hypertension
- Ask about renal disease (renal-retinal syndrome of diabetes).

Examination

- Background retinopathy, caused by microvascular leakage into the retina:
  - Microaneurysms, usually seen in the posterior pole temporal to the fovea
  - Dot and blot haemorrhages (Fig. 201.3B)

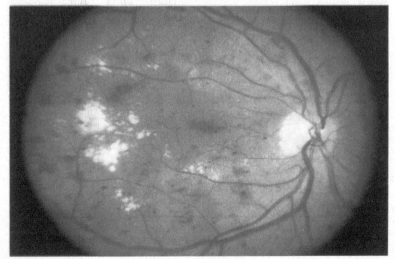

Fig. 201.1 Background retinopathy.

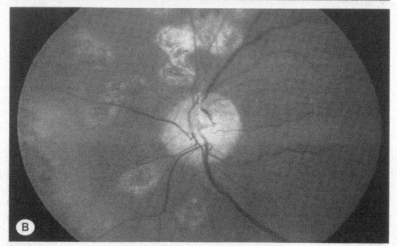

Fig. 201.2 Proliferative retinopathy.

- Hard exudates (Fig. 201.3C)
- Cottonwool spots (Fig. 201.3D).

DIAGNOSIS

This patient has dot and blot haemorrhages, and cottonwool spots (lesions), probably caused by diabetic retinopathy (aetiology), and good visual acuity (functional status).

QUESTIONS

What symptoms will this patient have?

The patient will be asymptomatic as the macula is spared.

How would you manage such a patient?

- Treat diabetes and associated hypertension
- Annual fundal examination.

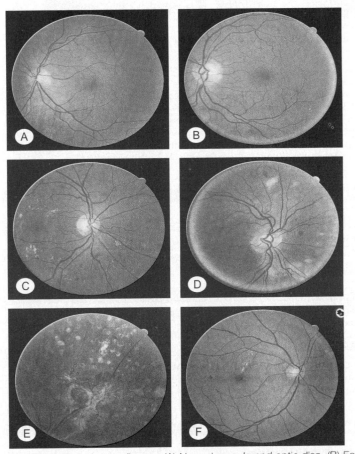

Fig. 201.3 Diabetic eye disease. (A) Normal macula and optic disc. (B) Early background retinopathy, dot and blot haemorrhages. (C) Early background retinopathy, plus hard exudates. (D) Preproliferative retinopathy, with multiple cotton-wool spots. (E) Proliferative retinopathy, with hallmark frond-like new vesicles. (F) Exudative maculopathy, with exudates within a disc-width of the macula.

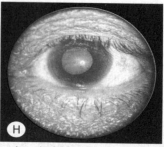

Fig. 201.3, cont'd (G,H) Central (G) and cortical (H) cataracts seen against the red reflex of the ophthalmoscope. (With permission from Kumar, Clark 2005.)

The Early Treatment of Diabetic Retinopathy Study (ETDRS) has established that early peripheral (panretinal) argon laser photocoagulation is not indicated for mild to moderate non-proliferative retinopathy. Early treatment in the form of argon laser photocoagulation applied directly to leaking microaneurysms, as well as grid photocoagulation applied to diffuse areas of leakage and thickening, is highly beneficial.

PATIENT 2

SALIENT FEATURES

Examination

- Signs of background retinopathy with hard exudates or oedema of the macula.

DIAGNOSIS

This patient has diabetic maculopathy, caused by the oedema and/or the hard exudates.

QUESTIONS

What symptoms may this patient have?
There will be a gradual impairment of central vision, such as difficulty in reading small print or seeing road signs.

PATIENT 3

SALIENT FEATURES

Examination

- Cottonwool spots
- Venous dilatation, beading, looping or sausage-like segmentation
- Arteriolar narrowing

- Haemorrhages: large dark blots
- Intraretinal microvascular abnormalities.

DIAGNOSIS

This patient has preproliferative retinopathy, which is uncommon and is caused by retinal hypoxia.

QUESTIONS

What symptoms may this patient have?
Asymptomatic if the macula is spared.

How would you manage this patient?
Semiurgent referral to the ophthalmologist for close follow-up to enable early detection and treatment of proliferative retinopathy.

PATIENT 4

SALIENT FEATURES

Examination

- Neovascularization around the disc or away from the disc; in early stages the vessels are bare and flat and easily missed. In later stages they are elevated and may be associated with a white fibrous component
- Presence of laser burns (in treated cases).

DIAGNOSIS

This patient has proliferative retinopathy caused by retinal hypoxia, usually seen in insulin-dependent diabetic retinopathy.

QUESTIONS

What symptoms may this patient have?
Asymptomatic in the absence of complications.

How would you manage this patient?
Urgent referral to an ophthalmologist for laser treatment.

What are the complications of proliferative retinopathy?
- Vitreous haemorrhage
- Traction retinal detachment
- Rubeosis irides
- Rubeotic glaucoma: some of these patients can have partial restoration of vision by microsurgery called pars plana vitrectomy.

ADVANCED-LEVEL QUESTIONS

What are the signs of macular oedema?
Macular oedema includes any of the following signs:
- Retinal thickening at or within 500 μm of the centre of the macula (Fig. 201.3F)

- Retinal thickening of one disc area or larger, in any part of the retina which is within the one-disc diameter from the centre of the macula
- Hard exudates at or within 500 μm of the centre of the macula.

How will you manage the patient with macular oedema?

Non-urgent referral to an ophthalmologist for photocoagulation, which will stabilize (seldom improve) visual acuity in 50% of patients. The ability to alter the course of visual loss in diabetic macular oedema favourably is a major advance but patients must be cautioned that the most likely result of treatment is stabilization, not improvement, of visual acuity.

What is the principal mechanism of visual loss in non-proliferative retinopathy?

The principal mechanism of visual loss in non-proliferative retinopathy is through macular oedema, which results from focal vascular leakage from microaneurysms in the macular capillaries, as well as from diffuse vascular leakage. With time, areas of leakage progress to macular thickening associated with hard exudates or cystoid changes.

What are the different types of clinical presentation of non-proliferative retinopathy?

Patients may present with no visual symptoms, paracentral scotomata or various degrees of central visual loss. Consequently, the diagnosis and management of macular oedema depend crucially on the determination of macular thickening by fundus examination. Ophthalmoscopy detects intraretinal haemorrhages and hard exudates but does not detect substantial retinal thickening. A critical evaluation of retinal thickening requires stereoscopic examination of the retina by slit-lamp biomicroscopy with lens for retinal visualization or stereoscopic fundus photography.

What is the prevalence of retinopathy in diabetes?

The overall prevalence is about 25%. It is 40% in type 1 (insulin-dependent) and 20% in type 2 (non-insulin-dependent).

What is the relationship between the duration of diabetes and retinopathy?

There is a close relationship: in patients diagnosed to have diabetes before the age of 30 years, the incidence of retinopathy is about 50% after 10 years and 90% after 30 years. It is unusual for retinopathy to develop within 5 years of onset of diabetes; however, 5% of patients with type 2 diabetes have background retinopathy at presentation. Sight-threatening retinopathy can be expected to develop in 50% of patients with type 1 diabetes and 30% of those with type 2; these patients will need intervention to reduce the risk of vision loss. Diabetic blindness can be reduced or prevented without preventing retinopathy. Systematic screening for diabetic retinopathy and preventive laser treatment for those who develop macular oedema or proliferative retinopathy reduces the rate of blindness to about 0·5% in the diabetic population (Acta Ophthalmol Scand 2007; 85:40–5) irrespective of the prevalence of retinopathy.

What associated systemic conditions worsen diabetic retinopathy?

- Pregnancy
- Hypertension
- Anaemia
- Renal failure.

What is the relationship between diabetic control and retinopathy?

The Diabetes Control and Complications Trial compared intensive treatment for blood glucose control with conventional treatment in patients with and without retinopathy at baseline who were followed for a mean of 6.5 years. Intensive treatment had profound benefits in both subgroups and was associated with a reduction in the incidence of both the development of new retinopathy and the risk of progression of existing retinopathy.

What is the relationship between diabetic retinopathy and pregnancy?

Retinopathy can progress rapidly in pregnant patients with diabetes; careful and more frequent evaluation is often indicated.

How often would you screen diabetic patients for retinopathy?

- Type 2 diabetics: annually
- Type 1 diabetics:
  - Newly diagnosed: no screening for the first 5 years
  - 5–10 years from initial diagnosis: annually
  - >10 years after initial diagnosis: every 6 months.

What is the earliest sign of retinal change in diabetes?

An increase in capillary permeability, evidenced by the leakage of dye into the vitreous humour after fluorescein injection, is the earliest sign.

What do you know about the pathogenesis of retinal new vessel formation?

It is not completely understood and current theories emphasize the production of angiogenic factors by areas of ischaemic and hypoxic retina. More recently vascular endothelial growth factor (VEGF) has been isolated from ocular fluid. It is increased in hypoxia and has been implicated in the neovascularization seen in diabetic retinopathy and retinal vein occlusion. Currently, four intravitreal inhibitors of VEGF for targeted non-surgical treatment of diabetic retinopathy are promising:

- Pegaptanib (Macugen; OSI/Eyetech, Melville, NY, USA) to reduce neovascularization
- Bevacizumab (Avastin; Genentech, South San Francisco, CA, USA), to reduce macular oedema
- Ranibizumab (Lucentis; Genentech) for treatment of macular oedema
- VEGF Trap-Eye (Regeneron Pharmaceuticals, Tarrytown, NY, USA) for treatment of macular oedema.

What is the role of the renin–angiotensin system blockade in diabetic retinopathy?

- The Diabetic Retinopathy Candesartan Trials (DIRECT) indicated that although candesartan reduced the incidence of retinopathy in type 1 diabetes it had no beneficial effect on retinopathy progression (Lancet 2008; 372:1394–1402). DIRECT also investigated whether candesartan treatment slows the progression or induces regression of retinopathy in type 2 diabetes. There is some indication that in type 2 diabetic patients it may improve mild to moderate retinopathy (Lancet 2008; 372:1385–93).
- The Renin–Angiotensin System Study (RASS) investigated the effect of renin–angiotensin system blockade with either an ACE inhibitor or an angiotensin receptor blocker on both renal and retinal morphology in

normotensive patients with type 1 diabetes and normoalbuminuria. Early blockade in patients with type 1 diabetes did not slow nephropathy progression but it did reduce the advancement of retinal changes by 60–70% compared with placebo, most likely independently of blood pressure reduction (N Engl J Med 2009; 361:40–51).

What do you know about photocoagulation?

Photocoagulation is a technique whereby several thousand lesions are produced over a 2-week therapy period with lasers. Panretinal photocoagulation reduces the risk of severe visual loss (50% in patients with severe diabetic retinopathy). The laser is used to ablate a portion of the retina and does not directly cauterize the neovascularization. It is believed that the regression of neovascularization results from destruction of ischaemic and hypoxic retina, thus reducing angiogenic factors. Photocoagulation decreases the incidence of haemorrhage or scarring in proliferative retinopathy. Photocoagulation is also useful in the treatment of microaneurysms, haemorrhages and oedema. Some loss of peripheral vision may be inevitable with this technique. The Early Treatment Diabetic Retinopathy Study showed that focal laser photocoagulation reduced the risk of moderate vision loss by 50–70% in patients with macular oedema.

What surgical technique may be used for a non-resolving vitreous haemorrhage and retinal detachment?

Pars plana vitrectomy may be used and is recommended for severe proliferative diabetic retinopathy when it is unresponsive to pan-retinal photocoagulation, is associated with severe vitreous haemorrhage or is associated with traction on the macula. However, it is often complicated by retinal tears, retinal detachment, glaucoma, infection, cataracts and loss of the eye.

202 HYPERTENSIVE RETINOPATHY

INSTRUCTION

Examine this patient's eyes.
Examine this patient's fundus.

SALIENT FEATURES

History

- Usually no ocular symptoms
- History of hypertension.

Examination

- Arteriovenous nipping (Fig. 202.1)
- Arteriolar narrowing
- Macular star
- Flame-shaped and blot haemorrhages (see Fig. 201.3B)
- Cottonwool exudates (see Fig. 201.3D)
- Papilloedema may or may not be present (Fig. 202.2).

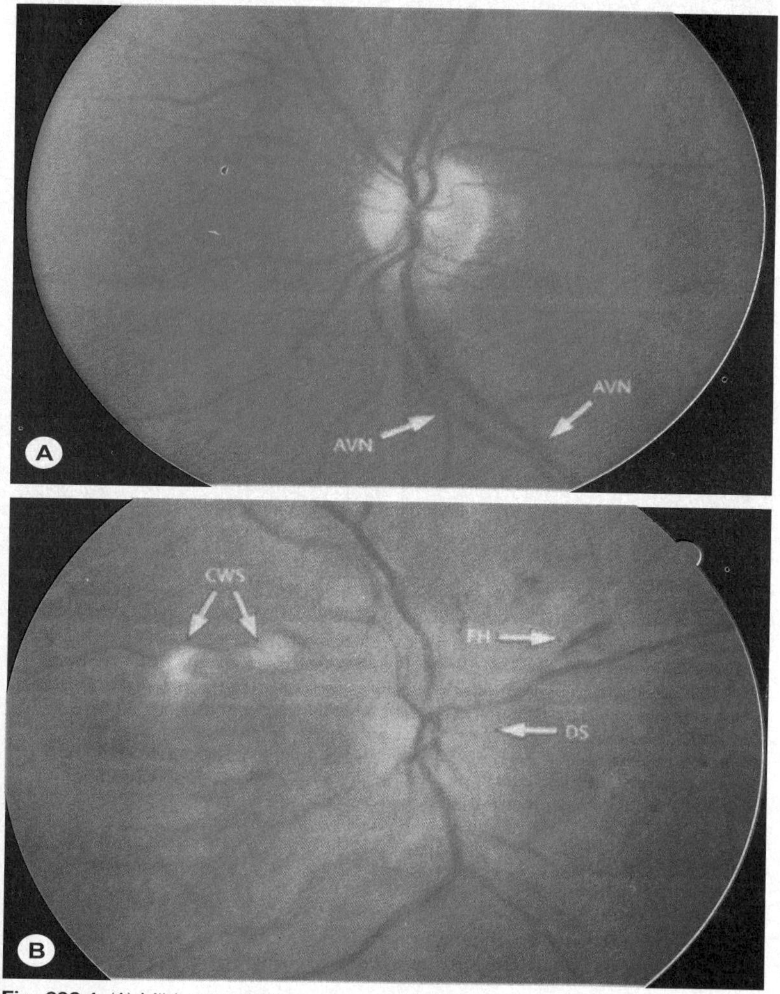

Fig. 202.1 (A) Mild retinopathy in an eye with ischaemic optic neuropathy. (B) Severe hypertensive retinopathy. CWS, cotton-wool spots; FH, flame-shaped retina haemorrhage; DS, swelling of the optic disc; AVN, arteriovenous nipping. (With permission from Wong, Mitchell 2007.)

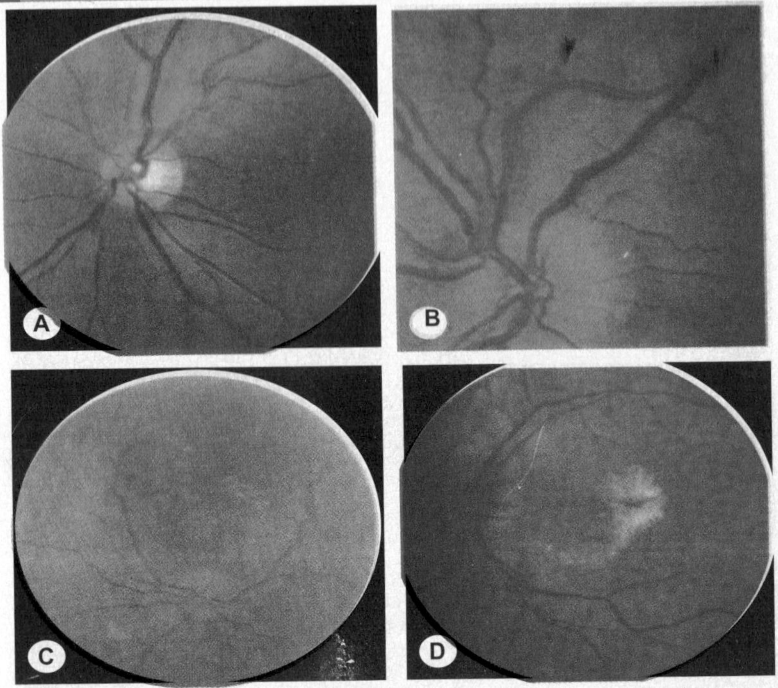

Fig. 202.2 (A) Grade 1: early and minor changes include increased tortuosity of a retinal vessel and increased reflectiveness (silver wiring) of a retinal artery (at 1 o'clock in this view). (B) Grade 2: increased tortuosity and silver wiring (arrowheads) plus 'nipping' of the venules at arteriovenous crossings (arrow). (C) Grade 3: as grade 2 plus flame-shaped retinal haemorrhages and soft 'cotton-wool' exudates. (D) Grade 4: swelling of the optic disc (papilloedema), retinal oedema and hard exudates around the fovea, producing a typical 'macular star'. (With permission from Forbes, Jackson 2003.)

Proceed as follows:
● Tell the examiner that you would like to:
  • check the BP
  • examine the urine for proteinuria
  • examine the heart for left ventricular hypertrophy.

DIAGNOSIS

This patient has flame-shaped haemorrhages with a macular star (lesions) caused by hypertension (aetiology).

ADVANCED-LEVEL QUESTIONS

How would you grade hypertensive retinopathy?

Keith–Wagener–Barker classification
This combines the clinical findings of hypertension and atherosclerosis:

- Stage I: arteriolar narrowing
- Stage II: irregular calibre of arterioles
- Stage III: cottonwool exudates; flame and blot haemorrhages, retinal oedema
- Stage IV: papilloedema.

Note: Subsequent studies have shown that the clinical features and prognosis of patients with stage III and stage IV disease were similar whether or not papilloedema was present; consequently the terms 'malignant' and 'accelerated' could be used interchangeably. Instead 'hypertensive crisis' is used to refer to the syndrome of raised BP complicated by end-organ damage (e.g. stroke, renal failure, myocardial ischaemia or infarction, stage III or IV hypertensive retinopathy).

- **Scheie classification** This separates the clinical findings of hypertension and atherosclerosis (Arch Ophthalmol 1953;49:117–38) (Fig. 202.2).
- **Hypertension**:
  Grade 0: no changes
  Grade 1: barely detectable arteriolar narrowing
  Grade 2: obvious arteriolar narrowing with focal irregularities
  Grade 3: grade 2 plus retinal haemorrhages and/or exudates
  Grade 4: grade 3 plus papilloedema.
- **Arteriolar sclerosis**:
  Grade 0: normal
  Grade 1: barely detectable light reflex changes
  Grade 2: obvious increased light reflex changes
  Grade 3: copper-wire arterioles
  Grade 4: silver-wire arterioles.

What is the significance of retinal arteriolar narrowing in normotensive individuals?

Retinal arteriolar narrowing might also be used to predict subsequent development of hypertension in individuals initially classified as normotensive (BMJ 2004; 329:79).

Mention some causes of cottonwool spots

- HIV infection per se
- Anaemias
- Infective endocarditis
- Leukaemias
- Diabetic retinopathy (p. 699).

Mention a few causes of hypertension

- In 90%, it is essential hypertension with no underlying cause and this may represent the 'normal' spread
- In 10%, there is an underlying cause:
  - Renal: renal artery stenosis, polycystic kidneys, chronic glomerulonephritis, polyarteritis nodosa, chronic pyelonephritis
  - Endocrine: Cushing syndrome, Conn syndrome, phaeochromocytoma, acromegaly, diabetes mellitus
  - Eclampsia and pre-eclamptic toxaemia of pregnancy
  - Coarctation of the aorta.

How would you investigate a patient with hypertension?

- Urine for protein, glucose, casts
- Midstream urine for microscopy and culture
- Urea and electrolytes, fasting lipids

- Chest radiography
- ECG
- Urine catecholamines
- Intravenous pyelography
- Renal artery digital subtraction angiography (DSA).

What is the relationship between morbidity and hypertensive retinopathy?

- Neurological link
- In a 3-year population-based cohort study of atherosclerosis risk, incident stroke events were more common in participants with signs of hypertensive retinopathy than in participants without retinopathy. When controlled for BP, diabetes, lipids and other risk factors, moderate signs of hypertensive retinopathy (cotton-wool spots, retinal haemorrhages and microaneurysms) were associated with a two- to four-fold higher risk of incident stroke. Weaker associations between signs of mild hypertensive retinopathy and risk of stroke were also present (Lancet 2001; 358:1134–40).
- Hypertensive retinopathy is also reported to be associated with cognitive decline, cerebral white-matter lesions identified by cerebral MRI, lacunar infarctions, cerebral atrophy and stroke mortality.

- Cardiovascular link
- Studies of the association between hypertensive retinopathy signs and heart disease have produced inconsistent results. However, hypertensive retinopathy has been linked with coronary artery stenosis and with incident coronary heart disease events.
- Some investigators suggest that moderate hypertensive retinopathy could be used to predict incident congestive heart failure, even in individuals without a previous history of myocardial infarction.

- Other links
- Retinopathy signs is also associated with indicators of target organ damage, such as microalbuminuria and renal impairment and left ventricular hypertrophy.

What are Elschnig's spots?

They are black flecks surrounded by yellow or red halos and occurs in advanced hypertensive retinopathy. They are caused by focal occulsion of the choroidal capillaries, which leads to necrosis and atrophy of retinal pigment epithelium. Acutely, these spots are punctuate tan-white lesions that leak on fluorescein angiography through breakdown in the blood–brain barrier.

How would you treat hypertension?

- Salt restriction
- Advise the patient to stop smoking
- First-line drug therapy:
  - In women and smokers: bendroflumethiazide
  - In non-smoking men: beta-blockers.

Further reading

Ahmed ME, Walker JM, Beevers DG, Beevers M: Lack of difference between malignant and accelerated hypertension, *BMJ* 292:235–237, 1986.

Dollery CT, Ramalho PS, Patterson JW, et al: Retinal microemboli: experimental production of 'cottonwool' spots, *Lancet* i:303, 1965.

Keith NM, Wagner HP, Barker NW: Some different types of essential hypertension: their course and prognosis, *Am J Med Sci* 197:332–343, 1939.

Anton Elschnig (August 22, 1863–1939) was an Austrian opthalmologist.

Marcus Gunn first described hypertensive retinopathy in the 19th century in a series of patients with hypertension and renal disease (Trans Ophthalmol Soc UK 1892;12:124–5).

In 1939, Keith, Wagner and Barker showed that the signs of retinopathy were predictive of death in patients with hypertension (Am J Med Sci 1939;197:332–43).

---

203 PAPILLOEDEMA

INSTRUCTION

Examine this patient's fundus.

SALIENT FEATURES

History

- Headache
- Transient visual disturbances
- Diplopia (from associated sixth cranial nerve palsy)
- History of hypertension, brain tumour
- History of ingestion of steroids, hypervitaminosis A (causes of benign intracranial hypertension).

Examination

- There is swelling of the optic disc (look for haemorrhages and soft exudates; Fig. 203.1).

Note: Common causes are:
- Intracranial space-occupying lesion
- Hypertensive retinopathy
- Benign intracranial hypertension.

DIAGNOSIS

This patient has bilateral papilloedema (lesion) and I would like to investigate for an intracranial space-occupying lesion (aetiology).

QUESTIONS

What do you understand by the term papilloedema?

Papilloedema is the swelling of the nerve head as seen on ophthalmoscopy. The colour of the disc becomes redder, approximating to that of the rest of the retina; its contour becomes blurred and the cup and cribrosa are filled in.

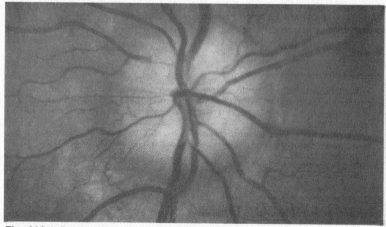

Fig. 203.1 Papilloedema.

What is the first manifestation of papilloedema?

The earliest manifestation of papilloedema is the engorgement of the veins.

What is the nature of the field defect in papilloedema?

Papilloedema is always associated with enlargement of the blind spot, with a consequent diminution of visual fields and gradual loss of visual acuity, but a fair degree of acuity may remain until papilloedema is marked.

ADVANCED-LEVEL QUESTIONS

Mention a few causes of papilloedema

- Raised intracranial pressure resulting from one of the following conditions:
  - Impaired circulation of the CSF in aqueduct stenosis
  - Meningitis
  - Subarachnoid haemorrhage.
- Cerebral oedema:
  - Following head injury
  - Following cerebral anoxia.
- Metabolic causes:
  - Carbon dioxide retention
  - Steroid withdrawal
  - Thyroid eye disease
  - Vitamin A intoxication
  - Lead poisoning.
- Increased protein in the CSF in:
  - Guillain–Barré syndrome
  - Spinal cord tumours
  - Any spinal block.
- Haematological and circulatory disorders:
  - Central retinal vein thrombosis
  - Superior vena caval obstruction

- Polycythaemia vera
- Multiple myeloma
- Macroglobulinaemia.

Mention a few conditions that simulate papilloedema

- Deep optic cup:
  - Nasal edge appears heaped up
  - Vessels plunge into the optic cup
  - Temporal edge is quite normal.
- Medullated nerve fibres: seen on the disc or even on the retina. The appearance is typically flared and on focusing will reveal fibres traversing the area. Field defects are the result of the retinal vessels being obscured. Since these are present from birth, the patient is unaware of the defect.
- Bergmeister's papilla: whitish elevation of the centre of the disc with venous and arterial sheathing. It is common and seen at all ages. There is an equal sex and racial incidence.
- Pseudopapilloedema: congenitally elevated discs secondary to hyaloid tissue (drüsen) or hyperopia.

Note: Elevation or swelling on the optic disc occurs in the following conditions:
- Papilloedema
- Papillitis
- Drüsen
- Infiltration of the nerve head by malignant cells.

What do you know about Foster Kennedy syndrome?

Unilateral papilloedema with or without 'secondary' optic atrophy on the other side suggests a tumour of the opposite side on the olfactory lobe or orbital surface of the frontal lobe or of the pituitary body.

What do you understand by the term papillitis?

- Demyelination of the optic nerve (multiple sclerosis)
- Inflammation
- Degeneration (Leber's optic atrophy)
- Vascular disorders of the nerve head
- Malignant infiltration.

How do you differentiate papillitis from papilloedema?

Papillitis	Papilloedema
Usually unilateral	Usually bilateral
Visual acuity is considerably reduced in relation to the degree of swelling of the disc	Visual acuity only slightly reduced until late stages
Visual field defect is usually central, particularly for red and green	Peripheral constriction or enlargement of the blind spot
Marcus Gunn pupil may be present	Marcus Gunn pupil is absent
Eye movements may be painful	Eye movements are never painful

Note: A Marcus Gunn pupil is one that shows better constriction to an indirect response than to direct light. Example is decreased constriction of both pupils when a light is shone into the left eye, indicating a relative afferent pupillary defect.

What are the stages of papilloedema?
- Stage I: increase in venous calibre and tortuosity.
- Stage II: optic cup becomes pinker and less distinct, the vessels seeming to disappear suddenly on the surface of the disc.
- Stage III: blurring of the discs on the nasal side. (In many normal discs, the nasal edge is less distinct and one of the most frequent false-positive signs is questionable blurring of the nasal disc margins.)
- Stage IV: the whole disc becomes suffused and slightly elevated. The margins may disappear and the vessels seem to emerge from a mushy swelling. The optic cup is filled and there are haemorrhages around the disc.

What are the features of benign intracranial hypertension?
Dandy's diagnostic criteria (Brain 1991;114:155–180):
- Patient is alert
- Clinical features of increased intracranial pressure
- No localizing neurological signs (except sixth cranial nerve palsy)
- Opening pressure of CSF during lumbar puncture is >20 cmH$_2$O and CSF is of normal composition
- Normal ventricles and normal study on CT or MRI.

What treatment options are available for pseudotumour cerebri?
- Discontinuation of steroids
- Weight loss
- Drugs: carbonic anhydrase inhibitors, diuretics
- Serial lumbar punctures, lumboperitoneal shunt
- Optic nerve fenestration, subtemporal decompression.

Foster Kennedy (1884–1952) was born in Belfast. He was Professor of Neurology at Cornell University. He described his syndrome in 1923.

---

204 OPTIC ATROPHY

INSTRUCTION

Examine this patient's eyes.
Examine this patient's fundus.

SALIENT FEATURES

History

- Visual loss: onset of symptoms depends on underlying aetiology
- History of multiple sclerosis
- History of glaucoma
- Optic nerve tumour

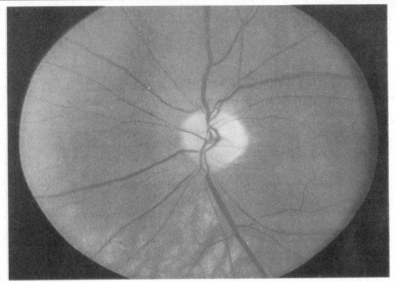

Fig. 204.1 Optic atrophy.

- Vitamin B$_{12}$ deficiency
- Paget's disease
- Exposure to toxins: lead, methanol, arsenic.

Examination

- Pale disc with sharp margins (Fig. 204.1)
- Intact consensual light reflex but impaired direct light reflex: Marcus Gunn pupillary response (seen in asymmetrical involvement of the two eyes)
- Central scotoma on testing of visual fields.

Proceed as follows:

- Tell the examiner that you would like to look for cerebellar signs (remember that multiple sclerosis is the commonest cause of optic atrophy).

DIAGNOSIS

This patient has primary optic atrophy (lesion) caused by multiple sclerosis (aetiology). I would like to check the visual fields for central scotoma (functional status).

QUESTIONS

What is the differential diagnosis?

- Demyelinating disorders (multiple sclerosis)
- Optic nerve compression by tumour or aneurysm
- Glaucoma
- Toxins: methanol, tobacco, lead, arsenical poisoning
- Ischaemia, including central retinal artery occlusion in thromboembolism, temporal arteritis, idiopathic acute ischaemic optic neuropathy, syphilis

- Hereditary disorders: Friedreich's ataxia, Leber's optic atrophy (sex linked, seen in young males)
- Paget's disease.
- Vitamin B_{12} deficiency
- Secondary to retinitis pigmentosa.

ADVANCED-LEVEL QUESTIONS

What is the difference between primary and secondary optic atrophy?

Primary	Secondary
White and flat with clear-cut edges	Greyish-white, edges indistinct
Visible lamina cribrosa	Cup filled and lamina cribrosa not visible
Arteries and veins normal	Arteries thinner than normal, veins may be dilated
Capillaries decreased in number	Capillaries decreased in number (fewer than seven): Kestenbaum's sign

What is consecutive optic atrophy?
Consecutive optic atrophy is a controversial term and is best avoided. Some use it as an equivalent or alternative for what has been described above as secondary optic atrophy, but others use the term to indicate an atrophy complicating retinitis or, rarely, Tay–Sachs disease or retinitis pigmentosa.

What is glaucomatous optic atrophy?
Glaucomatous optic atrophy denotes loss of disc substance, referred to as increased cupping.

How would you investigate a patient with optic neuropathy?
- FBC, ESR
- Blood glucose
- Serology for syphilis
- Serum vitamin B_{12} and B_1
- Skull radiograph of pituitary fossa, optic foramina and sinuses, or CT scan of the brain and orbit
- ECG
- Pattern-stimulated visual evoked responses
- Electroretinography.

R Marcus Gunn (1850–1909), a Scottish ophthalmologist who worked at Moorfields Eye Hospital, London.

T von Leber (1840–1917), Professor of Ophthalmology at the University of Heidelberg, Germany.

W Tay (1843–1927), a British ophthalmologist, Moorfields Eye Hospital, London.

BP Sachs (1858–1944), a German neuropsychiatrist who worked in New York. He described this condition independent of Tay.

205 RETINAL VEIN THROMBOSIS

INSTRUCTION

Examine these patient eyes, including the fundus.

SALIENT FEATURES

History

- Age: central retinal vein occlusions arise in 0·1–0·4% and branch retinal vein occlusions in 0·6–1·1% of adults aged ≥40 years
- Branched retinal vein occlusion: decreased vision, floaters suggest vitreal haemorrhage
- Central retinal vein occlusion: loss or decreased vision, headache (associated increase in intraocular pressure), floaters
- History of hypertension, diabetes, glaucoma, multiple myeloma or macroglobulinaemia.

Examination

- **Patient 1** Central retinal vein occlusion (Fig. 205.1), the occlusion is behind the cribriform plate:
  - Multiple retinal and preretinal haemorrhages surround the optic nerve head. there is marked dilatation and tortuosity of the veins, hyperaemia or oedema of the nerve head and soft exudates: 'blood and thunder' appearance
  - Visual acuity is only slightly reduced.

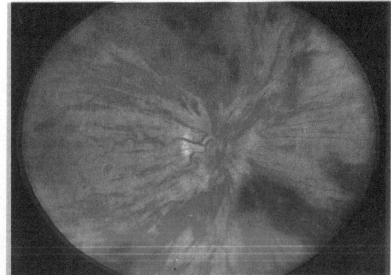

Fig. 205.1 Central retinal vein thrombosis.

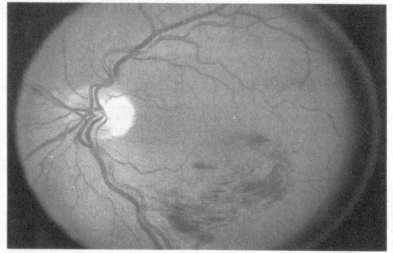

Fig. 205.2 Branch retinal vein thrombosis.

- Patient 2
- Branch vein occlusion (Fig. 205.2), the occlusion is in front of the cribri-form plàte:
  - Occlusion occurs just distal to the arteriovenous crossing and haem-orrhages can be seen surrounding the occluded vein; the superior temporal vein is most commonly involved
  - May cause a quadrantic field defect.

For both patients, proceed as follows:

- Tell the examiner that you would like to check for the following conditions:
  - Diabetes (urine sugar)
  - Hypertension (participants with hypertension were five times more likely to have a branch retinal vein occlusion than those without hypertension)
  - Chronic simple glaucoma
  - Hyperviscosity syndromes (Waldenström's macroglobulinaemia, multiple myeloma)
  - Haematological syndromes: hyperhomocysteinaemia, anticardioli-pin antibodies, protein S and C deficiencies, activated protein C resistance, and factor V Leiden mutation.

DIAGNOSIS

Patient 1 has multiple retinal haemorrhages (lesions) caused by central retinal vein occlusion with underlying diabetes mellitus (aetiology).

Patient 2 has branch vein occlusion (lesion). (**Note:** Visual prognosis is good if the haemorrhages do not extend to the macula with accompanying macular oedema.)

ADVANCED-LEVEL QUESTIONS

What are the usual sites of occlusion in branch retinal vein occlusion?

- At arteriovenous crossings, causing classical quadrantic or small macular occlusions
- Along the main veins, as in diabetes mellitus
- At the edges of the optic disc, resulting in occlusion of the hemisphere
- Peripherally, as in sickle cell disease.

What are the vascular responses to retinal vein occlusion?

- Dilatation of retinal capillaries
- Abnormal vascular permeability
- Retinal capillary closure.

What is the prognosis in branch retinal vein occlusion?

It varies from complete resolution with no residual visual deficits to a progressive deterioration resulting in permanent loss of vision.

What is the clinical course in central retinal vein occlusion?

- In mild cases, there is minimal dilatation of veins and haemorrhages with little or no oedema of the macula and no visual deficit.
- In severe instances, the vision may deteriorate to hand motions, with extensively deep and superficial haemorrhages with stagnation of blood in the markedly dilated veins and several cottonwool spots.

What are the complications of central retinal vein occlusion?

These include macular oedema, neovascularization of the retina, rubeosis iridis (usually visible by 1 month) and rubeotic glaucoma (usually by 3 months). Ophthalmic follow-up is needed to diagnose and prevent the two main complications of retinal vein occlusion: neovascularization and macular oedema.

How would you manage such eyes?

- Treat the underlying condition
- Fluorescein angiography to determine areas of retinal ischaemia
- Regular follow-up by the ophthalmologist as secondary neovascularization is a common sequel and may need laser therapy. Panretinal photocoagulation prevents the dreaded complications of neovascular glaucoma.

Randomized clinical trials have demonstrated that prophylactic panretinal laser treatment does not necessarily prevent neovascularization in ischaemic vein occlusions, and that laser treatment can be withheld unless the patient develops frank ocular neovascularization. Whereas, focal oedema from branch retinal vein occlusion, but does not seem to benefit macular oedema associated with central retinal vein occlusion.

What is the role of arteriovenous crossing sheathotomy?

Arteriovenous crossing sheathotomy is commonly used as an adjuvant to pars plana vitrectomy. Branch retinal vein occlusion typically occurs at arteriovenous crossings, where the artery and vein share a common adventitial sheath. Cutting the sheath around the vessels and physically separating them where they cross should improve blood flow through the vein.

Further reading

Weinstein R, Mahmood M: Case 6–2002: a 54-year-old woman with left, then right, central-retinal-vein occlusion, *N Engl J Med* 346:603, 2002.

JG Waldenström (1906–1996), Professor of Medicine, Uppsala University, Sweden.

206 SUBHYALOID HAEMORRHAGE

INSTRUCTION

Examine this patient's fundus.

SALIENT FEATURES

History

- Sudden, painless loss of vision
- Sudden appearance of floaters and black spots with or without flashing lights
- History of stroke (subarachnoid haemorrhage)
- History of diabetes, retinal tears, vitreous detachment, retinal vein occlusion
- History of trauma.

Examination

- A large, solitary subhyaloid haemorrhage (there may be no fluid level if the patient is lying flat) (Fig. 206.1)
- There may be associated retinal haemorrhage
- Mild papilloedema in 20%
- Comment on any obvious hemiplegia.

Note: When the subhyaloid (preretinal) haemorrhage extends into the vitreous humour it is called Terson syndrome (Fig. 206.2).

DIAGNOSIS

This hemiplegic patient has a subhyaloid haemorrhage (lesion) caused by subarachnoid haemorrhage (aetiology).

ADVANCED-LEVEL QUESTIONS

What is the commonest cause of subhyaloid haemorrhage?
Subarachnoid haemorrhage.

What are the other causes of haemorrhage into the vitreous humour?

- Local injury
- Blood diseases
- Hypertension
- Diabetes
- Idiopathic.

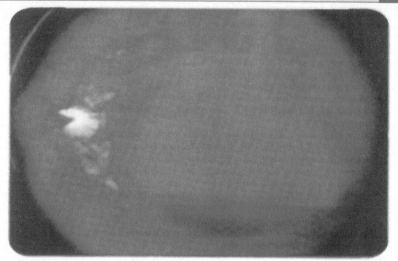

Fig. 206.1 Funduscopic photograph of a subhyaloid haemorrhage. (With permission from Field, Heran 2010.)

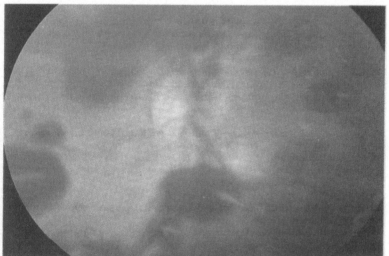

Fig. 206.2 Terson syndrome. (With permission from Yanoff, Duker 2008.)

Mention some causes of neck stiffness
- Subarachnoid haemorrhage
- Meningitis
- Posterior fossa tumours
- Local neck pathology, such as cervical spondylosis.

What is the cause of subarachnoid haemorrhage?
- Aneurysms are the cause of subarachnoid haemorrhage in 85% of cases (Lancet 2007; 369:306–18). Intracranial aneurysms are not congenital, as was once believed, but develop in the course of life.
- The best estimate of the frequency of aneurysms for an average adult without specific risk factors is 2.3% (95% confidence interval, 1.7–3.1); this proportion increases with age.
- Saccular aneurysms arise at sites of arterial branching, usually at the base of the brain, either on the circle of Willis itself or at a nearby branching point.
- Most intracranial aneurysms will never rupture. The rupture risk increases with the size of aneurysm, but paradoxically, most ruptured aneurysms are small (<1 cm); the explanation is that 90% of all aneurysms are small and even though only a small fraction of these rupture, this total outnumbers the greater fraction of the large aneurysms that rupture. The case fatality after aneurysmal haemorrhage is 50%; one in eight patients with subarachnoid haemorrhage dies outside hospital.

What are causes of deterioration in a patient with subarachnoid haemorrhage?
- Rebleeds
- Cerebral infarction as a result of reflex vasospasm of cerebral vessels (hence the rationale for using nimodipine)
- Secondary hydrocephalus.

How would you investigate such a patient?
CT head scan; if this rules out intracranial hypertension, then a lumbar puncture to diagnose minor leaks.

What is the management of subarachnoid haemorrhage?
- Rebleeding: occlusion of the aneurysm. Endovascular obliteration by means of platinum spirals (coiling) is the preferred mode of treatment, but some patients require a direct neurosurgical approach (clipping).
- Cerebral ischaemia: the risk is reduced with oral nimodipine and probably by maintaining circulatory volume.
- Hydrocephalus might cause gradual obtundation in the first few hours or days; it can be treated by lumbar puncture or ventricular drainage, dependent on the site of obstruction.

What are the indications of vitrectomy in Terson syndrome?
- Retinal detachment with vitreous haemorrhage
- Non-clearing vitreous haemorrhage in patient who is monocular
- Subfoveal haemorrhage
- Late complications of intraocular haemorrhage, such as epiretinal membrane formation (macular pucker)
- Occupational necessity for rapidly cleared vision.

Further reading
van Gijn J, Kerr, RS, Rinkel GJE: Subarachnoid haemorrhage, *Lancet* 369:306–318, 2007.

207   RETINITIS PIGMENTOSA

INSTRUCTION

Examine this patient's fundus.
Examine this patient's eyes.

SALIENT FEATURES

History

- Family history of blindness (can be autosomal recessive, which is more severe, or autosomal dominant, which is more benign)
- Decreased nocturnal vision
- Altered colour vision
- Loss of peripheral vision
- Blurry vision.

Examination

- Peripheral retina shows perivascular 'bone spicule pigmentation' and arteriolar narrowing (Fig. 207.1). The retinal veins (never the arteries) often have a sheath of pigmentation for part of their course. The pigment spots that lie near the retinal veins are seen to be anterior to them, and so they hide the course of the vessel. (In this respect, they differ from the pigment around the spots of choroidal atrophy in which the retinal vessels can be traced over the spots.)

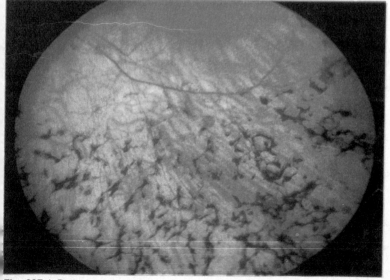

Fig. 207.1 Retinitis pigmentosa.

- Optic disc is pale
- Maculopathy which is atrophic or cystoid.

Proceed as follows:

- Look for polydactyly in the hands and feet (Laurence–Moon–Biedl syndrome)
- Comment on the white walking aid (if any) used by the registered blind
- Tell the examiner that you would like to check visual fields.

DIAGNOSIS

This patient is obese, has polydactyly and retinitis pigmentosa (lesion) caused by Laurence–Moon–Biedl syndrome (aetiology) and is registered blind (functional status).

QUESTIONS

What is the prognosis in retinitis pigmentosa?

Most patients are registered blind by the age of 40 years, with central field <20 degrees in diameter. Almost all patients lose central vision by the seventh decade.

What do you know about retinitis pigmentosa?

Retinitis pigmentosa is a slow degenerative disease of the retina. It occurs in both eyes, begins in early childhood, and often results in the loss of sight by middle or advanced age. The degeneration primarily affects the rods and cones, in particular the rods. Rods mediate achromatic vision in starlight or moonlight whereas cones are important for colour vision and fine acuity in daylight.

How may retinitis pigmentosa present?

It may present with defective vision at dusk (night blindness), which may occur several years before the pigment is visible in the retina.

ADVANCED-LEVEL QUESTIONS

Mention a few systemic disorders associated with retinitis pigmentosa

- *Laurence–Moon–Biedl–Bardet syndrome*, which is a recessively inherited disorder characterized by mental disability, polydactyly, syndactyly, hypogonadism, obesity and renal disease (structural abnormalities such as calyceal cysts or calyceal clubbing and blunting).
- *Bassen–Konzweig syndrome* (abetalipoproteinaemia), characterized by fat malabsorption, abetalipoproteinaemia, acanthocytosis and spinocerebellar ataxia (Ophthalmology 1984;91:991).
- *Refsum's disease* (phytanic acid storage disease), an autosomal recessive disorder characterized by hypertrophic peripheral neuropathy, deafness, ichthyosis, cerebellar ataxia, raised CSF protein levels in the absence of pleocytosis.
- *Kearns–Sayre syndrome,* a triad of retinitis pigmentosa, progressive external ophthalmoplegia and heart block (Br J Ophthalmol 1985;69:63).
- *Usher's disease,* a recessively inherited disorder characterized by congenital, non-progressive, sensorineural deafness (Arch Ophthalmol 1983;101:1367).
- *Friedreich's ataxia* (p. 267).

What do you know about the genetics of retinitis pigmentosa?

More than 45 genes for retinitis pigmentosa have been described. These genes account for only about 60% of all patients; the remainder have defects in as yet unidentified genes. Exceptions being the:

- *RHO,* gene for rhodopsin gene, which leads to about 25% of dominant retinitis pigmentosa
- *USH2A,* which might cause about 20% of recessive disease (including many with Usher syndrome type II)
- *RPGR,* which accounts for about 70% of X-linked retinitis pigmentosa.

Mutations in *RHO, USH2A,* and *RPGR* cause about 30% of all cases of retinitis pigmentosa in aggregate.

Which ocular conditions are associated with retinitis pigmentosa?

- Open-angle glaucoma
- Posterior subcapsular cataracts
- Myopia
- Keratoconus.

What is secondary retinitis pigmentosa?

Secondary retinitis pigmentosa is a sequela to inflammatory retinitis. It is often ophthalmoscopically indistinguishable from the primary condition, the electroretinographic and electro-oculographic responses are slightly subnormal unless the condition is far advanced. (In the primary type, the electroretinograph and electro-oculograph responses are markedly subnormal.)

What is retinitis pigmentosa sine pigmento?

A variety of retinitis pigmentosa but without visible pigmentation of the retina.

What is inverse retinitis pigmentosa?

Bone corpuscles are visible in the perifoveal area, whereas the retinal periphery is normal.

How would you manage this patient?

- Refer for genetic counselling
- Impaired vision training and aids for daily living
- Refer for job training
- Regular ophthalmology follow-up including visual fields, electro-retinography.

JZ Laurence (1830–1874), an English ophthalmologist.
   RC Moon (1844–1914), a US ophthalmologist.
   A Biedl (1869–1933), a Czech physician.
   G Bardet (b. 1885), a French physician.
   FA Bassen (b. 1903), physician, and AL Kornzweig (b. 1900), ophthalmologist, Mount Sinai Hospital, New York.
   S Refsum, a Norwegian physician.

208 OLD CHOROIDITIS

INSTRUCTION

Examine this patient's fundus.

SALIENT FEATURES

History

- Decreased vision, floaters, red eye
- History of HIV, sarcoidosis, TB.

Examination

- Old or inactive retinochoroiditis appears as white, well-defined areas of chorioretinal atrophy with pigmented edges (caused by proliferation of retinal pigment epithelium) (Fig. 208.1B)
- The retinal blood vessels pass over the lesions undisturbed.

DIAGNOSIS

This patient has areas of retinal atrophy with pigmented edges (lesion) caused by old choroiditis complicating cytomegalovirus infection (aetiology).

QUESTIONS

What may be the aetiology?

- Reactivation of congenital toxoplasmosis
- Cytomegalovirus infection
- HIV infection (Fig. 208.1A)
- Sarcoidosis
- TB
- Syphilis
- Behçet's disease.

What is the prognosis?

Prognosis varies according to the underlying aetiology. It is poor if the fovea is involved.

What does the presence of pigment on fundoscopy indicate?

A chronic lesion of the retina or choroid.

In which other conditions is the retinal pigment seen?

- Normally: racial (tigroid fundus)
- Retinitis pigmentosa
- Malignant melanoma.

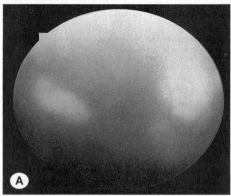

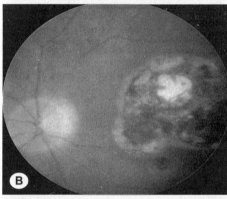

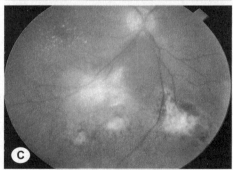

Fig. 208.1 Toxoplasmic chorioretinitis. (A) Active chorioretinitis with two lesions and vitreous haze in HIV infection. (B) Large inactive macular lesion typical of congenital disease. (C) Active chorioretinitis in an immunocompetent patient showing an inactive lesion on the right and the macular star, which is caused by an exudate around the macula. (With permission from Mandell et al. 2009.)

H Behçet (1889–1940), Professor of Dermatology in Turkey, described this syndrome in 1937 based on three patients he observed between 1924 and 1936.

209 CHOLESTEROL EMBOLUS IN THE FUNDUS

INSTRUCTION

Examine this patient's fundus.

SALIENT FEATURES

History

- Severe, acute and painless diminution or loss of vision
- History of atherosclerosis
- Risk factors of atherosclerosis: family history, diabetes, hypertension, ischaemic heart disease, peripheral vascular disease, cerebrovascular disease.

Examination

- Presence of a cholesterol embolus (Hollenhorst plaques) (Fig. 209.1) in one of the branches of the retinal artery.

Proceed as follows:

- Look for a cherry-red spot at the fovea (the ischaemic retina at the posterior pole becomes milky white and swollen, and the choroid is seen through the fovea as a cherry-red spot) (Fig. 209.2)
- Tell the examiner that you would like to check for visual field defects.

Remember: Retinal artery occlusion results in infarction of the inner two-thirds of the retina, reflex vasoconstriction of the retinal arterial tree and stasis in the retinal capillaries.

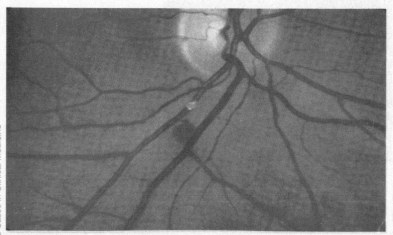

Fig. 209.1 Cholesterol crystal.

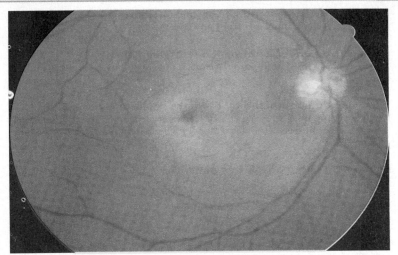

Fig. 209.2 Central retinal artery occlusion. (With permission from Wong, Mitchell 2007.)

DIAGNOSIS

This patient has a cholesterol embolus in one of the branches of the retinal artery (lesion) caused by underlying atherosclerotic disease (aetiology).

QUESTIONS

What are the complications of such an embolus?
Retinal artery occlusion causing field defects or loss of vision.

Where is the likely origin of this embolus?
The most likely origin is an atherosclerotic plaque in the carotid circulation. Reported to be associated with carotid stenting.

What are the causes of retinal arterial occlusion?
- Commonest cause: emboli arising from the major arteries supplying the head or from the left side of the heart; embolic particles consist of platelet clumps, cholesterol crystals or Hollenhorst plaques and others (mixed thrombus, calcific or septic material from cardiac valves, fat, myxoma, talc in intravenous drug abusers or silicone in those who receive injections for cosmetic purposes).
- Other causes:
  - Temporal arteritis
  - Collagen vascular diseases
  - Increased orbital pressure, e.g. retrobulbar haemorrhage, Graves' exophthalmos
  - Sickle cell disease
  - Acute arteriolar spasm caused by intranasal cocaine
  - Syphilis.

What do you understand by the term amaurosis?
Amaurosis means blindness from any cause.

What do you understand by the term amblyopia?
Amblyopia means that impaired vision is not caused by refractive error or ocular disease.

What do you understand by the term amaurosis fugax?
Amaurosis fugax is a retinal artery transient ischaemic attack that manifests with a painless, unilateral loss of vision that usually lasts a few minutes.

How would you manage this patient?
- Aspirin
- Ophthalmology opinion
- Ultrasonography of the carotid arteries
- Advise the patient to stop smoking
- Control of hypertension
- Carotid angiography with a view to performing carotid endarterectomy.

What is the effect of cholesterol crystals?
Cholesterol crystals rarely cause significant obstruction to the retinal arterioles.

What manoeuvre would you use to make the cholesterol crystals more apparent?
Mild lateral pressure on the globe may make the presence of unobtrusive crystals clearly visible when the retinal arteries pulsate.

How would you manage an acute occlusion of the retinal artery?
- Lie the patient in a supine position to ensure adequate circulation
- Intermittent ocular massage is applied for 15 min to dislodge the emboli, lower intraocular pressure and improve circulation
- Intravenous acetazolamide to lower intraocular pressure
- Inhalation of a mixture of 5% carbon dioxide and 95% oxygen
- Anterior chamber paracentesis.

If the investigation of a patient with amaurosis fugax comes up with no evidence of carotid artery disease, embolism or other recognized causes of the disorder, then the diagnosis by exclusion should be vasospasm. In such cases a calcium channel blocker should be tried.

What do you know about the 'purple-toe syndrome'?
This was first described with warfarin therapy by Feder and Auerbach in 1961 and was shown to be caused by showers of atheroemboli (Ann Intern Med 1961:55:911–917). Now, with the increasing use of coronary angioplasty and thrombolytic therapy in the elderly, cholesterol emboli are increasingly reported. They result in 'purple-toes' (Fig. 209.3), amaurosis fugax and atheroembolic disease of kidneys, skin and GI tract.

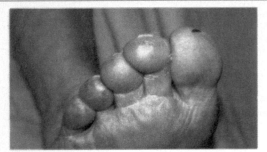

Fig. 209.3 Purple toes.

Further reading

N Engl J Med 329:427, 1993 (classic review)

210 VITREOUS OPACITIES

INSTRUCTION

Examine this patient's fundus.

SALIENT FEATURES

History

- History of diplopia (monocular diplopia)
- Floaters
- History of diabetes, hypertension.

Examination

- Small white opacities that are present in front of the retinal vessels
- The patient may complain of diplopia (monocular diplopia)
- Tell the examiner that you would like to:
  - test for monocular diplopia
  - check urine for sugar
  - check the BP.

DIAGNOSIS

This patient has vitreous opacities (lesions) with monocular diplopia (functional status), and has underlying diabetes mellitus (aetiology).

QUESTIONS

What are the causes of vitreous opacities?

- Blood: diabetes, retinal vein occlusion, trauma, subarachnoid haemorrhage, sickle cell retinopathy
- *Cholesterolosis bulbi:* where free floating, highly refractile crystals are seen in liquified vitreous humour in patients with severe intraocular disease

- *Asteroid hyalitis (Benson's disease):* where whitish yellow solid bodies containing calcium palmitate and stearate are suspended in normal vitreous. Prognosis for vision is good
- *Synchysis scintillans:* gold or yellowish-white particles made up of cholesterol located in the vitreous humour; they settle to the bottom of the eye through gravity. Associated with previous trauma or surgery to the eye
- Other: retinoblastoma, primary amyloidosis.

What are the other causes of monocular diplopia?
- Opacities in the lens
- Corneal opacities
- Retinal detachment.

211   MYELINATED NERVE FIBRES

INSTRUCTION

Examine this patient's fundus.

SALIENT FEATURES

History

- Asymptomatic.

Examination

- White, streaky patches that extend from the disc and terminate peripherally in a feather-like pattern. It may cover the retinal vessels (Fig. 211.1).

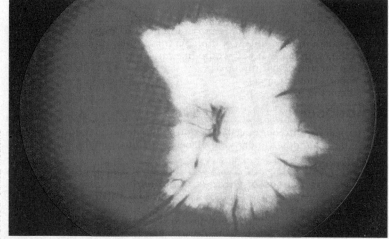

Fig. 211.1 Myelinated nerve fibres.

DIAGNOSIS

This patient has white streaky patches in a feather-like pattern (lesion); these are medullated nerve fibres (aetiology) and are benign (functional

QUESTIONS

What is the pathology?

Occasionally, the myelination of the optic nerve does not stop at the lamina cribrosa but extends on to nerve fibres surrounding the optic disc, terminating peripherally in a feather-like margin with fine striations from the course of the nerve fibre layer. It is a benign congenital abnormality, known as medullated or myelinated nerve fibres, caused by differential myelination. Myelinated retinal nerve fibres occur in 1% of the population and may mimic optic disc swelling or papilledema; an important differentiating feature is the absence of a feathery appearance in true optic disc swelling. The occurrence is bilateral in 17–20% of cases and is continuous with the disk in 81%. Usually, visual acuity is normal, and no particular ophthalmologic follow-up is required.

212   RETINAL CHANGES IN AIDS

INSTRUCTION

At a distance from the patient, the examiner will say that this patient has HIV, examine his fundus.

SALIENT FEATURES

History

- Floaters
- Red eye
- Impaired vision.

Examination

- Patient 1
- Cottonwool spots (Fig. 212.1)
- Tell the examiner that you would like to exclude diabetes and retinal vascular disease.

- Patient 2
- An area of retinitis with nerve fibre layer infarcts, haemorrhages, retinal opacification and perivascular sheathing: *'pizza-pie fundus'*.
- Tell the examiner that you would like to do a CD4 cell count (often $<50 \times 10^6$ cells/l in when acute cytomegalovirus infection occurs).

DIAGNOSIS

Patient 1 has cotton-wool spots (lesion) and Patient 2 has cytomegalovirus retinitis (lesion). Both patients are HIV positive and infection.

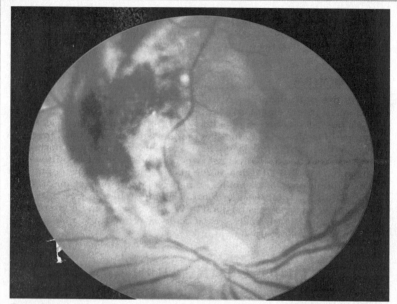

Fig. 212.1 Cotton-wool spots.

QUESTIONS

How would you treat these cotton-wool spots?
In a patient with known HIV infection, such infarcts require no specific therapy.

ADVANCED-LEVEL QUESTIONS

How would you treat retinitis?
- Therapy with intravenous ganciclovir or foscarnet is given lifelong to protect unaffected areas but does not restore functional areas already affected. The optimal treatment for patients with AIDS, normal renal function and cytomegalovirus (CMV) retinitis is foscarnet plus an antiretroviral nucleoside such as zidovudine. For similar patients with impaired renal function, ganciclovir would be the drug of choice, perhaps with an antiretroviral agent such as didanosine as it has few overlapping side effects. Late retinal detachment occurs despite therapy in 20% of these patients
- Sustained-release ganciclovir implant in the pars plana of the eye. Oral ganciclovir in conjunction with an implant reduces the incidence of a new CMV disease and delays the progression of retinitis (N Engl J Med 1999;340:1063–70)
- Intravitreal injections of ganciclovir or foscarnet.

What do you know about ganciclovir?
It is a derivative of aciclovir. It can cause bone marrow depression and hence should not be administered simultaneously with zidovudine.

What do you know about foscarnet?

It is an organic analogue of inorganic pyrophosphate. Its side effects include renal impairment, electrolyte imbalance and seizures. It can be safely administered with zidovudine.

What are the other retinal manifestations in patients with AIDS?

- *Toxoplasmosis retinochoroiditis:* usually nasal to the disc, characterized by extensive whitish infarction and inflammation, with minimal associated intraretinal haemorrhage (outer retinal involvement may show 'brush-fire' advancement of infection) (see Fig. 208.1A)
- *Pneumocystis jiroveci* (was *carinii*) choroiditis: characterized by scattered nodular yellowish-orange lesions deep in the retina, usually throughout the posterior pole
- *Acute retinal necrosis syndrome:* with severe peripheral retinal infarction and retinal vasculitis. Atrophic retinal holes appear later in these areas
- *Progressive outer retinal necrosis syndrome:* characterized by diffuse whitish opacification of the retina beneath the retinal vessels and a cherry-red spot in the fovea. It is associated with herpes zoster, and the prognosis for visual acuity is dismal
- Ocular presentations of syphilis include anterior and posterior uveitis, retinitis, retinal vasculitis and papillitis
- *Acute syphilitic posterior placoid chorioretinitis:* large placoid yellowish lesions at the level of the retinal pigment epithelium in the posterior retina with inflammation of the vitreous and loss of vision.

What diagnostic tests would you perform to detect retinal manifestations of AIDS?

- Careful clinical observations
- Serology: CD4 cell count (usually $<50 \times 10^6$ cells/l in presentation of untreated CMV retinitis)
- Culture
- Retinal biopsy by pars plana vitrectomy
- Fluorescein angiography: helpful in differentiating retinal lesions
- Sequential fundus photographs: for diagnosis and monitoring of lesions
- Testing of ocular fluid by PCR.

Mention some ocular non-retinal manifestations of AIDS

- Optic neuropathy
- Kaposi's sarcoma of the conjuctiva
- Orbital lymphoma
- Cranial nerve palsies
- Nystagmus.

213 RETINAL DETACHMENT

INSTRUCTION

Examine this patient's eye.

SALIENT FEATURES

History

- Patient complains of a dark curtain progressing across the visual field
- Floaters, flashes
- History of diabetes, hypertension
- History of kidney disease (diabetic renal-retinal syndrome).

Examination

- The retina has lost its pink colour and appears grey and opaque
- When the collection of subretinal fluid is large, the retina shows ballooning detachment with numerous folds (Fig. 213.1)
- Examine visual acuity and visual fields.

Proceed as follows:

- Tell the examiner that you would like to:
  - check urine for sugar
  - check the BP.
- Comment on any walking aid for the registered blind.

DIAGNOSIS

This patient has neovascularization and retinal detachment (lesion) caused by underlying diabetes mellitus (aetiology). She has a walking aid for the registered blind (functional status).

ADVANCED-LEVEL QUESTIONS

What is the pathology of retinal detachment?

It is a separation within the retina between the photoreceptors and the retinal pigment epithelium, characterized by collection of fluid or blood in this potential space.

What are the types of retinal detachment?

Rhegmatogenous retinal detachment. This is defined as the presence of a hole or break in the retina that allows fluid from the vitreous capacity to enter the subretinal space. It usually occurs spontaneously in those who have a predisposition to it following trauma to the eye or after intraocular surgery. Most of these patients develop symptoms. A break in the peripheral retina is associated with a sudden burst of flashing lights or sparks, which may be followed by small floaters or spots in the field of vision. When the retina detaches, the patient perceives a dark curtain progressing across the visual field, and when the fovea detaches central vision is abruptly diminished. It is treated surgically with a scleral buckling procedure.

Traction retinal detachment. This occurs when the intact retina is forcibly elevated by contracting membranes on the surface of the retina or by vitreous traction on areas of retinal neovascularization. Causes include diabetes, intraocular foreign body, perforating eye injuries and loss of

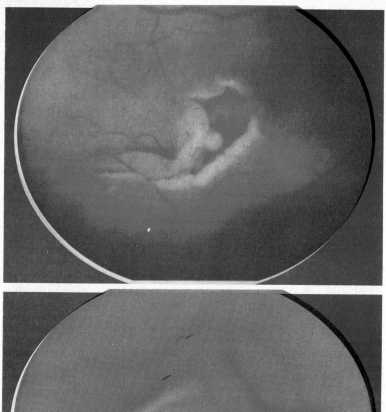

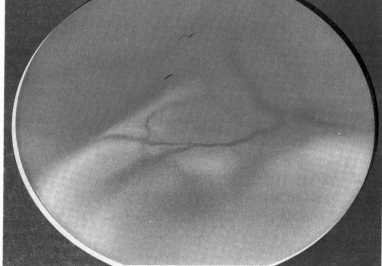

Fig. 213.1 Retinal detachment.

vitreous humour following cataract surgery. These retinal detachments are difficult to treat and pars plana vitrectomy is the only option.

Secondary retinal detachments: This occurs secondary to systemic disorders including hypertension, toxaemia of pregnancy, chronic glomerulonephritis, retinal venous occlusive disease and retinal vasculitis. Treatment is directed towards the underlying cause as these detachments are not amenable to scleral buckling surgery.

What surgical procedures are available for retinal detachment?

The three principal methods for reattachment of the retina are scleral buckling, vitrectomy and pneumatic retinopexy:

- *Scleral buckling* is an extraocular approach that indents the eye wall to restore contact with the detached retina. All retinal breaks are localized and adhesions between the choroid and retina are performed around the break with diathermy or a cryoprobe. After draining the subretinal fluid, the detached portion of the retina is indented towards the vitreous cavity by a scleral implant or explant. This pushs the retina towards the vitreous humour, causing closure of the retinal break (by the buckled sclera and choroid) and release of traction on the vitreous humour.
- *Pars plena vitrectomy* is an intraocular approach that relieves traction by removing the vitreous humour attached to the retinal breaks, permitting reapproximation to the retinal pigment epithelium, where the breaks are permanently closed with retinopexy.
- *Pneumatic retinopexy* closes retinal breaks using a small bubble of pure sulfur hexafluoride or perfluoropropane injected intravitreally; this allows the retinal pigment epithelium pump to reattach the retina. Gradual elution of gas from the eye coupled with permanent closure of the break by retinopexy leaves the retina reattached. The initial studies utilizing this procedure involved treatment of primary detachments with small breaks that were restricted to the superior two-thirds of the fundus.

There is a paucity of randomized trials comparing these approaches as treatment for primary retinal detachment.

Further reading

D'Amico DJ: Primary retinal detachment, *N Engl J Med* 359:2346–2354, 2008.

214 AGE-RELATED MACULAR DEGENERATION (SENILE MACULAR DEGENERATION)

INSTRUCTION

Look at this patient's fundus.

SALIENT FEATURES

History

- Often visual loss is detected when one eye is covered for testing visual acuity

- Loss of ability to read, recognize faces or drive a car; however, patients have enough peripheral vision to walk unaided
- Decrease in visual acuity (severe loss suggests choroidal neovascularization)
- Metamorphosia (distortion of the shape of objects in view)
- Paracentral scotoma
- Variable visual loss from atrophy of a large area of retinal pigment epithelium involving the fovea
- Family history
- History of smoking
- High BP (increases risk of choroidal neovascularization).

Examination

- Drüsen
- Disruption of pigment of the retinal pigment epithelium into small areas of hypopigmentation and hyperpigmentation (Fig. 214.1)
- Choroidal neovascularization.

Proceed as follows:

- Comment on the white walking aid by the bedside, which indicates the patient is registered blind.
- Check visual acuity and visual field (in most patients there is loss of central vision and maintenance of peripheral vision). Patients with only

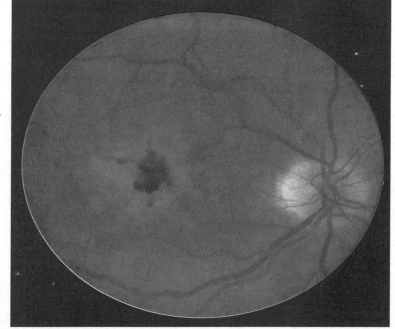

Fig. 214.1 Macular degeneration.

drüsen typically require additional magnification of text and more intense light to read small print text.

- Tell the examiner you would like to use Amsler grid to confirm your diagnosis.

Remember: Age-related macular degeneration is now the commonest cause of registrable blindness in the UK.

DIAGNOSIS

This patient has senile macular degeneration (aetiology) and is registered blind, as evidenced by the white walking aid (functional status).

QUESTIONS

What are drüsen?

Drüsen are pale yellow spots that occur individually or in clusters throughout the macula (Fig. 214.2). Nearly all individuals over the age of 50 years of age have at least one small drüsen (≤63 µm) in one or both eyes (Opthalmology 1992;14:130–42). They consist of amorphous material accumulated between the Bruch's membrane and pigment epithelium. Although the exact origin is not known, it is believed that drüsen occur from accumulation of lipofuscin and other cellular debris derived from cells of the retinal pigment epithelium that are compromised by age and other factors. Only eyes with large drüsen (>63 µm) are at increased risk for senile macular degeneration (Opthalmology 1997;104:7–21). The clinical hallmark and usually the first clinical finding of age-related macular degeneration is the

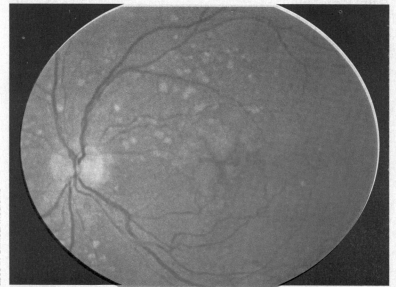

Fig. 214.2 Intermediate age-related macular degeneration with large drüsen. (With permission from Coleman et al. 2008.)

presence of drüsen. In most cases of age-related macular degeneration, drüsen are present bilaterally.

What are the types of age-related macular degeneration?

There are three types (Lancet 2008; 372:1835–45):

Early age-related macular degeneration. Multiple small drüsen (<63 μm) or intermediate drüsen (63–125 μm) with no evidence of advanced age-related macular degeneration.

Intermediate age-related macular degeneration. Extensive intermediate drüsen or large drüsen (≥125 μm) with no evidence of advanced age-related macular degeneration.

Advanced age-related macular degeneration. The presence of one or other of geographic atrophy or neovascular age-related macular degeneration:

Geographic atrophy. Presence of a discrete area of retinal depigmentation at least 175 μm in diameter with a sharp border and visible choroidal vessels in the absence of neovascular age-related macular degeneration in the same eye (Fig. 214.3). Geographic atrophy results from the continued loss of retinal pigment epithelium, with the eventual development of focal areas of total loss of the retina, retinal pigment epithelium and the small blood vessels directly under the epithelium. The disease is generally slowly progressive. Central geographic atrophy involves the centre of the macula.

Neovascular age-related macular degeneration. Serous or haemorrhagic detachment of either the retinal pigment epithelium or the sensory retina; the presence of subretinal fibrous tissue; or minimal subretinal fibrosis. Neovascularization develops under the retina, which can leak

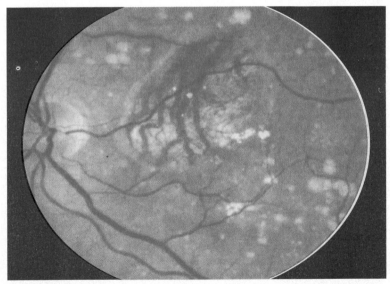

Fig. 214.3 Geographic atrophy involving the centre of the fovea, with sharply demarcated loss of normal retinal pigment epithelial cells and evidence of deeper larger choroidal vessels. (With permission from Coleman et al. 2008.)

fluid or bleed. Onset of vision loss is acute. This is the most common cause of severe central visual loss.

ADVANCED-LEVEL QUESTIONS

What do you know about neovascularization in these patients?
It leads to substantial visual loss as choroidal vessels proliferate across the Bruch's membrane under the retinal pigment epithelium and, in some cases, continue their extension into the subretinal space. Substantial leakage from these neovascular membranes can lead to retinal detachment. The most devastating consequence is haemorrhage, which resolves forming a disciform scar.

What are the risk factors for choroidal neovascularization in the other eye of a patient with disorder in one eye?
- Large drüsen (>63 μm)
- Drüsen number >5
- Focal hyperpigmentation of the retinal pigment epithelium.

What investigations are performed to detect choroidal neovascularization?
- Rapid-sequence fluoroscein angiography
- Retinal angiography using indocyanine green and infrared photography.

What are the risk factors for macular degeneration?
- Elderly
- Genetic factors
- A history of smoking within the past 20 years
- White race
- Obesity
- High dietary intake of vegetable fat
- Low dietary intake of antioxidants and zinc
- Complement factor H, Y402H variant
- *LOC387715/ARMS2*, A69S variant.

What therapies are available for age-related macular degeneration?
- Life style: cessation of tobacco, high dietary intake of beta-carotene, vitamins C and E and zinc, as well as high dietary intake of *n*3 long-chain polyunsaturated fatty acids and fish. Antioxidant vitamins and zinc can reduce the risk of developing advanced age-related macular degeneration by about a quarter in those at least at moderate risk.
- When visual loss is severe, low-vision devices such as electronic video magnifiers and spectacle-mounted telescopes, as well as low-vision rehabilitation services are available.
- Ranibizumab is a monoclonal antibody that inhibits all forms of vascular endothelial growth factor (VEGF). When ranibizumab is injected into the vitreous it has stabilized loss of vision and, in some cases, improved vision in individuals with neovascular age-related macular degeneration.
- Bevacizumab, a monoclonal antibody to VEGF used 'intravenously as an anticancer agent, is also increasingly being used off-label as intravitreal therapy for neovascular age-related macular degeneration.
- Photodynamic to reduce angiogenesis involves the use of an intravenously administered light-sensitive dye, verteporfin (Visudyne,

Novartis), that preferentially concentrates in new blood vessels and is activated with the use of a 689 nm laser beam focused over the macula. It causes localized choroidal neovascular thrombosis through a non-thermal chemotoxic reaction.

- Pegaptanib, an anti-VEGF therapy, appears to be effective.
- Triple therapy: intravitreal anti-VEGF agent, intravitreal dexamethasone and photodynamic therapy is also currently under investigation.
- Adenoviral vector-mediated intravitreal gene transfer of pigment-epithelium-derived factor (an antiangiogenic cytokine) appears to help to arrest the growth of choroidal neovascularization.
- Implantation of artificial intraocular devices (miniature telescopes) might improve the quality of life of patients with severe visual loss from end-stage disease.
- Implantation of electrical stimulated devices targeting the optic nerve and cortical, subretinal and epiretinal areas has led to the perception of phosphenes (discrete, reproducible perceptions of light) and is under investigation.

How is the neovascularization treated?

- Laser photocoagulation of regions outside the foveal avascular zone
- Subfoveal neovascularization: photocoagulated is associated with a treatment-induced visual loss immediately but in the long term is found to be beneficial. Treatment may have to be deferred in those with good initial visual acuity because a large scotoma occurs as a result of treatment
- Photodynamic therapy: with photosensitizers such as verteporfin
- Interferon-alfa: currently being evaluated
- Submacular surgery to remove the subfoveal choroidal neovascularization: reported to be useful, but the results are not as good as laser photocoagulation
- Zinc as a therapeutic agent for macular degeneration: has not been evaluated in a rigorous trial
- External beam radiation therapy
- Thalidomide
- Others: indocyanine green-guided laser treatment, retinal transplantation and transplantation of retinal pigment epithelium, retinal translocation, retinal prosthesis, gene therapy.

What is the difference between krypton and argon laser photocoagulation?

The krypton red photocoagulator is useful to treat when the neovascularization is closer than 200 μm but not under the fovea, because of its ability to spare the inner retina by its virtual lack of absorption by haemoglobin (unlike the argon laser). The conventional argon laser has blue and green wavelengths. The green wavelength is absorbed by haemoglobin and may damage the retina, while the blue wavelength is absorbed by the macular xanthophyll and results in foveal damage.

Argon laser photocoagulation therapy was once the most common therapy for neovascular age-related macular degeneration. It is now used only occasionally to treat choroidal neovascularization that extends by >200 μm from the centre of the macula, since this therapy can create a large retinal scar, which is itself associated with permanent visual loss.

Mention some drugs that can cause maculopathy

Chloroquine, thioridazine, chlorpromazine.

Miscellaneous
Examination of the foot

INSPECTION

- Comment on deformity: hallux valgus (Fig. IX.1A), pes cavus (Fig. IX.1B)
- Skin: comment on the colour, ulcers and gangrene, hair loss (remember that hair loss is not a reliable sign of ischaemia)
- Joint: comment on the swelling, e.g. ankle joint, first metatarsophalangeal joint in gout
- Palpation:
  - Ask the patient whether the foot is sore
  - Feel for temperature difference between the two feet
  - Pulses: dorsalis pedis and posterior tibials (compare with the other side)
  - Sensation: check light touch, pain and joint sensation
  - Check the plantar response and the ankle jerk.

WAGNER DIABETIC FOOT ULCER CLASSIFICATION SYSTEM

A: No ulcer but high-risk foot (e.g. deformity, callus, insensitivity).
B: Ulcer:
  1. Superficial full-thickness ulcer
  2. Deeper ulcer, penetrating tendons, no bone involvement
  3. Deeper ulcer, with bone involvement, osteitis
  4. Partial gangrene (e.g. toes, forefoot)
  5. Gangrene of whole foot.

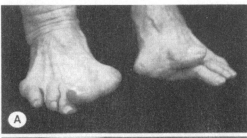

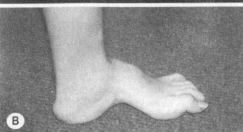

Fig. IX.1 (A) Hallux valgus. (B) Pes cavus. (A with permission from Canale, Beaty 2007; B with permission from Kliegman et al. 2007.)

215 DIABETIC FOOT

INSTRUCTION

Examine this patient's legs.
Examine this patient's feet.

NEUROPATHIC FOOT

SALIENT FEATURES

History

- Whether there is pain (usually painless neuropathy, but may be painful)
- Whether there is blistering (usually caused by an ill-fitting shoe)
- About a previous history of foot ulcers
- History of diabetes.

Examination

- Dry, warm and pink with palpable pulses
- Impaired deep tendon reflexes
- Reduced pinprick, light touch and vibration sensation
- Ulcers usually painless and plantar.

ISCHAEMIC FOOT

SALIENT FEATURES

History

- Ask whether there is pain (usually painful)
- Ask about rest pain and claudication
- History of diabetes.

Examination

- Skin is shiny and atrophic with sparse hair
- The foot is cold to touch
- Peripheral pulses are absent (calcified arteries may make pulse examination less reliable)
- Ulcers usually painful and present on the heels and toes
- Check all peripheral pulses.

NEUROPATHIC AND ISCHAEMIC FOOT PRESENTING TOGETHER

Examination

- Ulcer on the foot with callosities at pressure points
- Loss of the arch of foot
- Stocking distribution of sensory loss of all modalities
- Loss of dorsalis pedis and/or posterior tibial pulsations.

Proceed as follows:
- Tell the examiner that you would like to:
  - check the urine for sugar
  - do a simple neurologic examination of the lower extremities involving the use of a 10 g monofilament to test sensation.

Notes
- When asked to examine the feet, remember that the evaluation should include assessment of:
  - degree of neuropathy (clinically)
  - severity of ischaemia (clinically, Doppler, CT angiography)
  - bone deformity (clinically, radiograph, MRI)
  - infection (local swab, blood culture, radiograph, MRI).
- The common conditions affecting the feet are diabetes and atherosclerosis. Pay particular attention to the pulses and the skin.

DIAGNOSIS

This patient has features of both an ischaemic and neuropathic foot (lesion), which is caused by diabetes mellitus (aetiology); walking is limited by the plantar ulcer (functional status).

QUESTIONS

What are the types of diabetic foot?
- Neuropathic foot (Fig. 215.1)
- Ischaemic foot (Fig. 215.2).

Note: Features of both types often occur together.

ADVANCED-LEVEL QUESTIONS

What is the pathophysiology of the ischaemic foot?
Occlusive vascular disease involving both microangiopathy and atherosclerosis of large and medium-sized arteries.

Mention a few conditions in which neuropathic ulcers are seen
- Progressive sensory neuropathy
- Tabes dorsalis
- Leprosy
- Amyloidosis
- Porphyria.

How would you manage this patient?
- Patient education: avoid cigarette smoking, inspect the feet daily for blisters, no walking barefoot, avoid tight shoes and avoid cutting toenails straight across. 'The patient should be advised to take care of his foot as good as his/her face'
- Radiograph of the foot
- Antibiotics
- Removal of necrotic tissue
- Removal of weight bearing and friction from ulcerated areas; use appropriate footwear such as moulded insoles or plaster cast, instant total contact-cast or crutches to avoid weight bearing
- Control hyperglycaemia
- Chiropody

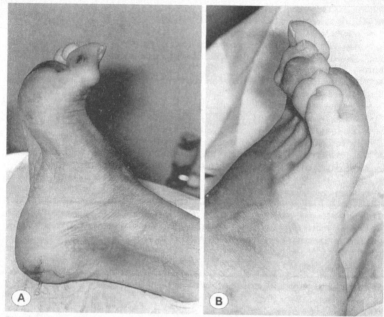

Fig. 215.1 The high-risk neuropathic foot: wasting of small muscles, clawing of the toes and marked prominence of the metatarsal heads. There is also ulceration. (With permission from Andersson, Svardsudd K 1995.)

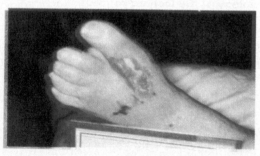

Fig. 215.2 Ischaemic diabetic foot: exposed tendon at the base of a left foot wound. (With permission from Auerbach 2007.)

- Surgical opinion and arteriography if reconstructive vascular surgery or angioplasty is considered. When irreversible arterial insufficiency occurs, it is often quicker and more humane for the patient to undergo early major amputation rather than be subjected to a series of debilitating conservative procedures
- Hyperbaric oxygen, platelet-derived growth factor and tissue-engineered skin; intermittent negative pressure applied to a wound to stimulate cellular proliferation; electrical stimulation and hydrotherapy.

How would you monitor a diabetic at annual review?

- Eyes: visual acuity, fundoscopy
- Sensory system: touch, pinprick and vibration sense
- Deep tendon reflexes
- Cardiovascular system: BP, peripheral pulses
- Biochemistry: urine and blood sugar, albumin, glycosylated haemoglobin, creatinine

What is the importance of the Neuropathy Disability Score?

The Neuropathy Disability Score is based in impairment of sensation. A score (for *both* feet) of ≥6 is predictive of foot ulceration. The annual risk of ulceration is 1.1% if the score is <6 and 6.3% if it is ≥6. A maximum of 5 points can be scored by each foot:

- Vibration threshold (apply 128 Hz tuning fork to apex of great toe):
  - Normal (can distinguish between presence and absence of vibration): 0
  - Abnormal: 1
- Temperature (to dorsum of foot, apply a tuning fork placed in a beaker of ice water or warm water):
  - Normal (can distinguish between hot and cold): 0
  - Abnormal: 1
- Pinprick (apply pin proximal to great toenail to barely depress skin):
  - Normal (can distinguish sharpness or lack of sharpness): 0
  - Abnormal: 1
- Achilles' reflex
  - Present: 0
  - Present with reinforcement: 1
  - Absent: 2

What do you know about measurement of cutaneous pressure perception?

Semmes–Weinstein monofilaments assess sensory perception. Individuals with normal feet can usually feel the 4.17 monofilament (~1 g linear pressure). Patients who cannot feel the 5.07 monfilament (~10 g of linear pressure) before it buckles are considered to have lost protective sensation. A seven-fold increase in the risk of ulceration has been reported in patients insensitive to the 5.07 monofilaments. However, up to 10% of persons who feel the monofilament before it buckles may still have cutaneous breakdown.

Professor Brian Frier, BSc (Hons), MD, FRCPE, FRCPG is a Consultant Physician in general (internal) medicine and diabetes at the Royal Infirmary of Edinburgh and is Honorary Professor of Diabetes in the University of Edinburgh. He graduated from the University of Edinburgh, trained in Scotland, and was a Clinical Research Fellow at the Cornell University Medical Center in New York. Professor Frier was previously a Consultant Physician in the Western Infirmary and Gartnavel General Hospital in Glasgow, Scotland (1982-87). He is currently Vice-President of the Royal College of Physicians of Edinburgh.

Professor Frier's principal research interest is the pathophysiology of hypoglycaemia in humans with particular relevance to diabetes.

Professor Miles Fisher, Consultant Physician Royal Infirmary Glasgow. He graduated from Glasgow University in 1979. He worked as a research fellow in the Department of Diabetes in Gartnavel General Hospital in the 1980s, where his interests were diabetes and the heart, and hypoglycaemia. He is Vice President of Royal College of Physicians and Surgeons of Glasgow.

216 SWOLLEN LEG I: DEEP VEIN THROMBOSIS

INSTRUCTION

Look at this patient's leg.

SALIENT FEATURES

History

- Recent history of immoblization including recent surgery, stroke, myocardial infarction
- Whether onset was acute or chronic
- Pain
- Past and family history of thromboses including deep vein thrombosis (DVT), pulmonary embolism
- Drug history: oral contraceptives
- Air travel; the evidence is circumstantial (BMJ 2001;322:188).

Examination

- Painful calf
- Redness
- Engorged superficial veins
- Unilateral swollen leg with pitting oedema (Fig. 216.1)
- Pain on the calf on dorsiflexion of the foot: Homans' sign (not diagnostic).

Proceed as follows:

- Check for pitting oedema on both sides (look at the patient's eyes while eliciting this sign to ensure that you are not hurting the patient).
- Compare the temperature of both the legs (use the dorsum of your fingers to elicit this sign).
- Check the arterial pulses in the leg.

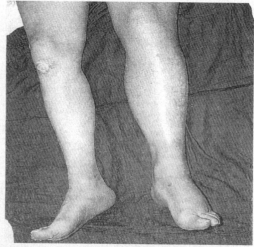

Fig. 216.1 Deep venous thrombosis: acutely swollen left leg with dilation of the superficial veins. (With permission from Forbes, Jackson 2003.)

- Comment on the heparin pump by the bedside.
- Remember to collect your thoughts when asked to examine the legs: do not rush in to grab the patient's legs.

DIAGNOSIS

This patient has a swollen leg resulting from deep vein thrombosis (lesion), which may be caused by the oral contraceptives she is taking (aetiology); the leg is oedematous and the patient is at risk of pulmonary embolism (functional status).

QUESTIONS

What are the complications of deep vein thrombosis?
- Pulmonary embolism
- Venous gangrene
- Pain, particularly in iliofemoral thrombosis.

What are the predisposing factors for venous thrombosis?
- Surgery (particularly of leg or pelvis, or after prostatectomy)
- Following cerebrovascular accident (about half of the patients develop DVT)
- Following myocardial infarction (one-third of patients have DVT)
- Obesity
- Malignancy (Lancet 1998;351:1077–80)
- Varicose veins
- Oral contraceptives
- Older age (exponential increase above the age of 50 years)
- Immobilization (paralysed limbs in stroke, paraplegia)
- Previous DVT (risk increases two- to three-fold)
- Pregnancy (risk increased in postpartum period)
- Hypercoagulable states: antithrombin III deficiency, protein C deficiency, protein S deficiency, antiphospolipid syndrome, excessive plasminogen activator inhibitor, polycythaemia vera, erythrocytosis
- Tissue trauma.

How would you investigate a patient with suspected deep vein thrombosis?
As clinical diagnosis is unreliable, it is essential to perform the following investigations to assess the extent of thrombosis:
- Duplex ultrasonography scanning and color Doppler studies
- D-dimer
- Venography: by injecting contrast into one of the leg veins.

What is the risk of pulmonary embolism in patients with below-knee thrombi?
The risk in such cases is low and many physicians refrain from prescribing anticoagulation to these patients.

How would you treat patients with below-knee thrombi?
- Pain relief
- Control of oedema
- Intermittent elevation of foot and elevation of foot during the night above the level of the heart
- Avoid long periods of standing
- Elastic support stockings from the midfoot to just below the knee, worn during the day.

The main aim is to prevent pulmonary emboli and restore venous patency and valvular function in order to prevent postphlebitic syndrome.

How would you treat patients with above-knee thrombi?

All patients with thrombi above the knee must receive anticoagulation therapy:

- Low-molecular-weight heparin has been shown to be more effective than unfractionated heparin in reducing size of thrombus and prevention of recurrence. It requires subcutaneous injection but does not require bolus or laboratory monitoring. Examples include enoxaparin, dalteparin or tinzaparin.
- Parenteral synthetic pentasaccharide analogues (e.g. fondaparinux) are factor Xa inhibitors that can also be used as first-line therapy.
- Unfractionated heparin is preferred in patients with iliofemoral thrombosis:
  - Initial therapy aims to maintain the activated partial thromboplastin time (APTT) at 1.5–2.5 times the normal value within the first 24 h. Failure to achieve this target APTT *within 24 h* increases the risk of recurrent venous thromboembolism by 15-fold. Heparin therapy is continued for about 5–10 days.
  - This is followed by warfarin therapy aiming to maintain the international normalized ratio (INR) at 2.0–3.0, which is recommended for the treatment of venous thromboembolic disease; however, substantially less intensive anticoagulation may be effective.

  Remember: Anticoagulants do not affect thrombus that is already present.
- When anticoagulation is contraindicated, inferior vena caval filters may be required when there is a high risk of pulmonary embolism.
- Thrombolysis should be considered when the thrombosis is 'limb threatening'.

There is no consensus on duration of therapy but the following are broad guidelines:

- 3–6 months with first episode
- 6 weeks to 3 months postoperatively if no other risk factors
- 6–12 months if persistent risk factors and recurrent venous thromboembolic events
- lifelong only rarely.

How would you prevent deep venous thrombosis?

- Subcutaneous low-dose heparin or low-molecular-heparin should be given to patients:
  - undergoing surgery to the leg, pelvis or prostatectomy
  - with myocardial infarction
  - with cardiac failure.
- Stop oral contraceptives prior to surgery
- Early ambulation within 72 h after surgery
- Encourage leg exercise following surgery
- Elastic supports to patients with a history of thrombosis or obesity
- Aspirin 160 mg every day reduces the risk of pulmonary embolism and DVT by at least a third particularly after hip surgery (Lancet 2000;355:1295–302).

ADVANCED-LEVEL QUESTIONS

How is bleeding risk from warfarin calculated?

The HEMORR$_2$HAGES score is computed by adding 1 point for each bleeding risk factor:

Hepatic or renal disease
Ethanol abuse
Malignancy
Older (age >75 years)
Reduced platelet count (<75 × 10^9/l) or function
Rebleeding risk (2 points for major bleed and 1 point for minor bleed)
Hypertension (uncontrolled), systolic BP >160 mmHg
Anaemia (hematocrit <30)
Genetic factors
Excessive fall risk
Stroke.

The risk of bleeding is then predicted by the following table (Am Heart J 2006;151:713–19):

HEMORR$_2$HAGES score	Bleeds per 100 patient-years warfarin (95% confidence interval)
0	1.9 (0.6–4.4)
1	2.5 (1.3–4.3)
2	5.3 (3.4–8.1)
3	8.4 (4.9–13.6)
4	10.4 (5.1–18.9)
≥5	12.3 (5.8–23.1)

What are causes of recurrent venous thrombosis?

- Pregnancy, surgery, trauma, oral contraceptives
- Abnormalities in antithrombin III, protein C, protein S, fibrinogen or factor V
- Acquired conditions such as anti-phospholipid antibody syndrome, occult cancer, myeloproliferative disorders, some vasculitides
- Potential abnormalities include thrombomodulin, tissue factor pathway inhibitor, vitronectin associated with heparin and antithrombin III and fibrinolytic receptors.

What do you know of the anti-phospholipid antibody syndrome?

The diagnosis of this syndrome requires that a patient have recurrent clinical events (such as thromboses or foetal loss) and an anti-phospholipid antibody (such as anti-cardiolipin antibody or lupus anticoagulant). The 'primary' syndrome has no accompanying autoimmune disease, whereas it is 'secondary' if the patient also has SLE or lupus-like disease. Many patients with this syndrome have livedo reticularis, thrombocytopenia and neurological symptoms (Lancet 1999;353:1348–53).

The clinical course of the secondary syndrome is independent of the activity and severity of the lupus, but the presence of anti-phospholipid antibody worsens the prognosis of the lupus. Warfarin therapy with an INR of ≥3 offers the best protection against recurrent thrombosis for patients who have a confirmed major thrombosis.

Note: The anti-phospholipid antibody can occur in certain drug reactions and infectious diseases, but only those that occur in patients with autoimmune disease are associated with the clinical syndrome.

Further reading

Gorman WP, Davis KR, Donnelly R: ABC of arterial and venous disease. Swollen lower limb 1: general assessment and deep vein thrombosis, *BMJ* 320:1453–1456, 2000 (review).

Prins MH, Büller HR: Deep-vein thrombosis, *Lancet* 353:479–485, 1999 (review).

J Homans (1877–1954) was an American surgeon who worked at Johns Hopkins Hospital with Cushing, initially on experimental hypophysectomy and later on vascular disease. He first reported venous thrombosis related to airtravel in a 54-year old physician who develop DVT after a 14-hour flight (N Engl J Med 1954;250:148–59).

GRV 'Hughes, contemporary London physician, Raynes Institute, St Thomas' Hospital, first described the anti-phospholipid antibody syndrome (N Engl J Med 1995;332:993–7).

---

217 SWOLLEN LEG II: CELLULITIS

INSTRUCTION

Look at this patient's leg.

SALIENT FEATURES

History

- History of fever and chills
- Diabetes
- Animal (or human!) bites
- Exposure to seawater (*Vibrio vulnificus*), fresh water (*Aeromonas hydrophila*) or aquacultured fish (*Streptococcus iniae*).

Examination

- Red, inflamed leg with a definite demarcation of erythematous area (Fig. 217.1)
- Oedema
- Increased temperature
- Crepitus: crepitant cellulitis is produced by either *Clostridia* sp. or non-spore-forming anaerobes (*Bacteroides* spp, peptostreptococci and peptococci).

Proceed as follows:

- Examine the peripheral pulses.
- Look for varicose veins (varicose eczema should be considered in the differential diagnosis of cellulites of the leg, BMJ 1999;318:1672–3).
- Look for superficial ulcers.

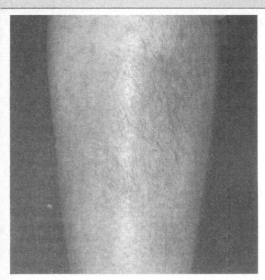

Fig. 217.1 Cellulitis. (With permission from Habif 2009.)

DIAGNOSIS

This patient has cellulitis of the leg (lesion) caused by pyogenic bacterial infection (aetiology) and the leg is acutely swollen and painful (functional status).

Remember: Cellulitis is a clinical diagnosis; it is a deep, subcutaneous infection characterized by warmth, swelling, tenderness and erythema and may be accompanied by lymphatic streaking. Pruritus is absent (unlike in contact dermatitis).

QUESTIONS

How would you manage such a patient?

- Cultures of aspirates and lesions
- Blood cultures: bacteraemia is uncommon in cellulitis but blood cultures are useful in those with lymphoedema
- Radiology: plain film radiography or CT is useful when accompanying osteomyelitis is suspected. Gallium-67 scintillography may aid in the detection of cellulitis superimposed on recently increasing, chronic lymphoedema of a limb
- Intravenous antibiotics: because most cases of cellulitis are caused by streptococci and *Staphylococcus aureus,* beta-lactam antibiotics with activity against penicillinase-producing *S. aureus* are the usual drugs of choice. Flucloxacillin can be used until microbe is identified
- Pain relief and pyretics
- Surgical referral
- Experimental: granulocyte-colony stimulating factor (G-CSF), particularly in diabetics.

What are the causes of bilateral swollen legs?

- Cardiac failure
- Renal failure
- Hypoproteinaemia (from cirrhosis or nephrotic syndrome).

What are the causes of an acutely swollen leg?

- Deep vein thrombosis
- Cellulitis
- Arterial occlusion
- Trauma
- Arthritis.

What are the causes of a chronically swollen leg?

- Venous causes: varicose veins, postphlebitic limb
- Lymphoedema: Milroy's disease, filariasis (in the tropics)
- Congenital.

WF Milroy (1855–1942) described familial lymphoedema of the legs in 1892.

---

218 CLUBBING

INSTRUCTION

Examine this patient's hands.

SALIENT FEATURES

History

- Lung conditions (bronchogenic carcinoma; fibrosing alveolitis; mesothelioma; suppurative lung disease such as bronchiectasis, lung abscess and empyema)
- Cardiac conditions (infective endocarditis, cyanotic heart disease)
- GI tract conditions (cirrhosis, ulcerative colitis, Crohn's disease)
- Thyroid disease (thyroid acropachy)
- Family history (hereditary clubbing).

Examination

- Increased curvature of the nails, obliteration of the angle of the nail. A positive Schamroth test is the absence of the normal diamond-shaped window created when the dorsal surfaces of the terminal phalanges of similar fingers are opposed (Fig. 218.1). (When in doubt, approximate the dorsal aspects of terminal phalanges of the fingers of both hands flexed at the interphalangeal joints. Normally, the angle between the nails does not extend more than halfway up the nail bed. In clubbing there is a wide and deep angle, Schamroth's sign.)
- Loss of Lovibond's angle (Fig. 218.2)
- The nails may have a drumstick appearance (see Fig. 106.1).

Proceed as follows:

- Look for the following signs:
  - Fluctuation at the nail bed
  - Nicotine (tar) staining of fingers

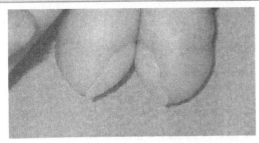

Fig. 218.1 Schamroth's sign. (With permission from Marrie, Brown 2007.)

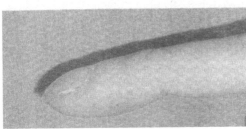

Fig. 218.2 Marked increase in the depth of the distal phalange, giving a ratio of the depth of the distal phalange to the depth of the interphalange of >1. Lovibond's angle is >180 degrees. (With permission from Marrie, Brown 2007.)

- • Central cyanosis
- • Clubbing of the toes.
- • Palpate the wrist joints for tenderness: hypertrophic pulmonary osteoarthropathy (HPOA); rapid painful clubbing is nearly always caused by bronchogenic carcinoma.
- • Tell the examiner that you would like to examine the following systems:
  - • Chest: bronchogenic carcinoma; fibrosing alveolitis; mesothelioma; suppurative lung disease such as bronchiectasis, lung abscess and empyema
  - • Heart: infective endocarditis, cyanotic heart disease; in infective endocarditis the fingers may be pale and their tips flushed ('pale hands, pink tipped')
  - • GI: cirrhosis, ulcerative colitis, Crohn's disease
  - • Thyroid: thyroid acropachy; ~20% of patients with thyroid dermopathy have thyroid acropachy, which manifests as clubbing of the fingers *and* toes.

DIAGNOSIS

This patient has marked clubbing of the fingernails (lesion) and tar staining, indicating that the condition may be caused by an underlying bronchial neoplasm (aetiology).

QUESTIONS

How is clubbing graded?

There are four grades:

I: increased glossiness and cyanosis of the skin at the root of the nail associated with increased fluctuation at the base of the nail bed

II: the normal angle between the base of the nail and the skin is obliterated (Lovibond's sign) and may even be reversed

III: hypertrophy of the soft tissue of the nail pulp and the nail curves excessively longitudinally to give a 'drum-stick' or 'parrot-beak' appearance ('doigts Hippocratique')

IV: bony changes involving the wrists and ankles, sometimes the elbows and knees (HPOA).

What do you know about pachydermoperiostitis?

This is an unusual variety of idiopathic familial HPOA, in which postpubertal clubbing and bone changes are accompanied by increased sweating of the palms and soles and marked thickening of the skin of the face, forehead and scalp.

What are the characteristics of pseudoclubbing?

Pseudoclubbing is distinguished clinically from clubbing by the preservation of the nailfold angle and bony erosion of the terminal phalanges on radiography.

ADVANCED-LEVEL QUESTIONS

What are the mechanisms for clubbing?

- Increased blood flow in clubbed fingers caused by vasodilatation rather than hyperplasia of vessels in the nail bed. The nature of the vasodilator is unclear and many contenders, such as ferritin, bradykinin, prostaglandin and serotonin (5-hydroxytryptamine (5-HT)), have been implicated. The vasodilator is probably inactivated in the lung in normal persons but when this inactivation is defective, or there is a right-to-left shunt, clubbing occurs.
- Increased growth hormone in disease states causes excessive cellular tissue in the nail bed.
- Clubbing occurs whenever organs supplied by the vagus are affected. It has been shown that, in bronchogenic carcinoma, vagotomy causes reversal of clubbing.
- Tumour necrosis factor has been implicated.
- Megakaryocytes and clumps of platelets may preferentially stream into blood vessels of the digits and release platelet-derived growth factor, vascular end growth factor (vascular endothelial growth factor). The resulting increased capillary permeability, fibroblastic activity and arterial smooth muscle hyperplasia could cause clubbing.

Further reading

Adams F: Hippocrates. The Book of Prognostics. The Genuine Works of Hippocrates, Vol. 1, London, 1849, Sydenham Society.

Burton MD, Wain JC: Clubbing and hypertrophic osteoarthropathy, *N Engl J Med* 329:1862, 1993 (classical pictures of these conditions).

Dickinson CJ: The aetiology of clubbing and hypertrophic osteopathy, *Eur J Clin Invest* 23:330–338, 1993.

Schamroth L: Clubbing of fingers: a method of assessment, *S Afr Med J* 50:297, 1976.

Digital clubbing was first described approximately 2400 years ago by Hippocrates.

In 1976, Leo Schamroth, an internationally recognized cardiologist from Johannesburg, South Africa, described the sign that bears his name. He had three episodes of infective endocarditis in 1975 and developed clubbing.

219 DUPUYTREN'S CONTRACTURE

INSTRUCTION

Look at this patient's hands.

SALIENT FEATURES

History

- Family history (there is a genetic predisposition)
- Cigarette smoking (J Bone Joint Surg 1997;79B:206–10)
- Alcohol intake (Arch Intern Med 1977;129:561–6)
- Chronic antiepileptic medications
- Systemic conditions: cirrhosis, diabetes, TB, epilepsy.

Examination

- Thickening of the palmar fascia, particularly along the medial aspect (feel for thickening before you comment on it).
- In almost all cases, the fourth finger is affected with associated involvement of fifth, third and second fingers in decreasing order of frequency (Fig. 219.1).
- Perform the *Hueston tabletop test*: if the patient is unable to lay his or her palm flat on a tabletop, the test is positive.
- Tell the examiner that you would like to:
  - check the feet for contracture of the plantar fascia (Fig. 219.2)
  - look for signs of alcoholism and cirrhosis.

DIAGNOSIS

This patient has Dupuytren's contracture (lesion) associated with chronic alcoholic liver disease (aetiology) and has developed disabling contractures (functional status). Be prepared to grade Dupuytren's contracture (see below).

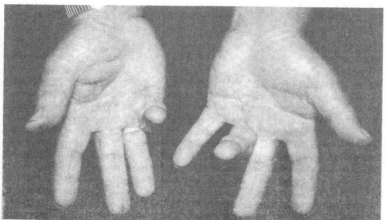

Fig. 219.1 Dupuytren's contracture.

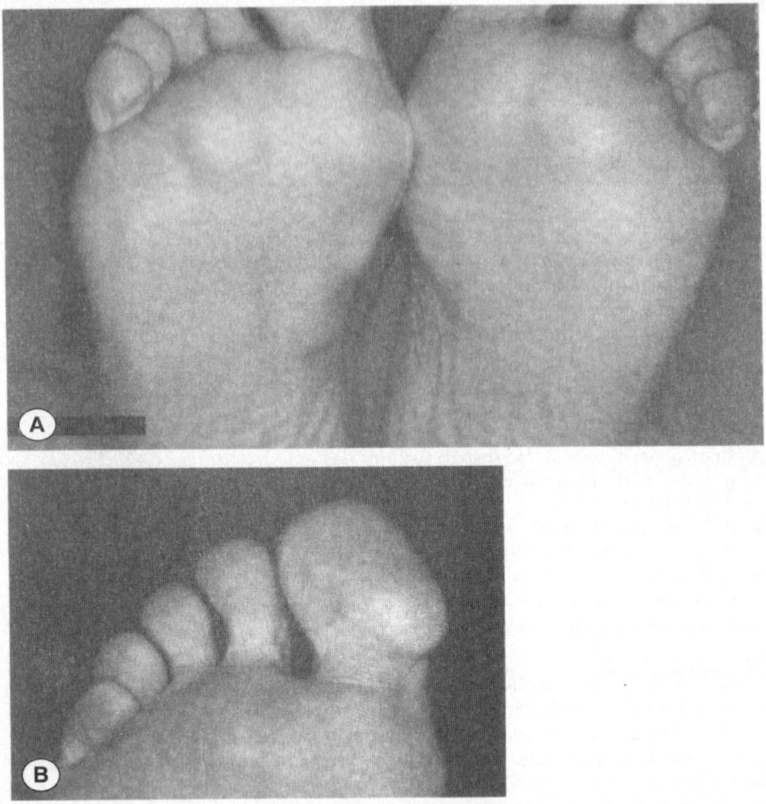

Fig. 219.2 Ectopic deposits. (A) Bilateral medial plantar and medial great toe involvement. (B) Right foot involvement. (With permission from Canale, Beaty 2007.)

ADVANCED-LEVEL QUESTIONS

What do you know about Dupuytren's contracture?

It is caused by the thickening and shortening of palmar fascia; the plantar fascia may also be affected. Fibrous nodules are often the earliest abnormality and reflect contracture of the proliferating fibroblasts in the superficial compartment of the palm. The nodules consist of mature-appearing fibroblasts surrounded by dense collagen. Ultrastructurally, many of these cells are myofibroblasts and so may be contractile.

What other structures are involved?

There does not appear to be any direct involvement of the muscles, joints, tendons (and their sheaths), nervous tissue or vascular tissue. However, the dermis is frequently invaded by fibroblastic cells, resulting in fixation to deeper structures.

What are the grades of Dupuytren's disease?

Grade 1 presents as a thickened nodule and a band in the palmar aponeurosis that may progress to skin tethering, puckering or pitting.

Grade 2 presents as a peritendinous band that limits extension of the affected finger.

Grade 3 presents as flexion contracture.

What is the natural history of this condition?

It is unpredictable, with little change or disability over a period of many years in some individuals. In others, the contraction of the fascia occurs rapidly, resulting in severe deformity and loss of hand function.

What do you know about the epidemiology of Dupuytren's contracture?

There may be a hereditary predisposition (usually autosomal dominant) and the disorder is about five times more frequent in men, more common in whites and in Europe. There is a gradual increase in the incidence with age.

With which other conditions is Dupuytren's contracture associated?

- Alcoholism
- Chronic antiepileptic therapy
- Systemic conditions such as cirrhosis, diabetes, epilepsy, TB
- Thickening of the corpora cavernosa of the penis (Peyronie's disease)
- Garrod's knuckle pads
- Retroperitoneal fibrosis.

Why is the deformity caused by this condition usually well tolerated?

Because it exaggerates the normal position of function of the hand.

How would you manage such patients?

Treatment depends on the severity of findings:

- Periodic examination of patients in early stages. If the palmar thickening is growing rapidly, local injections of triamcinolone into the growing nodule may be of benefit and reduce the need for surgery.
- Collagenase from *Clostridium histolyticum*, which lyses collagen and leads to disruption of contracted cords, is a new option for the therapy of advanced Dupuytren's disease. Collagenase clostridium histolyticum significantly reduces contractures and improves the range of motion in joints affected by advanced Dupuytren's disease. Therapy does not require anaesthesia. The collagenase is injected into the affected cord, and the treated joint is manipulated the next day to attempt cord rupture. Extensive hand therapy after treatment is not required (N Engl J Med 2009;361:968).
- Surgery is indicated when there are disabling flexion contractures (when the metacarpophalangeal joint contracture is >40 degrees or when the proximal interphalangeal joint contracture is >20 degrees), although recurrences are common (Lancet 1997;350:1568). The surgical procedures include open fasciectomy (the most common procedure), percutaneous or open fasciotomy, or needle fasciotomy.

F de la Peyronie (1678–1747), a French surgeon who influenced Louis XVI in his decision to issue an ordinance banning barbers from practising surgery.

Baron Guillaume Dupuytren (1777–1835), Surgeon-in-Chief, Hôtel-Dieu, Paris, is reported to have been the first to achieve successful removal of the lower jaw.

Sir AE Garrod (1857–1936), physician at St Bartholomew's Hospital, London, succeeded Osler as Regius Professor at Oxford.

220 CATARACTS

INSTRUCTION

Examine this patient's eyes.

SALIENT FEATURES

History

- Drug history (steroids, chloroquine, phenothiazines, chlorambucil, busulfan)
- History of gradual deterioration of vision
- History of diabetes
- Inquire about smoking (JAMA 1992;268:989–94) and alcohol consumption (Arch Ophthalmol 1993;111:1130) as both cigarette smoking and heavy alcohol consumption increase the risk of cataract formation
- Family history is important even in age-related nuclear cataract as it explains about 50% variation in the severity of disease (N Engl J Med 2000;342:1786–90).

Examination

- Bilateral cataracts (shine light obliquely across the lens; Fig. 220.1, see also Fig. 201.3).

Proceed as follows:
- Tell the examiner that you would like to check the urine for sugar.

DIAGNOSIS

This patient has premature bilateral cataracts (lesion) caused by diabetes mellitus (aetiology) and has had a gradual deterioration of vision (functional status).

QUESTIONS

Mention a few causes of cataracts

- *Common causes*:
  - Old age (look for arcus senilis). The Framingham study reported that 13% of people aged 65–74 years and about 40% of those over the age of 75 years had cataracts.
  - Diabetes mellitus (non-enzymatic glycosylation of lens protein is twice as high in diabetics as in age-matched controls and may contribute to the premature occurrence of cataracts).

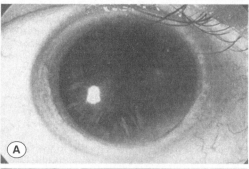

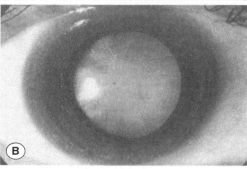

Fig. 220.1 Cataracts. (A) Early. (B) White mature cataract. (With permission from Kumar, Clark 2005.)

- *Uncommon causes:*
  - Trauma
  - Metabolic: Cushing syndrome, Wilson's disease (stellate cataracts), galactosaemia
  - Chromosomal disorders: dystrophia myotonica, Turner syndrome
  - Congenital infections (rubella or cytomegalovirus)
  - Drugs (see above)
  - Dermatological disorders: atopic dermatitis, ichthyosis
  - Radiation: infrared (glass-blower's cataract), X-ray, microwave radiation.

ADVANCED-LEVEL QUESTIONS

How are cataracts treated?

Cataract extraction is performed by removing the lens nucleus and cortex from within the lens capsule (extracapsular). In most adults, a plastic lens is implanted within the capsule. Multifocal intraocular lens implants in some instances have reduced the need for both reading and distance spectacles. Lens extraction improves vision in 95% of instances. In the remaining, prior retinal disease or postoperative complications such as haemorrhage, glaucoma, infection or retinal detachment may be the cause. There are data suggesting that there is substantial benefit from bilateral cataract eye surgery in that it improves stereoacuity (Lancet 1998;352:925–9).

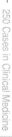

How is early cataract detected using direct ophthalmoscopy?

Examination of the red reflex with + 4 dioptres at approximately 20 cm from the patient will reveal a black opacity in the lens against the reddish hue of the reflex. If this opacity appears to move down on upward gaze, it is located in the posterior half of the lens, but if it appears to move up then it is located in the anterior half of the lens.

Is the use of inhaled steroids associated with cataracts?

The use of inhaled steroids is associated with nuclear and posterior sub-capsular cataracts (N Engl J Med 1997;337:8–14).

What do you know about calpains in the pathogenesis of cataracts?

The transparency and refractive capacity of the lens depend on the short-range interactions, concentration and configuration of water-soluble proteins, the crystallins, within the fibre cells of the lens. The calpains are calcium-dependent cysteine proteases (proteolytic enzymes with cysteine in the catalytic site) that cleave crystallins. In rats, m-calpain is the major calpain involved in the animal model of cataractogenesis and it is the only calpain active in human lenses. It cleaves the N-terminal region of the lens proteins α-crystallin and β-crystallin, producing truncated crystallin aggregates that resist additional proteolysis and form cataracts. Aging leads to post-translational modifications of crystallins that also result in progressive loss of solubility and a tendency to aggregate. The potential involvement of calpains in some types of human cataract has led to suggestions that calpain inhibitors may be possible therapy.

Jacques Divel of Bernay, a small town in Brittany, devised extracapsular extraction of cataracts in 1748.

Harold Ridley, who worked at St. Thomas's and Moorfields's Eye Hospital in London, was the first to champion the insertion of artificial lens after removal of a cataract in the 1950s (Lancet 1999;354:1912).

Controversy over process patents swelled after ophthalmologist Samuel Pallin was awarded a patent in 1992 for a method of performing cataract surgery that did not require stitches. The US Congress amended the Patent Act in 1996 to address these concerns.

---

221 ANAEMIA

PATIENT 1

INSTRUCTION

Would you like to ask this anaemic patient a few questions?

SALIENT FEATURES

History

- Ask about the following:
  - Blood loss such as bleeding per rectum, melaena, haematemesis
  - Menstrual blood loss: duration of periods, the occurrence of clots and the number of sanitary towels or tampons used

- Drug history: NSAIDs, phenytoin, chloramphenicol
- Associated symptoms such as weight loss, shortness of breath, chronic diarrhoea
- Diet: in vegans, alcoholics, elderly patients
- Past history of gastrectomy
- Family history.

DIAGNOSIS

This patient's anaemia is caused by severe melaena, which indicates bleeding in the upper GI tract and is probably the result of peptic ulcer or bleeding varices (aetiology). The patient is currently receiving a blood transfusion, indicating that the anaemia was severe (functional status).

PATIENT 2

INSTRUCTION

Would you like to examine this anaemic patient?

SALIENT FEATURES

Examination

- Examine:
  - nails for koilonychia or iron-deficiency anaemia and (rarely) for clubbing of infective endocarditis
  - tongue for pallor, atrophic glossitis and angular stomatitis of vitamin B_{12} deficiency (Fig. 221.1)

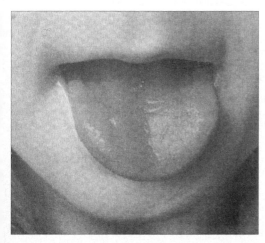

Fig. 221.1 Iron-deficiency anaemia leading to pallor of the face, lips and tongue plus atrophic glossitis and angular stomatitis. (With permission from Forbes, Jackson 2003.)

- mouth for angular stomatitis of severe malnutrition and ulcers of neutropenia
- lymph nodes in the neck, axillae and groin (secondaries, lymphoproliferative disorders)
- skin for bruising associated with bone marrow depression, seen in leukaemia and aplastic anaemia
- abdomen for hepatomegaly, splenomegaly and other masses
- legs for ulcers seen in haemoglobinopathies.
- Comment on the pallor of the face and conjunctiva, looking for the lemon-yellow hue of pernicious anaemia.
- Comment on the ethnic origin (thalassaemia).
- Tell the examiner that you would like to:
  - do a rectal examination and inspect the stool for occult blood
  - do an FBC including a peripheral smear and ESR.

DIAGNOSIS

This patient has koilonychia and anaemia indicating an iron-deficiency anaemia. I would like to exclude a GI cause for the blood loss (aetiology).

QUESTIONS

Mention a few causes of anaemia
- With a low mean corpuscular volume (MCV):
  - Iron-deficiency anaemia
  - Thalassaemia
  - Sideroblastic anaemia.
- With a high MCV:
  - Vitamin B_{12} deficiency: pernicious anaemia, vegans, alcoholics, coeliac disease
  - Folate deficiency: pregnancy, phenytoin, sprue, coeliac disease, malignancy, haemolysis
  - Other: myxoedema, liver disease, alcoholics.
- With a normal MCV:
  - Uraemia
  - Malignancy
  - Rheumatoid arthritis
  - Aplastic anaemia: myelofibrosis, chloramphenicol, phenylbutazone, gold, anticancer drugs.

What do you know about the Paterson–Kelly syndrome?
It comprises iron-deficiency anaemia and dysphagia from oesophageal webs in middle-aged women. The clinical significance of this syndrome is uncertain. It is also known as Plummer–Vinson syndrome.

What are the common causes of iron-deficiency anaemia?
Occult GI bleeding from the following:
- Peptic ulcer
- Carcinoma located anywhere in the GI tract
- Excessive anticoagulation
- Hereditary haemorrhagic telangiectasia
- Angiodysplasia of the colon.

How would you investigate microcytic anaemia?
- FBC
- Serum ferritin
- Faecal occult blood
- Upper GI endoscopy
- Barium enema, colonoscopy
- International normalized ratio (INR), prothrombin time and platelet count
- Haemoglobin electrophoresis in susceptible ethnic groups (Asians, Afro-Caribbeans).

How would you investigate macrocytic anaemia?
- Peripheral smear
- Vitamin B_{12} and red-cell folate and serum folate concentrations
- Serum ferritin, plasma iron and total iron-binding capacity (for associated iron deficiency)
- Schilling test
- Gastric parietal cell and intrinsic factor antibodies
- Upper GI endoscopy
- Reticulocyte count (a high MCV could be present when the reticulocyte count is >50%)
- Bone marrow examination.

When is a peripheral smear useful in the evaluation of anaemia?
When there is suspicion of:
- Sickle cell disease: dactylitis or sudden splenic enlargement and pallor in a young child, or limb, abdominal or chest pain in an older child or adult
- Thrombocytopenia (e.g. petechiae or abnormal bruising) or neutropenia (e.g. unexpected or severe infection)
- Lymphoma or other lymphoproliferative disorder (lymphadenopathy, splenomegaly): enlargement of the thymus (a mediastinal mass on radiology) or other lymphoid organs, skin lesions suggestive of infiltration, bone pain and systemic symptoms such as fever, sweating, itching and weight loss
- Myeloproliferative disease: splenomegaly, plethora, itching or weight loss
- Disseminated non-haematopoietic cancer: weight loss, malaise, bone pain
- Disseminated intravascular coagulation
- Infectious mononucleosis or other viral infection or inflammatory or malignant disease: general ill health, often with malaise and fever
- Bacterial or parasitic disease
- Acute or recent-onset renal failure or unexplained renal enlargement
- Retinal examination reveals haemorrhages, exudates, signs of hyperviscosity, optic atrophy
- Unexplained jaundice, anaemia or both.

RF Schilling (b. 1919), Chairman of the Department of Medicine and haematologist at the University of Wisconsin.

222 LYMPHADENOPATHY

INSTRUCTION

Perform a general examination.
Examine this patient's neck.

SALIENT FEATURES

History and examination

Use the mnemonic ALL AGES to approach a patient with lymphadenopathy:

ALL:
  Age at presentation (e.g. infectious mononucleosis is commoner in younger age groups, Hodgkin's disease has a bimodal peak)
  Location(s) of enlarged lymph nodes: those outside the inguinal regions, enlarged for >4 weeks and measuring 1 cm^2 or larger without an obvious diagnosis should be considered for biopsy (Semin Oncol 1993;20:570–82)
  Length of time the lymph nodes are present.

AGES:
  Associated symptoms and signs including fever ('B' symptoms: temperature >38°C, drenching night sweats, unexplained weight loss >10% body weight)
  Generalized lymph node enlargement
  Extranodal organ involvement
  Splenomegaly: consider infectious mononucleosis, lymphoma, chronic lymphocytic leukaemia, and acute leukaemia; rare in metastatic cancer (Cancer 1987;60:100–2).

● As soon as you feel a group of lymph nodes, examine drainage areas for obvious pathology. For example:
  • Inguinal lymph nodes: examine the lower limbs and external genitalia
  • Axillary lymph nodes: examine the chest, breasts and upper limbs
  • Upper cervical lymph nodes: examine the chest, breast and upper limbs; also, perform an ear, nose and throat (ENT) examination for nasopharyngeal carcinoma
  • Lower cervical and supraclavicular lymph nodes: examine the thyroid, chest, abdomen for gastric carcinoma (Virchow's nodes) and testis.

● Examine other lymph node areas in a systemic manner: submental, submandibular, deep cervical (upper and lower), occipital, posterior triangle, supraclavicular, axillary, epitrochlear and inguinal.

● Examine the mouth for the following signs:
  • Tonsillar lymph nodes
  • Palatal petechiae and pharyngitis (glandular fever)
  • Neoplastic tumours or ulcers.

● Examine the abdomen for liver and spleen.

● Examine the chest and do a chest radiography: for bronchogenic carcinoma, TB.

DIAGNOSIS

This patient has generalized lymphadenopathy, probably a lymphoma—either Hodgkin's or non-Hodgkin's (aetiology)—and has severe disease, as evidenced by alopecia, presumably caused by chemotherapy (functional status). I would like to discuss other causes of generalized lymphadenopathy.

QUESTIONS

What are the causes of regional lymphadenopathy?

Cervical lymphadenopathy. Causes include infections and malignancies. Infectious causes include bacterial pharyngitis, dental abscess, otitis media, infectious mononucleosis, cytomegalovirus, gonococcal pharyngitis, toxoplasmosis, hepatitis and adenovirus. Malignancies include non-Hodgkin disease, Hodgkin disease and squamous cell carcinoma of head and neck.

Virchow node (anterior left supraclavicular lymph node; also known as Troiser's ganglion). Enlargement suggests the presence of a thoracic or abdominal neoplasm (Am J Surg 1979;138:703). Common causes include carcinoma of breast; bronchus, lymphomas and GI neoplasms.

Delphian node (a midline prelaryngeal lymph node). Heralds thyroid disease, laryngeal malignancy or lymphoma.

Axillary lymphadenopathy. Causes include infections and malignancies. Infectious causes include staphylococcal, streptococcal infections of the arm, cat-scratch fever, tularaemia and sporotrichosis. Malignant causes, including Hodgkin's disease, non-Hodgkin lymphoma, carcinoma of breast and melanoma, are common.

Epitrochlear lymphadenopathy. The most common causes are lymphoma/chronic lymphatic leukaemia and infectious mononucleosis. Other diagnoses include HIV, sarcoidosis and connective tissue disorders. In developing countries, secondary syphilis, lepromatous leprosy, leishmaniasis and rubella are important causes.

Inguinal lymphadenopathy. In adults, some degree of lymph node enlargement is not uncommon. In those who walk outdoors with footwear, benign reactive lymphadenopathy is common. Malignant causes include lymphoma, malignant melanoma, carcinoma of external genitalia. Benign causes include cellulitis, syphilis, chancroid, genital herpes and lymphogranuloma venereum.

Node of Cloquet (also known as *Rosenmüller node*). A deep inguinal lymph node located near the femoral canal. When palpable it may be mistaken for an inguinal hernia.

What are the causes of generalized lymphadenopathy?

- Lymphomas, chronic lymphatic leukaemia, acute lymphoblastic leukaemia
- Glandular fever, cytomegalovirus
- HIV infection, toxoplasmosis
- SLE, rheumatoid arthritis, sarcoid
- Chronic infections such as TB, secondary syphilis, brucellosis
- Drugs: phenytoin

(Use the mnemonic CHICAGO: **c**ancers, **h**ypersensitivity, **i**nfections, **c**onnective tissue disorders, **a**typical lymphoproliferative disorders, **g**ranulomatous disorders, **o**ther unusual causes.)

What do you understand by the term Hodgkin's disease?

Hodgkin's disease is a group of neoplasms characterized by Reed–Sternberg cells in an appropriate reactive cellular background. It is divided into several subtypes histologically: lymphocyte predominance, nodular sclerosis, mixed cellularity and lymphocyte depletion. The Reed–Sternberg cell is a giant cell with two or more nuclear lobes and huge eosinophilic inclusion like nucleoli. The classic Reed–Sternberg cell has a symmetrical, mirror image nucleus that creates an 'owl-eye' appearance.

ADVANCED-LEVEL QUESTIONS

What is the cause of egg-shaped calcification in hilar lymph nodes?

Silicosis.

What do you know of Sister Joseph's nodule?

It is a classic sign of gastric adenocarcinoma i n the umbilical area and may represent a metastatic deposit or an enlarged anterior abdominal wall lymph node (Fig. 222.1).

What is the mode of presentation of Hodgkin's disease?

- Usually as a painless lymphadenopathy
- Other presenting symptoms include systemic symptoms such as fever, weight loss, drenching night sweats, generalized pruritus or pain in the affected lymph node following the ingestion of alcohol.

How is Hodgkin's disease staged?

The staging system has four stages (I–IV) plus a system of letters to indicate symptoms, bulk, lymph node involvement.

Stage I: one lymph node region involved

Stage II: more than two lymph node regions involved on one side of the diaphragm

Stage III: lymph nodes involved on both sides of the diaphragm

    3.1 with splenic hilar, coeliac or portal nodes

    3.2 with para-aortic, iliac or mesenteric nodes

Stage IV: involvement of extranodal sites(s) beyond that designated as 'E' below.

Systemic symptoms:

A: absent

B: significant weight loss >10% in six months, fever or night sweats.

Disease bulk and spread:

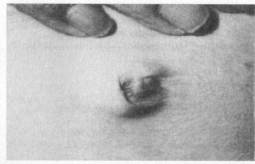

Fig. 222.1 Sister Joseph's nodule. (With permission from Leow, Lau 2008.)

X: bulky disease: greater than a third widening of mediastinum, >10 cm maximum diameter of nodal mass

E: involvement of single, contiguous or proximal extranodal site.

Clinical stage (CS) is determined by history, physical examination, radiological studies, isotope scans, laboratory tests of urine and blood, and the initial biopsy results.

Pathological stage (PS) relates to the tissue sampled and the results of histopathological examination.

How is a patient with Hodgkin's disease treated?

- Localized disease (i.e. stages IA, IIA) is treated with radiotherapy. Five-year cure rates are in excess of 80% and relapses are treated with chemotherapy.
- Disseminated disease (stages IIIB, IV) is treated with combination chemotherapy with the ABVD regimen (adriamycin, bleomycin, vincristine, dacarbazine) alternating with the MOPP regimen (mechlorethamine, oncovin, procarbazine and prednisolone). Five-year survival rates are about 50%. Patients who relapse after initial chemotherapy may be cured with autologous bone marrow transplantation.
- In stages IIB and IIIA, optimal management is controversial but current evidence suggests an advantage to combination chemotherapy (N Engl J Med 1993;328:560).

What do you understand by the term non-Hodgkin's lymphomas?

These are a heterogeneous group of cancers of lymphocytes. They are variable in their presentation and natural history, varying from a slow indolent course to a rapidly progressive illness (N Engl J Med 1993;328:1023).

How are non-Hodgkin's lymphomas classified?

A working classification is as follows.

Low grade or favourable. There is a slow, indolent course with good response to minimal therapy and long survival. These include small lymphocytic, plasmocytoid, follicular small cleaved cell and follicular mixed cell. Patients are usually treated with alkylating agents such as chlorambucil or a CVP regimen (cyclophosphamide, vincristine and prednisolone).

High grade or unfavourable. This includes immunoblastic, small non-cleaved (Burkitt's and non-Burkitt's), lymphoblastic and true histiocytic lymphoma. The mainstay of therapy is combination chemotherapy; traditionally the CHOP regimen (cyclophosphamide, doxorubicin, vincristine and prednisolone) is used. In highly aggressive lymphomas, autologous bone marrow transplantation may increase the chances of cure.

Intermediate grade. Follicular large cell, diffuse small cleaved cell, diffuse mixed cell, diffuse large cell.

Others. Cutaneous T cell (mycosis fungoides, adult T cell leukaemia/lymphoma).

What symptoms of Non-Hodgkins's lymphoma merit urgent referral to an oncologist?

Symptoms of non-Hodgkin lymphoma needing urgent referral include (Lancet 2003; 362:139–46):

- lymphadenopathy (>1 cm persisting for 6 weeks)
- hepatosplenomegaly
- three or more of the following symptoms:

- Fatigue
- Night sweats
- Weight loss
- Itching
- Breathlessness
- Bruising
- Recurrent infection
- Bone pain.

What are the risk factors in localized Hodgkins' lymphoma?

European Organisation for the Research Treatment of Cancer risk factors in localized disease (Lancet 2003; 361:943–51):

- *Favourable*: patients must have all features:
  - Clinical stage 1 and 2
  - Maximum of three nodal areas involved
  - Age younger than 50 years
  - ESR <50 mm/h without B symptoms or ESR <30 mm/h with B symptoms
  - Mediastinal/thoracic ratio <0.35
- *Unfavourable*: patients have any features:
  - Clinical stage 2 with involvement of at least four nodal areas
  - Age >50 years
  - ESR >50 mm/h if asymptomatic or ESR >30 mm/h if B symptoms
  - Mediastinal/thoracic ratio >0.35.

What are the poor prognostic factors of advanced Hodgkin's lymphoma?

Hasenclever index is an international prognostic score including the following seven factors:

- Age >45 years
- Male sex
- Serum albumin <40 g/l
- Haemoglobin concentration <105 g/l
- Stage IV disease
- Leukocytosis (white cell count greater than or equal to 15_109/l
- Lymphopenia (<0.6 × 10^9/l or <8% of the total white-cell count).

These factors individually reduced predicted 5-year freedom from progression rate by around 8% (Lancet 2003; 361:943–51).

What are the late effects of Hodgkin's lymphoma and its treatment?

- Second malignancies
- Cardiac disease
- Endocrine dysfunction
- Psychological trauma
- Lung damage (usually subclinical)
- Hyposplenism (after splenectomy or splenic irradiation)
- Dental caries.

(See Lancet 2003; 361:943–51.)

What are the investigations done before initiation of treatment on non-Hodgkins's lymphoma?

Essential procedures (Lancet 2003; 362:139–46):

- A full history, recording growth rate, symptoms present, performance status

- A detailed physical examination, with special attention to all node-bearing areas including Waldeyer's ring
- Adequate surgical biopsy specimen, allowing immunophenotyping and examined by a skilled pathologist
- Laboratory procedures:
  - FBC, including ESR
  - Serum lactate dehydrogenase, calcium, uric acid, proteins and electrophoresis, alkaline phosphatase
  - Assessment of renal and liver function
- Radiological studies:
  - Chest radiograph
  - Thoracic and abdominal-pelvic CT scan.
- Bone marrow aspirate and trephine, to include molecular genetic analysis if available.

Optional procedures, depending on clinical picture:

- β_2-microglobulin
- Endoscopy, e.g. for gastric MALT lymphoma
- Plain radiographs, bone scan or MRI
- Positron electron tomography (PET)
- Head or spinal MRI for neurological symptoms
- CSF analysis in patients at risk.

Thomas Hodgkin (1798–1866), an English physician at St Thomas's Hospital, London. He was the Curator of the Pathology Museum at Guy's Hospital before this.

RLK Virchow (1821–1902), successively Professor of Pathology at Würzberg and Berlin. He also described Virchow cell (lepra cell), Virchow space (perivascular space of Virchow–Robin) and Virchow triad of the pathogenesis of thrombosis.

Dorothy Reed (1874–1964) graduated from Johns Hopkins Hospital, Baltimore, and worked successively in New York and Wisconsin.

K Sternberg (1872–1935), an Austrian pathologist who described the cells in 1898. Burkitt's lymphoma was described by Dennis Burkitt in children in West Africa who presented with a lesion in the jaw, extranodal abdominal involvement and ovarian tumours. Most patients have Epstein–Barr antibodies in the serum.

The disease was first described in China in 1937 by Kim and Szeto but became more widely known as Kimura disease after a description in 1948 by Kimura and co-workers.

---

223 CROHN'S DISEASE

INSTRUCTION

These patients have chronic diarrhoea.
Examine this patient's face (Patient 3).
Examine this patient's abdomen (Patients 1 and 2).
Comment on this patient's perianal area (Patient 4).

SALIENT FEATURES

History

- Loose stools or diarrhoea which is not usually bloody
- Abdominal discomfort or pain
- Anorexia, malaise and weight loss
- Perianal inflammation and pain (Fig. 223.1)
- Joint pains, eye complaints, skin changes.

Examination

- Mass in the right iliac fossa (Patient 1)
- Multiple fistulous openings in the right iliac fossa (Patient 2)
- Swollen lips (Patient 3)
- Multiple perianal fistulous tracts (Patient 4).

Proceed in all four patients by examining:
- The mouth for:
  - Aphthous ulcers
  - Uveitis
  - Anaemia
  - Arthropathy.
- Skin lesions (erythema nodosum, pyoderma gangrenosum)
- Liver disease.

Remember: Crohn's disease may affect any part of the GI tract from the mouth to the anus but has a tendency to involve the terminal ileum. The inflammation is transmural (extending through all layers of bowel) with relatively normal bowel in between (skip lesions).

DIAGNOSIS

Patients 2 and 4 have multiple anal fistulae (lesions) caused by Crohn's disease (aetiology), indicating that the disease is active (functional status). Patients 1 and 3 also have Crohn's disease.

QUESTIONS

Mention some complications

- Toxic megacolon (Fig. 223.2)
- Iritis
- Arthritis

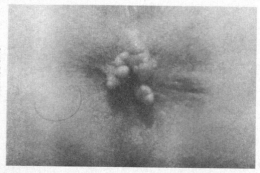

Fig. 223.1 Perianal skin tags. (With permission from Sohn et al. 2010.)

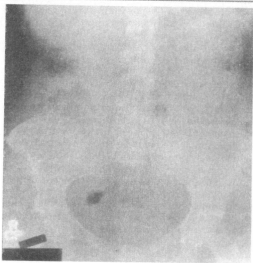

Fig. 223.2 Abdominal radiograph in toxic megacolon, showing oedematous haustral folds (thumbprinting) and a dilated transverse colon. (With permission from Marrero et al. 2008.)

- Erythema nodosum
- Pyoderma gangrenosum.

Mention some associated diseases
- Ankylosing spondylitis (HLA-B27 positive)
- Sacroiliitis
- Cholangitis, hepatitis, cirrhosis.

ADVANCED-LEVEL QUESTIONS

Mention some ocular features of Crohn's disease
Eye lesions are seen in about 5% of cases:
- Common: conjunctivitis, anterior uveitis
- Rare: scleritis, keratitis, keratoconjunctivitis sicca, choroiditis, retinal vasculitis, optic neuritis and orbital pseudotumour.

How would you investigate a patient with Crohn's disease?
- FBC, ESR, C-reactive protein, liver function tests, serum iron, vitamin B_{12}, red cell folate
- Sigmoidoscopy and rectal biopsy
- Small bowel enema
- Capsule endoscopy to determine extent of small bowel involvement
- Barium enema (rarely used): 'Cobblestone' pattern, 'rose-thorn' ulcers, colon strictures with rectal sparing
- Colonscopy to determine extent of disease (preferred to barium enema)
- MRI of pelvis to determine pelvic involvement and fistulae
- MRI of small bowel to determine disease activity and strictures.

How would you treat Crohn's disease?
- Sulfasalazine or rectal steroids for colonic disease
- Oral steroids for small bowel disease
- Metronidazole for perianal disease and fistulae

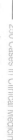

- 6-Mercaptopurine and azathioprine may be useful in severe cases
- Tumour necrosis factor-α inhibitors such as adalimumab and infliximab. A recent study reported that infliximab plus azathioprine or infliximab monotherapy was more likely to result in corticosteroid-free clinical remission than azathioprine monotherapy (N Eng J Med 2010;362:1383–95)
- Surgery is reserved for intestinal fistulae and intestinal obstruction that does not respond to medical management. Proctocolectomy and ileostomy is the standard operation. (**Note**: Ileorectal anastomosis or ileoanal anastomosis should be avoided in Crohn's disease.)
- Empirical clinical experience suggests that antibiotics are useful in the treatment of subgroups of patients. Metronidazole can be effective in those who have perianal fistulae. Ciprofloxacin and clarithromycin have been advocated as alternatives to metronidazole. The effectiveness of non-specific antibiotics and experimental evidence of the central role of the luminal flora for the development of disease has led to the use of probiotic bacteria (the administration of 'healthy' bacteria). Patients with pouchitis or active Crohn's disease who were treated with a mixture of commensal bacteria had a positive therapeutic response. Local treatment with interleukin-10-secreting *Lactococcus lactis* is undergoing clinical evaluation.

What is the role of macroautophagy in this disease?

In Crohn's disease, there is an inability to eliminate intestinal bacteria by macroautophagy. The defect may be the primary cause of *ATG16L1*-associated Crohn's disease. Defective autophagy-related protein 16-1 in Paneth cells and reduced lysozyme in the intestinal lumen results in an increase in intestinal inflammation.

Macroautophagy is accompanied by the formation of double-membrane cytosolic vesicles (autophagosomes) that sequester cytoplasmic contents and deliver them to the lysosome for subsequent degradation. The process involves membrane expansion, which allows sequestration of particles of almost any size. The ability to remove invasive bacteria is probably an important role for these epithelial and immune cells that encounter a heavy microbial load (N Engl J Med 2009;360:1785).

Burrill Bernard Crohn (1884–1983) was a physician in Mount Sinai Hospital, New York; he described the condition in 1932 and pointed out the non-tuberculous aetiology (Crohn BB, Ginzburg L, Oppenheimer GD. Regional ileitis: a pathologic and clinical entity. JAMA 1932;99:1323–9).

Anne Ferguson, formerly Professor of Gastroenterology at the Western General Hospital in Edinburgh, whose chief interest was inflammatory bowel disease. Sir Richard Thompson, President of Royal College of Physicians of London trained in natural sciences and medicine at Oxford and St Thomas' Hospital Medical School. His chief interest was nutritional gastroenterology.

---

224 DYSPHAGIA

INSTRUCTION

This patient has difficulty in swallowing; would you like to ask her a few questions and examine her?

SALIENT FEATURES

History

- Ask about the following:
  - The duration of symptoms: progressive dysphagia over months or weeks suggests the presence of organic narrowing (carcinoma esophagus, stricture from ongoing reflux esophagitis)
  - Whether the difficulty is in swallowing liquids or solids, or both. (liquids first then motility disorder, solids first then suspect oesophageal stricture)
  - Nasal regurgitation
  - Whether or not the patient coughs on swallowing
  - Is it difficult to make the swallowing movement (bulbar palsy)
  - Is the swallowing painful: odynophagia (oesophageal ulcer, spasm or cancer)
  - Is it intermittent (spasm of oesophagus)?
  - The level at which the food sticks (suprasternal notch or midsternal)
  - Does the neck distend or gurgle on swallowing (pharyngeal pouch)?
  - Associated heart burn
  - Weight loss.

Examination

- Examine:
  - Mouth for ulcers, thrush and pallor
  - For the gag reflex
  - Neck for lymph glands and goitres
  - For scleroderma
- for an underlying neurological deficit (evidence of stroke, motor neuron disease, myasthenia gravis).

DIAGNOSIS

This patient with dysphagia is recovering from a stroke (aetiology) and his functional status is best determined by videofluoroscopy and assessment by a speech therapist.

QUESTIONS

Mention a few causes of dysphagia

- Benign oesophageal stricture: occurring in reflux and producing slowly progressive dysphagia for solids in the absence of anorexia and weight loss
- Schatzki's ring (Fig. 224.1B): narrowing of the lower part of the oesophagus by a ring of mucosal or muscular tissue; it produces either intermittent, non-progressive dysphagia for solids or acute food impaction in the absence of anorexia or weight loss
- Carcinoma of the oesophagus (Fig. 224.1C): producing rapidly progressive dysphagia for solids in association with both anorexia and weight loss
- Peptic ulcer of the oesophagus
- Achalasia cardia
- Pharyngeal pouch
- Retrosternal goitre, bulbar palsy, myasthenia gravis, Plummer–Vinson syndrome (Paterson–Kelly syndrome).

250 Cases in Clinical Medicine

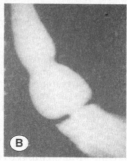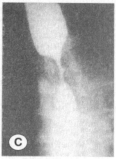

Fig. 224.1 Barium oesophagograms in dysphagia for solids. (A) Peptic stricture. (B) Schatzki's ring. (C) Malignant stricture. (With permission from Feldman M, Shiller R 1997.)

Remember: Oesophgeal dysphagia results from either mechanical narrowing or a motor disorder affecting normal peristalsis.

How would you investigate such a patient?

● FBC, ESR
● Barium swallow and video fluoroscopy (Fig. 224.1)
● Gastroscopy.

What do you understand by the term presbyoesophagus?

It is a condition that occurs in the elderly, characterized by impaired motor function of the oesophagus.

HS Plummer and PP Vinson, both physicians at the Mayo Clinic, Rochester, Minnesota.
DR Paterson and A Brown Kelly, both British ENT surgeons.

225 DIARRHOEA

PATIENT 1

INSTRUCTION

This patient has diarrhoea; would you like to ask him a few questions?

SALIENT FEATURES

History

● Ask about the following:
  • Onset
  • Duration of diarrhoea
  • Frequency
  • Whether or not it is nocturnal

- Blood (seen in ulcerative colitis, shigellosis, diverticulitis, carcinoma of the colon) and mucus in the stools; blood on the toilet paper
- Nature of the stools (pale and bulky and difficult to flush away in steatorrhoea)
- Associated pain in the abdomen
- Appetite (increased in thyrotoxicosis)
- Weight loss (marked in chronic diarrhoea)
- Associated nausea and vomiting
- Drug ingestion (including antibiotics and laxatives)
- Foreign travel.

PATIENT 2

INSTRUCTION

This patient has diarrhoea, would you like to examine her?

SALIENT FEATURES

Examination

- Look for the following signs:
  - Anaemia
  - Clubbing
  - Aphthous ulcers
  - Abdominal tenderness, abdominal masses.
- Tell the examiner that you would like to do a rectal examination and check for faecal occult blood.

DIAGNOSIS

This patient has chronic diarrhoea with aphthous ulcers and abdominal tenderness indicating that she has inflammatory bowel disease (aetiology).

QUESTIONS

What do you understand by the term diarrhoea?
It implies passing of increased amounts of loose stool (stool weights >250 g/day).

How would you investigate a patient with diarrhoea?
- FBC, ESR
- Serum albumin
- Sigmoidoscopy
- Stool chart, stool cultures, faecal cultures
- Barium enema, small bowel barium studies.

ADVANCED-LEVEL QUESTIONS

What are the mechanisms of diarrhoea?
- Osmotic diarrhoea: the mucosa of the gut acts as a semipermeable membrane; the diarrhoea stops when the patient fasts (e.g. diarrhoea from magnesium sulfate, lactulose, malabsorptive states)
- Secretory diarrhoea: there is active secretion of intestinal fluid (e.g. *Escherichia coli* diarrhoea)

250 Cases in Clinical Medicine

- Inflammatory diarrhoea: there is mucosal damage (e.g. shigellosis, ulcerative colitis)
- Increased gut motility (e.g. irritable bowel syndrome).

What are the poor prognostic factors in ulcerative colitis?
Anaemia (haemoglobin <100 g/l), raised ESR (30 mm/h), fever (37.5°C), increased frequency of stools (>6/day), tachycardia (>90 beats/min) and hypoalbuminaemia (<30 g/l).

226 MARFAN'S SYNDROME

INSTRUCTION

Look at this patient.
Examine this patient's heart.

SALIENT FEATURES

History

- Family history.

Examination

- Disproportionately long limbs compared with the trunk: the arm span will exceed the height.

Proceed by examining:

- hands for hypermobile joints and spidery fingers or arachnodactyly; confirmed by:
  - *thumb sign (Steinberg test; Fig. 226.1):* asking the patient to clench his thumb in his fist; the thumb should not exceed beyond the ulnar side of the hand in normal subjects but because of hypermobility and laxity of the joint in Marfan's disease the entire thumbnail projects beyond the border of the hand
  - *wrist sign (Walker–Murdoch sign; Fig. 226.2):* when the wrist is grasped by the contralateral hand, the thumb overlaps the terminal phalanx of the fifth digit by at least 1 cm in 80% of patients (Arch Intern Med 1970;126:276).
- eyes, for iridodonesis or ectopia lentis (subluxation upwards): the patient may be wearing thick spectacles; blue sclera
- head, for long-headedness: dolichocephalic with bossing of frontal eminences and prominent supraorbital ridges
- palate for high arched palate
- skin for small papules in the neck (*Miescher's elastoma*)
- chest for pectus excavatum, cystic lung disease (Thorax 1984;39: 780–4)
- heart for mitral valve prolapse, aortic aneurysm and aortic regurgitation
- spine for scoliosis and kyphosis.

Remember: Every patient should be referred for ophthalmic examination, annual echocardiography and genetic counselling to maximize the preventive potential in this disease.

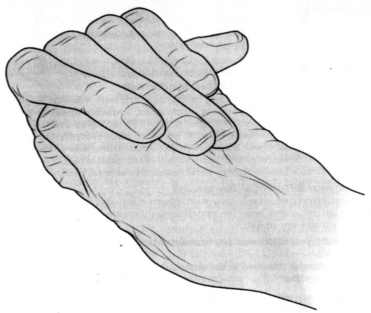

Fig. 226.1 Steinberg test or thumb sign.

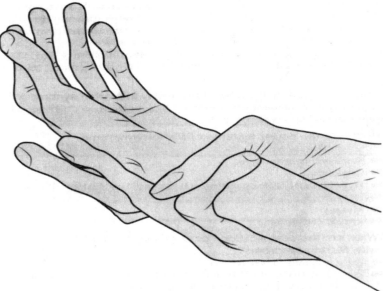

Fig. 226.2 The Walker Murdoch test or wrist sign.

DIAGNOSIS

This patient has Marfan syndrome and aortic regurgitation (lesion) and is limited by cardiac failure (functional status).

QUESTIONS

What are the criteria for Marfan syndrome?

- People with no family history require, apart from skeletal features (including pectus carinatum or excavatum, reduced upper-to-lower segment ratio, arm-span-to-height ratio >1.05, scoliosis and reduced elbow extension), involvement of at least two other systems and one of the major criteria (these include ectopia lentis, dilatation of the aortic root or aortic dissection and lumbosacral dural ectasia by CT or MRI).
- Patients with a family history need features in at least two systems.

What is your differential diagnosis?

Homocystinuria (recessively inherited inborn error of amino acid metabolism caused by a deficiency of cystathionine β-synthetase) in which the skeletal features are similar.

How would you differentiate homocystinuria and Marfan syndrome?

In homocystinuria, the lens is dislocated downwards and there is homocystine in the urine.

ADVANCED-LEVEL QUESTIONS

Why do these patients need annual echocardiography?

To monitor aortic diameter and mitral valve function. Prophylactic replacement of the aortic root with a composite graft when the diameter reaches 50–55 mm (normal <40 mm) prolongs life. Untreated patients commonly die in the fourth or fifth decade from dissection of the aorta or from cardiac failure caused by aortic regurgitation. Chronic beta-blockade to produce a negative inotropic effect retards the rate of aortic dilatation (N Engl J Med 1994;330:1335–41). Also, patients should be advised regarding infective endocarditis prophylaxis.

What is the common cause of mortality in Marfan syndrome?

Cardiovascular complications cause 95% of deaths in such patients and reduce mean life expectancy by 40%.

What are the ocular features of Marfan syndrome?

- Subluxation of lens
- Small and spherical lens
- Glaucoma
- Hypoplasia of dilator pupillae, making pupillary dilatation difficult
- Flat cornea
- Myopia
- Retinal detachment.

What are the complications of pregnancy in women with Marfan syndrome?

- Early premature abortion
- Risk of maternal death from aortic dissection. Pregnancy is not dangerous when the aortic diameter is <40 mm.

Is there a gene implicated in Marfan syndrome?

Marfan syndrome appears to be caused by mutations in a single gene *FBN1* on chromosome 15 and encoding fibrillin (N Engl J Med 1992;326:905, Genomics 1993;17:468–75). Fibrillin is a glycoprotein produced by fibroblasts that aggregates alone or with other proteins in the extracellular matrix to form microfibrillary fibres on which elastin can be deposited. These fibres are particularly abundant in the ciliary zonules that support the lens, in ligaments and in the aorta. Dilatation of the aorta occurs as a result of cystic medionecrosis.

One study has suggested that the angiotensin II type 1 receptor antagonist losartan antagonizes the action of transforming growth factor-β in preventing aortic dilatation in mice with mutant fibrillin-1. Therapy for 6 months stopped progression of aortic dilatation and elastin fragmentation in the aortic wall, a histologic hallmark of Marfan syndrome. A beta-blocker, currently the therapy of choice for Marfan syndrome, was also effective but not as effective as losartan. In a small cohort study ($n = 18$), the use of an angiotensin II receptor antagonist in patients with Marfan syndrome significantly slowed the rate of progressive aortic root dilation (N Engl J Med 2008;358:2787). Another small study reported that perindopril reduced both aortic stiffness and aortic root diameter in patients with Marfan syndrome (JAMA 2007;298:1539–47). The US National Institutes of Health is sponsoring a clinical trial that will compare losartan with beta-blocker therapy in children and young adults with Marfan syndrome and aortic aneurysm.

American President Abraham Lincoln is suspected to have had Marfan syndrome.

B-J Antoine Marfan (1858–1942), a French paediatrician, wrote his paper in 1896. He was appointed Foundation Professor of Hygiene at the Clinic of Infantile Diseases in Paris in 1914. He was elected honorary fellow of the Royal Society of Medicine, UK in 1934.

Victor McKusick, contemporary Professor of Medicine at Johns Hopkins Hospital, Baltimore, whose chief interest is genetics.

---

227 NEPHROTIC SYNDROME

INSTRUCTION

Look at this patient.

SALIENT FEATURES

History

- History of diabetes (N Engl J Med 1998;338:1202–11)
- Hypertension
- History of acute glomerulonephritis, streptococcal sore throat
- Medications: NSAIDs, captopril, street heroin, gold, pencillamine, lithium, chlorpropamide, rifampin, tolbutamide
- History of SLE, vasculitides, amyloidosis
- Neoplasms: Hodgkin's and other lymphoma, solid tumours

- Familial history: sickle cell disease, partial lipodystrophy (p. 611), Alports syndrome
- Parasites: malaria, toxoplasmosis, schistosomiasis.

Examination

- Generalized oedema: puffiness of face, pitting oedema of legs and hands
- Look at the nails for ridges of hypoproteinaemia
- Comment on the pallor
- Tell the examiner that you would like to examine:
  - the abdomen for ascites
  - the urine for protein and sugar.

Note: Urine microscopy may show oval fat bodies, which consist of degenerating tubular epithelial cells having cholesteryl esters; these appear as 'grape clusters' with light microscopy and have a 'Maltese-cross' appearance under polarized light.

DIAGNOSIS

This patient has nephrotic syndrome (lesion) caused by diabetes mellitus (aetiology), and has developed gross anasarca indicating hypoalbuminaemia and marked urinary protein loss (functional status).

QUESTIONS

What do you understand by the term nephrotic syndrome?

It consists of albuminuria (>3.5 g/day) and hypoalbuminaemia accompanied by generalized oedema, hyperlipidaemia (caused by increased hepatic production) and lipiduria.

What causes this syndrome?

- Glomerular disease: minimal change glomerulonephritis, membranous glomerulonephritis, proliferative glomerulonephritis.
- Systemic disease: diabetes mellitus, SLE, amyloidosis, drugs (captopril, gold, penicillamine, street heroin), Hodgkin's disease, syphilis, malaria, HIV, cancer, hepatitis B, multiple myeloma, renal primary (AL) amyloidosis.

How would you investigate these patients?

- Creatinine clearance, 24-hour urinary protein, urine electrophoresis
- FBC, ESR
- Urea and electrolytes, serum creatinine, albumin
- Serum cholesterol (dyslipidaemia is caused by both overproduction and impaired catabolism of apolipoprotein B-containing lipoproteins)
- DNA antibody, anti-nuclear factor, complement levels
- Renal biopsy.

What complications may such a patient suffer?

- Thromboembolic events, including renal vein thrombosis and deep vein thrombosis (caused by loss of antithrombin III and other proteins involved in the coagulation and fibrinolytic cascade)
- Protein malnutrition
- Acclerated atherosclerosis
- Infection.

ADVANCED-LEVEL QUESTIONS

What is orthostatic proteinuria?

It is usually seen in adolescents and occurs when standing and resolves on lying down. The long-term prognosis is good.

What do you know about Tamm–Horsfall protein in the urine?

Normal individuals excrete <150 mg/day protein. Of this, about 5–15 mg is albumin and the remainder consists of different plasma proteins and glycoproteins derived from renal cells. Tamm–Horsfall mucoprotein is the most abundant protein that is not derived from plasma but from the cells of the ascending limb of the loop of Henle; it is excreted at the rate of 50–75 mg/day. Pathological proteinuria occurs when daily excretion exceeds 150 mg protein.

What is the treatment of patients with nephrotic syndrome?

- Diuresis: furosemide (acts in the ascending thick loop of Henle) with thiazides (reduce sodium absorption in the distal nephron) and potassium-sparing diuretics
- Prevention of thromboemboli: heparin, anticoagulants and support stockings when patients have nephrotic proteinuria, an albumin level <20 g/l or both
- Infusion of hyperoncotic albumin should only be tried if symptomatic hypovolaemia is present
- Plasma ultrafiltration in severe cases
- Renal ablation by bilateral nephrectomy or embolization of the renal artery may be indicated to avoid serious risks of severe hypoproteinaemia and hypovolaemia
- Pneumococcal vaccine
- ACE inhibitors or angiotensin receptor blockers is indicated even in normotensive patients to reduce proteinuria
- Colchine in familial Mediterranean fever
- Interferon-alfa in hepatitis B-associated nephrotic syndrome, hepatitis-C associated membranoproliferative glomerulonephritis and cryoglobulinaemia
- Prednisone, 8-week course, in minimal change nephropathy.

Nephrotic syndrome was clearly described by R Bright (1789–1858), an English physician. He qualified from Edinburgh and worked at Guy's Hospital, London. Chronic nephritis is known as Bright's disease. Three of his renal specimens are still preserved at Guy's Hospital.

I Tamm, scientist, Rockefeller University, New York.

FL Horsfall, Professor of Microbiology, Sloan Kettering Institute and Cornell University, New York.

---

228 URAEMIA

INSTRUCTION

Would you like to ask this uraemic patient some questions and perform a relevant examination?

SALIENT FEATURES

History

- Loss of appetite, anorexia, nausea, vomiting and hiccups
- Fatigue, malaise, loss of energy
- Polyuria, nocturia, dysuria, haematuria, difficulty in passing urine
- Swelling of the face and feet
- Shortness of breath (from secondary left ventricular failure)
- Itching
- Restless legs (overwhelming need to frequently alter position of legs)
- Paraesthesia from either hypocalcaemia (associated tetany) or peripheral neuropathy
- Bone pain (from metabolic bone disease)
- Drug history, in particular NSAIDs, tetracycline
- History of diabetes, hypertension, recurrent urinary tract infections
- Family history of renal disease, in particular polycystic kidneys
- Tell the examiner that you would like to take a history for impotence in men and ameonorrhoea in women.

Examination

- Pallor (from anaemia)
- Comment on short stature (indicates uraemia from childhood)
- Examine the nails (for Lindsay's 'half-and-half' nails where the proximal portion is whitish while the distal portion is brownish red; the lunula is usually obscured)
- Comment on the lemon tinge of the skin, the pallor and scratch marks. Rarely, there may be 'uraemic frost': increased photosensitive skin pigmentation
- Examine the arms for asterixis (flapping tremor), haemodialysis fistula
- Comment on the vascular shunts, if any
- Comment on hyperventilation of Kussmaul's respiration secondary to metabolic acidosis
- Examine the abdomen for palpable kidneys (hydronephrosis, polycystic kidneys) and palpable bladder
- Check for pitting leg oedema
- Tell the examiner that you would like to proceed as follows:
  - Check the BP (hypertension, hypotension)
  - Look for pericardial friction rub
  - Look for evidence of peripheral neuropathy (glove and stocking sensory loss)
  - Do a rectal and vaginal examination if urinary obstruction is suspected
  - Examine the urine for sugar, albumin, specific gravity, microscopy
  - Examine the retina in diabetics.

DIAGNOSIS

This patient has chronic renal failure (aetiology) caused by diabetes mellitus (aetiology), and is currently requiring dialysis, as evidenced by the arteriovenous fistula in the arm (functional status). Be prepared to determine which stage of chronic kidney disease the patient is at if asked (see below).

QUESTIONS

How would you investigate a patient with renal failure?

- Urine: glucose, microscopy, specific gravity, creatinine clearance, 24-hour urinary protein, urine electrophoresis
- Blood: FBC, ESR
- Serum: urea, electrolytes, creatinine, protein, calcium phosphate, uric acid
- Ultrasonography of the abdomen for kidneys, bladder
- Special investigations: pyelography, protein electrophoresis, complement components, autoantibody screening, serum cryoglobulins, kidney biopsy.

What do you understand by the term azotaemia?

Azotaemia indicates a raised level of urea and creatinine without symptoms (glomerular filtration rate (GFR) about 20–35% of normal).

What do you understand by the term uraemia?

Uraemia implies a deterioration of renal function associated with symptoms (GFR <20% of normal).

Note: Chronic renal insufficiency is defined by a serum creatinine concentration of 15–30 mg/l (133–265 μmol/l); chronic renal failure is >30 mg/l.

What is the classification of chronic kidney disease?

Chronic kidney disease (CKD) is classified based on clinical parameters and the GFR.

Stage	Description	Estimated GFR (ml/min per 1.73m²)
1	Normal or increased GFR, with other evidence of kidney damage	≥90
2	Slight decrease in GFR, with other evidence of kidney damage	60–89
3	Moderate decrease in GFR, with or without other evidence of kidney damage	30–59
4	Severe decrease in GFR, with or without other evidence of kidney damage	15–29
5	Established in renal failure	<15

What are the common causes of chronic renal failure?

Glomerulonephritis
Diabetes mellitus
Hypertensive nephropathy
Pyelonephritis
Polycystic kidney disease
Analgesic nephropathy.

ADVANCED-LEVEL QUESTIONS

Mention a few drugs that you would avoid in renal failure

Aminoglycosides, furosemide with cephalosporins, potassium salts, tetracycline.

What are the consequences of renal failure?

- Metabolic: sodium imbalance, hyperkalaemia, metabolic acidosis, hyperuricaemia, hypocalcaemia, hypermagnesaemia, hyperphosphataemia
- Cardiovascular: left ventricular hypertrophy (LVH), cardiac failure, hypertension, accelerated atherosclerosis, pericarditis. (Pericarditis is either uraemic pericarditis or dialysis pericarditis.) LVH in large part results from hypertension, expansion of extracellular volume and anaemia. The LVH may be accompanied by left ventricular remodelling and fibrosis, and these changes, with or without coronary artery disease, may lead to cardiac failure, myocardial infarction or sudden death
- Haematological: anaemia, clotting disorders, leukocyte abnormalities
- Skin: itching, hyperpigmentation, bruising
- Nervous system: encephalopathy, peripheral neuropathy, autonomic neuropathy
- GI: anorexia, nausea, vomiting, peptic ulcer, diarrhoea, constipation (particularly in patients on continuous ambulatory peritoneal dialysis
- Endocrine: vitamin D disorders, secondary hyperparathyroidism, impotence, amenorrhoea, glucose intolerance.

What are the mechanisms underlying the progression from early-stage to advanced chronic kidney disease?

- Progressive glomerulosclerosis and interstitial fibrosis result in the progression from early CKD to advanced CKD.
- Loss of renal mass results in haemodynamic adaptations, activation of the renin–angiotensin–aldosterone system, systemic hypertension, proteinuria and hyperlipidaemia.
- These adaptations result in increased inflammation and oxidative stress, with upregulation of proinflammatory cytokines and growth factors, their receptors, or both; the increased inflammation and oxidative stress stimulate cell hypertrophy and proliferation and inflammatory-cell infiltration.
- Some of these early adaptations (such as haemodynamic and hypertrophic responses) become maladaptive and eventually contribute to the structural and functional changes in the kidney that are characteristic of advanced CKD.

What is the management of stage 4 chronic kidney disease?

- Therapy with an angiotensin receptor blocker or an ACE inhibitor, with the medication adjusted to achieve a BP below 130/80 mmHg (reduction of BP to this level slows the rate of decline in GFR even in patients with advanced CKD). A thiazide diuretic should be replaced by a loop diuretic; if the targeted BP is not reached, a beta-blocker, a calcium channel blocker, or both should be added
- Dietary protein should be limited to approximately 0.8 to 1.0 g per kilogram/day
- Treatment of hyperlipidaemia with a statin and aspirin therapy to reduce the likelihood of cardiovascular disease
- Tobacco cessation
- Anaemia: target haemoglobin concentration of 110–120 g/l. Iron deficiency should be assessed and treated
- Serum phosphate levels should be monitored; if >46 mg/l (1.5 mmol/l) a phosphate binder should be added to the therapeutic regimen

- Low-dose active vitamin D analogue will help to control secondary hyperparathyroidism
- Serum bicarbonate <20 mmol/l and systemic acidaemia should be treated with sodium bicarbonate
- Patients should be educated about methods of renal replacement therapy, and efforts should be made to preserve the venous circulation in the upper extremities in order to maintain vascular access in those patients who opt for haemodialysis.

When would you consider dialysis?
- Hyperkalaemia (potassium concentration >7 mmol/l)
- Bicarbonate concentration <12 mmol/l
- Urea level greater than 20 mmol/l
- Creatinine concentration greater than 500μmol/l.

Patients must be referred for dialysis before the above features are present because those managed close to or at end-stage renal failure have a much poorer prognosis than those managed for at least 3 months before needing dialysis or transplantation (Am J Kid Dis 1995;25:276–80, Nephrol Dial Transplant 1998;13:246–50).

What is the best measure of efficiency of dialysis?
Efficiency of dialysis is best measured by blood urea nitrogen (BUN). Serum creatinine is a poor measure of dialysis efficacy. Each treatment is adjusted to achieve a urea reduction ratio (URR) of at least 65%, with most treatments lasting 3–4 h.

What are the bone changes in chronic renal failure?
- Osteomalacia (renal rickets)
- Osteitis fibrosa cystica (secondary hyperparathyroidism): subperiosteal erosions, especially of the skull (pepperpot skull), phalanges, long bones and distal end of clavicles
- Osteosclerosis: enhanced density of the bone in the upper and lower margins of vertebrae (rugger-jersey spine).

Is there any benefit in restricting dietary protein in chronic renal disease?
A large randomized controlled trial suggested no benefit from protein restriction.

How are the beneficial effects of angiotensin converting enzyme inhibitors in renal disease produced?
They probably result from a combination of antihypertensive effect and antiproteinuric effect (Ann Intern Med 1 97;127:337). A randomized multicentre trial demonstrated that ACE inhibitors lead to less renal failure than other antihypertensive in renal disease (N Engl J Med 1998;334:939–45).

What criteria are used to assess acute renal failure?
- **The RIFLE criteria** Based on GFR or urine output or both plus urine output on a body weight basis:

Risk: serum creatinine increase 150%, GFR decrease <25%, urine output <0.5 ml/h per kg over 6 h

Injury: serum creatinine 200%, GFR decrease <50%, urine output <0.5 ml/h per kg over 12 h

Failure: serum creatinine 300%, GFR decrease <75%, urine output <0.3 ml/h per kg over 24 h or anuria for 12 h

Loss: complete loss for >4 weeks
End-stage renal disease: complete loss >12 weeks

- **The AKIN criteria** The Acute Kidney Injury Network (AKIN) modifies the RIFLE scheme to exclude GFR:
  - I: serum creatinine increase $\geq 150\%$ (>3.0 mg/l)
  - II: serum creatinine increase $\geq 200\%$
  - III: serum creatinine increase >300% or >40 mg/l in the setting of an increase of ≥ 50 mg/l.

I is equivalent to risk, II to injury and III to failure on the RIFLE scale.

What is Bricker's trade-off hypothesis?
Early in the course of renal failure, the kidney fails to excrete phosphorus, causing a rise in body levels. To normalize the rise in serum phosphorus and calcium, parathyroid hormone is released, which leads to bone disease (osteitis fibrosa cystica). This is the basis for secondary hyperparathyroidism in renal failure.

What is the intact-nephron hypothesis?
There is increased solute excretion per nephron particularly when there is depletion of extracellular fluid resulting in impaired ability of the kidney to concentrate urine. Because nephrons are functioning at maximum capacity, the ability to adjust to low and high intake of sodium, water, potassium and other dietary solutes is impaired.

PG Lindsay, an American physician.
  Neil S Bricker, a US nephrologist.

---

229 PAGET'S DISEASE

INSTRUCTION

Examine this patient's face.
Examine this patient's legs.

SALIENT FEATURES

History

- Ask the patient whether there is an increase in hat size
- Bone pain
- Joint pain (from osteoarthritis secondary to bone disease)
- Painless bowing of the bone can be the first symptom
- Hearing loss
- Fractures with minimal trauma
- Nerve entrapment syndromes including paraparesis and radioculopathy when the spine is affected.

Examination

- *Face*:
  - Comment on the hearing aid, if any; test hearing and determine whether the deafness is a conduction defect (from involvement of the ossicle) or neural (from compression of the eighth nerve)

- Typical appearance of the skull and increased skull diameter (>55 cm is abnormal)
- Tell the examiner that you would like to examine the fundus for optic atrophy or angioid streaks.
- *Neck*:
  - Look for platybasia
  - Raised JVP (cardiac failure in Paget's disease is caused by hyperdynamic circulation).
- *Spine*:
  - Deformity of the spine: kyphosis
  - Auscultate over the vertebral bodies for bruits
  - In up to one-third of patients the third and fourth lumbar vertebrae are involved, and in 20% the lower thoracic vertebrae are involved.
- *Legs*:
  - Comment on the anterior bowing of the tibia (Fig. 229.1D) and the lateral bowing of the femur
  - Feel the bone for warmth
  - Tell the examiner that you would like to examine the joints for osteoarthritis (limitation of hip movement, in particular abduction, and fixed flexion deformity of the knees).
- Proceed by tell the examiner that you would like to:
  - Do a urine analysis (high incidence of renal stones)
  - Measure the patient's height (for serial follow-up)
  - Compare the patient's appearance with a previous photograph
  - Ask the patient whether there is an increase in hat size.

Remember: Paget's disease is a remodelling disease of isolated areas of the skeleton.

DIAGNOSIS

This patient has Paget's disease (lesion) with hyperdynamic cardiac failure and sensorineural deafness (functional status).

QUESTIONS

What are complications of Paget's disease?
- Diminished mobility
- Fractures
- Basilar invagination can lead to a *'Tam O'Shanter'* deformity
- Cord compression from basilar invagination
- Narrowing of basal foramina, producing cranial nerve lesions, especially deafness, and occasionally compression of the medulla oblongata or upper spinal cord
- Root lesions as a result of vertebral damage
- Hypercalcaemia
- High-output cardiac failure
- Sarcomatous changes are seen in <2% of patients.

ADVANCED-LEVEL QUESTIONS

Mention the neurological complications of Paget's disease
- Headache
- Fits
- Platybasia

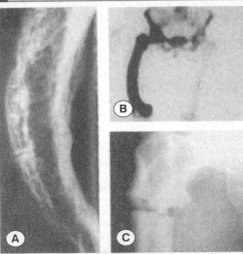

Fig. 229.1 (A) Radiograph of tibia, showing bone deformity, expansion and alternating areas of osteosclerosis and osteolysis with a pseudofracture on the convex aspect of the tibia. (B) Radionuclide scan showing increased tracer uptake in affected femur. (C) Pathological fracture through affected femur. (D) Severe tibia deformity. (With permission from Ralston et al. 2008.)

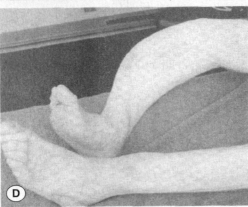

- Hydrocephalus
- Cerebellar signs
- Cranial nerve palsies
- Cord compression.

What are the mechanisms of hearing loss in such patients?
- It is usually caused by the disease process involving the ossicles
- Less commonly it is caused by the progressive closure of the skull foramina compressing the eighth cranial nerve.

What is the basic defect in bone metabolism?
Increased osteoclastic activity resulting in bone resorption and increased osteoblastic activity.

What are the radiological manifestations of this disease?

- Skull: 'honeycomb' appearance with underlying osteoporosis circumscripta, 'cottonwool' appearance
- Pelvis: thickening of the iliopectineal line 'brim-sign', enlargement of ischial and pubic bones
- Long bones: increased trabeculation and localized bone enlargement
- Vertebra: sclerotic margins giving a 'picture frame' appearance.

Remember: A bone scan is more sensitive than a radiograph in determining the extent of disease.

What is the prevalence of Paget's disease?

The exact prevalence is not known but several reports indicate a 3% prevalence in those >40 years of age and this increases with age to reach a maximum of 10% by the ninth decade. Males predominate by a ratio of about 2:1.

What factors have been implicated in the aetiology of Paget's disease?

- Slow viral infection: measles syncytial virus, paramyxovirus (canine distemper)
- Genetic factors: mutations have been identified in at least four genes. The most important of these is *SQSTM1,* encoding sequestosome 1, a scaffold protein in the nuclear factor NF-κB signalling pathway. Patients with *SQSTM1* mutations have severe Paget's disease of bone and a high degree of penetrance with increasing age
- Other potential triggers include deficiency of dietary calcium and repetitive mechanical loading of the skeleton.

Note: Juvenile Paget's disease, a genetic bone disease characterized by accelerated bone turnover, results from inactivating mutations in the gene encoding osteoprotegerin (an important modulator of osteoclastogenesis). Osteoprotegerin is a member of the superfamily of tumour necrosis factor receptors (TNFRSF11B) and is a receptor activator of NF-κB RANK ligand (RANKL).

What are the biochemical features of this disease?

- Serum calcium concentration is normal (except in prolonged immobilization or malignancy).
- Increased bone serum alkaline phosphatase, indicating increased osteoblastic activity.
- Increased urinary hydroxyproline secretion, indicating increased bone resorption.

Which drugs are commonly used in the treatment of this disease?

- Bisphosphonates, which inhibit osteoclast-mediated bone resorption (aledronate)
- Calcitonins, which acts by reducing osteoclastic activity.

To which patients would you offer therapy?

Treatment is offered to patients with any of the following symptoms:

- Agonizing bone pain, headache with skull involvement, fissure fracture
- Prior to surgery such as potential hip replacement
- Severe deformity
- Hypercalcaemia
- Cardiac failure.

Sir James Paget (1814–1899), Surgeon at St Bartholomew's Hospital, London. He also described Paget's disease of the nipple (carcinoma involving the areola and the nipple), Paget's disease of the skin (skin cancer involving the apocrine glands) and Paget–Schroetter syndrome (venous thrombosis of the axillary veins, of unknown cause). (Paget J. On a form of chronic inflammation of bones (osteitis deformans). Med Chir Trans 1877;60:37).

Stuart Ralston, FRCP is Professor and holds the ARC Chair of Rheumatology at the University of Edinburgh has written extensively on Paget's disease.

230 PAROTID ENLARGEMENT

INSTRUCTION

Look at this patient's face.

SALIENT FEATURES

History

- Ask the patient whether the parotids are painful and dry mouth
- Ask the patient about dry eyes or use of artificial tears
- History of sarcoidosis
- History of lymphoma, leukaemia.

Examination

- Bilateral parotid enlargement (Fig. 230.1).
Proceed as follows:
- Look for the following conditions:
  - Dry mouth
  - Lupus pernio
  - Rheumatoid arthritis.
- Tell the examiner that you would like to know whether the patient has gritty eyes or dry mouth.

Remember: Unilateral parotid enlargement with associated facial nerve palsy is more likely to be malignant tumour of the parotids; it is very rare for facial weakness to occur with benign tumours.

DIAGNOSIS

This patient has parotid enlargement, which is painless, and has a dry mouth (lesion) probably caused by Sjögren syndrome (aetiology). The dry mouth is making swallowing difficult (functional status).

QUESTIONS

What are the causes of painless bilateral parotid enlargement?
- Sarcoidosis
- Sjögren syndrome or keratoconjunctivitis sicca
- Lymphoma and leukaemia.

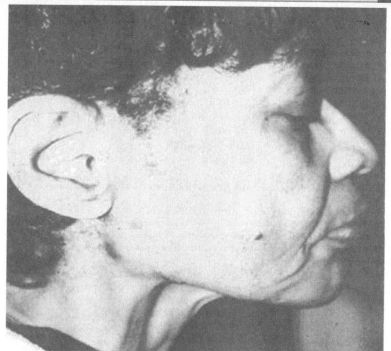

Fig. 230.1 Sjögren syndrome with moderate parotid swelling. (With permission from Firestein et al. 2008.)

How would you test objectively for dry eyes?

Schirmer's test: filter paper is hooked over the lower eyelid; in normal people at least 15 mm is wet in 5 min whereas a value of <5 mm is seen in sicca syndrome.

What do you know about keratoconjunctivitis sicca?

It is a condition characterized by decreased production of tears by lacrimal glands.

ADVANCED-LEVEL QUESTIONS

Mention a few causes of keratoconjunctivitis sicca

- Primary keratoconjunctivitis sicca is common and characterized by involvement of the lacrimal gland alone.
- Primary Sjögren syndrome is an autoimmune disorder that is usually positive for rheumatoid factor, anti-nuclear antibodies and hypergammaglobulinaemia. Less frequently, autoantibodies to DNA, salivary gland, smooth muscle and gastric parietal cells are present. There may be associated dry mouth and bronchial epithelium, and the vagina may also be affected. Histopathogically the glands show intralobar ductal epithelial hyperplasia and lymphocytic infiltration of the gland.

- Secondary Sjögren syndrome is the presence of keratoconjunctivitis sicca in association with a systemic disorder such as the following:
  - Rheumatoid arthritis
  - Psoriatic arthritis
  - Connective tissue disorder
  - Sarcoidosis
  - Crohn's disease.

How would you manage such patients?

- Artificial tears (e.g. hypromellose) are instilled frequently for dry eyes
- Artificial saliva for dry mouth.

Which are the other salivary glands?

These include submandibular, sublingual and minor salivary glands in the oral cavity, pharynx and larynx.

What do you know about superficial anatomy of the salivary gland?

The gland lies on the lateral surface of the ramus of the mandible and folds itself along the posterior mandibular border. It is usually not palpable as a discrete structure. Clenching the teeth tenses the masseter and makes the anterior border of the gland more prominent (as the gland lies just behind the masseter muscle).

How are parotid secretions carried into the oral cavity?

By Stensen's duct, which opens just opposite the upper second molar tooth.

What is Mikulicz's disease?

It is the enlargement of salivary and lacrimal glands (caused by sarcoidosis, lymphoma or TB) associated with dry mouth and dry eyes but not arthritis.

Which neoplasm may be associated with Sjögren syndrome?

Usually B cell-derived non-Hodgkin's lymphoma.

OWA Schirmer (1864–1917) a German ophthalmologist.

J von Mikulicz-Radecki (1850–1905) was successively Professor of Surgery at Könisberg and Breslau.

HSC Sjögren (1899–1986), Swedish Professor of Ophthalmology in Gothenburg.

N Stensen (1638–1686), Danish anatomist and Professor of Anatomy at Copenhagen. He was then appointed the Catholic Bishop of Titioplis in 1677 and was an international authority on geology. He described the tetralogy of Fallot before Fallot, in 1672.

---

231 SUPERIOR VENA CAVAL OBSTRUCTION

INSTRUCTION

Look at this patient.

SALIENT FEATURES

History

- Headache
- Dysphagia
- Dyspnoea
- Wheezes
- Blackouts
- Oedema of the face.

Examination

- Tortuous, visible and dilated veins on the chest wall and neck (Fig. 231.1).
- The neck veins are non-pulsatile
- The face may be plethoric and suffused. The patient may be short of breath
- Look for signs of Horner syndrome and for radiation marks
- Tell the examiner that you would like to examine for signs of bronchogenic carcinoma, i.e. clubbing, tar staining, lymph nodes and chest signs.

DIAGNOSIS

This patient has superior vena caval obstruction (lesion), which is usually caused by bronchogenic carcinoma (aetiology), and is tachypnoeic at rest (functional status).

QUESTIONS

What are the causes of superior vena caval obstruction?

- Bronchogenic carcinoma is the commonest cause (in 70%)
- Lymphoma: in young adults
- Other causes:

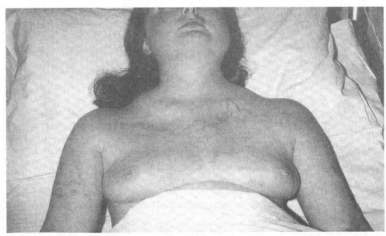

Fig. 231.1 Superior vena cava obstruction in bronchial carcinoma. Note the swelling of the face and neck and the development of collateral circulation in the veins of the chest wall. (With permission from Forbes, Jackson 2003.)

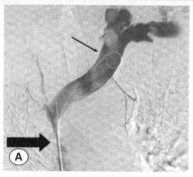
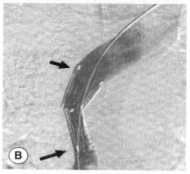

Fig. 231.2 Superior vena cava venogram. (A) Venogram made after a right femoral venous approach, with insertion of a catheter (thin arrow) into the left brachiocephalic vein; there is severe stenosis (thick arrow). (B) A double-Z stent placed in the portion of the stenotic vena cava (arrows) immediate restored normal blood flow. (With permission from Walsh 2008.)

- Aortic aneurysm
- Mediastinal goitre
- Mediastinal fibrosis (from methysergide, histoplasmosis or TB)
- Constrictive pericarditis.

How would you manage this patient?

This condition is a medical emergency and an urgent CT scan or MRI of the chest should be requested (Chest 1993;103(suppl 4):394S). Emergency treatment consists of:

- intravenous furosemide to relieve the oedematous component of vena caval compression
- intravenous anticancer chemotherapy, e.g. cyclophosphamide
- mediastinal irradiation within 24 h (the majority of the tumour types causing the superior vena cava syndrome are sensitive to radiotherapy, but tissue diagnosis is required prior to radiotherapy)
- more recently, expandable metal stents have been used to relieve the obstruction (Fig. 231.2)
- mechanical thrombectomy with an Amplatz thrombectomy device (BMJ 1994;308:1697–9).

How are the venous collaterals formed?

Blood flows through a collateral vascular network to the lower body and the inferior vena cava or the azygos vein when the superior vena cava is obstructed. It usually takes several weeks for these venous collaterals to dilate sufficiently to accommodate the blood flow. The cervical venous pressure is usually increased to 20–40 mmHg (normal range, 2–8 mmHg). The severity of the symptoms depends on the degree of narrowing of the superior vena cava and the rapidity of the onset of the narrowing.

> Obstruction of the superior vena cava was first described in 1757 by William Hunter in a case of syphilitic aortic aneurysm.

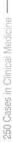

232 GLASS EYE

INSTRUCTION

Look at this patient's fundus.
Examine this patient's eyes.
Check this patient's vision or visual fields.

SALIENT FEATURES

History

- History of trauma.

Examination

- Glass eye, which is obvious
- The patient is blind on the affected side
- The light reflex is absent.

Note: Suspect malignant melanoma if asked to examine the abdomen and the liver is palpable (from metastases).

DIAGNOSIS

This patient has a glass eye (lesion) that is secondary to trauma in childhood (aetiology).

ADVANCED-LEVEL QUESTIONS

What is sympathetic ophthalmitis?

It is inflammation that attacks the sound eye after injury (usually perforating wound) to the other. It is almost always a plastic iridocyclitis; rarely it manifests as neuroretinitis or choroiditis. It never occurs after excision of an injured eye unless it has already commenced at the time of operation. Steroids have improved the prognosis if such treatment is commenced early.

What fungus can invade the globe?

Rhizopus mucormycosis, originating in the paranasal sinuses and nose, occurs predominantly in patients with poorly controlled diabetes mellitus, malignancy, organ transplantation and those who are receiving long-term desferrioxamine therapy. This fungus can invade the globe or ophthalmic artery to cause blindness.

From which tissues do ocular melanomas arise?

They arise from a variety of ocular tissues including the conjuctiva, uveal tract (iris, ciliary body and choroid), eyelid, orbit and nasolacrimal ducts. Iris melanomas rarely metastasize, whereas ciliary body and choroidal melanomas readily disseminate.

What is the histology of ocular melanomas?

Unlike cutaneous melanomas, the ocular type consists of two distinct cell types: spindle and epithelioid. Lesions composed of completely or predominantly spindle cells have low aggressiveness, do not tend to metastasize and are associated with a 75% survival rate at 15 years. Consequently, enucleation is usually avoided. The epithelioid type is associated with only a 35% survival rate despite enucleation, because of late metastases.

233 TURNER SYNDROME

INSTRUCTION

Look at this patient.

SALIENT FEATURES

Examination

- Webbing of the neck in a female patient
- Abnormal angulation of both elbows: increased carrying angle (cubitus valgus; Fig. 233.1)
- Dwarfism
- Receding chin
- Low-set ears
- Epicanthal folds, double eyelashes, strabismus occurs in 18%, and ptosis in 13%
- Low hairline over the back of the neck
- Shield-shaped chest: nipples are widely separated with microthelia
- Multiple pigmented naevi
- Short fourth metacarpal

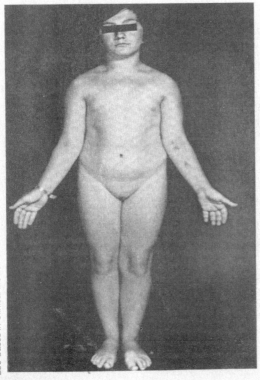

Fig. 233.1 A 15-year-old girl exhibiting failure of sexual maturation, short stature, cubitus valgus and a goitre. There is no webbing of the neck. (With permission from Kliegman et al. 2007.)

- Lymphoedema of the hands and feet
- Check for radiofemoral delay (coarctation of the aorta) and aortic stenosis.

Proceed as follows:

- Tell the examiner that you would like to:
  - examine genitalia for infantilism
  - measure serum follicle-stimulating hormone (FSH) and luteinizing hormone (LH) (these will be high, confirming primary hypogonadism)
  - check thyroid-stimulating hormone (hypothyroidism occurs in 15 to 30%)
  - order a renal ultrasound (kidney malformations, including horse-shoe kidney and duplication of the collecting system, are found in up to 40%)
  - echocardiogram: as physical examination may be inadequate to detect a bicuspid aortic valve
  - request for a formal assessment of learning disability (~70% have learning disabilities affecting non-verbal perceptual motor and visuospatial skills).

DIAGNOSIS

This patient has Turner syndrome (lesion), which is caused by the absence of one of the X chromosomes (aetiology). She has amenorrhoea and skeletal abnormalities (functional status).

QUESTIONS

What constitutes a web?
Either a fan-like fold of skin extending from the shoulder to the neck or an abnormal splaying out of the trapezius.

ADVANCED-LEVEL QUESTIONS

Which other cardiovascular lesions are associated with webbing of the neck?
Noonan syndrome or Ullrich syndrome with pulmonary stenosis.

What are the facial features of Turner syndrome?
Ptosis, micrognathia, low-set ears, epicanthal folds.

What are the renal abnormalities associated with Turner syndrome?
Horseshoe kidney, hydronephrosis.

Is pregnancy possible in these patients?
Only in mosaic individuals with a normal 46XX cell line; in this group sufficient follicles may persist postnatally to initiate pubertal changes and, therefore, cause ovulation and consequently pregnancy.

How would you manage such patients?
The treatment is supportive and includes replacement hormone therapy on attaining puberty, primarily to prevent osteoporosis and induce sexual maturation and menses.

What is the chromosomal defect in Turner syndrome?
It is caused by the absence of one of the X chromosomes (blood karyotype showing 46,XO). Other variants of the syndrome include 46,X (with abnormal X), 45,XO/46,XX mosaics and 45,XO/46,XY mosaics. Although this is

the single most common chromosomal disorder, >95% of the foetuses are aborted, which results in an incidence of ~1 in 4000 newborns. Women with a 45,X/46,XX karyotype and a preponderance of 46,XX cells may have all the findings of the disorder.

Loss of *SRY* on the short arm of the Y chromosome (e.g. 46,X,del(Yp)) encoding a testis-determining factor, also leads to the phenotype of Turner syndrome, even without a 45,X cell population.

Is there a correlation between karyotype and phenotype?

There are some correlations between karyotype and phenotype, but note that phenotypic predictions for a given patient that are based on karyotype may not be reliable (e.g. women with a 45,X karyotype have conceived).

- Growth failure
- Loss of interstitial or terminal long-arm material of the X chromosome (Xq) can result in short stature and primary or secondary ovarian failure.
- Deletions distal to Xq21 appear to have no effect on stature.
- Loss of the short arm (Xp) results in the full phenotype.
- Very distal Xp deletions are compatible with, but do not ensure, normal ovarian function. Loss of this region usually confers short stature and the typical skeletal changes, in part as a result of haploinsufficiency of the short stature–homeobox (*SHOX*) gene, located in the pseudoauto-somal region of Y and Xp. (*SHOX* is probably not the only gene that determines skeletal features.)
- Aneuploidy itself may contribute to growth failure.
- Women with mosaicism for 45,X/46,XX are marginally taller than other women with Turner syndrome.

- Neurocognitive defects
- Loss of a region at Xp22.3 appears to be associated with the neurocognitive problems.
- The presence of a ring or marker chromosome confers an increased risk of mental retardation and atypical phenotypic features.

- Lymphoedema
- A region on Xp11.4 has been postulated to be important for the development of lymphoedema.
- Infants with a 45,X karyotype are the most likely to have congenital lymphoedema.

- Reproductive organs
- A karyotype of 45,X/46,XX or 45,X/47,XXX is most likely to be associated with spontaneous menarche and fertility.
- Girls with mosaicism for a cell population with a Y chromosome are at increased risk for gonadoblastoma (risk, 7–30%) in their streak gonads.

Hypothyroidism and inflammatory bowel disease

- The presence of an isochromosome Xq suggests an increased risk for hypothyroidism and inflammatory bowel disease.

What do you know about Lyon's hypothesis?

In 1961, geneticist Mary Lyon outlined that only one of the X chromosomes is genetically active, the other being inactive. The inactivation of either the maternal or paternal X chromosome occurs at random among all the cells of the blastocyst around the 16th day of embryonic life, and inactivation of the same X chromosome persists in all cells derived from each precursor cell.

More recent studies, however, have shown that many genes escape X chromosome inactivation and that both X chromosomes are important for normal growth, as evidenced by severe abnormalities in Turner syndrome with a monosomy of X chromosome. It is now believed that a gene that maps to Xq13 serves as a master switch which is critical for 'switching-off' most of the genes on the active chromosome 13. This gene is known as X-inactive-specific transcript gene (*XIST*).

Henry H Turner (1892–1970), an American endocrinologist, described this condition in 1938.

Mary Lyon (b. 1925), geneticist who worked for the Medical Research Council in Oxford.

There are several support groups for patients with Turner syndrome and their families.

Turner Syndrome Society of UK is such a support group; 12 Irving Quadrant, Hardgate, Clydebank G81 6AZ, UK; telephone +44(0)1389–380385; fax +44(0)1389–380384; e-mail Turner.Syndrome@tss.org.uk; or see www.tss.org.uk/contact.html. It provides:

- free growth charts for patients with Turner syndrome.
- publications at cost (e.g. Reiser PA, Underwood LE. Turner syndrome: a guide for families, 1992, Rosenfeld RG. Turner syndrome: A guide for physicians, 1992).
- videotapes of their annual conferences, available for a fee.

---

234 YELLOW NAIL SYNDROME

INSTRUCTION

Look at this patient's hands.

SALIENT FEATURES

History

- Ask about past history of sinusitis
- History of chronic cough, bronchiectasis, pleural effusion, recurrent lung infections
- History of lymphoedema
- Ask about associated disorders:
  - Malignancy: melanoma, carcinoma of larynx, lung and breast, Hodgkin's disease
  - Thyroid disease: Hashimato's thyroiditis, hypothyroidism, thyrotoxicosis
  - Hypogammaglobulinaemia
  - Rheumatoid arthritis.

Examination

- Yellow discoloration of all the nails. The nails are often smooth, thickened and overcurved. There is no involvement of the skin.

Proceed as follows:

- Tell the examiner that you would like to:
  - examine the chest (for pleural effusion, bronchiectasis)
  - examine the legs for lymphoedema.

Remember: Yellow nail syndrome is the differential diagnosis of chronic pleural effusions that has been present for >1 year, for bronchiectasis and rhinosinusitis.

DIAGNOSIS

This patient has yellow nail syndrome (lesion) complicated by severe bronchiectasis (functional status).

ADVANCED-LEVEL QUESTIONS

What is the pathogenesis?

The pathogenic mechanism underlying the yellow nail syndrome has not been defined. Abnormality of lymphatic vessels was suggested as the cause by Samman and White in their original description of the syndrome (Br J Dermatol 1964;76:153–7). This theory is supported by lymphangiographic findings which in most patients showed few, hypoplastic or dilated, deficient lymphatics. Electron microscopy in two cases noted dilated but otherwise normal lymphatics (J Am Acad Dermatol 1983;10:187–92).

What is the treatment?

Therapy (Chest 2008;134:375–381) includes:
- Bronchopulmonary hygiene (e.g. postural drainage)
- Symptomatic exacerbations: inhaled steroids and antibiotics
- Pleural effusions: serial thoracocentesis or pleurodesis
- Lymphoedema: compression stockings, postural therapy, low-salt diet and diuretics
- Yellow nails: often improves spontaneously; treatment with vitamin E has been proposed.

This syndrome was first described in 1964 by PD Samman and WF White.

---

235 OSTEOGENESIS IMPERFECTA

INSTRUCTION

Look at this patient's eyes.

SALIENT FEATURES

History

- Ask about previous fractures
- Ask whether or not the condition runs in the family.

Examination

- Blue sclera
- Look for the following signs:
  - Hearing loss as a result of otosclerosis
  - Signs of old fractures
  - Defective dentine formation in the teeth

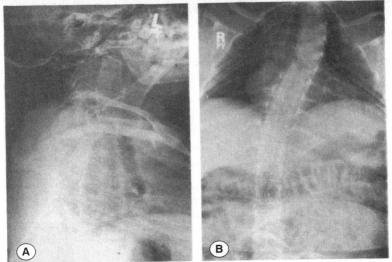

Fig. 235.1 Lateral (A) and anteroposterior (B) radiographs showing in typical findings in osteogenesis imperfecta: diffuse osteopenia, scoliosis, compression of several cervical vertebral bodies, and a focal kyphosis at the midcervical level. (With permission from Song, Maher 2007.)

- Kyphosis and scoliosis (Fig. 235.1)
- Joint hypermobility
- Hernias
- Aortic regurgitation.

DIAGNOSIS

This patient has blue sclera with abnormalities of skeleton and teeth (lesion) caused by osteogenesis imperfecta tarda (aetiology), and is disabled by the condition (functional status).

QUESTIONS

Why is the sclera blue?
Because the choroid pigment is visible.

Mention other conditions in which the sclera is blue
- Marfan syndrome
- Ehlers–Danlos syndrome.

ADVANCED-LEVEL QUESTIONS

What is the inheritance?
Usually autosomal dominant, although it may be autosomal recessive. The gene defects are in the two genes, COL1A1 or COL1A2, that encode the procollagen chains of type I collagen. Mutant type I collagen results in autosomal dominant osteogenesis imperfecta. Mutations affecting either of two components of the collagen prolyl 3-hydroxylation complex

(cartilage-associated protein and prolyl 3-hydroxylase 1) cause the auto-somal recessive form with rhizomelia (shortening of proximal segments of upper and lower limbs) and delayed collagen folding (N Engl J Med 2010;362:521–8).

What is the characteristic pathology?

The most characteristic pathology is a primary reduction in bone matrix with secondary mineralization.

What are the clinical types?

The Sillence classification is into four types (I–IV):

I: nearly normal stature, imperfect dentition, blue sclera, fractures of variable number and minimal deformity

II: usually foetuses die in utero or shortly after birth; multiple fractures of ribs and long bones with little mineralization of calvarium and pulmonary hypertension

III (osteogenesis imperfecta congenita, foetal type): stature markedly diminished as a result of multiple fractures and deformity of long bones in utero; blue sclera, imperfect dentition and hearing loss

IV (osteogenesis imperfecta tarda): stature usually reduced, bone deform-ity and fractures common; sclera bluish to normal; imperfect dentition; may or may not have loss of hearing.

How would you manage this patient?

- Genetic counselling
- Calcium, vitamin D
- Bisphosphonates may improve bone density and growth in children (N Engl J Med 1998;339:947)
- Bone marrow transplantation to correct mesenchymal defect in children (Nat Med 1999;5:309–13).

236 DOWN'S SYNDROME

INSTRUCTION

Look at this patient.

SALIENT FEATURES

History

- Ask the mother at what age she delivered the child (it occurs once in 1550 live births in women under the age of 20 years, in contrast to 1 in 25 live births for mothers over the age of 45 years).

Examination

- Collapse of the bridge of the nose
- Low-set ears
- Epicanthic folds
- Look at the iris for Brushfield's spots: yellow speckles seen in young children
- Tell the examiner that you would like to:
  - examine the hands for simian palmar crease (Fig. 236.1)
  - examine for short inward curving of the little finger (Siegert's sign)

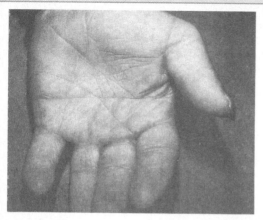

Fig. 236.1 Simian crease.

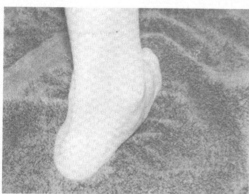

Fig. 236.2 Ankle pronation, loss of arch as a result of ligamentous laxity and pes planus. (With permission from Davidson 2008.)

- examine the heart for murmur of mitral regurgitation (endocardial cushion defects) and atrial septal defect (ASD; ostium primum type)
- check mental status quotient (MSQ) and formal IQ testing (80% have an IQ between 25 and 50)
- examine the foot for ankle pronation and pars planus (Fig. 236.2).
- Tell the examiner that you would like to check for hypothyroidism and thyroid antibodies

DIAGNOSIS

This patient has features of Down syndrome (lesion), which is usually caused by trisomy 21 (aetiology) and is associated with a reduced life expectancy (functional status).

QUESTIONS

What complications can be seen in such patients?
- Increased incidence of acute leukaemia
- Presenile dementia of Alzheimer type (occurs in the fourth and fifth decades and reduces life expectancy)

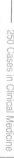

- Atlantoaxial subluxation
- Duodenal atresia in children.

What are the broad management principles of such a patient?

- *Evaluation*:
  - Echocardiography
  - Sight
  - Hearing.
- *Prevention*:
  - Obesity
  - Periodontal disease.
- *Monitoring*:
  - Coeliac disease
  - Thyroid function.
- *Vigilance*:
  - Diabetes
  - Leukaemia
  - Arthritis
  - Obstructive sleep apnoea
  - Seizures
  - Atlantoaxial subluxation.
- *Other*:
  - Sexual and reproductive health
  - Skin problems
  - Behaviour problems
  - Development.

ADVANCED-LEVEL QUESTIONS

Mention two chromosomal abnormalities seen in this condition

- Trisomy 21 (N Engl J Med 1991;324:872)
- Mosaicism (46,XY/47,XY, +21). Approximately 1% are mosaics from mitotic non-dysjunction.

What are the underlying genetic mechanisms?

- Non-dysjunction (occurs during meiosis, particularly in the ovum, and correlates with maternal age)
- De novo translocation
- Familial translocation, usually robertsonian translocation of the long arm of chromosome 21 to another acrocentric chromosome, e.g. 22 or 14.

A 41-year-old woman, gravida 1, seeks prenatal care at 8 weeks of gestation. Her family history and medical history are unremarkable. What would you advise regarding her risk of foetal chromosomal abnormalities such as Down syndrome and her options for prenatal screening and diagnosis?

- First trimester screening:
- Measurements of two biochemical markers: pregnancy-associated plasma protein A (PAPP-A) and human chorionic gonadotrophin (hCG)
- Measurement of nuchal translucency
- Non-visualization of the nasal bone on ultrasonographic examination in the first trimester has been associated with an increased risk of Down syndrome and other aneuploidies.

- **Second trimester screening** Quadraple screening: maternal α-fetoprotein levels, hCG, unconjugated oestriol, inhibin A. Trisomy 21 is associated with high maternal levels of hCG and inhibin A and low levels of α-fetoprotein and unconjugated oestriol. Quadraple screening has a detection rate of 80% for trisomy 21 at a positive screening rate of 5% (a rate at or below this level is considered to be acceptable for aneuploidy screening).

- **Stepwise sequential screening during trimesters one and two** Stepwise sequential screening keeps the false positive rate low and provides early results to women with a positive test, but it combines the results of both the first-trimester and the second-trimester measurements into a final second-trimester risk assessment.

  If a woman prefers to know with certainty that the foetus does not have Down syndrome or another form of aneuploidy, she may decide to bypass screening and choose either chorionic-villus sampling at 10 to 12 weeks of gestation (if available) or amniocentesis at 15 and 20 weeks of gestation.

Which maternal serum markers are used for prenatal screening of Down syndrome?
Serum α-fetoprotein, hCG and oestriol.

J Langdon Down (1828–1896) wrote an article in Clinical Lectures and Reports of the London Infirmary (now the Royal London Hospital) in 1866 entitled 'The ethnic classification of idiots'. The extrachromosome was discovered by Lejeune in 1959.

T Brushfield (1858–1937), a British physician.

Ferdinand Siegert (1865–1946), a German paediatrician.

Mitchell in 1876 observed the increased incidence with maternal age and Penrose in 1933 confirmed it statisitically.

Hyman Isaac Goldstein (1887–1954), an American physician, described Goldstein's sign, which is a wide space between the great toe and the adjoining toe seen in Down syndrome.

---

237 LATE CONGENITAL SYPHILIS

INSTRUCTION

Look at this patient.

SALIENT FEATURES

History

- Hearing loss
- Arthritis from Clutton's joints
- Eye pain (from intersititial keratitis).

Examination

- Collapsed bridge of the nose (saddle nose or Zaufal's sign) (Fig. 237.1)
- Corneal opacity (interstitial keratitis)

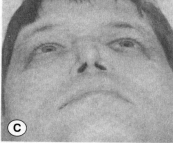

Fig. 237.1 Saddle nose deformity. (A) Type 0. (B) Type I. (C) Type II. (D) Type III. (E) Type V. (With permission from Pribitkin EA, Ezzat WH. Classification and treatment of the saddle nose deformity. Otolaryngolc Clin North Am 2009;42:437–61.)

- Rhagades (linear scars at the angles of the mouth)
- Peg-shaped incisors (Hutchinson's teeth): the central incisors are widely spaced, have a central notch and tapered like a peg
- Mulberry molars: first molars dwarfed by a small occlusal surface; characterized by roughened lobulated hypoplastic enamel (leading to caries)
- Perforation of the palate
- Frontal bossing.

Proceed as follows:
- Check for deafness (nerve deafness)
- Look at the shins for sabre tibia
- Look for Clutton's joints (bilateral knee effusions)
- Look at the fundus for optic atrophy.

Remember:
Cardiovascular manifestations have not been observed in this condition. Late congenital syphilis is defined as congenital syphilis of >2 years' duration.

DIAGNOSIS

This patient has a saddle nose and peg-shaped incisors (lesions) caused by congenital syphilis; this has resulted from maternal *Treponema pallidum* infection (aetiology).

ADVANCED-LEVEL QUESTIONS

What is Hutchinson's triad?
- Interstitial keratitis
- Deafness
- Typical dental change, i.e. peg-shaped incisors (Hutchinson's teeth).

What are the ocular features of congenital syphilis?
- Interstitial keratitis
- Retinopathy: fine pigmentation, 'salt and pepper fundus'.

How is saddle nose classified?
Daniel and Brenner introduced a more detailed classification system in 2006 that classified saddle nose deformities into six different types based on clinical features and pathophysiologic processes (Fig. 237.1).

0: pseudosaddle deformity as a result of overresection of the cartilaginous middle vault

I: minor saddle nose deformity from decreased septal support but greater supratip depression and columellar retraction

II: more advanced; progressive weakening of the septal support wall leads to collapse of the cartilaginous middle vault, reduced tip support and retracted columella; internal nasal valve collapse is common

III: total loss of cartilage vault integrity and flattening of the nasal lobule; there can be nasal septal perforation, obvious flattening and depression of the middle vault and rotation of the nasal tip

IV: progressive involvement of the bony vault, leading to a pinched internal nasal valve, columellar retrusion, deprojection of the nasal tip and a short nose

V: castastrophic deformity with associated orbital and facial deformities; the tip cartilage is preserved but deformed by the relentless middle and upper vault collapse.

Sir Johnathan Hutchinson (1828–1913) was simultaneously a surgeon at The London Hospital (now the Royal London Hospital), an ophthalmologist at Moorfields Hospital and a dermatologist at Blackfriars Hospital (now closed).

H Clutton (1850–1901), an English surgeon who worked at St Thomas's Hospital, London.

Emanuel Zaufal (1833–1910), a Czechoslovakian rhinologist.

238 ARTERIOVENOUS FISTULA

INSTRUCTION

Look at this patient's arms.

SALIENT FEATURES

History

- History of trauma to the limb
- History of haemodialysis and artificial arteriovenous fistula.

Examination

- Hypertrophy of the affected arm
- Prominent, dilated, tortuous veins
- Continuous thrill over the fistula; listen for continuous bruit
- Collapsing pulse; increased pulse pressure indicating hyperdynamic circulation.

Proceed as follows:

- Look for signs of cardiac failure.
- Elicit Branham's sign: slowing of the pulse on occluding the feeding vessel of the fistula.
- If the fistula is in the upper limb, then perform Allen's test: the radial and ulnar arteries are occluded at the wrist and the hand is exercised; the arteries are then released one at a time to establish which is the dominant feeding vessel.
- Look for signs of chronic renal failure.

Note: An arteriovenous fistula is a *direct subcutaneous anastomosis of an artery and vein without prosthetic material*, and is the preferred means of vascular access for haemodialysis.

DIAGNOSIS

This patient has an arteriovenous fistula (lesion) that has been surgically created (aetiology) for haemodialysis and is functioning well.

ADVANCED-LEVEL QUESTIONS

How are arteriovenous malformations classified?

Angiographically, as follows:

- Group 1, predominantly arterial or arteriovenous lesions: present with pain, hypertrophy of the digit or limb, deformity, distal ischaemia, venous hypertension; large lesions can cause symptoms and signs of cardiac failure

- Group 2, lesions affecting tiny vessels including capillaries: for example port-wine stain, epistaxis in hereditary haemorrhagic telangiectasia, GI haemorrhage with colonic dysplasia
- Group 3, predominantly venous lesions: local oedema, pain and venous ulceration; there may be a history of trauma.

How would you manage a patient with an arteriovenous malformation?

- Referral to a vascular surgeon
- Doppler ultrasonography
- Angiography.

When and how is an arteriovenous malformation treated?

Arteriovenous malformations are treated when they cause discomfort, disfigurement and danger to the patient. The patient should be jointly assessed by a vascular surgeon and an interventional radiologist for embolization. The temptation to ligate the feeder vessel should be resisted as subsequent embolization may be difficult. Complete exicision of the fistula is accepted treatment in resistant cases.

Why are fistulae preferred to prosthetic grafts?

Fistulae have a far lower risk of failure and a reduced requirement for revision compared with prosthetic grafts. In 2005, the Center for Medicare and Medicaid Services recommended a goal of arteriovenous fistula formation in 66% of all new patients undergoing haemodialysis in the breakthrough initiative that has become known as 'Fistula First'. Unfortunately, a substantial number of patients lack suitable veins for the creation of autogenous fistulae and require placement of prosthetic grafts.

What the alternatives, when a fistula cannot be formed in patient requiring long-term haemodialysis?

Placement of synthetic grafts subcutaneously or of a long central line into a great vein.

What is the leading cause of failure of a prosthetic arteriovenous haemodialysis-access graft?

The leading cause of failure of a prosthetic arteriovenous haemodialysis-access graft is venous anastomotic stenosis (Fig. 238.1). Balloon angioplasty, the first-line therapy, has a tendency to lead to subsequent recoil and restenosis. Percutaneous revision of venous anastomotic stenosis in patients with a prosthetic haemodialysis graft is improved with the use of an expanded polytetrafluoroethylene endovascular stent graft, which appears to provide longer-term and superior patency and freedom from repeat interventions than standard balloon angioplasty (N Engl J Med 2010;362:494–503).

HH Branham, an American surgeon in the nineteenth century.
   EV Allen (1900–1961), Professor of Medicine at the Mayo Clinic, Rochester, Minnesota, introduced coumarin anticoagulants into clinical practice and edited one of the first comprehensive textbooks on peripheral vascular disease.

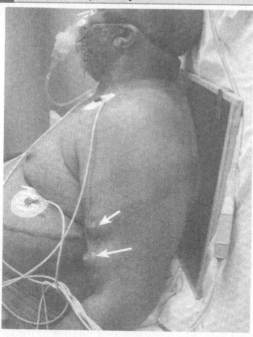

Fig. 238.1 Older dialysis fistula, showing multiple aneurysms (arrows) from multiple time use. (With permission from Roberts, Hedges 2009.)

239 CAROTID ARTERY ANEURYSM

INSTRUCTION

Examine this patient's neck.

SALIENT FEATURES

History

- History of hypertension
- History of diabetes
- History of smoking
- History of transient ischaemic attacks or an embolic stroke (a neurologic event was the presenting symptom in 37.5–100% of cases in one reported series).

Examination

- Pulsatile swelling along the course of the carotids, usually unilateral (the swelling may be firm) and at the base of the neck.

Proceed as follows:

- Auscultate over the mass for a bruit
- Look for Horner syndrome
- Tell the examiner that you would like to examine:
  - all peripheral pulses
  - the heart and BP
  - the fasting blood sugar.

DIAGNOSIS

This patient has a carotid artery aneurysm (lesion) caused by atherosclerosis (aetiology), and may require surgery before the lesion ruptures (functional status).

ADVANCED-LEVEL QUESTIONS

How would you manage this patient?

- All patients must be referred to a specialist for either open surgery (a venous conduit, usually the proximal greater saphenous vein is used for arterial continuity) or endovascular approach
- Check urine for sugar
- Serum lipids
- Duplex ultrasonography
- Intravenous carotid digital subtraction angiography or CT angiography (Fig. 239.1).

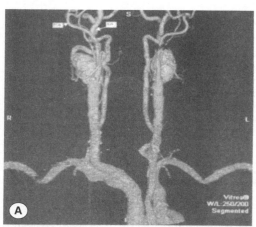

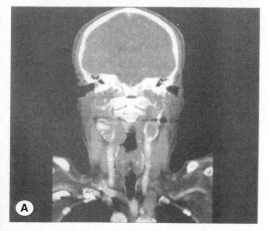

Fig. 239.1 Bilateral aneurysms of the internal carotid arteries (ICA). (A) CT angiography showing aneurysms between the artery origins and the base of the skull. The left aneurysm is thrombosed and the right has a very tortuous distal vessel beyond. (B) Coronal CT angiography shows extensive calcification and atheroma bilaterally with thrombosed left aneurysm. ECA, external carotid artery; S, superior. (With permission from Roche-Nagle 2009.)

240 RETRO-ORBITAL TUMOUR

INSTRUCTION

Examine this patient's eyes.

SALIENT FEATURES

History

- History of atherosclerosis
- History of hypertension
- History of diabetes
- History of trauma to the eye or head.

Examination

- Unilateral exophthalmos (proptosis; Fig. 240.1)
- Impaired extraocular movement (from either muscle or nerve involvement)
- Chemosis, conjunctival oedema
- Radiation marks may be present.

Proceed as follows:

- Examine the visual acuity and visual fields.
- Look for pulsations over the globe.
- Palpate the orbital margin for erosion of the underlying bone.
- Auscultate over the globe for bruit.

DIAGNOSIS

This patient has a retro-orbital tumour with a bruit over the globe (lesion), indicating a pulsatile structure such as an arteriovenous fistula in the orbit (aetiology). The tumour is causing considerable distress to the patient (functional status).

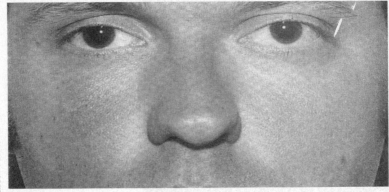

Fig. 240.1 Proptosis of the left eye from a retro-orbital tumour. (With permission from Yanoff, Fine 2002.)

ADVANCED-LEVEL QUESTIONS

What is your differential diagnosis?
- The commonest cause of unilateral exophthalmos is Graves' disease.
- Other causes are:
  - retro-orbital tumour (primary or metastatic)
  - arteriovenous fistula (carotico-cavernous fistula)
  - cavernous sinus thrombosis
  - orbital cellulitis.

What investigations would you do?
- Throxine, thyroid-stimulating hormone (TSH), free thyroxine
- Orbital ultrasonography
- Cranial MRI, in particular the orbits.

How would you manage such a patient?
- Ophthalmology opinion
- Therapy: radiation to the orbit and steroids, and surgical decompression, depending on the underlying aetiology.

What are the causes of a unilateral pulsating proptosis?
- Arteriovenous fistula between the carotid artery and cavernous sinus: stops with pressure.on the artery in the neck
- Aneurysm of the ophthalmic artery
- Cirsoid aneurysm of the orbit
- Vascular neoplasms in the orbit growing rapidly.

241 ACHONDROPLASIA

INSTRUCTION

Look at this patient.

SALIENT FEATURES

History

- Family history (autosomal dominant inheritance; however, 80% are new mutations)
- Paternal age (increases in frequency with increasing age of father at child's birth).

Examination

- Dwarfism
- Bulging forehead
- Depression of the root of the nose
- Midface hypoplasia
- Shortened proximal extremities with hands have a 'trident' shape
- Trunk of normal size
- Exaggerated lumbar lordosis.

DIAGNOSIS

This patient with short stature and normal trunk size has achondroplasia (lesion), which is caused by mutation of the gene for the fibroblast growth factor receptor (aetiology).

QUESTIONS

Is the lifespan reduced in these subjects?

No, they have a normal lifespan, although this has been disputed (Lancet 1998;352:1950).

How is the IQ affected in these patients?

IQ is normal.

Is the reproductive status affected?

Reproductive status is normal.

What are the complications of this condition?

- Hydrocephalus or compression of brainstem, spinal cord or nerve roots
- Impingement by an osteophyte or disc on the small spinal canal can cause neurological disturbance.

ADVANCED-LEVEL QUESTIONS

What do you know about the genetics of achondroplasia?

- It is inherited as an autosomal dominant trait with complete penetrance. The gene *FGFR3* on human chromosome 4, encoding fibroblast growth factor receptor 3, is mutated at location 1138, leading to replacement of guanine by adenine or cytosine (Cell 1994;78:335–42, Nature 1994;371:252). The change causes increased function of the gene, resulting in decreased endochondral ossification, inhibited proliferation of chondrocytes in the growth plate cartilage, decreased cellular hypertrophy and decreased cartilage matrix production.
- Severe mutations in *Trip11*, which encodes a Golgi-associated microtubule-binding protein (thyroid receptor-interacting protein 11 or GMAP-210) causes a form of achondroplasia in mice, with defective glycosylation and cell transport of several proteins. *TRIP11* mutations have now been found in humans with achondrogenesis type 1A (N Engl J Med 2010;362:206–16).

What do you know about idiopathic short stature?

Idiopathic short stature (also referred to as normal-variant short stature or short stature of undefined cause) is a diagnosis of exclusion. Growth hormone deficiency, intrauterine growth retardation, genetic or syndromic causes of short stature and other factors compromising growth, such as depression or psychosocial deprivation, should be excluded before making the diagnosis. Recombinant human growth hormone therapy was approved by the US Food and Drug Administration in 2003 for idiopathic short stature; the anticipated average height gain being 4 to 7 cm after several years of daily injections.

What do you know about Crouzon syndrome?

Crouzon syndrome is an autosomal dominant condition characterized by premature fusion of the cranial sutures (craniosynostosis); it has been shown to map to chromosome 10 and is associated with mutations of the gene for fibroblast growth factor receptor 2.

> This syndrome has been depicted by aritists in several paintings, including the painter Velasquez in his portrait of Don Sebastian de Morra, a courtier of the Spanish King Phillip V.

242 BREAST LUMP

INSTRUCTION

Examine this patient's breasts.

SALIENT FEATURES

History

- History of weight loss
- History of a palpable mass in breast and/or axilla
- Breast pain (present in 10% of breast cancer patients) and unrelated to menstrual cycle
- Nipple discharge, erosion, enlargement or itching of the nipple
- Back or bone pain, jaundice or weight loss (indicate systemic metastases)
- Family history (20% of breast cancer have family history)
- Some forms of mammary dysplasia
- History of cancer in the other breast
- History of endometrial cancer
- Nulliparous or late first pregnancy.

Examination

- Breast lump that is non-tender and has poorly delineated margins. Asymmetry of the breasts and retraction or dimpling of the skin can often be accentuated by having the patient raise her arms overhead or press her hands on her hips to contract the pectoralis muscle.

Remember: Breast examination is performed with the patient supine and arm abducted (hand is behind the head).

Proceed as follows:
- Examine axillary and supraclavicular lymph nodes
- Look for oedema of the ipsilateral arm (as a result of metastatic infiltration of regional lymphatics)
- Examine the chest (metastases, lymphangitis carcinomatosa)
- Examine for hepatomegaly (metastases); breast cancer spreads to the bones, lungs, brain and liver.

Remember: All patients should undergo 'triple assessment':
- Clinical examination
- Imaging: ultrasound <35 years of age, mammography and ultrasound >35 years
- Cytology and histology: ultrasound-guided core biopsy and occasionally fine needle aspiration.

Note: Be prepared to discuss breast anatomy.

DIAGNOSIS

This patient has a breast lump that is infiltrating the skin and axillary lymph nodes (lesion), indicating malignant breast carcinoma (aetiology).

QUESTIONS

How would you investigate such a patient?
- FBC and ESR (ESR is consistently raised)
- Urea and electrolytes, liver function tests (hypercalcaemia, raised alkaline phosphatase level indicates bone or liver metastases)

- Ultrasound of breast
- Biopsy: large needle-core biopsy, fine-needle aspiration or open biopsy under local anaesthesia
- Carcinoembyronic antigen (CEA) could be a marker for recurrence
- Imaging for metastases:
  - Chest radiograph for lung secondaries
  - CT scan of liver or brain when metastasis is suspected in these areas
  - Bone scanning if patient has bone pain or raised alkaline phosphatase level.

ADVANCED-LEVEL QUESTIONS

How would you investigate a patient with a suspicious mammogram but no clinical evidence of mass?

Although a mass cannot be palpated, the patient should undergo a mammographic localization biopsy.

What are the histological types of breast cancer?

They are of two main types, which may be invasive or in situ.

- Ductal: arising from the epithelial lining of large or intermediate-sized ducts. Most arise from intermediate ducts and are invasive (e.g. invasive ductal, infiltrating ductal). When ductal carcinoma has not invaded extraductal tissue, it is intraductal or in situ ductal.
- Lobular: arising from the epithelium of the terminal ducts of the lobules.

How are patients with breast cancer managed?

- **Surgery**
- Breast-conserving surgery (lumpectomy, axillary dissection and radiation therapy) is usually offered to patients with single tumours <4 cm in diameter because the cosmetic outcome of excising larger tumours is poor. However, in 80% of patients with large tumours and in 25% of those with locally advanced breast cancers, breast conservation is possible if the size of the tumour is reduced by a course of primary systemic treatment (such as combination chemotherapy and hormonal therapy).
- Modified radical mastectomy (total mastectomy, removal of the overlying skin, nipple as well as the underlying pectoralis fascia with axillary lymph node dissection). The major advantage is that radiation is not necessary, but many patients suffer from the psychological trauma of breast loss.

- **Adjuvant therapy**
- CMF regimen (cyclophosphamide, methotrexate and fluorouracil)
- MMM regimen (mitozantrone, methotrexate and mitomycin C)
- Doxorubicin and cyclophosphamide
- Tamoxifen
- Trastuzumab, a monoclonal antibody against the human epidermal growth factor receptor type 2 (HER2), is associated with an improvement of approximately 50% in disease-free survival among the 15–20% of women with HER2-positive disease
- Weekly paclitaxel after standard adjuvant chemotherapy with doxorubicin and cyclophosphamide improves disease-free and overall survival in women with axillary lymph node-positive or high-risk, lymph node-negative breast cancer.

- Palliative therapy
- Radiotherapy is indicated for most patients who undergo breast-conserving surgery for invasive disease. The one subgroup of patients for whom breast-conserving surgery without radiation can be considered an appropriate option is women who are at least 70 years of age who are treated with surgery and hormonal therapy for oestrogen receptor-positive stage I breast cancer. In this cohort, the risk of local recurrence without radiation therapy is <10%. Accelerated, hypofractionated, whole-breast irradiation is useful in selected women with node-negative breast cancer after breast-conserving surgery. Accelerated partial-breast irradiation is delivered with double-plane or balloon-based radioactive implants and through conformational three-dimensional external-beam treatment. Radiation may be complicated by brachial plexus neuropathy.
- Hormonal treatment (tamoxifen, diethylstilbestrol, megestrol acetate, aminoglutethimide), chemotherapy (doxorubicin, paclitaxel, docetaxel, trastuzamab or herceptin).

- Breast reconstruction
- Implants, latissmus dorsi flaps, TRAM flap (transverse rectus abdominus myocutaneous flap).

Which breast cancers are suitable for treatment by conservative breast surgery?
- Single clinical and mammographic lesion
- Tumours <4 cm in diameter (or those >4 cm in a large breast)
- No sign of local advancement.

Which patients are best treated by mastectomy?
- Those who prefer mastectomy
- Those in whom breast conservation would produce an unacceptable cosmetic result
- Those with either clinical or mammographic evidence of more than one focus of cancer in the breast.

What factors are associated with increased rates of local recurrence after mastectomy?
Axillary lymph node involvement, lymphatic or vascular invasion by cancer, grade III carcinoma or tumours ≥4 cm in diameter.

What are the prognostic factors in 'node-negative' breast cancer?
- Tumour type and size
- Oestrogen and progesterone receptor status
- Histological grade
- Percentage of cells in the S phase (i.e. synthesizing DNA)
- The HER-2/neu (c-erbB2) oncogene. The HER-2/neu (c-erbB2) oncogene is expressed by 25% of breast cancers and is associated with a poorer prognosis but a better response to doxorubicin and herceptin therapy.

Which 6.195 ptpatients are more likely to respond to hormone therapy?
- Women with high levels of oestrogen receptors in the tumour
- When there is a long interval from initial surgery to time of relapse
- Those with metastatic disease in bone and soft tissue (unlike those with liver or lymphangitis carcinomatosa).

Are women with fibroadenomas at increased long-term risk of breast cancer?

Not all patients with fibroadenomas are at increased risk, but those with a family history of breast cancer, complex fibroadenomas or proliferative disease have an increased long-term risk of breast cancer.

What is the role of implants for breast augmentation?

In breast cancer, silicone gel implants were used for augmentation, but with new evidence that these may cause autoimmune reactions or connective tissue disorders, their use has been stopped. Saline implants do not work well for reconstruction after surgery for breast cancer or for very thin women. If silicone gel implants are removed from the market, these patients will have no alternative.

Which genes have been implicated in familial breast cancer?

There may be more than five genes causing familial breast cancer; the most important of these is *BRCA1* located on the long arm of chromosome 17. BRCA1 helps to repair damaged DNA and small ubiquitin-like modifier (SUMO) proteins are responsible for transporting the BRCA1 protein to DNA breaks. The gene *p53* on the short arm of chromosome 17 has been implicated in the rare breast cancer family syndrome (the Li Fraumeni syndrome, in which breast cancer occurs at a younger age associated with soft tissue sarcoma, osteosarcoma, adrenal tumours, gliomas and other childhood tumours). The two most important breast-cancer genes, *BRCA1* and *BRCA2*, confer a risk of breast cancer among carriers that is 10 to 30 times higher than the risk among women in the general population. Although *BRCA1* and *BRCA2* mutations are rare (occurring in approximately 1 of 400 persons), they are common in the Ashkenazi Jewish population, in which 1 of 40 persons carries one of three main disease-causing mutations. Less frequent mutations associated with a relative risk of breast cancer of ≥2.0 have also been identified and these account for <1% of cases of breast cancer.

What is the role of gene-expression profiling?

Gene-expression profiling distinguishes four main molecular classes of breast cancer using a single assay; these subgroups correspond fairly well to clinical characterization on the basis of oestrogen receptor (ER) and HER2 status, as well as proliferation markers or histologic grade.

Basal-like breast cancers. These mostly correspond to tumours that are negative for ER, progesterone receptor (PR) and HER2 mutations (hence, 'triple-negative' tumours). Although these are biologically aggressive, they can still have an excellent outcome with breast-conserving surgery and whole-breast irradiation. These cancers are *BRCA1*-related cancers and are difficult to detect by mammography. Therefore, screening for these cancers with MRI is warranted. The risk of contralateral breast cancer among carriers of *BRCA1* and *BRCA2* is significant (~3% per year), requiring more vigorous breast surveillance with MRI or even prophylactic mastectomies.

Luminal-A cancers. These are mostly ER positive and histologically low grade. (The one subgroup of patients who can be offered breast-conserving therapy without irradiation as the standard of care are those who are at least 70 years of age who have stage I, ER-positive disease treated with adjuvant hormonal therapy.)

Luminal-B cancers. These are also mostly ER positive but may express low levels of hormone receptors and are often high grade.

HER2-positive cancers. These show amplification and high expression of *ErbB2* and several other genes of the *ErbB2* amplicon.

What are the factors associated with increased rates of local recurrence after mastectomy?

Axillary lymph node involvement, lymphatic or vascular invasion by cancer, grade III carcinoma, tumour >4 cm in diameter.

What are the theories of cancer spread?

● *The 'Halstedian' theory* proposed that breast cancer begins as a strictly local disease and that tumour cells spread over time in a contiguous manner away from the primary site through lymphatics; consequently, even distant metastases are the result of direct extensions of local involvement (affecting the breast, the chest wall, axillary and supraclavicular lymph nodes, or any combination of the sites). This concept therefore required aggressive local therapy for control of disease in the breast, chest wall and regional lymph nodes as this should have a substantial effect on survival. These ideas also provided basis for evermore radical breast cancer surgery.

● *The 'systemic' theory* proposed by Bernard Fisher and others considers breast cancer as a systemic disease that can be divided into two distinct groups: tumours that have the ability to metastasize to distant sites and those that lack this ability (Cancer Res 1980;40:3863–74). According to this concept, if distant metastases were destined to develop, they would already exist at the time of diagnosis of the breast tumour. As the length of a patient's overall survival is a function of distant disease, this theory hypothesized that therapies that improve local control would have little or no effect on patient's survival. Therefore, the emphasis was on the importance of effective systemic therapy in breast cancer therapy.

  ● *The 'spectrum theory'* proposed by Hellman and others synthesized aspects of the two above approaches (J Clin Oncol 1994;12:2229–34), seeing breast cancer as a heterogeneous disease with '...a spectrum of proclivities extending from a disease that remains local throughout its course to one that is systemic when first detectable'. This view holds that there is a time when tumour cells have not metastasized to distant sites for many breast cancers, but it is generally not known whether this time has passed at the point of diagnosis. According to this theory, failure to achieve initial local control will allow some tumours to disseminate later to distant sites, reducing a patient's chance for long-term survival. The spectrum theory is in agreement with the concept that the greater the likelihood that systemic spread (now known to occur primarily through direct haematogenous routes) has occurred at the time of diagnosis in a patient, the lower the likelihood that local treatment will affect survival.

In 1896, George Beatson published his seminal report that bilateral oophorectomy resulted in the remission of breast cancer in premenopausal women (Beaston GT. On the treatment of inoperable cases of carcinoma of the mamma: suggestions for a new method of treatment, with illustrative cases. Lancet 1896;2:104–7).

In 1894, William Halsted published his seminal report on radical mastectomy for the cure of cancer of the breast.

243 GINGIVAL HYPERTROPHY

INSTRUCTION

Look at this patient's mouth.

SALIENT FEATURES

History

- Drugs (phenytoin, ciclosporin, nifedipine) (Fig. 243.1)
- Leukaemia (myelomonocytic leukaemia) (Fig. 243.2)
- Wegener's granuloma (Fig. 243.3).

Examination

- Hypertrophy of the gums.
Proceed as follows:
- Look for other features of chronic phenytoin therapy: coarsening of facial features, hypertrichosis, hirsutism, generalized lymphadenopathy, rash, cerebellar syndrome, peripheral lymphadenopathy.

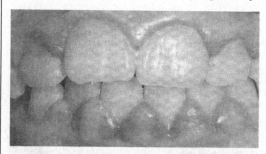

Fig. 243.1 Fibrous gingival enlargement associated with phenytoin treatment.

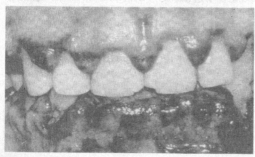

Fig. 243.2 Myelogenous leukaemia with neoplastic cellular infiltration of the gingiva and ecchymosis.

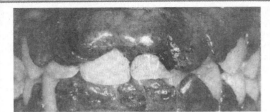

Fig. 243.3 Wegener's granulomatosis with necrotizing vasculitis and granulomatous infiltration of gingiva.

DIAGNOSIS

This patient has poor oral hygiene and gingival hypertrophy (lesion) caused by chronic ingestion of phenytoin (aetiology).

QUESTIONS

What are the other long-term side effects of phenytoin?
Coarsening of facial features, rashes, SLE, blood dyscrasias, generalized lymphadenopathy, induction of hepatic microsomal enyzmes, folic acid deficiency, peripheral neuropathy, cerebellar syndrome (ataxia, nystagmus and dysarthria), hypertrichosis, osteomalacia and encephalopathy.

When taken during pregnancy, phenytoin may result in cleft lip and palate in the child.

In which types of seizure is phenytoin generally used?
Generalized clonic–tonic seizures.

244 HAEMOPHILIA A

INSTRUCTION

Examine this patient's knee (or elbow) joint; he has a bleeding disorder.

SALIENT FEATURES

History

- Family history of bleeding (X-linked recessive disorder): draw the family tree
- Recurrent bleeding into the joints
- Intramuscular haematomas (after trauma, such as injections)
- Retroperitoneal bleeds
- Bleeding from mucous membranes
- Haematuria, haemospermia
- Intracranial bleeds (second most common cause of death in haemophiliacs after HIV)
- History of spontaneous bleeds (suggests severe disease).

Examination

- Male patient
- Fixed deformity of the joint (haemarthrosis causes bone and joint destruction).

Proceed as follows:

DIAGNOSIS

This patient has a fixed deformity of the elbow (lesion) caused by bleeding into the joint as a complication of haemophilia A (aetiology). The joint is now undergoing osteoarthritic changes (functional status).
Note: Be prepared to discuss the coagulation cascasde.

QUESTIONS

What is the inheritance of haemophilia?
One-third are sporadic and the rest are X-linked (defects include deletions, point mutations and insertions on the X chromosome).

What is deficient in haemophilia?
It is factor VIII:C, the clinical manifestations depend on its level. Levels <1% are associated with spontaneous bleeding, whereas patients with levels <5% have severe bleeding after trauma and occasionally spontaneous bleeding. When levels are >5%, bleeding occurs after trauma.

ADVANCED-LEVEL QUESTIONS

How are bleeding episodes treated?
- Factor VIII concentrates:
  - For minor bleeding, factor VIII concentrates should be raised to 20–30% of normal
  - For severe bleeding factor VIII is raised to at least 50%
  - For major surgery, factor VIII should be raised to 100% and maintained at over 50% until healing has occurred.
- Patients can stock Factor VIII in domestic refrigerators for self-administration to start treatment immediately on bleeding. It is given twice daily and intravenously.
- Desmopressin (DDAVP), administered intravenously, can increase factor VIII levels depending on the initial level.

What are the complications of haemophilia?
- Complications of the disorder
- Recurrent joint bleeding:
  - Chronic arthropathy, pain and loss of function
  - Crippling arthritis: recombinant factor VIII can prevent joint damage and decrease the frequency of joint and other haemorrhages in young boys with severe haemophilia A (N Engl J Med 2007;357:535–44).
- Death from haemorrhage.

- Complications related to treatment
- Transfusion-transmitted infections (risk reduced with virally inactivated concentrates; risk probably eliminated with recombinant products)
- Development of antibodies (inhibitors). Black patients with haemophilia A (factor VIII deficiency) are twice as likely as white patients to produce inhibitors against factor VIII proteins given as replacement therapy.

What is the commonest cause of death?
Currently, it is HIV infection, transmitted by contaminated factor VIII concentrate administered in the past. HIV-associated immune thrombocytopenia may worsen the bleeding tendency.

In 1803, John Conrad Otto emphasized its inheritance as an X-linked disorder in his description of a New Hampshire family.

Queen Victoria's descendants are said to have suffered from haemophilia (BMJ 1995;311:1106–7). She was a clinically normal carrier; she had one son, Leopold, who had haemophilia, and two daughters, Alice and Beatrice, who were carriers and who, in turn, transmitted the disease to the Russian, Prussian and Spanish royal families.

In 1964 Pool and co-workers discovered that factor VIII is concentrated in cryoprecipitate.

In 1984 the gene for factor VIII was cloned and expressed in tissue culture.

Robert Gwyn Macfarlane, Professor at Oxford, did pioneering work on the care of haemophiliacs and was the first to propose the cascade hypothesis of blood coagulation.

245 KLINEFELTER SYNDROME

INSTRUCTION

Examine this patient and give us your diagnosis.

SALIENT FEATURES

History

- Infertility (commonest cause of male infertility)
- Mentally subnormal
- Ask about sensation of smell (to exclude Kallman syndrome).

Examination

- Male patient with eunuchoid body habitus with abnormally long legs (Fig. 245.1)
- Elongated body with an increase in length between the soles and pubic bone
- Lack of a beard, and the voice is not masculine.

Proceed as follows:

- Tell the examiner that you would like to:
  - examine the external genitalia (small atrophic testes, lack of male distribution of pubic hair)
  - test the IQ: usually lower than normal, although mental disability is uncommon
  - check for hypo-osmia (Kallman syndrome).

DIAGNOSIS

This patient has Klinefelter syndrome (lesion) caused by an excess of X and Y chromosomes (aetiology), and has infertility (functional status).

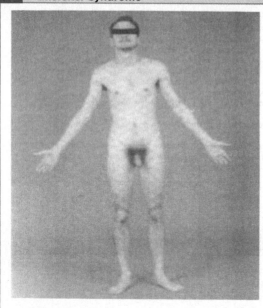

Fig. 245.1 Patient with Klinefelter syndrome after several months of testosterone therapy. Note eunuchoidal body proportions, lack of muscular development and scant body hair after several months of testosterone therapy. Gynaecomastia has been surgically corrected. (With permission from Rayman 2000.)

QUESTIONS

How would you investigate such a patient?

- Plasma gonadotrophins: follicle-stimulating hormone is consistently raised
- Plasma testosterone concentration: variably reduced
- Plasma oestradiol: raised
- Chromosomal analysis (two or more X chromosomes and one or more Y chromosomes). Cytogenetic arrays (or genomewide assessment of copy-number alterations (deletions and duplications) by means of high-density array technologies) should allow identification of microdeletions.

What is the commonest karyotype?

Eighty-two per cent of patients have 47,XXY, which results from non-dysjunction during meiosis in one of the parents.

Are the patients fertile?

No. However, some men have chromosomal mosaicism (46,XY/47XXY) and are fertile. One report has suggested that in vitro fertilization using intracyoplasmic injection of sperm may be possible for men with non-mosaic Klinefelter syndrome (N Engl J Med 1998;338:588).

ADVANCED-LEVEL QUESTIONS

What is Kallman syndrome?

It is idiopathic hypogonadotrophic hypogonadism with involvement of the hypothalamus. Patients have hypoosmia and other defects of the rhinencephalon (cleft lip/palate, congenital deafness and blindness).

Replacement therapy with both gonadotrophins and gonadotrophin-releasing hormone (GnRH) ensures fertility in many of the affected individuals.

What do you know about the *DAX1* gene?

DAX1 is linked to the X chromosome and encodes a member of the nuclear receptor family of proteins that inhibits testicular differentiation. It has been hypothesized that in Klinerfelter syndrome the presence of two X chromosomes, although in different cells (one from 45,XO and the other from 46,XY) may be sufficient to prevent sustained growth and differentiation of the testis by providing excessive DAX1 (or another inhibiting molecule), which suppresses testicular development.

> Harry F Klinefelter (1912–1990), an American physician who worked at Johns Hopkins Hospital in Baltimore. He described this syndrome with Fuller Albright (1900–1969) and Edward Reifenstein while he was a visiting fellow at Massachusetts General Hospital and Harvard Medical School (Klinefelter HF Jr, Reifenstein EC Jr, Albright F. Syndrome characterized by gynaecomastia, aspermatogensis with a Leydigism and increased excretion of follicle stimulating hormone, J Clin Endocrinol 1942;2:615–27).
>
> Albright described Albright syndrome and was stricken with Parkinson's disease at the age of 36 years, and was rendered invalid in 1953 following surgical attempts to improve his Parkinson's disease. 15 years after their description A Jacobs and JA Strong confirmed the association between the extra X-chromosome and Klinefelter syndrome (Nature 1959;183:302–03, Lancet 2000;356:333–35).

Information can be obtained from the Klinefelter Organisation (www.klinefelter.org.uk).

246 MACROGLOSSIA

INSTRUCTION

Examine this patient's mouth.

SALIENT FEATURES

History

- Ask whether there is any difficulty in breathing or swallowing
- Look for an underlying cause such as hypothyroidism or acromegaly.

Examination

- Protrusion of the resting tongue beyond the teeth or alveolar ridge. The impressions of the teeth may be obvious along the edges of the tongue on either side (Fig. 246.1).

DIAGNOSIS

This patient has macroglossia (lesion), the cause of which is not obvious by clinical examination (aetiology); it is complicated by heavy breathing (functional status).

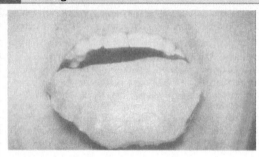

Fig. 246.1 Macroglossia in AL amyloidosis. (With permission from Firestein et al. 2008.)

QUESTIONS

What do you understand by the term macroglossia?
It is a resting tongue that protrudes beyond the teeth or alveolar ridge. It is usually used to indicate long-term painless enlargement rather than the rapid growth of acute parenchymatous glossitis.

What are the types of macroglossia?
- True macroglossia: definitive histopathological findings:
  - Primary: characterized by hypertrophy or hyperplasia of tongue muscles
  - Secondary: the result of infiltration of normal tissue with anomalous elements.
- Pseudomacroglossia: relative enlargement secondary to a small mandible with no histological abnormalities.

ADVANCED-LEVEL QUESTIONS

What are the causes of true macroglossia?
- In children:
  - Hypothyroidism
  - Lymphangioma
  - Haemangioma
  - Idiopathic hyperplasia
  - Metabolic disorders
  - Beckwith–Wiedmann syndrome.
- Secondary macroglossia:
  - Amyloidosis
  - Acromegaly
  - Angioedema
  - Lymphoma
  - Chronic infections: TB, syphilis
  - Space-occupying lesions: cystic hygroma, cysts in lingual thyroglossal ducts, rhabdomyosarcoma.

What are the causes of pseudomacroglossia?
- Down syndrome
- Pierre Robin syndrome
- Cerebral palsy.

What are the complications of macroglossia?

- Prolonged exposure can cause ulceration and necrosis of the mouth and tip of the tongue
- Noisy breathing, drooling and unsightly appearance, particularly in children
- Maxillofacial defects such as anterior open bite, prognathism
- Difficulty in swallowing and, as a consequence, poor weight gain
- Difficulty in the articulation of consonants requiring the tip of the tongue to be in contact with the alveolar ridge or roof of the mouth
- Airway obstruction, which can be life threatening.

- **How would you manage macroglossia?**
- Medical:
  - Treatment of the underlying systemic cause, e.g. thyroxine in hypothyroidism, bromocriptine in acromegaly
  - Steroids: in life-threatening airway obstruction or postoperative oedema.
- Surgical:
  - Reduction glossectomy for symptomatic macroglossia
  - Excision for neoplastic lesions.
- Rehabilitation of physical and psychological problems:
  - Secondary orthodontic care and speech therapy
  - Psychological and psychiatric support.

Further reading

Murthy P, Laing MR: Macroglossia, *BMJ* 309:1386, 1994.

247 OSTEOPOROSIS OF THE SPINE (DOWAGER'S HUMP)

INSTRUCTION

Examine this patient's spine.

SALIENT FEATURES

History

- History of back pain (usually the onset is sudden with severe pain in the dorsal spine)
- Spontaneous fractures and loss of height
- Long-term corticosteroid, heparin therapy or proton pump inhibitors (>7 years of last) (CMAJ 2008;179:319–26)
- Postmenopausal or has had an oopherectomy
- Smoker or consumes alcohol (>3 units/day)
- Is there a family history particularly in a parent
- What is the patient's weight (body mass index (BMI) <22 kg/m^2 is associated with osteoporosis)
- Associated conditions: rheumatoid arthritis, uncontrolled diabetes mellitus, Crohn's disease, ankylosing spondylitis, multiple myeloma, Cushing syndrome, thyrotoxicosis, oestrogen deficiency in women and

androgen deficiency in men, Marfan syndrome, Ehlers–Danlos syndrome, homocystinuria.

Examination

- Elderly patient (usually a woman)
- Marked kyphosis (Fig. 247.1)
- Loss of height
- Protuberant abdomen
- Look for spinal tenderness, demonstrate straight-leg rising sign.

DIAGNOSIS

This elderly patient with marked kyphosis (lesion) has postmenopausal osteoporosis (aetiology) complicated by frequent fractures and loss of height (functional status).

QUESTIONS

What do you understand by the term osteoporosis?

It is 'a systemic skeletal disorder characterized by low bone mass and microarchitectural deterioration of bone tissue, with a consequent increase in bone fragility and susceptibility to fracture.' (Am J Med 1993;94:646–50). NICE (UK National Institute for Health and Clinical Excellence) defines a diagnosis as a T score of −2.5 or below on dual-energy X-ray absorptiometry (DEXA) scanning (see below), although it says that women aged over 75 with two or more risk factors for fracture or low bone density can be assumed without a scan to have osteoporosis.

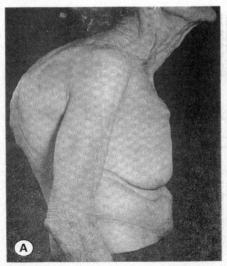 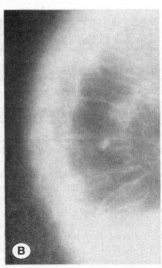

Fig. 247.1 Dowager's hump. (A) Marked thoracic kyphosis caused by multiple osteoporotic fractures. (B) Corresponding radiograph. (With permission from Hochberg et al. 2003.)

ADVANCED-LEVEL QUESTIONS

What is the pathology of osteoporosis?

It is characterized by a decrease in the amount of bone present, so that the structural integrity of the skeleton is compromised. The rate of bone formation is normal but the rate of bone resorption is increased. This results in greater loss of trabecular bone than compact bone, accounting for the clinical features of the disease.

What are the types of osteoporosis?

- Type I results from accelerated bone loss, particularly trabecular bone, and is probably caused by oestrogen deficiency. It typically results in fractures of vertebral bodies and the distal forearm in women in their 60s and 70s.
- Type II results from age-related bone loss and is much slower. It occurs in both sexes and typically results in fracture of the proximal femur in the elderly.
- Secondary osteoporosis: accounts for about 20% of cases in women and 40% of cases in men.

What are the typical sites of fracture in osteoporosis?

Vertebrae, neck of femur and distal radius (Colles' fracture).

What are the clinical consequences of osteoporosis?

Increased mortality rate (increases by 20% in the first year after hip fracture), pain, deformities (kyphosis, loss of height and abdominal protrusion) and loss of independence.

What are the risk factors for osteoporosis?

- *Independent of bone mineral density*: age, previous fragility fracture, maternal history of hip fracture, corticosteroid therapy, smoking, alcohol intake >3 units/day, rheumatoid arthritis, BMI <22 (thin body type in women), falls, organ transplantation
- *Depending on bone mineral density*: untreated hypogonadism (secondary amenorrhoea), anorexia nervosa, malabsorption, endocrine disease (hyperthyroidism, primary hyperparathyroidism), chronic renal disease, chronic liver disease, chronic obstructive pulmonary disease, immobility, medications (aromatase inhibitors, androgen deprivation therapy).

How would you investigate such a patient?

- Radiographs and bone scans looking for fractures and to exclude metastases
- Serum calcium and phosphates, alkaline phosphatase and creatinine (remember osteoporosis is not a disorder of calcium metabolism)
- Urinary calcium and creatinine excretion: 24-h samples
- Urinary Bence Jones protein concentration and serum protein electrophoresis
- Thyroid-stimulating hormone concentrations
- Serum testosterone level in men
- DEXA scanning, which determines bone density, is the gold standard test.

What is the T score for bone mineral density?

The WHO classifies bone mineral density on the basis of the T-score: the difference in standard deviations between the patient's bone density measured by DEXA and the mean bone mineral density of a young adult reference population. T scores are:

−1.0 or higher: normal
−1.0 to −2.5: osteopenia
−2.5 or greater: osteoporosis
−2.5 or greater plus a fragility fracture: severe osteoporosis.

What are the recommendations to measure bone mineral density?

Bone mineral density measurements are recommended for the following indications where assessment would influence management:

- Radiographic evidence of osteopenia and/or vertebral deformity
- Loss of height, thoracic kyphosis (after radiographic confirmation of vertebral deformity)
- Previous fragility fracture
- Prolonged corticosteroid therapy (prednisolone >7.5 mg daily for 6 months or more)
- Premature menopause (age <45 years)
- Prolonged secondary amenorrhoea (>1 year)
- Primary hypogonadism
- Chronic disorders associated with osteoporosis
- Maternal history of hip fracture
- Low BMI (<19).

Is screening the general population recommended?

Screening for osteoporosis in not recommended until issues about long-term treatment are resolved (BMJ 1999;319:1148–9) but it may be considered in patients with a high 10-year probability of fracture risk.

How would you estimate the 10-year probability of fracture risk in this patient?

FRAX is an electronic clinical tool (www.shef.ac.uk/FRAX/), developed by Professor John Kanis, that is used to determine fracture risk using seven clinical risk factors (previous fracture, hip fracture, current smoking, glucocorticoid use, rheumatoid arthritis, secondary osteoporosis, ingestion of ≥3 units of alcohol daily); the patients age, gender, height and weight; and bone mineral density of the femoral neck. This clinical tool derives an algorithm that estimates the 10-year probability of hip fracture and the 10-year probability of a major osteoporotic fracture (hip, spine, proximal humerus or distal forearm).

How would you prevent osteoporosis?

- The goal of therapy is to half the risk of fracture
- Life-style advice: exercise, stop smoking and reduce alcohol consumption
- Regular weight-bearing exercise
- Replacement oestrogen therapy in postmenopausal women should be administered for at least 5 years
- Raloxifene (a selective oestrogen receptor modulator) is indicated in the prevention or treatment of osteoporosis in postmenopausal women. Lasofoxifene (a non-steroidal selective oestrogen receptor (ER) modulator), in postmenopausal women, was associated with reduced risks of non-vertebral and vertebral fractures, ER-positive breast cancer, coronary heart disease and stroke with no increase in the risk of endometrial cancer but an increased risk of venous thromboembolic events (N Engl J Med 2010;362:686–96). The results of this trial suggest that lasofoxifene offers no major clinically important benefits over raloxifene for the skeleton, breast, heart or reproductive tract

- Dietary calcium intake increased to 1.5 g/day (with no more than 500–600 mg in a single dose because of limited absorption with higher doses) and vitamin D_3 800–1000 IU/day with a goal of achieving serum 25-hydroxyvitamin D of 30 µg/l (75 nmol/l) or higher
- Alendronate, a new bisphosphonate, is 1000 times more potent than etidronate in inhibiting bone resorption and hence is able to provide effective inhibition at a dosage that does not affect mineralization. It is indicated only in the prevention and treatment of postmenopausal osteoporosis and in the treatment of glucocorticoid-induced osteoporosis and osteoporosis in men
- Residronate significantly reduces the risk of hip fracture among elderly women with confirmed osteoporososis (N Engl J Med 2001;344:333–40). Risedronate (dosed daily, weekly or monthly) and zoledronate (dosed annually) are indicated for prevention and treatment of postmenopausal and glucocorticoid-induced osteoporosis and in treatment of osteoporosis in men
- Ibandronate (oral or intravenously) is indicated only for treatment of postmenopausal osteoporosis
- Calcitonin nasal spray results in decreased bone resorption and is indicated only for treatment of postmenopausal osteoporosis
- Sodium fluoride
- Denosumab, a human monoclonal antibody to the receptor activator of NF-κB ligand (RANKL), inhibits the development and activity of osteoclasts, decreasing bone resorption and increasing bone density
- Teriparatide (recombinant parathormone) as a subcutanous injection daily for up to 2 years is approved for the treatment of osteoporosis in postmenopausal women and in men who are at high risk for fracture. Teriparatide labelling in the USA carries a black-box warning for osteosarcoma. There is also a risk of renal malignancy
- Future treatments: vitamin D analogues, strontium salts, iprifiavone, calciomimetic drugs that stimulate intermittent production of parathyroid hormone, inhibitors of sclerostin (a protein produced by bone that is a negative regulator of bone formation) and its signalling pathway, testosterone in men with hypogonadism.

What are the precautions needed with bisphosphonates?
- An oral bisphosphonate should be avoided in patients with a history of oesophageal stricture but an intravenous bisphosponate may be considered.
- Bisphosphonate-associated osteonecrosis of the jaw is rare and most cases have been noted in cancer patients who received high doses intravenously (BMJ 2006 333:982–3).
- There is increased risk of clinical vertebral and hip fractures after bisphosphonates are discontinued, and, therefore, a drug holiday is not the best choice in those patients with a high risk of fracture.

A Colles (1773–1843), Professor of Anatomy and Surgery at the College of Surgeons (Ireland).

Prof. John A. Kanis received his medical degree from the University of Edinburgh. After a MRC Clinical Research Fellow position at the Nuffield Orthopaedic Centre he became Wellcome Senior Research Fellow at the

University of Oxford. He was initially appointed Reader in Human Metabolism and Clinical Biochemistry at the University of Sheffield, where he is currently the Emeritus Professor in Human Metabolism and the Director of the WHO Collaborating Centre for Metabolic Bone Diseases. He spearheaded the WHO initiative on the FRAX model.

248 PRESSURE SORES (BEDSORES)

INSTRUCTION

Look at this leg.

SALIENT FEATURES

History

- Prolonged bed rest
- Diabetes mellitus
- Anaemia
- Malnutrition
- General debility.

Examination

- Pressure sore over the sacrum (Fig. 248.1).

Proceed as follows:

- Look for pressure sores elsewhere, particularly the skin overlying the occiput, ears, elbows, hips and ankles.
- Comment on any obvious paralysis or incontinence (the latter contributes to ulcers in the sacral areas).
- Comment on skin traction or any orthopaedic splints (as 70% are orthopaedic patients).
- Tell the examiner that you would like to culture and biopsy the ulcer if it has not been healing properly or looks suspicious.

DIAGNOSIS

This patient has a large non-healing ulcer (lesion) over the sacral region caused by pressure (aetiology) and requires special nursing care to allow the pressure sore to heal (functional status).

QUESTIONS

What are the causes of pressure sores?

- Loss of sensation and when circulation or nutrition to the skin and underlying tissue are compromised: diabetes mellitus, malnutrition, peripheral vascular disease, oedema, arthritis, anaemia, general debility.
- Other: sedation, urinary or faecal incontinence, sedation and anaesthesia.

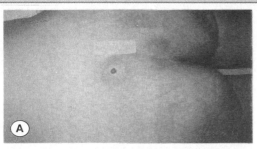

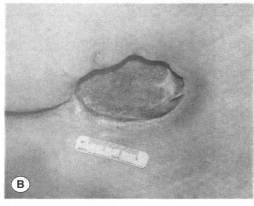

Fig. 248.1 (A) Pressure ulcer at first visit. (B) Clean sacral pressure sore. (With permission from Levi, Rees 2007.)

ADVANCED-LEVEL QUESTIONS

How are pressure sores graded?

Grade I: erythema, skin intact

Grade II: skin loss, epidermis or dermis (abrasion, blister, shallow crater)

Grade III: full thickness loss and damage to subcutaneous tissues

Grade IV: extensive destruction, tissue necrosis or damage to the underlying muscle or bone.

How are pressure sores best prevented?

- Good nursing care, nutrition and maintenance of skin hygiene
- Moribund, paralysed patients should be turned frequently (at least every hour) and pressure points should be inspected for areas of redness and tenderness
- Water-beds, alternating pressure mattresses and sheep skins are useful.

Professor Hans Ludwig Frankel, MB, OBE developed the Frankel
classification for spinal injuries. Following his medical education at University
College and University College Hospital in London, he was recruited by Sir
Ludwig Guttmann to work at the National Spinal Injuries Centre, Stoke
Mandeville Hospital, Aylesbury, where he dedicated his career to the care of
persons with spinal cord injury. Sir Guttmann was the first to show that
pressure sores were preventable.

249 SICKLE CELL DISEASE

INSTRUCTION

Examine this patient's hands who has recurrent episodes of abdominal
pain, precipitated by infection.

SALIENT FEATURES

History

- Bone pain
- Past history of strokes, fits
- Priapism
- Family history of similar problem
- Precipitating factors (infection, dehydration, cold, acidosis or hypoxia)
- Recurrent painful episodes.

Examination

- Afro-Caribbean patient
- Anaemia
- Digits of varying lengths (may be painful) (Fig. 249.1)
- Tell the examiner that you would like to examine the:
  - urine for haematuria (renal papillary necrosis)
  - leg for arterial ulcers
  - abdomen for hepatomegaly
  - heart for cardiomegaly and hyperdynamic circulation
  - retina for neovascularization (which may cause blindness) (Fig. 249.2).

DIAGNOSIS

This black African patient has evidence of old dactylitis (lesions) caused
by sickle cell anaemia (aetiology), which has caused severe deformity of
the hand. She has difficulty buttoning her clothes (functional status).

QUESTIONS

What is the abnormality in this patient?

This patient has a structural abnormality of the haemoglobin chain (producing haemoglobin S (HbS)). A single base mutation from adenine to
thymine results in substitution of valine for glutamine at the sixth residue
of the β-globin chain. HbS polymerizes on deoxygenation and this results
in the characteristic sickle appearance of haemoglobin. Sickling can

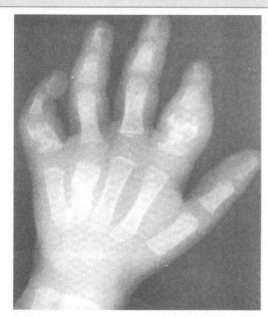

Fig. 249.1 Sickle-cell disease. Infarction in several of the metacarpals and proximal phalanges has resulted in bone destruction and swelling of the soft tissues. (With permission from Adam et al. 2008.)

produce a shortened red cell survival and impaired passage of cells through the microcirculation, leading to obstruction of small vessels and tissue infarction.

What do you know about the genetics of this syndrome?
In the homozygous state (sickle cell anaemia), both genes are abnormal (HbSS), whereas in the heterozygous state (sickle cell trait), only one chromosome carries the gene (HbAS). The disease does not manifest until the foetal form of haemoglobin (HbF) decreases to adult levels at about 6 months of age.

Does the haemoglobin level fall during a sickle cell crisis?
The patient has 'steady-state' anaemia and the haemoglobin level does not fall unless there is parvovirus-induced bone marrow aplasia, drug-induced haemolysis or sequestration of sickle cells in the liver and spleen.

Is the spleen enlarged in these patients?
The spleen may be enlarged in childhood as a result of haemolysis; in adult life, patients often undergo autosplenectomy (from infarcts), which increases their susceptibility to infection by *Streptococcus pneumoniae* (pneumonia, meningitis) and salmonella osteomyelitis.

What are the other complications of this disease?
Chronic leg ulcers (from ischaemia), pigmentary gallstones (from persistent haemolysis), chronic renal failure, aseptic necrosis of femoral heads, chronic renal disease, acute chest syndrome and pulmonary hypertension (appears to be a complication of chronic haemolysis, is resistant to hydroxyurea therapy and confers a high risk of death).

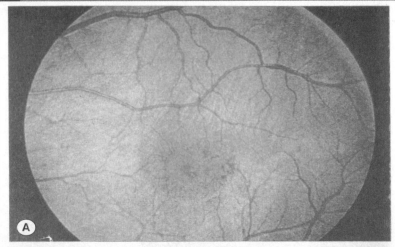

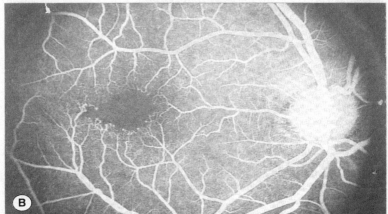

Fig. 249.2 Sickle-cell disease. (A) Macular ischaemia with the macular depression sign and perifoveal vascular remodelling. (B) Fluorescein angiogram of the same patient demonstrating an irregular and moth-eaten perifoveal capillary network and vascular telangiectasia. (With permission from Yanoff, Duker 2008.)

How would you investigate these patients?

- FBC: haemoglobin 60–80 g/l, with raised reticulocyte count
- Blood smear shows signs of hyposplenism (Howell–Jolly bodies, target cells)
- Sickling of red cells can be introduced by sodium metabisulfite but does not differentiate HbSS from HbAS
- Haemoglobin electrophoresis: there is no HbA, 80–95% HbSS and 2–20% HbF. High HbF levels are associated with a more benign progress. The parents of the patient will show features of sickle cell

trait (remember that sickle cell trait protects against *Plasmodium falciparum* malaria).

How would you manage an acute sickle cell crisis?

Supportive therapy with intravenous fluids, oxygen, antibiotics and analgesia. Folic acid is given for those with severe haemolysis.

Is there any long-term treatment?

- Hydroxyurea and erythropoietin are given to increase synthesis of HbF.
- Allogenic bone marrow transplantation is being investigated as a possible 'cure' in severely affected individuals.
- Experimental therapy: induction of HbF by short-chain fatty acids, membrane-active drugs and other experimental treatments.

What is the role of blood transfusion in these patients?

- Steady-state anaemia requires no treatment and regular blood transfusions are given only when the anaemia is severe or if the patient has frequent episodes of crisis, particularly during pregnancy (to suppress endogenous production of HbS).
- Exchange transfusion is used for intractable pain crises, priapism and stroke.

What is the prognosis of this condition?

It is variable, with some having a normal lifespan while others succumb in the first few years of life to infection or episodes of sequestration. Median age of death is 42 years for homozygotes. The acute chest syndrome is the leading cause of death and its cause is unknown. The syndrome is precipitated by fat embolism and infection, particularly community-acquired pneumonia (N Engl J Med 2000;342:1855–65).

WH Howell (1860–1945), Professor of Physiology at Johns Hopkins Hospital, Baltimore, who also discovered and isolated heparin.
JMJ Jolly (1870–1953), French Professor of Histology.

---

250 THRUSH

INSTRUCTION

Look at this patient's tongue.

SALIENT FEATURES

History

- Ask the patient about dysphagia (oesophagitis)
- Diabetes mellitus
- Leukaemia, anticancer therapy or immunosuppressive drugs (cause neutropenia)
- Drugs (steroids, broad-spectrum antibiotics and oral contraceptives)
- HIV infection.

Examination

- Superficial white patches or large fluggy membranes that are easily detachable (e.g. by a tongue depressor), leaving underlying erythema (Figs 250.1 and 250.2)

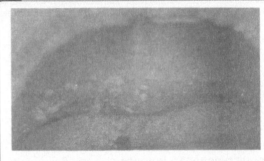

Fig. 250.1
Pseudomembranous candidiasis of the palate demonstrating multiple areas of Candida colonization. (With permission from Lerman MA, Laudenbach J, Marty FM. Management of oral infections in cancer patients. Dental Clin North Am 2008;52:129–53.)

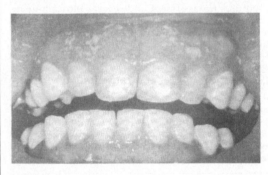

Fig. 250.2 Candida albicans. (With permission from Habif 2009.)

- Erythema, transverse fissuring and maceration may be seen at the angles of the mouth (perleche) as an associated finding.

Proceed as follows:
- Look for other sites of candidal infection (eczematoid lesions in moist areas of the skin, such as inframammary folds, inguinal creases, between the fingers and toes).
- Look for id reactions (which are hypersensitivity cutaneous reactions remote from the site of infection).
- Ask the patient about dysphagia (oesophagitis).
- Tell the examiner that you would like to investigate for underlying:
  - diabetes mellitus
  - neutropenia (secondary to chronic granulomatous disease, leukaemia, anticancer therapy or immunosuppressive drugs)
  - drug use: steroids, broad-spectrum antibiotics and oral contraceptives
  - HIV infection
  - polyendocrine deficiencies (including hypoparathyroidism, hypoadrenalism and hypothyroidism).

DIAGNOSIS

This patient has oral thrush or candidal infection (lesion), which is a complication of the use of the broad-spectrum antibiotic tetracycline (aetiology), and has dysphagia (functional status).

QUESTIONS

What is the most common species that causes human infection?
Candida albicans.

How would you confirm your diagnosis?
- Wet preparation of a smear with potassium hydroxide will confirm spores and may show non-septate mycelia
- Biopsy will show intraepithelial pseudomycelia.

With which type of antibiotics is candidal infection common?
Broad-spectrum antibiotics, e.g. tetracycline, chloramphenicol.

Which candidal species usually colonizes skin?
C. parapsilosis.

How would you treat candidal infection?
- Effective antifungal therapy may be achieved with fluconazole, ketoconazole, clotrimazole or nystatin. Amphotericin lozenges may be useful in oral candidal infection. Itraconazole may be substituted when there is concomitant dermatophyte disease.
- Sexual partners of oral or vaginal disease should be screened and appropriately treated.

What are the features of disseminated candidiasis?
- Disseminated candidiasis manifests with systemic features including fever, toxicity, pulmonary involvement, endocarditis and retinal abscesses. Very rarely, it may cause focal manifestations including pustular skin abscesses, osteomyelitis, myositis, brain abscess or meningitis. It often causes sepsis associated with intravenous catheterization.

How is disseminated candidiasis treated?
- Patients with blood cultures with *Candida* should receive intravenous amphotericin B. For candidaemia in those with renal failure, fluconazole is an alternative because of the absence of restrictions on intravenous administration in patients with a creatinine clearance <50 ml/min.
- Echonocandins and newer generation azoles may be considered if fluconazole fails or patients are intolerant to amphotericin B. The echinocandins (caspofungin, anidulafungin, micafungin) have a broad spectrum of activity against a variety of *Candida* spp. and, therefore, may be preferred when *C. glabrata* or *C. krusei* is identified or suspected. The choice of an echinocandin, as opposed to an azole, for initial therapy of candidaemia in a patient who does not have neutropenia is not well established. The echinocandins are not well absorbed orally and must be administered intravenously. Renal insufficiency does not require dose adjustment.

What is the role of the β-glucan receptor dectin-1 in candidiasis?
Chronic mucocutaneous candidiasis may also be caused by a genetic defect of the β-glucan receptor dectin-1. Dectin-1 deficiency increases susceptibility to mucocutaneous but not systemic fungal infections. Deficient type 17 helper T cell responses in patients with dectin-1 deficiency (N Engl J Med 2009;361:1760–7), and a similar defect in persons with defective CARD9 (caspase recruitment domain-containing protein 9) suggests that impaired T cell immunity (N Engl J Med 2009;361:1727–35) may have a role in the development of candidiasis.

In 1923 Christine Marie Berkhout named the fungus that we now know as *Candida albicans* for the white robe, *toga candida*, worn by Roman senators and senatorial candidates.

Index

Page numbers followed by 'f' indicate figures, 't' indicate tables, and 'b' indicate boxes.